Stress and Health

Third Edition

Phillip L. Rice
MOORHEAD STATE UNIVERSITY

D1438503

Brooks/Cole Publishing Company

I(T)P® An International Thomson Publishing Company

Pacific Grove • Albany • Belmont • Bonn • Boston • Cincinnati • Detroit • Johannesburg • London
Madrid • Melbourne • Mexico City • New York • Paris • Singapore • Tokyo • Toronto • Washington

Sponsoring Editor: *Marianne Taflinger*
Editorial Assistant: *Scott Brearton/Rachael Bruckman*
Production Editor: *Tessa A. McGlasson*
Marketing Team: *Michael Campbell/Deanne Brown/Jean Thompson*
Manuscript Editor: *Mark Vining*
Permissions Editor: *May Clark*

Interior Design: *Paul Uhl*
Interior Illustration: *Lori Heckelman*
Cover Design: *Roger Knox*
Art Editor: *Jennifer Mackres*
Photo Editor: *Robert J. Western*
Typesetting: *Carlisle Communications, Ltd.*
Printing and Binding: *Malloy Lithographing, Inc.*

For more information, contact:

BROOKS/COLE PUBLISHING COMPANY
511 Forest Lodge Road
Pacific Grove, CA 93950
USA

International Thomson Publishing Europe
Berkshire House 168-173
High Holborn
London WC1V 7AA
England

Thomas Nelson Australia
102 Dodds Street
South Melbourne, 3205
Victoria, Australia

Nelson Canada
1120 Birchmount Road
Scarborough, Ontario
Canada M1K 5G4

International Thomson Editores
Seneca 53
Col. Polanco
México, D. F., México
C. P. 11560

International Thomson Publishing GmbH
Königswinterer Strasse 418
53227 Bonn
Germany

International Thomson Publishing Asia
60 Albert Street
#15-01 Albert Complex
Singapore 189969

International Thomson Publishing Japan
Hirakawacho Kyowa Building, 3F
2-2-1 Hirakawacho
Chiyoda-ku, Tokyo 102
Japan

Printed in the United States of America

10   9   8   7   6

Library of Congress Cataloging-in-Publication Data

Rice, Phillip L., [date]
    Stress and health / Phillip L. Rice. — 3rd ed.
        p.   cm.
    Includes bibliographical references and index.
    ISBN 0-534-26502-2
    1. Stress (Psychology)   2. Medicine, Psychosomatic.   I. Title.
BF575.S75R53   1998
155.9′042—dc21
                                        98-7726
                                        CIP

For Ruth,
*   For soon, the dream becomes reality*

Brief Contents

Contents

CHAPTER 2

STRESS RESEARCH: LOGIC, DESIGN, AND PROCESS 32

BEING SCIENTISTS AND BEING CONSUMERS 33

MODES OF THINKING IN SCIENCE 34

PART 4 Coping, Relaxation, and Imagery 283

CHAPTER 10

COPING STRATEGIES: CONTROLLING STRESS 285

APPENDIX

RELAXATION INSTRUCTIONS 425

Preface

In the short life of stress research, the notion that unmanaged stress has a negative effect on health seems to have passed from the realm of interesting hypothesis to the arena of demonstrated fact. The personal significance of this notion cannot be underestimated. Although many details of the stress process remain to be identified, it is now part of conventional wisdom that people need to learn stress management techniques to maintain a high quality of life and to reduce their risk for illness. With this increased awareness, a growing need exists for information on the many faces of stress, and there is especially a heightened demand for accessible guides to coping skills. This book was written to provide both a concise summary of what science has learned about stress, and to enable people to learn the basic skills needed to manage stress effectively.

Perhaps the most significant change in this third edition is that more self-study exercises have been incorporated throughout to help readers make connections between the principles being discussed and their own stress experiences. Further, the World Wide Web has provided a hi-tech means for distributing different types of information packaged sometimes in very novel ways. This edition includes special end-of-chaper sections with addresses for some of the better Web sites for stress facts and skill learning. Some chapters have assignments using the Web to analyze a specific health risk. For example, Chapter 5 suggests a multimedia tour that provides information on behavioral risks for AIDS.

Of course, appropriate attention has been given to updating research and theory as well. Many references come from the most recent two or three years so that readers will be up-to-date on the most important developments in the field. Although currency is important in a rapidly changing field, I have tried to include new information without sacrificing important historical perspectives. There still are many controversial issues in stress theory, not the least of which is the status of the concept itself. My effort has been to balance basic principles and practice throughout the book. Still, I am inclined to ask the reader to critically examine the issues involved in understanding a notion so complex as stress and health without, I hope, getting bogged down in endless intricacies.

PEDAGOGIC FEATURES

This book has several important pedagogic features, some of which are new to this edition:
- Each chapter opens with an outline of the chapter and a list of critical questions to help the reader focus on and examine important issues.
- Chapter summaries have been rewritten to provide a point-by-point recap of the most important concepts of the chapter.
- Most chapters now have multiple self-study exercises to help the reader examine aspects of their own stressors and coping skills.
- Each chapter ends with a list of Websites to help interested readers pursue more information. One of the most important reasons to learn to use the Web may be the ability to maintain currency. Those who want to know the latest in regard to stress research and skills may find it readily available at their fingertips.
- More material has been included reflecting cultural diversity issues in stress and health. For example, Chapter 8 has a new section on race and socioeconomic status and their relationship to stress and health. Chapter 14 has a section on stress among minority and international university students.
- Issues of concern to women are also strengthened both in Chapter 6 on the family and in Chapter 8 on stress in the work place.
- Chapter 8 includes a new section on religion and coping with stress. This has been almost a taboo topic, but the rapid increase in thoughtful papers and the rudiments of controlled research suggest that this could be one of the more exciting arenas of work in the coming years.
- Chapter 14 is now rewritten to reflect on student stress and coping. Special emphasis is given to issues of loneliness and test anxiety.
- More current news stories have been incorporated to illustrate specific issues. For example, Chapter 9 revisits the Estonia ferry capsizing and the Oakland firestorms as examples of environmental disasters. These stories have helped students better understand the process that people go through in dealing with such catastrophes. Chapter 15 retells the story of Kelly Perkins, a young woman from California who restored her strength and her confidence in herself by climbing 14,000-foot mountains shortly after surviving a heart transplant.

THE BOOK'S PLAN AND A PREVIEW

Part 1
The first chapter introduces the concept of stress and examines problems in defining stress. The chapter also examines several of the rival theories that attempt to explain the stress process. Chapter 2, first added in the second edition, introduces the reader to several problems in research design—problems that require critical thinking whether one is a research designer or a consumer. Further, I introduce the terminology and procedures of epidemiological research. This approach is not typically taught in traditional courses on behavioral science research. Health researchers use epidemiological procedures extensively to answer questions about the relationships between lifestyle and disease and between therapeutic interven-

tions and improved health. The importance of epidemiological procedures cannot be overlooked or minimized.

Part 2

The three chapters that make up Part 2 are the foundations for understanding stress in a biopsychological context. Chapter 3 on cognitive processes includes material on the Health Belief Model, as well as conceptual notions derived from Seligman's *attribution model* of learned helplessness. Many research studies have begun to examine how cognitive attributions may influence the course of illness. New material has been added on the *hot and cold memory systems* based on evidence that the distortions in cognitive-memory processes associated with post-traumatic stress disorder may be related to differences in this system.

Chapter 4 examines a variety of issues on personality and stress, including the notion of biotypes. Research on the Type A behavior pattern suggests that the toxic core may well be anger and hostility, especially inward directed anger. The development of this line of thinking is chronicled in both logical and empirical detail. Still, there are many lingering concerns and controversies that question the alleged link between coronary risk and Type A behavior. As the chapter shows, it may be more prudent to talk about a general disease-prone personality rather than a specific personality-disease connection.

Chapter 5 considers the very complex issue of brain-behavior connections and the physiological mechanisms that govern the stress response. I struggled again with the issue of placement of this chapter. Still, it seemed wiser to have the more basic psychological foundations in place (which can be presented with a minimum of neuroanatomy) before moving into the myriad details of neuroanatomy that must still be connected to behavioral expressions.

Part 3

Part 3 is organized to reflect increasingly molar systems that extend from the personal to the impersonal. Thus, Chapter 6 focuses on the family, Chapter 7 on work, Chapter 8 on social systems, and Chapter 9 on environmental stressors. The chapter on family process reflects increased attention to cognitive and systems models of family stress. New information is presented on family violence and abuse, and positive models for coping with family stress are presented. Chapter 7 reviews common sources of stress at work, and considers new potential sources of stress in the growing cottage industry and among telecommuters. Gender differences in work stress are discussed. Chapter 8 on social stress includes new material on road rage, ethnic and socioenocomic variables in stress, and the role religion plays in coping with stress. A tremendous amount of research on natural and technological disasters has occurred in the time since the last edition. Several highly publicized disasters, including the San Francisco earthquake, the Oakland fire storms, and the Estonia ferry capsizing have been featured in such research. Several of these projects have added important details to our understanding how survivors deal with such catastrophic events.

Part 4

Chapter 10 provides a general overview of coping theory, research, and skills. This provides a framework for introducing the more important coping skills in subsequent chapters. In this chapter, we grapple with issues in defining coping, and discuss how specific types of coping may be useful for certain situations. Chapter 11 introduces one of the most general and powerful coping skills, the technique of progressive relaxation. More recent theoretical and empirical data have been added to these skills chapters, but their structure remains much the same. One significant addition is the treatment of eye movement desensitization and reprocessing in Chapter 12. This treatment program has been pushed almost as the new elixir of clinical intervention, but the claims for its power may be exaggerated. Caution is urged in considering its claims even as it is still relevant to consider its potential usefulness in this area.

Part 5

The final chapters do not fit as easily into the general structure of coping skills. However, I have been impressed by the wide range and seriousness of stressors that students confront in their quest for the degree. To this end, Chapter 14 has been substantially revised to include a focus on several of the more important student stressors. Unfortunately, the material on this area is vast (entire books have been devoted to this topic), so I have had to be highly selective. This, of course, always leaves open the possibility of second-guessing my choices, but I must accept responsibility for those choices. A section on time management has been retained as a significant part of this chapter since time management remains one of the most important general stress management skills whether at home, in school, or on the job. The final chapter on nutrition and exercise has been updated to reflect new information and some changing ideas. Most of these changes are based on nationally formulated health goals and refinements in information about the relationships between diet and wellness, and between exercise and wellness.

TO THE INSTRUCTOR

As with previous editions, the third edition of *Stress and Health* is intended to be an introductory text for a variety of psychology, health, and education courses. It is, I believe, as rigorous as the second edition, but the added dimension of self-study exercises will, I hope, make the book easier to use for those wanting a more applied type of course. I have no illusion that the book will meet all instructors' biases. It is not a how-to manual in the strictest sense, though the skills chapters will provide most readers with what is necessary to develop a base of coping skills. Neither is it a compendium of research and theory. The field is simply too expansive and the body of literature too immense for any single book to make that kind of claim. Still, it is gratifying to see the many different niches this book has filled in the years since the first edition.

If time permits using the entire book, the course will provide a fair balance between the principles and the practice of coping and wellness. If time does not permit covering all the topics in the book, some choices obviously must be made based on the needs of the typical student and the objectives of the course.

The book has been organized to permit the instructor to teach either a *principles syllabus* or an *applied syllabus*. The principles syllabus covers major content areas of stress and health. The chapters that are intended to serve this focus include Chapters 1 through 10 and Chapter 15, which cover the following topics:

Chapter 1: Stress Concepts, Theories, and Models

Chapter 2: Stress Research

Chapter 3: The Cognitive Stress System

Chapter 4: Personality and Stress

Chapter 5: The Physiology of Stress

Chapter 6: Stress in the Family

Chapter 7: Job Stress

Chapter 8: Social Sources of Stress

Chapter 9: Environmental Stress

Chapter 10: Coping Strategies

Chapter 15: Behavioral Health Strategies

The applied syllabus covers the major techniques that enable an individual to cope more effectively with stress, eliminate high-risk behaviors, and maintain better total health. The chapters that serve this purpose are Chapters 1, 6, 7, and 10 through 15. These chapters cover many topics and techniques central to a self-help orientation, as indicated by this list of topics:

Chapter 1: Stress Concepts, Theories, and Models

Chapter 6: Stress in the Family

Chapter 7: Job Stress

Chapter 10: Coping Strategies

Chapter 11: Progressive Muscle Relaxation

Chapter 12: Cognitive and Imagery Techniques

Chapter 13: The Concentration Techniques

Chapter 14: Student Survival Skills

Chapter 15: Behavioral Health Strategies

An instructor's manual with test-item file is available. The test-item file is also available on computer disk in ASCII format for both IBM and MAC formats.

ACKNOWLEDGMENTS

I am grateful to the numerous instructors who have forwarded suggestions for making this a better text. In addition, several people reviewed the manuscript, lending their expertise and insights to help refine the chapters in several ways. A very special thanks, then, to the reviewers of the current edition: Jill M. Black, Cleveland State University; Lisa Bohon, California State University, Sacramento; Joel E. Grace, Mansfield University of Pennsylvania; Malcolm Kahn, University of Miami Counseling Center; Charles Kaiser, College of Charleston; Lawrence R. Murphy, Xavier University; Philip Singer, Oakland University; and Ronald K. White, The University of Albany.

I have continued to benefit from the support, patience, and encouragement of my family, friends, and colleagues. My research assistants, Tammi Fortney and Dan Buchin, have kept the doors of the library spinning and the electronic databases hot with many hours of searching and retrieving hundreds of articles and books for this revision. I am most grateful to Marianne Taflinger for her support, prodding, and many useful suggestions that have been incorporated into this edition. I am also grateful for the efforts of all the great people at Brooks/Cole, who seem to find ways to make the task of producing a book as much fun as such an arduous task can be. I am indebted to Tessa McGlasson, production editor, both for seeing me through the last lengthy project and for continuing on to this project in so short a time. I'd also like to thank Mark Vining, copyeditor; May Clark, who managed the many details of permissions; Jennifer Mackres and Bob Western, who managed the art and the photo programs; and Vernon Boes for coordinating the cover and interior design. Thanks again to all of you.

Phillip L. Rice

NOTE ON WEBSITES FEATURE

At the end of each chapter, a list of Internet sites is provided. This is to help in furthering the reader's study of stress and health, but it will also serve to guide individuals who would like more help in developing coping skills. Many sites related to stress and health are now either tutorial or interactive. The interactive sites allow the user to provide relevant information and get immediate feedback. This is especially true in the diet and exercise area where, for example, a person can get an exact calculation of Body Mass Index (BMI) or have a complete nutrition analysis done on current diet with proposed changes for weight control. Other stress sites provide a variety of assessments—for example, current level of stress or job stressors. It is hoped that these Internet resources will prove valuable in many ways beyond the confines of the classroom.

The Internet is rapidly becoming a major professional resource with online journals and databases covering almost any topic imaginable. It is already prompting questions about how to reference citations from the Internet for APA reports whether for the classroom or for formal publication. The APA has a Webpage (listed in the following table) devoted to this issue with examples for citing different types of articles obtained from the Web. You could make this your first simple Internet exercise: access the APA website and print the guide for citing the web. (Hint: Look for the Frequently Asked Questions under Student Information.) When in doubt, ask your instructors for guidance on their preferences for citation.

A few words are in order regarding the selected sites. First, the amount of information on the Internet is now so voluminous that the issue is not whether you can find something, but how to narrow the choices. Beware of sites that read like "Annie's Anxiety Outlet" or "Billy's Stress Express." Many of these sites are little more than one person's ventilation of some frustration or cutesey material with little relevance. Sticking with major professional organization sites (such as the APA) is usually a safe bet. Alternatively, using a web search engine that allows a user to search for only ranked high quality sites can reduce the likelihood of ending up with Internet garbage.

Second, in most cases I have opted for link sites rather than a long listing of individual sites. Link sites provide automated connections to many other sites with a common interest. Third, I tried to verify the operational integrity and currency of each site. At the same time, the Internet is a dynamic enterprise where some sites can disappear almost as fast as you find them, or they can be functional one day but not the next, or they are not maintained by their authors and thus become dated. There is no guarantee, then, that the sites will be functional or current by the time you read this. Still, if you learn some simple search strategies, you can generate your personal list of favorite, important sites very quickly.

To this end, the list on the next page shows some of the most powerful search engines available for searching the web. It also notes resources for individuals with disabilities. The Yahoo engine allows you to search by categories (such as health). Alta Vista tends to produce very broad searches. This is not very helpful when the topic is well represented on the Internet. You will not be very charmed to see that your search results in 67,252 sites on a single topic! Still, Alta Vista can be very helpful when you are having difficulty getting a lead. The Magellan site (mckinley.com) and the Lycos site (lycos.com) are my personal favorite starting points because they both allow you to search only on rated (for example, the top 5% or top 20%) sites if desired. This can produce a focused list of high-quality sites very quickly. In many cases, this is all that is needed to get started.

One point in regard to addresses is very important. Some URL addresses can get very long, and this has made it difficult to always keep the address on a single line (the Blind Links address, for example). Just remember that you type in a URL address on a single extended line with no spaces or hard returns. Also, every character, including capitals or small case letters, must be typed in as shown or it will lead to an error in accessing the site.

WEBSITES for internet access

URL ADDRESS	SITE NAME & DESCRIPTION
http://www.yahoo.com	☆A general purpose, powerful search engine. Use the **Health** category to find virtually anything of interest
http://www.altavista.digital.com	Altavista's powerful but general search engine
http://www.lycos.com	☆The Lycos Search engine—allows search of the top 5% rated sites
http://searcher.mckinley.com	☆Magellan—powerful search engine with access to top-rated sites
http://www.excite.com	☆Excite—powerful search engine allows listing by Web address
http:/www.apa.org	The American Psychological Association
http://seidata.com/~marriage/rblind.html	Blind Links—comprehensive list of resources for the blind
http://www.deafworldweb.org/	Deaf World Web—the Central Deaf Point on the Internet
http://www.c-cad.org/	Resource page for people with disabilities—links to disability websites and adaptive software

PART ONE

Principles and Issues:

The Background

CHAPTERS

CHAPTER 1

Stress Concepts, Theories, and Models

I'm an old man and have known a great many troubles, but most of them never happened.

MARK TWAIN

QUESTIONS

- How should we define stress?
- What are the formal or scientific definitions of stress?
- How is stress distinguished from states such as anxiety, conflict, and frustration?
- How do we distinguish disease from illness behavior, and sickness from health?
- What is a theory?
- What is the biological view of stress?
- What is the distinction between predisposing and precipitating factors?
- How does the cognitive transactional model explain stress?
- What are the key ingredients of social, holistic, and systems theories of stress?

The concept of stress is somewhat like the illusive concept of love: everyone knows what the term means, but no two people would define it the same way. Common-sense definitions, dictionary definitions, and formal scientific definitions all point in the same general direction but continue along different paths. Hans Selye, the grand master of stress research and theory, said that "Stress, like relativity, is a scientific concept which has suffered from the mixed blessing of being too well known and too little understood" (1980, p. 127).

Our first task in this chapter, therefore, will be to impose some order on the confusing array of stress terms. Then we will review major theories of stress that have evolved in the last few years. This will lay the foundation for an in-depth study of stress sources in later chapters. Before proceeding to read the next section, though, take a moment to respond to Self-Study Exercise 1-1. Feedback on the exercise is provided at the end of the chapter.

SELF-STUDY EXERCISE 1-1

What Do You Think About Stress?

Respond to the following true-or-false statements before reading the rest of Chapter 1. For each statement, try to give the first response that comes to mind without internal editing and do not worry about being right or wrong. After responding, look for information on the issues addressed as you continue reading. Some information about the quiz and the answers and comments about the exercise appear at the very end of the chapter.

1.	Stress is related only to major catastrophes like a death in the family or financial ruin.	T or F
2.	All stress is necessarily bad stress.	T or F
3.	Stress can be objectively identified and defined.	T or F
4.	Life for teenagers is more stressful today than it was 30 years ago.	T or F
5.	The body reacts the same to good stress as it does to bad stress.	T or F
6.	We all experience stress the same way.	T or F
7.	The only meaningful solution is to eliminate stress completely.	T or F
8.	I do not need to worry about stress until the symptoms get really severe.	T or F

COMMON SENSE AND NOT-SO-COMMON DEFINITIONS OF STRESS

When most people talk about stress, it is usually in terms of pressure they are feeling from something happening around them or to them. Students talk about being under stress because of poor exam performance or an impending deadline for a major paper. Parents talk about the strain of raising teenagers and the financial burdens of running a household. Teachers talk about the pressure of maintaining professional currency and research while still managing to keep up with teaching and advising. Doctors, nurses, and lawyers talk about meeting the endless demands of their patients and clients.

In each case, it is obvious that several other terms could be substituted easily for the term **stress.** Two such terms, **pressure** and **strain,** were already substituted in the preceding paragraph without any forewarning. Most readers probably would not notice anything unusual about the substitutions. Yet *Webster's New Twentieth Century Dictionary* uses precisely those two terms in its definition: that stress is "strain; pressure; especially . . . force exerted upon a body, that tends to strain or deform its shape." This variation in terminology suggests that stress wears many masks.

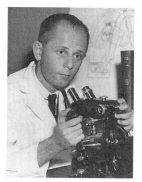

Hans Selye, the grand master of stress research and discoverer of the General Adaptation Syndrome.

Stress or Distress: The Negative View

Many people use *stress* and **distress** as though they are interchangeable terms. Perhaps this is because common sense suggests that stress is something bad. To avoid this dilemma, Selye introduced the terms *distress* and **eustress.** According to Selye (1974), distress is "damaging or unpleasant stress" (p. 31). Expressed in these terms, stress is much the same as a state of anxiety, fear, worry, or agitation. The core of the psychological experience is negative, painful, something to be avoided.

Stress or Eustress: The Positive View

Pleasurable, satisfying experiences come from what Selye (1979) calls *eustress.* Participating in a wedding ceremony, anticipating competition in a major sports event, and performing in a theatrical production are examples of eustress. This is positive stress. We even hear of the "joy of stress," a phrase some use to emphasize the good that can come from stress (Hanson, 1986).

Eustress heightens awareness, increases mental alertness, and often leads to superior cognitive and behavioral performance. Eustress may supply the arousing motivation for one individual to create a work of art, another an urgently needed medicine, another a scientific theory. It is, in other words, challenge—stress to be sought out and used as an ally for personal and professional growth.

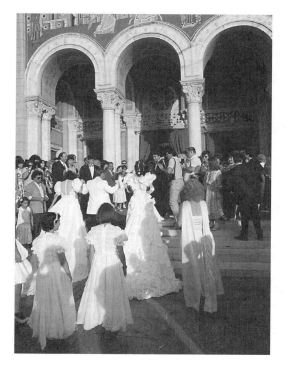

In one view, even pleasant events such as a wedding can produce stress for the people involved.

FIGURE 1-1
Effects of amount of stress or arousal on efficiency of performance.

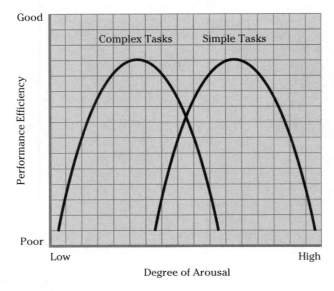

The relationship between arousing stress and performance is not a simple one, though. The **Yerkes-Dodson Law** was the first attempt to summarize this relationship (Yerkes & Dodson, 1908). The law states that, *up to a point,* performance will increase as arousal increases. Performance is best when arousal is optimum (not maximum). Beyond the optimal level of arousal, performance begins to deteriorate. A graphic illustration of this relation appears in Figure 1-1.

With exceptionally high levels of tension, performance may be as bad as when a person is not aroused at all. Compare the performance efficiency of someone about to fall asleep because of fatigue or boredom with the performance efficiency of someone who is hysterical. Both are generally inefficient and nonproductive.

People perform best with at least some pressure. Too little stress is just as bad as too much. *The aim of stress management, then, is not to eliminate stress entirely but to control it so an optimal level of arousal is present.* Selye (1974) said that "Complete freedom from stress is death" (p. 32). It is only extreme, disorganizing stress that we want to avoid, manage, or reduce. (Take a moment to identify your most common stressors. A worksheet for this purpose is provided in Self-Study Exercise 1-2.)

FORMAL DEFINITIONS OF STRESS

Walter Cannon (1932), a noted Harvard physiologist, probably introduced stress terminology to the scientific community. Cannon contributed the idea of **homeostasis,** the tendency of organisms to maintain a stable internal environment. Homeostasis is not a steady state, though. It is a dynamic oscillatory state; that is, it exhibits pendulum swings

---

SELF-STUDY EXERCISE 1-2

What Are Your Personal Stressors?

In the following worksheet, identify your most common stressors. Do not be concerned about giving an exhaustive list here, just the few that you regard as the most important. When you are finished, check some of your listed stressors against the brief information on common stressors provided at the very end of the chapter.

PERSONAL STRESSORS	WORK OR SCHOOL STRESSORS	ENVIRONMENTAL STRESSORS

---

between need and fulfillment (Goldstein, 1995). Cannon also investigated mechanisms of emergency preparedness, the fight-or-flight response. He showed that this response involves a complex interaction between sympathetic nervous system arousal and hormonal secretions from the adrenal glands. Still, the key to Cannon's use of the term stress may have been his observation that organisms tend to "bounce back" or "resist" deforming influences from external forces (Hinkle, 1974a). In other words, the organism tries to maintain balance when it is confronted with stress.

In contemporary scientific literature, stress has at least three distinct meanings. First, it may refer to any event or environmental stimulus that causes a person to feel tense or aroused. In this sense, stress is something *external.*

Second, stress may refer to a subjective response. In this sense, stress is the *internal* mental state of tension or arousal. It is the interpretive, emotive, defensive, and coping processes occurring inside a person. Such processes may promote growth and maturity. They also may produce mental strain. The particular outcome depends on factors that will be explained later in the cognitive model of stress.

Finally, stress may be the body's *physical reaction* to demand or damaging intrusions. This is the sense in which both Cannon and Selye used the term. Demand promotes a natural arousal of the body to a higher level of activity. The function of these physical reactions is probably to support behavioral and psychological efforts at coping (Baum, 1990). Conditions of chronic stress may bring about negative states, including exhaustion, disease, and death. On the positive side, it is clear that some good can come from physiological challenge. This comes from evidence that repeated exposure to arousing stressors may lead to **physiological toughness.** Dienstbier (1989) defines physiological toughness as "increased capacity for responding to stress plus increased resistance to the potential physical damage that stress can produce."[1]

---

[1]Chapter 5 will elaborate on this idea.

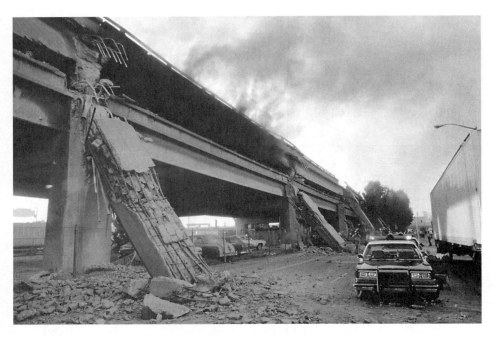

When a powerful earthquake ravaged the San Francisco Bay Area, many people were exposed to extreme negative stress, like those trapped in cars on this interstate.

Stress as External Cause

When speaking of stress as an external stimulus, it is more appropriate to talk of **stressors.** The concept of stressors is similar to the notion of force in engineering. An engineer might calculate the force exerted by cars on a bridge or the pressure of wind against a skyscraper. The demands we experience daily are the forces that wear on us: too much work, too little money, too many creditors, the arrival of a baby, the excitement of a new job, and so on. These are stressors, not stress. Just as a bridge must withstand the load of cars and trucks, we must have some means of meeting or resisting the pressure of external stressors. We do this through coping strategies or defensive reactions.[2]

Stress as Psychological Resistance and Tension

You can respond outwardly to stress passively or actively. But the mental processes involved in meeting external demands are in some sense always active, energy-consuming, and tension-producing.[3] Emotional reactions are likely to be more volatile, marked by

---

[2]Chapter 10 will present an overview of coping strategies.

[3]Tension should be taken here in the most neutral sense of the term—that is, simply "aroused and straining." When you get involved in a TV murder mystery, you may actively try to figure out who did it. You are in a state of mental tension. This does not necessarily mean extreme strain, such as a rope stretched to the breaking point.

increased irritability, explosiveness, and displacement of anger and frustration (Berkowitz, 1990). Perceptual processes involved in interpreting external stimuli may be distorted. It is even very possible that no objective threat exists at all, that the problem is solely due to how the person has interpreted mental events. Situations previously treated as humorous or nonthreatening become ominous and threatening. Even with the best intentions, rational planning and decision-making processes may deteriorate or fail to function at all.

Although the focus is on internal states, people still use a variety of physical terms to report their personal batting average against stress. They may talk about being on the verge of a physical or emotional collapse, or they may suggest that they are ready to snap or break. When cognitive, physical, and behavioral coping resources have been taxed to the limit, they may say things like, "This is beyond me," or "I just can't take this (pressure) anymore." Some may even reach a point where they say, "I just feel like giving up." These are signs of the cracks in the defensive armor, reflections of the strain that accumulates while enduring stress.

Just as the term *stressor* refers to forces bearing down on a person, *strain* refers to the effect of that pressure within the person. According to Selye (1974), though, strain occurs whether the stressor is pleasant or unpleasant. All that "counts is the intensity of the demand for readjustment or adaptation" (pp. 28–29). Whether it is distress or eustress, the demand on coping resources is the same. Further, whether strain fosters growth through challenge or is detrimental to physical and mental health depends on personal appraisals of demands and resources (Lazarus & Launier, 1978). It is also important to note that no one typically regards positive stress as a problem (Orman, 1991). While eustress may place demands on the body, then, it is not processed in the same way mentally and emotively that distress is processed.

Stress as Bodily Defenses

The third definition of stress emphasizes the global biological reaction to stress. Selye (1974) stated that *"Stress is not merely nervous tension"* (p. 30). Stress is *"the nonspecific response of the body to any demand made upon it"* (p. 27). The body has multiple systems that control the stress response. One system, called the **HPA** complex, includes the **H**ypothalamus (neural control) and the **P**ituitary and the **A**drenal glands (glandular-hormonal control). The second system, the **SAM** complex, includes the **S**ympathetic division of the autonomic nervous system and the **A**drenal **M**edulla. When subjected to chronic stress, the body may undergo several negative changes. Selye (1993) observed a prototypic three-part (triadic) body reaction to stress, including (1) enlarged adrenal glands, (2) shrinkage of the thymus and lymph nodes, and (3) ulcers. One weakness in Selye's theory was that he rarely dealt with the psychosocial side of stress. In response to Selye, then, we can say that *stress is not merely physical arousal.*

To summarize, a stressor is an external force, real or perceived. Strain is the wear and tear that result from resisting pressure. In this view, the stressor is the cause and strain is the combined psychological and physiological effect. When the term *stress or strain* occurs without qualification, then, think of this combined psychological and physiological arousal.

DISTINGUISHING STRESS FROM OTHER EMOTIVE STATES

Several related terms appear frequently in discussions of stress, sometimes almost as though they are interchangeable. These include **anxiety, conflict,** and **frustration.** Some clarification of their usage in stress literature may be helpful.

Anxiety: Apprehension and Impending Doom

According to Lazarus (1993), "the core relational theme of anxiety is facing an existential threat, . . . a threat to our being and to the essential meanings that comprise it" (p. 31). The most serious anxiety reactions are panic attacks. These attacks involve a "sudden onset of intense apprehension, fearfulness, or terror, often associated with feelings of impending doom" (American Psychiatric Association, 1994, p. 393).

Anxiety differs from fear in that anxiety is a general state of apprehension, and fear has a specific object. A person is afraid of spiders or snakes or heights, for example. Anxiety, on the other hand, does not seem related to anything in particular, at least, not that the person can point to directly.

Distinguishing anxiety from stress, though, is nearly impossible. In one entire volume devoted to the topic, the authors never distinguish between stress and anxiety (Kutash, Schlesinger, & Associates, 1980). Thus, stress and anxiety can both refer to the subjective psychological result of environmental pressure.

Conflict: The Lesser of Two Evils

Competition between two goals results in conflict. The fact that conflict can produce ulcers in rats (Sawrey & Weiss, 1956) is another indicator that negative emotion has the potential to harmfully influence health. There are three types of conflict (Lewin, 1948; Miller, 1944). **Approach-approach conflicts** occur when two equally desirable goals compete and only one goal can be obtained. Assume that a high school graduate applies to two equally attractive universities—say Harvard and Yale. Upon admission to both, the graduate may go through some degree of conflict before making a decision. Choosing whether to buy a new car or a new boat also may entail conflict when only one can be purchased. In general, though, these are the type of problems most of us would love to have; we would not regard them as aversive and undesirable.

Avoidance-avoidance conflicts occur when two goals have equally unattractive values. The choice of having to either rake the leaves or wash all the windows in the house illustrates this type of conflict. Deciding whether to study for an important exam or go to the library and work on a term paper that is due could also raise this type of conflict.

Approach-avoidance conflicts exist when the same goal has both positive and negative features. Marriage provides permanence and stability in one's primary intimate relationship, a sense of teamwork and sharing, and the prospect of family. It also may contain negatives such as the perception of loss of freedom and independence, overwhelming responsibility, and an uncertain yet seemingly irreversible commitment to one person. Most of life's day-to-day pressures are probably of an approach-avoidance variety.

Frustration: Immovable Barriers

When some barrier comes between a person and attainment of a goal, frustration occurs. A student who works hard to get into medical school may be frustrated by earning poor grades on an entrance exam. Someone who wants to begin a small business but cannot save enough money to get started may experience frustration. Similarly, a person who wants to impress a boss or a potential lover but finds someone else constantly interfering will likely feel frustration.

One possible, though not inevitable, outcome of frustration is aggression. Berkowitz (1990) provided evidence that a primary negative emotion, such as frustration, works through a sequence of body-arousal and cognitive attributions to increase the likelihood of aggression. A person wanting to start a business may decide to steal the needed money. A person thwarted in an attempt to impress the boss or lover may become verbally or physically aggressive toward the person who interferes.

Hamilton (1979) believed that anxiety "is the major and most fundamental source of strain in the person" (p. 86). He also suggested that "the greater the load from these sources [conflict, frustration, and anxiety], the greater the number and the severity of the stressors and the farther the movement towards a limit of 'stress' tolerance" (p. 80).

IN SICKNESS AND IN HEALTH: HEALTH STATUS AND SOCIAL ROLES

A major concern today is the nature of the relationship between stress and health. This concern is based on both clinical and laboratory observations of stress symptoms. In general, we can identify four different types of stress symptoms: behavioral, emotive, cognitive, and physical (Vlisides, Eddy, & Mozie, 1994). The presence of physical disturbance in response to stress most often raises questions about the stress and health connection.

Behavioral Symptoms: Changed Behavior Patterns

Among the many behavioral signs of stress are procrastination and avoidance, withdrawal from friends and family, loss of appetite and energy, emotional outbursts and aggression, beginning or dramatically increasing the use of drugs, changes in sleep patterns (especially restless or agitated sleep), neglect of responsibilities, lower productivity in personal and professional pursuits, absenteeism from classes and/or job, and accident proneness. Other behavioral symptoms include crying, pacing and agitation, and excessive nail-biting. Some people show an overall lower activity (energy) level, but this may be due to two factors. First, stress can easily lead to appetite loss and lower nutritional integrity. Second, stress can drain energy through constant inner turmoil and struggle.

Emotive Symptoms: Volatile or Depressed Feelings

The most common emotive symptoms of stress are anxiety, dread, irritability, and depression. Other symptoms may include denial, fear, a sense of frustration, feelings of uncertainty, and feelings of loss of control. On the job, stress may translate to a loss of morale and lower job satisfaction.

Cognitive Symptoms: Mind's Miscalculations

Among the most common mental symptoms of stress are loss of motivation and concentration. It may appear that a person has lost the ability to focus on needed tasks and lost the ability to bring tasks to successful conclusion. Typically, this is because the mind is using too many resources for dealing with the stress situation and does not have enough resources left to deal with day-to-day activities. Other mental symptoms include excessive worry, loss of recall, misperceptions and misattributions, confusion, reduced capacity for decision making, poor problem-solving capacity especially during a crisis, self-pity, and loss of hope. One final mental trait is an escape mentality, also likened to a "bunker" or "fox-hole" mentality. The term "bunker" literally refers to a wartime defense structure. When soldiers came under siege, their mind-set was often one of escape translated in commonsense terms as "I wish I were anyplace but here."

Physical Symptoms: The Body Language of Stress

As noted earlier, a great amount of attention has focused on body language and stress because these symptoms are often correlates of disturbances that are either the prelude to or direct expressions of some type of disease process (Williams, 1995). Among the most commonly noted physical symptoms are fatigue and physical weakness, migraine and tension headaches, backaches including lower back pain, and muscle tension that can translate as tremors and even spasms. In the cardiovascular system, stress is often reflected by accelerated heart rate, hypertension, and exacerbation of atherosclerotic process. The respiratory system typically responds with rapid but often shallower breathing, and in extreme situations, hyperventilation may occur. In addition to these symptoms, certain syndromes are also noted to be correlates of stress. Such syndromes include grinding teeth (bruxism), irritable bowel syndrome, and chronic fatigue syndrome (Farrar, Locke, & Kantrowitz, 1995). More serious breakdowns may also occur, such as ulcers, cancer, cardiac arrhythmias, and cardiac events leading to death. However, it should be noted that the most serious events not only are rare, but they also have a significant biomedical history that has led to vulnerability independent of the stress.

The Stress-Illness Connection: Disease, Illness Behavior, and Health

At the start of this section, I noted that there is great interest in how stress may be related to increased vulnerability to sickness. To consider this connection, we must ask some basic questions. What does it mean to be sick or to have a disease? When one displays illness behavior, is that the same as sickness? Is health the opposite of being sick? How does health behavior relate to being healthy? These terms—disease, health, illness behavior, and health behavior—are discussed briefly in this section.

Disease and Sickness

Disease refers to a physical condition that results from a body malfunction. It may be due to a breakdown in a body organ or a malfunction in one of the body's systems. Disease is most often explained by the germ model; that is, a toxic microorganism invades the body, causing alterations in body tissue leading to observable symptoms of distress. Sickness and illness are equivalent terms that refer to a state of suffering from a disease.

Illness Behavior

Symptoms are the first visible signs of disease. When they appear, you probably run through an internal check that evaluates and attaches meaning to the symptoms. In the process, you form a plan of action that may involve family members, and you may take a trip to the doctor's office.

Upon reaching the clinic, you complain about your discomfort and describe your symptoms. You seek medical remedies and signs of support from medical staff, family, and friends. This process—evaluating symptoms, seeking medical help to bring relief, and seeking support from family—is the core of **illness behavior** (Mechanic, 1966).

Illness behavior can occur with or without physical indicators of disease. It is appropriate when a medical diagnosis or obvious symptoms (such as vomiting) occur. It is deviant, or at least frowned on, when it occurs in the absence of a diagnosed illness. Thus, *disease* refers to a physical condition of the body, while *illness behavior* defines a social role with expectations for both the sick and the healer (Parsons, 1951).

An important characteristic of illness behavior is that it often brings **secondary gains,** rewards or benefits obtained through the sick role. These gains include increased sympathy and attention, special favors such as being waited on, and release from duties at school or work.

When conducting research on stress and health, we must not confuse the social role of illness behavior (including unverified reports of sickness) with physical disease. This could lead to the erroneous conclusion that stress causes disease, when it may only increase people's tendency to engage in illness behavior.

Health: The Opposite of Sickness?

We could define **health** as the absence of disease. Most people, though, would easily recognize the weakness in this definition. One can be free of disease but still not enjoy a full, wholesome, satisfying life. Health entails valuations of the quality of physical and mental vigor. The World Health Organization defined health as "a state of complete physical, mental, and social well-being and not merely the absence of disease or infirmity" (cited in Seeman, 1989, p. 1100). On the physical side, the definition means that the person enjoys a robust life with the energy needed to engage in satisfying pursuits and explorations of the environment. Simultaneously, the healthy person enjoys emotional fulfillment and self-esteem, both signs of positive mental health. Finally, social well-being is shown by the formation of close personal relationships, involvement in community, and interest in the well-being of others.

Health Behavior

Kasl and Cobb (1966) defined **health behavior** as activity undertaken by a person who believes himself or herself to be healthy for the purpose of preventing disease. It is estimated that 50% of premature deaths are a result of lifestyle risks and that lifestyle contributes 54% of the variability to cardiovascular disease (Institute of Medicine, 1979; Wilson, 1989). Health behavior may include reducing or eliminating high-risk behaviors such as smoking or eating poorly. The person also may adopt positive behaviors such as exercising regularly. Finally, health behavior may involve adhering to a distasteful though necessary medical regimen, such as taking a medicine or going through chemotherapy with unpleasant side effects.

BUILDING THEORIES: THE EXPLANATORY STORIES OF SCIENCE

Many theories have been developed to explain what stress is, how it works, and how it relates to health. Though the term *theory* sounds very formal, theories are really the explanatory stories of science. Theories summarize a body of data. They provide an organized, coherent picture of some part of nature or some aspect of human behavior. When a theory can generate new, testable hypotheses that fill more gaps in our knowledge, the theory is said to have heuristic value and power. Theories are never fully verified; some leap of inference is always made between the theory and the data that support it. Finally, theories are never complete. They evolve and change as new data accumulate and new techniques allow more sophisticated tests of relevant hypotheses.

TABLE 1-1
Comparison of key features of stress models

STRESS MODEL	DEFINITION OF STRESS	SOURCE(S) OF STRESS	MODEL'S STRENGTHS	MODEL'S WEAKNESSES
General Adaptation Syndrome	Nonspecific demand on body— disturbs body equilibrium	Various environmental pressures— chronic—depletes energy reserves	Empirically derived and extensively tested	Extreme biological emphasis Treats good and bad stressors in the same way
Diathesis-stress model	No specific definition provided	Mismatch between biological endowment and environmental stressors	Interaction model Gives equal weight to internal and external factors	Ignores cognitive-social factors in stress Indirect evidence rather than direct tests Difficult to give terms operational reference
Psychodynamic theory	Defined primarily by reference to anxiety	Signals of danger and intrapsychic conflict	Uses few constructs with great power Intuitive appeal	Inadequate in scope Little or no consideration of biological or social factors Difficult to test
Learning theory	Faulty conditioning causing conditional emotional responses	Presence of any conditional stimuli and/or reinforcing stimuli	Empirically derived Clear operational definitions for basic terms and procedures Attempted explanation of related coping actions	Scope is limited Largely ignores any biological factors Limited use of social-context factors Ignores or denies importance of cognitive process

Some theories, such as Selye's physiological theory, attempt to explain the way the body responds to stress. Psychological theories attempt to understand the ways in which personality, expectations, and interpretations turn a personal or social event into a stressful situation. They try to build plausible explanations of the way behavior changes because of stress. Further, psychological theories try to explain how coping behaviors may reduce the impact or prevent the reappearance of stress. Social theories provide explanations of stress based more on group conflict and the unequal distribution of power and wealth. Holistic health theories espouse a set of social and personal values based on the idea that body and mind must be treated in unified fashion. Finally, systems theory attempts to explain how organisms engage in self-regulation even when embedded in more complex self-regulating systems.

Table 1-1 summarizes the key features and the strengths and weaknesses of the major theories. It may be helpful to refer to the table periodically while reading the remainder of this chapter.

TABLE 1-1 *continued*

STRESS MODEL	DEFINITION OF STRESS	SOURCE(S) OF STRESS	MODEL'S STRENGTHS	MODEL'S WEAKNESSES
Transactional theory	Relationship between demand and coping sources	Real or perceived psychosocial pressures	Compatible with both the biological and social models Large and growing body of supporting evidence	Criticized for its circularity Some constructs not well-defined Does not explicitly suggest how the mind influences body process
Social stress theory	Pressures to conform or adapt to social systems/norms	Social conflict and coercion Social change and living conditions Lack of access to resources	Incorporates many plausible social factors related to stress	Very broad and ill-defined Difficult to give terms operational reference Ignores biological variables Ignores individual difference
Control theory	Disturbance between reference (normal) value and comparator value in feedback loop	Any data that produce disequilibrium in the system	Has potential to include all the different systems that influence stress reactions	Difficult to operationalize and test
Holistic health theory	No specific definition provided	Implies that stress results from failure to treat the person as a functional whole	Scope is global Tacit acceptance of interaction between biological, psychological, and social factors	Not a formal theory Lacking in formal operational definitions Lacking in specific supporting research

VARIETIES OF BIOLOGICAL STRESS THEORIES

While many biological theories of stress exist, only two such theories will be discussed here. The first is Hans Selye's **General Adaptation Syndrome** (1974, 1979); the second is genetic-constitutional theory.

The General Adaptation Syndrome

Selye's theory may be summarized in four general statements:

1. All biological organisms have an innate drive to maintain a state of internal balance, or equilibrium. The process that maintains an internal balance is homeostasis. As it turns out, maintaining homeostasis is a lifelong task.
2. Stressors, such as germs or excessive work demands, disturb internal equilibrium. The body responds to any stressor, whether pleasant or unpleasant, with a nonspecific physiological arousal. This reaction is defensive and self-protective.

3. Adjustment to stress occurs in stages. The time course and progress through the stages depends on how successful the resistance is in relation to the intensity and duration of the stressor.
4. The organism has a finite reserve of adaptive energy. When depleted, the organism lacks the ability to cope with continued stress, and death may follow.

The pioneer research program that led to this theory was already under way in the 1950s and 1960s. Selye (1956) studied laboratory animals exposed to chronic severe stressors. The animals reacted with signs of physical stress, up to and including acute traumatic ulcers of the stomach and subsequent death.

Many studies supported Selye's conclusions, but one study will be discussed in detail—the classic executive monkey study (Brady, Porter, Conrad, & Mason, 1958). This study illustrates some of the complexities of designing research to provide unequivocal answers to important questions. It will show, further, how other explanations may be proposed and tested.

In the Brady study, four pairs of monkeys learned how to press a lever to avoid a punishing shock. Each monkey in the pair faced a completely different situation. The executive monkey could engage in an avoidance response that would prevent the punishment from being delivered to both himself and his *yoked-control* partner, who could do nothing to avoid the shocks. The partner's safety and comfort depended solely on the alertness and decision process of the executive monkey.

The outcome of this story has been widely publicized. The four executive monkeys charged with the responsibility to act developed ulcers and died. The four monkeys with

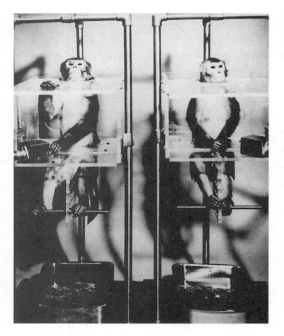

Executive monkeys with responsibility to press a lever to avoid shock for themselves and their yoked control partners.

no responsibility suffered no ill effects. It seemed that the demands of work, the responsibility placed on the *executives,* produced the stress and, ultimately, death.[4]

A major flaw in the procedure, however, was not as widely publicized. That flaw had to do with a simple principle of experimental design: the monkeys were not randomly assigned to be executives or controls. Instead, when the monkeys first received shocks, the first member of the pair to respond became the executive, and the other one became the yoked-control member. It is possible that the monkeys who responded first were more emotional or hyperreactive. This, in turn, suggests that physiological differences existed between the pairs, such as increased autonomic reactivity and gastric motility. If so, the executive monkeys would be more susceptible to ulcers because of preexisting differences in temperament and constitution. This biological explanation would be as acceptable under the circumstances as the responsibility explanation.

The responsibility explanation became even less acceptable when subsequent studies did not replicate Brady's findings (Weiss, 1968, 1971). Indeed, most subsequent findings are in direct opposition to Brady's—that is, helpless animals generally develop more ulcers than controlling animals. Control theory suggests that organisms generally fare better under threat when they have some response available that will be instrumental in dealing with the threat (Wiener, 1961). What might account for this discrepancy?

One possible explanation concerns the type of control the executives had. In the Brady study, the executives lacked feedback about success. Fisher (1988) argued that such control is more stressful and may have contributed to the outcome of this study. This brief excursion into a classic study should alert the reader to the importance of sound research design. It should also encourage an attitude of healthy skepticism and critical analysis of the details in published reports of research, especially when the report is made through the mass media.

Selye's research program led him to propose the existence of a three-stage process called the General Adaptation Syndrome, or GAS (Figure 1-2). The syndrome can be summarized as follows.

1. **Alarm.** The alarm reaction occurs at the first appearance of a stressor. For a short period, the body has a lower than normal level of resistance. Short-term increases in gastrointestinal disturbances and elevated blood pressure may result. Then the body quickly marshals defensive resources and makes self-protective adjustments. If the defensive reactions are successful, the alarm subsides and the body returns to normal activity. During this period, often dubbed an *acute* stress reaction, many stresses are resolved.

2. **Resistance.** If a stressor becomes *chronic*—that is, it continues over a longer time because of factors outside the organism's control or because the first reaction did not remove the emergency—the body will call for full-scale mobilization. The problem is that the body has to expend many resources to win this war, which generally results in decreased resistance over time. In addition, more serious physical symptoms, such as ulcers or atherosclerosis, may develop. These physical symptoms may reduce resistance even more.

---

[4]Investigators attempting to follow up on Brady's executive monkey study made an interesting discovery. They found that it was while off duty—in other words, during vacation time—that the ulcers developed in the executive monkeys, not during the working time.

FIGURE 1-2
The three stages of Selye's General Adaptation Syndrome (GAS): Alarm, resistance, exhaustion.
SOURCE: Hales (1997).

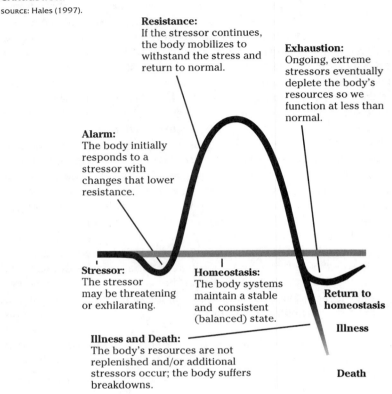

Resistance:
If the stressor continues, the body mobilizes to withstand the stress and return to normal.

Exhaustion:
Ongoing, extreme stressors eventually deplete the body's resources so we function at less than normal.

Alarm:
The body initially responds to a stressor with changes that lower resistance.

Stressor:
The stressor may be threatening or exhilarating.

Homeostasis:
The body systems maintain a stable and consistent (balanced) state.

Return to homeostasis

Illness

Illness and Death:
The body's resources are not replenished and/or additional stressors occur; the body suffers breakdowns.

Death

3. **Exhaustion.** If the stressor is unusually severe or drawn out, the body further depletes or exhausts its reserves of energy. Resistance breaks down altogether, and death may follow shortly thereafter (Selye, 1980).

Influential as Selye's theory has been, its narrowness is not compatible with current views of stress. One major weakness is that it does not encompass the psychosocial factors of critical importance to understanding human stress. It does not address the cognitive processes that influence the point when demand becomes challenge or when demand becomes threat. Further, it does not consider the selection of strategies to combat stress or the effectiveness of coping strategies.

Genetic-Constitutional Theories

The ability to resist stress depends on the coping strategies applied in the face of a current emergency. In addition, several factors related to individual genetic history, called **predisposing factors,** affect resistance. They influence resistance through preset organ weaknesses, by increasing risk for diseases, or by setting response sensitivities (irritability). Predisposing factors may be likened to threshold or tolerance factors.

Genetic–constitutional research attempts to establish a link between genetic makeup (genotype) and some physical characteristic (phenotype) that lowers a person's general ability to resist stress. Genetic factors may reduce resistance in several ways. Genetic makeup influences balance in the autonomic nervous system (ANS). The ANS helps to balance body processes between the quiet restorative side and the active aroused side or the so-called fight-or-flight emergency reaction system. General temperament is also genetically determined in part. **Temperament,** a very broad term, refers to three differences in initial response patterns. First, activity levels vary on a continuum from active to passive. Second, emotional responses range from pleasant to unpleasant. Finally, reactivity to stimuli varies from hypersensitive to hyposensitive (Fuller & Thompson, 1978).

Genes also control the codes for the structure and function of organs and body systems. Of most importance to stress resistance are the kidneys, the cardiovascular system (risks for coronary, high blood pressure, arteriosclerosis), the digestive system (risks for stomach and duodenal ulcers), and the nervous system (imbalance in the autonomic system).

THE DIATHESIS-STRESS MODEL

For decades, scientists have debated the relative contribution of inheritance and environment (nature and nurture) to personality and intelligence. While the debate is far from over, one thing seems clear. We do not have to choose between two competing processes. Instead, as the **diathesis-stress model** suggests, heredity and environment are complementary processes that interact to influence biological structures and functions.

This theory suggests there is an interplay between predisposing and **precipitating factors.** A person's genetic map contributes predisposing factors, as discussed in the preceding section. A lower threshold for stress or an organic weakness makes the person vulnerable to illness. Whether that weakness ever shows up or not depends on the amount of stress—the precipitating force—the person experiences. In a somewhat sheltered and *stressless* environment, even a very vulnerable person might never show signs of the strain. Conversely, a person under severe, continuous strain might respond poorly even though genetic predispositions are strong. Parsons (1988) also suggests that evolutionary change continues to work in selecting for behaviors that enable organisms to adapt to stressful environments.

VARIETIES OF PSYCHOLOGICAL STRESS THEORIES

Major psychological theories include the psychodynamic, learning, cognitive, and general systems models. There are several cognitive models, but Richard Lazarus and his associates proposed the most influential model (Lazarus & Launier, 1978). One extension of the cognitive approach is the **conservation-of-resources model** proposed by Steven Hobfoll (1989). Finally, Carver and Scheier (1981, 1982) and Gary Schwartz (1982, 1983) constructed general systems models, generally called control theories.

The Psychodynamic Model

Sigmund Freud's theory is undoubtedly the accepted standard among psychodynamic models. Freud described two kinds of anxiety: *signal* and *traumatic* anxiety. **Signal anxiety** occurs when an objective external danger is present. It corresponds most closely to the stressor-strain (danger-anxiety) relationship. The second kind, **traumatic anxiety,** was the dominant form of anxiety in Freud's theory. It refers to instinctual, or internally generated, anxiety. Examples include anxiety aroused when coping with repressed sexual drives and aggressive instincts. Anxiety puts a strain on psychic functioning. The resulting symptoms are the 11 "psychopathologies of everyday life," to use Freud's (1966) term. The notion of **conversion** was also important. Essentially, conversion is a process that takes the energy from a psychic conflict and turns it into a relatively harmless, physical symptom, such as a facial tic.

The Learning Theory View

As an explanation of stress, learning theory generally uses either the **classical conditioning** (Pavlovian) model, the **operant** (Skinnerian) model, or a combination of the two. Russian Nobel laureate Ivan Pavlov pioneered development of the classical conditioning model.

To illustrate classical conditioning, consider the famous (or infamous) experiment conducted by the father of behavioral psychology, John Watson. Watson showed 11-month-old Albert a pet rat. Initially, Albert displayed no fear of the animal. Later, Watson arranged that Albert saw the rat immediately followed by a loud noise. Predictably, Albert responded with fear to the loud sound. After just seven repetitions, Albert was afraid of the rat even when no loud sound was present. Fear was also present with a variety of other objects similar to the rat, such as a rabbit, a sealskin coat, and a Santa's mask (Watson & Rayner, 1920). Figure 1-3 illustrates this conditioning process.

In classical conditioning, loud noise is one of a general class of stimuli called **unconditional stimuli** (UCS).[5] These are biologically powerful unlearned signals related to survival needs of the organism. When an unconditional stimulus occurs, it evokes an unlearned reflex, or **unconditional response** (UCR). The rat was one of another class of signals called **conditional stimuli** (CS). Before any experience, conditional stimuli may be regarded as novel or neutral stimuli (NS). To have any power, they first must be associated with powerful unconditional stimuli. When a conditional stimulus brings about the response previously produced only by the UCS, it is now a learned reflex or **conditional response** (CR).

Two aspects of the conditioning process are important for stress theory. First, emotional responses, such as fear and anxiety, are complex and include (1) behavioral, (2) psychological, and (3) physiological components. Escape and/or avoidance behaviors keep a person as far away as possible from stressful stimuli. Subjectively, the person experiences a state of internal tension when confronting a feared object or event. The body becomes physiologically aroused, as reflected by increased blood pressure, heart rate, and body temperature. When conditioning occurs, as in Albert's case, all three

---

[5]Instead of using the mistranslated "conditioned," as is conventional, it is more accurate to say "conditional," and the meaning is clear: "unconditional" means "not dependent upon," and "conditional" means "dependent upon." Thus, the UCS does not depend on anything for its power while the CS depends on prior associations with the UCS for power.

FIGURE 1-3
Classically conditioned fear illustrated with the case of Little Albert.
SOURCE: Goldstein (1994).

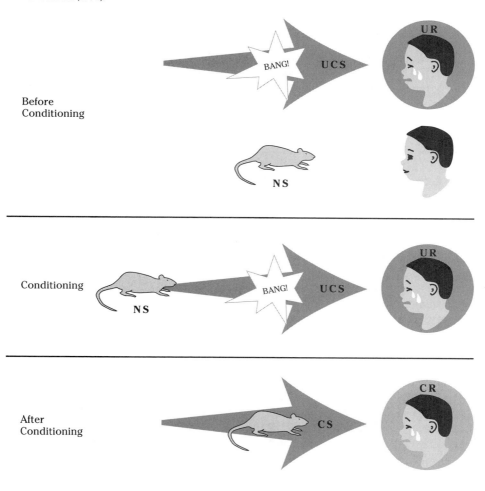

components are conditioned to the CS (the rat). Later, even very low levels of the stimulus (a picture of a rat) can result in subjective tension and physiological arousal, although the person may not show it outwardly.

Second, anxiety may become anticipatory after the original conditioning has occurred. Anxiety can be aroused just by talking or thinking about the feared stimulus, even when there is no immediate pressure to confront it. Imagine someone afraid of snakes. A friend reports watching an interesting documentary on reptiles. With the mention of snakes, the person may visibly tense, shudder, and redirect the conversation to another topic. If the person cannot control the anxiety while confronting a frightening situation, the anxiety has the potential to be disabling, keeping the individual from enjoying normal pleasures.

Operant theory proposes that behavior changes because it produces either good or bad outcomes. When a behavior produces pleasant outcomes, or rewards, the behavior increases. When a behavior produces unpleasant outcomes, or punishment, the behavior decreases. Explanations of stress from an operant perspective place most emphasis on the acquisition of avoidance behavior and the discriminative control of symptomatic behavior.

Avoidance behavior is an operant response that serves to reduce learned fear or anxiety. For Albert, associating the rat with the loud noise conditioned a fear response to the rat. Fear is an unpleasant emotion that increases internal tension. People generally try to reduce or remove unpleasant tension. Because running away from the rat reduces tension, running away is strengthened. If the rat appears again, the most likely response is flight. In general, any stressful situation that produces high or unmanageable levels of anxiety is likely to motivate some form of escape or avoidance.

The Cognitive Transactional Model of Stress

People perceive and label events, store information about their experiences, and retrieve and use that information in different ways. How this influences new encounters is important to the arousal of stress and to the coping strategies employed to deal with stress. Cognitive researchers attempt to understand stress mechanisms in terms of the way in which the brain processes information through its many pathways and way stations.

Cognitive theorists assume that humans are active, reasoning, and deciding beings. They also assume that people construct **schemata,** or mental blueprints. Schemata[6] represent things learned about the world, how it works, and how to relate to it. Certain schemata may be almost universal, such as the schema for gravity. Others always show a high degree of personal uniqueness, such as a schema for teacher/student relationships.

Several cognitive transactional theories have appeared over the years. The most prominent is the model developed by Richard S. Lazarus (Lazarus & Launier, 1978). This theory is previewed here but developed more fully in Chapter 3. As explained by Lazarus, the theory has roots in several scientific soils. These include the cognitive sciences, personality theory, attitude research, social research, health research, and behavioral medicine. Lazarus assumes that stress and health have reciprocal influences. That is, stress can have a powerful impact on health, and conversely, health can influence a person's resistance or coping ability.

The central point of the transactional model is that stress is "neither an environmental stimulus, a characteristic of the person, nor a response, but a relationship between demands and the power to deal with them without unreasonable or destructive costs" (Coyne & Holroyd, 1982, p. 108). It is apparent that a *relational* analysis is the key to this theory. There are some important implications to be drawn from this.

First, the same environmental event may be interpreted as stressful by one person but not stressful by someone else. This suggests that most external stimuli cannot be defined in any absolute sense as stressful. Instead, it is a personal cognitive appraisal that makes the event stressful or not stressful. It is important to note that personal appraisals are embedded in the person's cultural and gender assimilation contexts (Leadbeater, Blatt, & Quinlan, 1995; Slavin, Rainer, McCreary, & Gowda, 1991). Second, the same person may interpret an event as stressful on one occasion but not on an-

---

[6]*Schemata* is plural, while *schema* is singular.

other. This may be due to changes in physical condition or changes in psychological states. The person might be physically relaxed and rested on one occasion but tense and tired on another. Emotional and motivational states differ across time, which can also affect the appraisal process.

HASSLES: THE STRAWS OF STRESS Richard Lazarus also suggested that we should substitute the term **hassles** for the frequently used and oft-abused *stress*. In everyday conversation, the term *hassles* conveys the sense that pressures are piling up ("I don't need this hassle") or that someone is pressing too hard ("Don't hassle me"). More formally, hassles are "the irritating, frustrating, *distressing* demands that in some degree characterize everyday transactions with the environment [italics added]" (Kanner, Coyne, Schaefer, & Lazarus, 1981, p. 3). Parallel to Selye's eustress, there are also *uplifts*, positive experiences such as loving relationships, finishing a job, and being healthy.

Hassles are less intense than catastrophic types of stress, but they are persistent, nagging thorns in the flesh. The types of events used to illustrate hassles come from everyday life. They include losing the car keys, bills piling up with no end in sight, constant interruptions, not enough time for leisure, and the shoelace that breaks when you're in a hurry. In comparing hassles with life changes such as divorce or death of a spouse, Lazarus and his colleagues showed that hassles and illness are more strongly related than life changes and illness. This finding has been confirmed cross-culturally as well (Nakano, 1989).

SELF-STUDY EXERCISE 1-3

What Are Your Methods of Coping?

For the following exercise, try to focus on the coping strategies that you most often use to confront and relieve stress. Do this for each of the stressors that you identified in the previous worksheet (Self-Study Exercise 1-2). Later in this work, you will have a chance to study a variety of different coping strategies. It is often helpful to compare what you have been doing intuitively against the way experts suggest that you handle certain stressful situations.

PERSONAL STRESSORS	WORK OR SCHOOL STRESSORS	ENVIRONMENTAL STRESSORS

Critique of Transactional Theory and an Alternative

Although the cognitive-transactional theory continues to evolve and mature, it has encountered numerous criticisms. Steven Hobfoll (1989) argued that the model is "tautological, overly complex, and not given to rejection" (p. 515). He says that it is tautological because demand and coping capacity are not defined separately. Whether an event is demanding or not depends on coping capacity, and whether coping capacity is adequate is dependent on demand. Refuting the theory is difficult also because both positive and negative instances of coping can be taken as consistent with the model.

In place of the transactional model, Hobfoll argued for a conservation-of-resources model of stress. According to Hobfoll, people possess resources they value and wish to protect or conserve. These include object resources (a home or business), condition resources (seniority, power, marriage), personal characteristics (self-efficacy and self-esteem), and energies (time, money, and knowledge). Psychological stress occurs when there is a real or perceived net loss of resources or when there is lack of gain after investment of resources.

Although Hobfoll criticized weaknesses of the transactional model, he used similar cognitive concepts. He tried to suggest one quantifiable marker—loss—that may make stress theories more testable. Still, there does not appear to be a significant difference in the precision, or quantifiability, of loss as opposed to Lazarus's concept of harm (R. S. Lazarus, personal communication, August 13, 1991). While it is important to keep in mind potential weaknesses in a theory, we cannot and should not quickly abandon a strong and well-researched one on the basis of speculation alone.

VARIETIES OF SOCIAL STRESS THEORIES

Several **social stress theories** focus on integration of the individual into society and tensions that are part of any society. These are **conflict theories.** A major source of tension is that society has to engage in some degree of coercion to get members to comply with social norms. One conflict theorist believes that a crucial problem is affording members of society more life chances or opportunities for growth (Dahrendorf, 1979). Stress occurs when people cannot obtain work, homes, education, or technical retraining, or cannot participate in the political process. Conflict theories also look at the stability of social relationships, the distribution of economic goods and services in society (Dooley & Catalano, 1984), and the distribution of interpersonal power and personal control. These conflict variables are related to stress in fairly obvious ways. Theoretically, stress is the inevitable outcome of less stable social relationships, poverty and lack of access to necessary social services, and low power and personal control.

Lesley Slavin and his colleagues (1991) extended the cognitive-transactional theory of Lazarus into the social arena by proposing a multicultural model of stress. They suggest that membership in cultural groups can affect the nature and frequency of certain stressors. Being a member of a minority group can increase frequency of stressful events. Belonging to an oppressed group increases the likelihood that members will experience acts of discrimination. Those who are poor and those who lack political power face stressors such as evictions and jailings that more advantaged groups do not face. In many ways, then, culture will affect primary appraisals of harm-loss and threat. Culture will also influence secondary appraisals of resources—including personal, familial, and social—that are available to deal with the stressor. Finally, social customs unique to the person's culture will also influence the form and direction of coping efforts. Although the model is offered as a speculative extension of the cognitive-transactional theory, it may prove useful in conceptualizing the perceptual filters that influence the person's interpretation of events as stressful or not.

Evolutionary theory views social change and tension as the inevitable results of social development. People must accept the fact of social change and accommodate to it instead of fighting against it. Environmental–ecological theory explains stress in terms of conditions such as crowding, pollution, health hazards from industrialization, and environmental accidents. Finally, **life-change theory** explains stress by reference to life changes that require major adaptations by the person. Death of a spouse, bankruptcy, loss of a job, or life-threatening illness fit the definition of major events that require substantial personal adjustment.

The Holistic Health Model

Holistic theory has many faces. It is a movement with political and economic overtones. It is a pseudoreligion of lifestyle and self-sufficiency practiced with evangelistic zeal by a group of true believers (Alster, 1989). It is a humanistic philosophy with anti-scientific sentiments. Finally, it is a reaction to biological reductionism and medical specialization in Western medicine.

In the health arena, holistic theory suggests that it has a new paradigm of health care to offer (Capra, 1982). The intensity with which its values are expressed conveys the impression of a counterculture with antimedical establishment themes. This is most evident when it suggests that Western medicine is dehumanizing and devalues the role of mental processes in health and healing. Still, holistic health presents itself as a synthesizing movement trying to regain a sense of humane medical treatment and respect for the whole person (Sobel, 1979). Treatment of the whole person is a valued medical tradition that has existed without interruption since ancient times, most visibly in Eastern medical tradition.

According to Burstein and Loucks (1982), there are three trademarks of the holistic health movement. These are "(1) a recognition of human complexity and diversity, (2) an emphasis on the importance of mental events and personal value systems, and (3) a recognition of the desirability of responsibility for oneself" (p. 179). Girdano and Everly (1979) stated that *holistic* is "the concept underlying an approach to controlling stress and tension that deals with the complete lifestyle of the individual, incorporating intervention at several levels—physical, psychological, and social—simultaneously" (p. 20).

While there is research to support the holistic model, the model does not generate research itself. Further, it does not have the formal properties of a scientific theory. Alster (1989) is blunt when she suggests that holistic health is a movement without a theoretical framework. She concludes also that the movement has not defined its basic terms and relies on slogans for its support.

Control Theory: A Systems Model of Stress

Each of the preceding theories tried to explain stress and health by focusing on a limited though promising set of variables. Selye focused on the physiological response system but left out social and psychological detail. Learning theory used narrow conditioning constructs with little concern for physiological processes and slight attention to social systems. Cognitive theory emphasized the information processing system, a system that must deal with data from the external social environment as well as from the internal biopsychological environment. Still, cognitive theory gives little detail on physical parameters of stress and health, and it does not explicitly entertain social constructs. Social theory focused almost exclusively on large-scale factors such as poverty, crowding, and rate of social change. Each view has its unique strengths but also its inherent weaknesses.

An alternative to these theories is systems theory. Systems theory is an outgrowth of the attempt to understand self-regulating systems. The origins of systems theory usually are traced to Norbert Wiener's (1961) classic work on **cybernetics.** Cybernetic concepts usually depend on feedback mechanisms and goal-seeking behavior in more or less self-contained units. General systems theory (GST) considers complex, dynamic interactions in multivariate systems, where systems may be hierarchically enmeshed with other systems (von Bertalanffy, 1968). Cybernetic theory, then, is a subset of general systems theory (Schwartz, 1982).

Cybernetics, also called "control theory," suggests that self-regulating organisms compare their current state to some reference to maintain a match. An often-used example is the thermostat. An organism obtains information about current conditions (room temperature) through sensory input (thermometer). If the comparator detects a discrepancy between the current state (68°) and the reference (70°), the organism engages in some act to reduce the discrepancy (switches the furnace on). This will continue until new information provided to the comparator shows a match with the reference standard. The loop is called a *negative feedback loop* because it attempts to negate the difference between current and reference conditions. An elementary feedback loop is shown in Figure 1-4.

Probably the most widely known cybernetic system is homeostatic control. With reference to stress, external stressors are disturbances that carry information to the system. When a disturbance produces a discrepancy (extreme tension) from the reference (ideal or moderate tension), the system will engage in self-regulating behavior to restore the ideal state. These are coping actions to reduce or eliminate the source of stress. A

FIGURE 1-4
A simple systems model for feedback of a disturbance from the environment.
SOURCE: Carver & Scheier (1982).

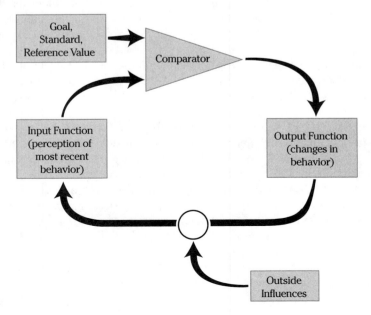

more subtle negative feedback loop is found in the regulatory mechanisms of the immune system (Dantzer & Kelley, 1989).

Feedback processes are reactive. Human organisms also engage in feed forward, or proactive self-regulation (Ford, 1990). That is, they act to make good things happen as well as to prevent bad things from happening. This is especially important in reducing existing stress or preventing potential stressors. It is also important in maintaining positive health and preventing ill health.

Charles Carver and Michael Scheier (1981, 1982) applied control theory to health psychology, a discipline concerned with the ways in which behavior can influence health for better or for worse. Carver and Scheier view the person as a self-contained health-care system that engages in behavior to reduce discrepancies in feedback loops. They suggested that good health is a high-order reference value used to regulate behavior. Good health, though, is related to many different body systems, each with their own low-order reference values. Symptoms are low-order bits of information that tell us something is wrong in a body system.

For example, we monitor a variety of body signals, such as weight, temperature, and blood pressure. If weight becomes undesirably high, we diet and/or exercise to reduce weight. We know that a high temperature may be symptomatic of a cold or flu attack. When this happens, we take appropriate countersteps, such as taking aspirin, fluids, and bed rest. We seek professional help to monitor weak body signals such as blood pressure and hypertension, the silent illness. Then we take prescribed medications to reduce symptoms. All these behaviors are control processes that seek to match a current state (presence of body symptoms) with a reference value (normality in the body system) and ultimately with the value of good health.

Gary Schwartz (1982, 1983) and Julius Seeman (1989) argue for a general systems approach in the discipline of behavior medicine. Schwartz's model is called the "biopsychosocial model," even though it has its roots in general systems theory.[7] This is a multicausal and multieffect model of health and illness. It proposes that medical diagnosis should consider the matrix of biological, psychological, and social factors represented in the patient's history and current condition. Further, it suggests that treatment must consider the treatment's interaction with other treatments as well as with the psychosocial system of the patient.

Whether we consider any given stress response to have a health consequence or not, stress is embedded in a multivariate system. Stress has the potential for multiple effects in systems that range from the function of the body, to the function of psychological processes, to the harmony of home and job. It remains to be seen whether systems theory will be able to generate supporting data, or whether it will function more as a metatheory, which integrates the results of smaller but more testable theories.

MAKING SENSE OF THE CONFUSION

After reading this assortment of stress and health theories, the reader may feel more confused than enlightened. What is one to think when science can't make up its mind? As a first step, we can borrow the classic parable from Eastern literature of the dermis probe. Three blind men felt an elephant and each gave their impressions. Each had a different

---

[7]Schwartz appropriately credits Engel (1977) with the first application of GST to medicine.

image of reality derived from examining the small area they could reach. If they could combine their solitary sources of information, they might end up with a more complete picture of the elephant.

The science of stress is somewhat like the dermis probe. Many different disciplines are engaged in stress research, each with a slightly different perspective. These different contributions, then, reflect contact with different domains of stress. No one theory has provided a complete picture. Still, each provides important pieces of information that help round out the picture.

As a second step, we should consider the issue of compatibility and compensation. To borrow an analogy from marital relations, strong relations usually come from being compatible. Couples may be strong because they have similar (redundant) competencies and values, or they may be strong because one partner's strengths compensate for the other's weaknesses. The cognitive model of stress and the biological model of stress are compatible in a nonredundant sense. They may turn out to be good partners because each compensates for the other's oversights. Current work shows subtle connections between the cognitive system and body responses that supports this view.

Finally, where does the systems view fit in this scheme? There is nothing inherently incompatible or competitive between the biological model, the cognitive model, and the systems model. The biological subsystem has a job to do in keeping a physical balance, but it interacts with the cognitive system. The cognitive system is the primary self-referent control system that monitors signals and processes information from the biological subsystem and from family, job, and social systems. It works to preserve a psychological balance. Finally, the family system is enmeshed in the larger social system. Each has its job to do in regulating functions within their respective spheres. Each tries to maintain a steady state or balance within its domain. Instead of viewing these theories as competitive, then, we should view them as complementary and compensatory. In this book, I refer to the cognitive system as the self-referent control system that integrates information and orchestrates responses between external social systems and internal physiological systems.

SUMMARY

At the outset, I noted that stress is an illusive concept. At the same time, it is necessary to have some agreed-on definitions. This chapter provided the basic working definitions that will be used throughout the book. In addition, several theories commonly encountered in stress and health research were reviewed. This review was selective and brief rather than exhaustive and intensive. Still, it will help to know some of the varied points of view that scientists hold about the stress process. The following reflects a summary of some of the more important points.

- The external source or cause of stress was defined as the *stressor.*
- The internal tension, be it psychological tension (such as anxiety) or a physical defense reaction, was defined as *stress* or *strain.*
- Homeostasis is the tendency of a body to try to maintain an internal state of equilibrium. Stressors tend to disturb internal equilibrium and require a defensive reaction to restore balance.
- The efforts to manage stress are called coping.
- Good stress is called *eustress* while bad stress is called *distress.*

- We sometimes confuse other emotional states with stress, but some distinctions are important. Anxiety is a feeling of apprehension, a feeling of impending doom.
- Conflict occurs when we must choose between two competing goals, and frustration occurs when a barrier is imposed between us and a goal.
- Efforts to identify connections between stress and health are complicated by the fact that illness behavior does not correspond perfectly with sickness. Disease is a physical condition (or pathology) that results from germs or toxins or body malfunction. Illness behavior is the process of evaluating symptoms and seeking medical or family support.
- Health is more than the absence of disease; it is a positive state of physical, mental and social well-being. Health behaviors are the actions we take to preserve health and prevent disease.
- A theory is an explanatory story of science. It attempts to draw together a wide range of data to present a coherent picture of a phenomenon.
- Selye's theory of stress is largely biological. It emphasizes the nonspecific physical reaction of the body to demands. Selye also proposed the General Adaptation Syndrome, a three-phase reaction to prolonged stress involving alarm, resistance, and exhaustion. It is important to note that coping efforts often reduce or eliminate stress before the body ever reaches the exhaustion stage.
- The diathesis-stress theory suggests that predisposing factors (biological or constitutional variables) set a threshold somewhere on the continuum from weak to strong. Whether a person actually will break down under stress depends on whether or not the stress has exposed (exceeded) the person's particular weakness.
- Psychological theories vary from the psychodynamic to the conditioning views.
- Probably the most influential theory to date is the cognitive transactional theory proposed by Richard Lazarus. This theory suggests that stress only occurs when we judge that our coping skills are inadequate to meet the current demand.
- In contrast to Selye's notion of distress and eustress, Lazarus focused on the little things: the hassles that pile up everyday and irritate us, or the uplifts that are positive and encouraging.
- Holistic theory tries to counter the reductionistic models of medicine, and to some extent psychology, by emphasizing that the person must be treated as a whole, whether we are dealing with physical, mental, or spiritual illness.
- Systems models focus on self-regulation and suggest that the person is simply one system embedded in a hierarchy of systems from the molecular to the astronomical plane.

CRITICAL THINKING AND STUDY QUESTIONS

1. How should we define stress? What factors need to be taken into account in order to have a general definition, in other words, one that does justice to the complexity of the process?
2. What is the difference between distress and eustress? In Selye's theory, did one have more importance for stress than the other? Be able to answer this in some detail.
3. What is a theory? What are the general criteria for a good theory?

4. What are the major principles of the stress theories reviewed in this chapter? Be able to compare and contrast each theory. From your perspective, what are the strengths and weaknesses of each theory? Granted that the review was brief, which theory do you feel does the best job?

5. How do hassles and uplifts compare with distress and eustress?

KEY TERMS

alarm reaction	diathesis-stress model	predisposing factors
anxiety	distress	pressure
approach-approach conflict	eustress	resistance
approach-avoidance conflict	exhaustion	schemata
	frustration	secondary gain
avoidance-avoidance conflict	General Adaptation Syndrome	signal anxiety
	hassles	social stress theory
classical conditioning	health	strain
conditional response	health behavior	stress
conditional stimulus	holistic theory	stressor
conflict	homeostasis	temperament
conflict theory	illness behavior	traumatic anxiety
conservation of resources model	life-change theory	unconditional response
	operant conditioning	unconditional stimulus
conversion	physiological toughness	Yerkes-Dodson Law
cybernetics	precipitating factors	

WEBSITES stress concepts, theories, and models

URL ADDRESS	SITE NAME & DESCRIPTION
http://imt.net/~randolfi/StressLinks.html	☆Links to Stress-Related Resources. Single most comprehensive set of stress links
http://www.apa.org	☆American Psychological Association. Use the **PsychCrawler** search engine for leads on many, many topics.
http://www.psych-web.com	PsychWeb, containing an extensive listing of links to many psychology resources
http://freud.apa.org/divisions/div38/	Health Psychology, Division 38
http://socbehmed.org/sbm/sbm.htm	Society of Behavioral Medicine
http://www.fisk.edu/vl/Stress/	Virtual Library on Stress with several Stress-Related Links
http://www.hir.com/	Holistic Internet Resources, including learning resources and web links

NOTE: URL addresses are typed in continuous line with no spaces or returns.

ANSWERS AND COMMENTS ON SELF-STUDY EXERCISE 1-1

1. F—Little irritants or hassles can put a strain on us.
2. F—Even some good things put stress on us. However, we tend to respond to eustress differently, and we certainly do not tend to regard it as problematic.
3. F—Stress is in the eye of the beholder. The mind can construct some distasteful pressures that do not exist in any objective sense.
4. T—Possibly, but each generation has had its own measure of stress. The pressures of modern technological society are probably increasing for everyone, not just teenagers.
5. F—Even though Selye thought it did, there is evidence that bodily reaction depends on a number of factors. In general, although eustress may require coping energies, it does not have the negative consequences that distress has.
6. F—Due to our unique developmental histories and personalities, we each may experience stress in at least a slightly different way.
7. F—Some stress cannot be eliminated completely; it can only be managed and reduced.
8. F—Even when there are subtle signs of distress, the body is likely in a state of activation. If chronic arousal occurs, the body can be experiencing unnoticed internal changes that can have long-term negative health consequences.

COMMENTS ON SELF-STUDY EXERCISE 1-2

As we proceed in Chapters 2 to 9, we will learn about many specific stressors. Several research projects have endeavored to identify what stressors are reported most commonly by distinct subgroups of the populace.

Among working adults, the most commonly identified stressors are (1) financial pressures; (2) marital pressures including nonacceptance by a spouse, lack of reciprocity in give and take, and lack of equitable division of labor in the family; (3) parental pressures including conflicts with children over rules, family values, and lack of respect for parents; and (4) occupational pressures including lack of adequate income, lack of intrinsic rewards from the job, work overload, and poor quality work environment.

Among college students, the most common stressors include transitional stressors having to do with leaving home and breaking or greatly reducing connections with siblings and friends. Once in the university setting, there are many pressures having to do with making new friends, interspersed with difficult periods of loneliness and managing romantic relationships. On the academic side, the most common stressors have to do with time management, financial pressures, class (assignment) pressures, test anxiety, and grade pressures.

This is a selective list of the most common stressors, but as you read through the next few chapters, you may find it instructive to refer to the list of your most personal stressors.

CHAPTER 2

Stress Research:

Logic, Design, and Process

It is difficult to imagine ...a small speck of creation truly believing it is capable of comprehending the whole.

MURRAY GELL-MANN

The death of A. Bartlett Giamatti on September 1, 1989, sent shock waves through the academic and sports communities. These two seemingly disparate groups had become strange bedfellows, wedded by the personality of Giamatti and his great love of America's game. Giamatti became president of Yale at the awesome age of 40, but when he was asked to become the National League's president, the lure of baseball proved irresistible. Later, because his service to the league was as illustrious as his work in academia, he was asked to serve as baseball's commissioner.

For those who were close to him, the one and only problem was how to deal with the grief of sudden loss. For others, Giamatti's death at 51 prompted a predictable round of speculation about causes. He was overweight, and he chain-smoked three to four packs each day. For at least the five months preceding his death, he apparently worked 22 hours a day, getting only two hours sleep per night. He also had to deal with an immense pressure: confronting Pete Rose, one of the great sports legends, who had just been charged with betting on baseball. There were even rumors of threats against Giamatti's life if he went through with sanctions against Rose. Some speculated it might have been this monumental stress that killed him. Some suggested that whatever stress he felt, it was only the last straw added to the other risk factors. Others said that stress had nothing to do with it at all.

For a group of scientists whose profession is epidemiology, the job is to untangle the web of causes—the etiology or origins of disease. How does one go about untangling such complex webs as risk factors for cardiovascular disease? How do we go about tracing the complex links between psychosocial stress and immune system suppression? This chapter is concerned with how science goes about assembling its body of knowledge, including the research methods used to investigate connections between stress and health. Space limitations dictate brevity, but those who want to pursue more reading in depth will find specialized discussions in Kasl and Cooper (1987), Karoly (1985), and Cohen, Kessler, and Gordon (1995).

BEING SCIENTISTS AND BEING CONSUMERS

At the outset of a study of this nature, there may be a temptation to want only what is useful for personal self-help to cope with stress and make positive decisions for a better lifestyle. There may be as well a temptation to think that studying research methods is at least tedious, if not unnecessary. Still, the study of research methods may, in its own right, help you as an information consumer to better understand the many claims made in the popular press. The mass media inundates us with new seemingly important information from various sciences concerning medicine, technology, and lifestyle choices. Sometimes good details about a study's design are presented. Unfortunately, this is not always the case, as can be seen in self-serving advertising segments where information is presented in the best possible light solely to persuade the consumer to buy. The contents of this chapter, therefore, serve a twofold purpose: first, to help you understand the scientific basis of stress and health research as presented in later chapters, but second, to help you as a consumer learn how to exercise critical and analytical thinking when claims about health and lifestyle issues are made. As a prelude, take a moment to consider some of the claims presented in Self-Study Exercise 2-1.

Critical Thinking About Health Research Claims

The following advertising claims have been made in regard to certain health products. What critical questions should be asked in response to these claims? Stated in other words, what problems do you see in these claims?

1. One advertisement suggests that if you are suffering from some type of sleep disturbance, you should take melatonin, a substance found naturally in the brain that is responsible in part for regulation of sleep cycles. Often, an advertising claim will point to a scientific study without citing its exact source or nature to support the biomedical basis of the claim. It will cite a study, for example, showing that adults with disturbed sleep have markedly improved results after taking the advertised 3 mg melatonin caplets.
2. Many manufacturers of food and snack products claim that their products have very low fat and low amounts of or no cholesterol. The implication seems to be that the product is a food that the health-conscious consumer can eat without concern.
3. Many food and snack products claim to have reduced fat from a previous version. One snack bar is advertised as having reduced fat by 60%. Once again, the implication seems to be that the food must be healthy if there has been that much fat reduction.
4. A variety of therapies are available for quitting smoking. An advertisement in a local paper provides testimonials from people who have received help at a hypnosis clinic and successfully given up the habit.
5. Another use of the testimonial is in regard to natural vitamins and herbal medicines as substitutes for synthetic drugs. After fen-phen was withdrawn from use because of the heart-valve risks it posed, ads began to appear with claims such as: St. John's Wort helped me lose 60 pounds in 6 weeks.

Comments on these claims are provided at the end of the chapter.

MODES OF THINKING IN SCIENCE

We should not assume that science approaches theory building with uniformity. Our theories of health and illness show great diversity. Gary Schwartz (1982) discussed four ways of thinking about nature:[1] formistic, mechanistic, contextual, and organistic. **Formistic thinking** is categorical, either-or thinking. It does not admit middle categories or a series of categories. In this way of thinking, you are either sick or well; Type A or Type B; alcoholic or non-alcoholic. Although formistic thinking is necessary to categorize relevant events for scientific study, it can only lead to overly simplistic, if not primitive, models of environment-behavior relations.

    Mechanistic thinking assumes that cause-effect chains are singly determined. That is, there is one cause linked to one effect. To the mechanistic mind, a specific germ causes a certain disease. A specific stressor has one and only one effect. A lifestyle choice will produce one fixed outcome. The notion of multiple causes contributing to an effect or multiple outcomes owing to a single cause is foreign to this way of thinking.

    Contextual thinking takes the view that any effect depends on context. It is relational and multicausal thinking. In addition, the context of the observer may provide alternate though equally plausible explanations of an event. Stress may be good or bad

[1]Schwartz credits these to Pepper's (1942) notion of world hypotheses.

depending on how you view it. Disease may be caused by a set of interconnected factors, including decisions to engage in high-risk behaviors that lead to exposure or lowered resistance. Disease may be related as well to attitudes toward preventive behavior and compliance with medical regimens.

Finally, **organistic thinking** is systems thinking. The healthy functioning of an organism results from the interplay of numerous components both within the organism and between the organism and its environmental context. The interactions are complex, resulting in interactive multicausal, multieffect models. Contextual thinking and organistic thinking are clearly compatible, and provide, according to numerous authors, the framework within which satisfactory models may be developed that explain how psychosocial forces contribute to maintaining health or increasing risk for illness.

It is important to note that research on stress and health has to deal with proximal and distal causes. **Proximal causes** are events hypothesized to operate in the recent past. Acute infections, respiratory disorders, injury, or a serious car accident (an acute stressor) are typically treated as proximal causes. **Distal causes** are those presumed to act from some remote time past. Rheumatic fever in childhood may be the cause of heart problems in adulthood. It is all the more difficult to untangle the causal web between stress and health when the matrix of biopsychosocial variables must be considered across long time-spans.

Further, we distinguish between precipitating factors and predisposing factors. **Precipitating factors** are insults, physical or psychosocial, that immediately precede the onset of a breakdown. These are similar to proximal causes, but this distinct terminology is introduced for reasons that will become clear momentarily. **Predisposing factors** are biological-genetic factors that influence organic or constitutional weakness, and probably also determine stable personality traits. They may be at work, sometimes in very imperceptible ways, over long time periods. These two sets of variables have been integrated in the diathesis-stress theory as described in Chapter 1. Theory and method in health science research has increasingly sought to incorporate this intermix of variables to provide more powerful explanatory models of health and illness.

THE LOGIC OF SCIENTIFIC METHOD

Scientific method is a serial process that seeks to establish cause-effect relationships. The cause is the independent variable (IV), while the effect (or outcome) is the dependent variable (DV). In the social-behavioral sciences, the independent variable is usually an environmental stimulus and the dependent variable is some sort of behavior. In design terms, the **independent variable** is the treatment condition manipulated by the investigator, while the **dependent variable** is the behavior that is measured. For example, it is widely assumed that chronic distress causes a decline in health. Distress is the independent variable, while decline in health is the dependent variable.

However, in health research, the variables selected as cause and effect can differ markedly (Rodin & Salovey, 1989). Stated in other terms, what is cause and what is effect depends on where we decide to cut into the chain of events. This is illustrated in Figure 2-1.

For this discussion, it is helpful to think of the organism as a complex system influenced by information from external events as well as feedback from its own behavior. Stimuli may be external physical or psychosocial events. They also may be internal

FIGURE 2-1
Possible stimulus-response sequences that structure stress and health research.

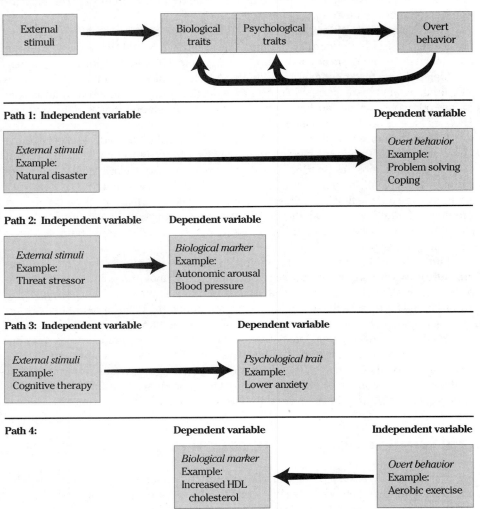

biological or psychological processes. Outcomes may be internal-biological, internal-psychological, or overt-behavioral. Adding further to the complexity, behavior itself can function as a stimulus that alters the person's internal biological and psychological states.

Independent Variables: Biomedical Versus Psychosocial Stimuli

A social psychologist might study variations in the type of social support systems (intimate-extended versus impersonal-limited) that people have and how that support protects against the effects of stress. Environmental psychologists might compare reactions to different physical stressors (natural disasters versus technological). Clinical health care personnel might be concerned about how different therapies (relaxation versus cognitive restructuring) alter subjective reports of stress or the feeling of tension. In each case, the independent variable is some aspect of the external environment.

Alternatively, we might focus on internal differences in the host organism. For example, we might categorize people in regard to autonomic reactivity (hyperreactive versus hyporeactive) and how this influences stress reactions. We could test for differences in levels of trait anxiety and categorize people from high to low on this personality variable. Then we could assess differences in stress reactions related to this trait. In each of these examples, it is an internal personal trait that is used as the independent variable. In the first case, we selected a biological characteristic, in the second, a psychological trait.

Finally, we might take differences in behavior patterns as the stimulus event. For example, we might classify people in terms of the frequency and intensity of exercise. We could then look at several different dependent measures, such as changes in the cardiovascular system, alterations in physical fitness, improvements in level of depression, or differences in subjective reports of stress.

Dependent Variables: Measuring Outcomes

Dependent variables are also defined primarily by their point in the chain. Janice Kiecolt-Glaser and her colleagues wanted to know if immune competence changes following relaxation training as compared to social support or to no contact at all (Kiecolt-Glaser et al., 1985). Their dependent variable was change in natural killer-cell activity. Others are concerned about the origins of the Type A personality. Does it result from genetic factors, or does it result from familial patterns of discipline? Here, Type A is measured as an outcome variable. In another context, it might be a stimulus variable similar to trait anxiety. Finally, we might be concerned that coronary risk relates to a mood state such as chronic intense hostility. In this case, the dependent variable is a cardiovascular measure such as blood pressure or serum cholesterol and the independent variable is an internal psychological mood.

A variety of dependent measures focus on internal biological changes. This focus reflects the notion that biomedical measures somehow are more real than psychosocial or behavioral measures. Robert Kaplan (1990) made a compelling argument for behavior as the central outcome of health research. He noted that numerous interventions result in clinical improvement, such as reducing blood pressure, but quality-of-life indicators are unchanged. Further, Kaplan cited the highly touted study showing that aspirin reduced deaths from myocardial infarction. The rest of the story was not publicized. Total coronary deaths did not decrease. Aspirin only changed the distribution of deaths among the categories. As Kaplan noted, though, families are rarely as much concerned with how their loved one died as they are that death occurred.

Taking the Measure of Health: Issues in Assessment

It is clear from the foregoing that stress researchers must use assessment methods frequently to establish levels of an independent variable or to measure a dependent variable. Assessment issues thus have become so important that entire books now devote attention to assessment techniques (biomedical, psychosocial, or behavioral), to assessment in special populations (women and minorities, for example), and to assessment for different health conditions (heart health, cancer, or pain, for example; Bellack & Hersen, 1988; Blechman & Brownell, 1988; Karoly, 1985, 1988).

Identifying Research Variables

In the following exercise, I have listed in a variety of forms several hypotheses as they may be made by investigators. Your task is to identify the independent variable and the dependent variable for each hypothesis. As one clue to guide you, I have restricted these hypotheses to studies in which no more than two variables of either type is possible.

1. One research group wanted to know if exercise was related to blood cholesterol levels. They grouped people according to self-reported level of exercise into sedentary, low-exercise, and intense exercise groups. Over a period of several weeks, they monitored both good cholesterol (HDLs) and bad cholesterol (LDLs).
2. Problem-focused coping is a more effective coping strategy for interpersonal stress, whereas emotion-focused coping is more effective when dealing with natural or technological disasters. In a study of these differences, investigators grouped people according to type of coping strategy used in response to one of two types of stress. Then they measured levels of currently reported stress.
3. One study focused on the hypothesis that Type A behavior pattern, as compared to Type B behavior, is associated with higher risk for coronary disease.
4. In a large-scale epidemiological study, investigators wanted to know if vitamin E was related to risk for cancer. They grouped people according to high doses, low doses, or no supplemental vitamin E use, over the past two years. Then, with permission, they obtained medical records on the incidence of cancer in the three groups.
5. One focus of stress research has been on the role of social support in buffering the effects of stress. One group looked at levels of stress in relationship to the type of social support women received during and after two types of surgery (radical mastectomy versus lumpectomy) for breast cancer.

When investigators need a psychosocial test, there are usually two choices: either find a currently available standardized test that has been developed for the target situation and clientele, or develop the test from scratch. When we say a test is **standardized,** we mean it is built with specific rules so it can be, indeed must be, administered the same way every time (Anastasi, 1988). If investigators must develop the measure, then they must test it before basing clinical or research judgments on it. Testing the test basically means determining how reliable and valid it is.

The Reliability Criterion: Issues of Accuracy

Since so much rides on the outcome of tests, the instruments must themselves be subjected to careful scrutiny to ensure that they yield accurate results. This is no less true when the test in question is biomedical than when it is psychosocial. The technical sophistication and the appearance of quantitative precision that accompany most biomedical tests may lead to a premature judgment that the tests are both reliable and valid, when in fact the measures have not been thoroughly tested (Kaplan, 1990). The same is true of computerized clinical psychological tests and interpretations (Matarazzo, 1986). Psychology has developed extensive procedures for testing the tests, procedures that we can only discuss briefly.

Good tests must meet two fundamental criteria; that is, they must have reliability and validity. **Reliability** means that the test measures consistently. Reliability is measured as the correlation (Pearson r) between two scores obtained from the same person on two occasions. **Validity** means that the test measures what it is supposed to measure.

Test designers recognize three major types of reliability: test-retest, alternate forms, and split-half (also called internal consistency) reliability. In **test-retest** reliability, a test is administered at one time and then at a second time. If it gives approximately the same scores both times, it has test-retest reliability. **Alternate-forms** reliability requires two separate tests that are nearly equivalent in content. Perhaps the most common measures of reliability, however, are internal consistency measures.[2] One such measure, **split-half** reliability, uses two scores from a single test—for example, one score from the odd-numbered items and one score from the even-numbered items. Reliability is the correlation between the two halves of the test. Internal consistency measures are often used because they are the quickest and simplest to compute.

The Validity Criterion: Issues of Credibility

Reliability is of little value if the test does not measure what it is supposed to measure. Suppose that I set out to construct a personality test that measures as many meaningful facets of personality as possible. Further, suppose that it yields precisely the same score for the same person every time it is given. Still, a colleague points out that my test is measuring only one, very narrow facet of personality, say hysteria. In this case, no matter how reliable my test is, it is not a valid general measure of personality. At the same time, it is impossible to determine the validity of a test unless it is also reliable. In this sense, reliability sets the upper limit for validity.

There are three major types of validity: content validity, criterion-related validity, and construct validity. **Content validity** requires that the test content fairly represents the behavior domain to be measured. It is not a statistical analysis, but an exercise in expertise and logic resulting in the systematic selection of items for inclusion in the test. Content validity is often confused with **face validity,** which is a simple intuitive judgment that test items look like they tap what the scale claims to measure. **Criterion-related validity** is obtained by checking the test against a relevant performance-based measure. For example, we might check a graduate entrance exam against a composite academic-performance index near the end of a person's graduate program.

One of the most important forms of validity is **construct validity,** which is concerned with whether the test measures the specific trait or theoretical construct of concern. To illustrate this notion, consider the construct of trait anxiety. When we say that a test measures anxiety, we should provide evidence that this trait is precisely what the test measures. We may do this by checking the test against other tests of anxiety with known track records. Further, we may use physiological measures of anxiety obtained in the laboratory under distinct conditions designed to induce varying degrees of anxiety. Under conditions of high threat, a highly anxious person should obtain a high score on the test as well as show a strong physiological response. If these cross-checks are all positive, we may conclude that the anxiety test is a valid measure of the trait anxiety construct.

Testing Causal Connections: Educated Guesses

To return to the steps in scientific method, the common strategy is to test the truth value of a hypothesis by directly manipulating the causal variables presumed to influence behavior. A **hypothesis** is a tentative answer to a research question. It is a prediction of what behavior we expect under specified conditions.

---

[2]Several internal consistency measures are used. Besides split-half reliability, Kuder-Richardson and Cronbach's alpha are frequently used, but are beyond the scope of this book.

We will use a prototypic experiment to illustrate the process. Suppose a research group wants to know if relaxation training will reduce migraine headaches. As a first step, they inspect the methods and results of previous research. Their goal is to become familiar with migraine and its treatment. Based on this review, they state a plausible hypothesis: Relaxation training (IV) will be effective in reducing both the frequency (DV_1) and severity (DV_2) of migraine attacks.

The team then obtains a volunteer group of migraine sufferers. They review medical records (only with client permission) to ensure that each subject fits the definition of migraine. If they included nonmigraine pain patients (for example, chronic low-back pain patients), that inclusion would confuse interpretation of results.

Then, the investigators randomly assign subjects to one of two groups, the **experimental group** or the **control group. Random assignment** permits the assumption that no differences exist between the groups except that introduced by the independent variable. Unfortunately, random assignment is not always possible. People cannot be randomly assigned to disease categories, such as coronary heart disease. They cannot be assigned randomly to behavioral or personality profiles, such as the Type A behavior pattern (Friedman & Booth-Kewley, 1987). Because of this limitation, the investigator must use a quasi-experimental design (Cook & Campbell, 1979). *Quasi* literally means "resembling." A **quasi-experimental design** is one that resembles a true experiment in most respects, but still falls short. The resemblance is that both true and quasi-experiments have treatments, outcome measures, and sampling units (Rosenthal & Rosnow, 1991). The difference is that quasi-experimental designs cannot assign subjects to the treatment conditions completely at random.

The experimental group receives training in relaxation while the **control group** receives no training. This difference between the two groups represents manipulation of the independent variable. In reality, there are very few times when the control group receives nothing. More often than not, the control group receives an **attention placebo.** An attention placebo may be given during a series of nonspecific informational meetings. These meetings would be roughly equal to the contact time the experimental group receives but without training in relaxation.

Over time, subjects provide data on the frequency and intensity of their headaches. These two measures are the dependent variables. **Baseline,** or pretreatment, data will tell the experimenters where the behavior was before treatment and whether the experimental and control groups were equivalent at the outset. After treatment, the data will allow the investigators to either refute or confirm the hypothesis that relaxation changed frequency and intensity of headaches. If the groups were not equivalent in headache measures at the beginning, then any favorable change in the dependent variable could not be assigned reliably to the relaxation treatment. Similarly, if the treatment and control groups were still equal in headaches at the end of the experiment, even if headache rates for both were significantly lower, the investigators could not be confident that relaxation provided an effective treatment.

We should take steps to protect against the chance that subjects know or guessed the research hypothesis. This could bias the results (Rosenthal, 1966). To control for this, a special group of collaborators may collect and tabulate the data. They are special because they do not know the purpose of the experiment nor do they know to which group the subjects belong. In technical terms, this is a **double-blind** control. If they were blind to group membership but knew the hypothesis of the experiment, then it is a **single-blind** control. A recent meta-analysis of modeling procedures to prepare children for surgical operations revealed the importance of this control. That is, treatment effects all but disappeared in experiments using adequate blind-control procedures, but treatment effects remained quite strong (almost three times the effect size) in experiments not using blind-control procedures (Saile, Burgmeier, & Schmidt, 1988).

Using Subjects for Research: Ethical Dilemmas

An important criterion for conducting responsible research is that subjects receive information about the basic procedures and any personal risks involved from their participation. Researchers provide this information in an **informed consent** form. Subjects read and sign the informed consent form to show they understand the procedures and risks and agree to participate.

Ethical issues in research can be very complicated. Any agency that uses federal monies must form an **Institutional Research Board** (IRB) to review projects and ensure that investigators comply with ethical guidelines. When deception is involved, the investigator must be certain that such deception is necessary to test the hypothesis. After the project, subjects must receive **debriefing** to explain what the deception was and to remedy any ill-effects that might result. Another serious dilemma (exemplified in our prototype experiment) occurs when one group receives a treatment that may be helpful but treatment is withheld from the control group. Investigators may ask their subjects to sign the informed consent knowing that they may be assigned to the control group. Kiecolt-Glaser's group used this procedure in the study of relaxation versus social support mentioned earlier. Investigators typically offer the treatment to the control group after completing the study.

Making Sense of the Numbers: Inferences and Confidence Levels

It is very easy to be confused by numbers, even intimidated by statistics. Helen Taft, wife of William Taft, the 27th American president, said, "I always find that statistics are hard to swallow and impossible to digest. The only [statistic] that I can ever remember is that if all the people who go to sleep in church were laid end to end, they would be a lot more comfortable." (Cited in Jaccard & Becker, 1997.)

In spite of this tongue-in-cheek assessment, scientists see statistical techniques as most helpful allies in their quest to understand nature. When the migraine headache project is complete, for example, investigators must try to make sense of the numbers. In order to reduce the chance that personal bias will influence interpretation, scientists use numerous statistical tools. In this hypothetical project, the team would compute the average number of headaches and the mean intensity ratings for the experimental and control groups. If the relaxation group showed a sizable decrease in headaches or greatly reduced pain, the hypothesis is confirmed. The problem is to know what makes a sizable decrease or change in severity of pain. It is possible that decreases reflect nothing more than uncontrolled chance factors.

We use **inferential statistics** to enable us to state with mathematical precision how confident we can be that the results can be attributed to the experimental treatment. To be safe, the team sets a confidence level (or level of significance) before the project begins. The **confidence level** defines a statistically significant result by reference to a probability so rare that the results are not likely to have occurred by mere chance. Scientists typically use confidence levels around $p = .05$ or $p = .01$. A confidence level of .05 states that the results could occur by chance no more than 5 times in 100. A confidence level of .01 states that the results could occur by chance no more than 1 time in 100. Chance factors usually refer to a combination of sampling error, measurement error, or experimental error. If the decrease in frequency or severity of headaches is reliable by statistical test, then the investigators say that the hypothesis is true.

There is, of course, always a small chance that when we say the experimental hypothesis is true, it is in fact false. This is so since the decision itself is dependent on the statistics of chance. Stated in other terms, when we say the results could not occur by chance more than 5 times in 100, we have no way of knowing whether this result is one of the 5 chance outcomes that could occur, or one of the nonchance outcomes that means our experimental hypothesis is confirmed.

Two types of decision errors may occur. One is the **Type I error** just described. That is, when we say that our experimental manipulation is responsible for the observed changes in behavior but it was really just chance operating, we have made a Type I error. The likelihood of making a Type I error is exactly the confidence level we have set. The second decision error is a **Type II error.** This occurs when we overlook a meaningful experimental outcome. In this case, we say that chance was operating when in fact our experimental manipulation did have an effect.

Typically, investigators do not want to make Type I errors when they are far into a program of research and when they are refining theory. Conversely, they do not want to make a Type II error when they are just beginning a new research program of discovery, or when their work is applied and the results have the potential to benefit a lot of people.

Operational Definitions and Repeatability

Scientists take steps to ensure that the procedures used to test hypotheses are explicit and repeatable. They must make certain that special constructs and terms are stated clearly and precisely. A research project may appear elegant in design. But if its central constructs are fuzzy, interpretation of results will be an exercise in futility. Some terms, such as heart rate, are concrete and have well-defined referents. Other terms, such as stress or ego, are more abstract or theoretical (Clark & Paivio, 1989).

When ambiguity exists because a term has several connotations (for example, pain, stress, anxiety, or headache), then scientists use an operational definition. **Operational definitions** are statements about the procedures the researcher used to establish levels of an independent variable or to measure a dependent variable. To illustrate, pain might be defined qualitatively as a particular type of pain—lower-back as opposed to headache pain. Then the pain might be quantified as a score on a standardized pain scale. The investigator may want to look at differences in cognitions and attitudes between high-pain and low-pain groups. The high-pain group might be defined as the top 40% on the pain scale and the low-pain group the bottom 40%. This provides an operational definition of pain.

Finally, the end of data analysis does not necessarily mean the end of responsibility for subjects. If the results support the contention that relaxation was effective, the team would provide relaxation training to the control group. Typically, this action would satisfy the investigator's ethical obligations to subjects. Still, we are reminded that various ethical issues confront investigators involved in this type of research (O'Leary & Borkovec, 1978).

This statement represents the bare essentials in the logic of experimental design. We now turn to research strategies used in health psychology research. Table 2-1 summarizes the more common strategies. It may be helpful to refer to this table as you read about each design.

CASE STUDIES: THE INTENSIVE ANALYSIS OF ONE

The **case-study method** has a long and venerable history in clinical circles. Originally, it signified an intensive examination of a single client. Any and all facets of the client's medical, psychological, familial, educational, and social backgrounds could provide information crucial to treatment. The case-study method also proved useful to open new areas of inquiry, such as behavior modification research. This led to formal methods for single-subject designs and the experimental analysis of behavior, a technique that will be described later. The major limitation of the case-study method is that it cannot directly test hypotheses.

John Carton and Julie Schweitzer (1996) reported a case study in which they wanted to increase compliance during hemodialysis in a 10-year-old male. Patients with chronic renal (kidney) failure have to go through complicated medical regimens that include dietary and fluid restrictions, medications, and hemodialysis 3 times each week. Hemodialysis itself is not a pleasant procedure, since it may last 3 to 4 hours while blood is purified. During this time, the patient must be relatively passive. While some patients may find the procedure only mildly aversive, others may find it very stressful and refuse to comply. In this case, the boy engaged in a variety of noncompliant behaviors— screaming at, kicking, and hitting the nurses—that slowed down the procedure.

Carton and Schweitzer used a classic single-subject method called the ABAB design. They first took a baseline (A) of noncompliant behavior over 6 successive 4-hour sessions. If noncompliant behavior occurred during any 30-minute interval, that interval was counted as a noncompliant interval. Thus, a maximum undesirable score of 8 could occur in any 4-hour session. Baseline measures revealed that the boy averaged about 7.3 noncompliant intervals each of the 6 days of baseline. Treatment (B) consisted of receiving a token for any 30-minute interval with no noncompliant behavior. At the end of the hemodialysis sessions, the tokens could be turned in for baseball cards, comic books, or small toys. Over 9 treatment sessions, noncompliant intervals dropped to 1.0. When the token system was withdrawn, in other words returning to baseline conditions (A), noncompliant intervals rose to 3.8. Finally, when the token economy was resumed (B), noncompliant intervals again dropped to .22 intervals per session. This case study showed that a simple behavioral intervention could be used to reduce troublesome behavior that was interfering with health treatments.

Field Studies: Constructing Plausible Explanations

Think for a moment about how you might try to find answers to these questions. What are the mental and physical health outcomes for victims of a natural catastrophe, such as hurricane Andrew, which ravaged Florida and Louisiana in August 1992? Can we provide any information to patients waiting for painful medical procedures that will minimize their anguish and promote recovery? Are air traffic controllers at increased risk of nervous breakdowns and physical health problems? Does high caffeine consumption increase coronary risk? What is the relationship between physical fitness and coronary risk?

TABLE 2-1
Comparison of key features of research designs

TYPE OF DESIGN	DEGREE OF CONTROL	METHOD OF ANALYSIS	DESIGN STRENGTHS	DESIGN WEAKNESSES
Case-study method	No control over any variables, whether experimental or extraneous	Subjective (clinical) interpretation Possible comparison to normative data when using standard psychometric exams	Extensive data about the individual May be of heuristic value when it leads to testable hypothesis May be the only way to document rare cases/disorders	Subject to bias of the observer Cannot test causal hypotheses Cannot be repeated Limited generality
Reversal designs	Direct control over experimental or treatment variables Limited or no control over extraneous variables	Graphical—comparison of treatment period to baseline May include some statistical analysis with multiple groups or baselines	Weak causal connections may be inferred Study is repeatable Especially useful in early development of clinical treatments	Usually carried out with very small n Limited generality Cannot eliminate many sources of contamination
Field studies	No direct control over most variables Statistical control over demographic variables	Statistical—yields descriptive values such as means and normative data Comparisons between subgroups with inferences about differences	Potential to obtain quantitative data on many variables from many subjects Establish norms and/or trends May be of heuristic valueMay provide data on social/ecological phenomena that cannot be studied in the laboratory Can be repeated with most survey studies	Cannot test causal hypotheses May be subject to reporting biases such as selective memory, failures in memory, or expectancies about the nature of the studyNot repeatable with disaster events

TABLE 2-1 *continued*

TYPE OF DESIGN	DEGREE OF CONTROL	METHOD OF ANALYSIS	DESIGN STRENGTHS	DESIGN WEAKNESSES
Correlational studies	Statistical control over demographic variables	Statistical—results in correlation coefficient and estimate of variance	Identify relations between any number of variables Identify potentially interesting causal variables for controlled study	Cannot determine causal connections Significance of the coefficient does not reveal the amount of variance explained
Pre-post designs	Direct control over experimental or treatment variables Added levels of control depend on type of control group(s) used	Statistical—comparison of target behavior after treatment to pretreatment levels Comparison to control groups to eliminate competing explanations for change	Stronger inferences of causal link as controls become better More generality than reversal designs (this depends on sampling and n Repeatable	Limited causal inferences with no control group or weak controls Potential ethical questions with untreated controls
Experimental designs	Direct control over hypothesized causal variables Potential to control most important extraneous variables	Statistical—both descriptive and inferential Comparison between groups	Most powerful design to establish causal links Multicausal links Interactions can be established with extended (factorial) designs Repeatable Generality good but related to sampling and task demands	Criticized for using artificial tasks Can be difficult to interpret with large number of variables Cannot manipulate some variables for ethical reasons Ethical issues with untreated controls

TABLE 2-1 *continued*

TYPE OF DESIGN	DEGREE OF CONTROL	METHOD OF ANALYSIS	DESIGN STRENGTHS	DESIGN WEAKNESSES
Epidemiological studies	Varies with specific type of design but potentially very good control Many variables must be controlled by selection rather than by direct manipulation	Statistical—both descriptive and inferential Comparisons between treatment conditions Comparisons between groups exposed to different risk factors	Usually conducted in natural environment Useful for issues of disease etiology and lifestyle disease links Repeatable Generality good	Difficult to obtain good control over many variables Costly in terms of time and effort Outcomes are often still subject to more than one interpretation Ethical issues with untreated controls
Meta-analysis	Only decisional control over how to select and combine studies	Statistical—aggregate effect size Comparison of effect sizes in subsets of studies	Resolves issues from conflicting results Resolves disputes due to disparate methodologies Resolves disputes between competing theoretical models Repeatable	Must work with existing data no matter how clean or dirty the data are Potential bias of using only published studies

Each of these questions is important and deserves to be answered. Each situation presents a problem, though, in where and how to observe whatever stress-health connection may be present. Hurricanes are natural disasters. Surgery takes place in hospitals, not in research labs. Air traffic controllers may face very different work conditions, depending on size of city and density of airport traffic. Those conditions cannot be recreated in a laboratory. Caffeine consumption and physical fitness are behaviors whose effects on coronary health may not show up for years. For these questions, investigators often depend on a family of designs called field studies. Included in this group are **survey research, ex-post-facto designs,** and **correlational designs.**

Survey Research: Sampling at Large

Survey research is a widely used procedure that seeks to discover typical attitudes or behaviors in large representative samples. Surveys require extensive time for face-to-face interviews or require respondents to fill out lengthy questionnaires. The most elaborate survey research is the United States census that occurs every ten years. Other visible examples are Gallup polls and Roper polls, which tap attitudes on social and political issues. They assess changes in behavior tendencies such as religious affiliation, sexual mores and conduct, and health behaviors. Although a Gallup (1984) poll on fitness suggested that the habit of exercise had nearly doubled over the previous 20 years, a more recent Harris (Facts on File, 1993) poll showed that an increasing number of Americans are giving up healthy lifestyles.

Surveys are helpful in indicating trends in attitudes and behaviors, but they also suffer from several limitations. Since survey data is self-reported, we must be concerned with the credibility of that report. Most surveys expend little effort to verify data. Surveys often ask people to report blood pressure or other biomedical statistics without cross-checks. The investigator also must hope that respondents interpret questions in a consistent way. Surveys also may suffer a reactivity effect. That is, the respondent may change as a result of being a subject. The respondent may have no opinion before the interview, but form an opinion on the spot to satisfy the social-demand characteristics of the interview. Finally, surveys do not allow the investigator to manipulate causal variables or to control for confounding variables.

EX-POST-FACTO STUDIES: LOOKING BACK

One special type of field study is the ex-post-facto design. This design is unique because the investigator must select variables to study after the event has already happened. Natural and technological disasters call for an ex-post-facto study. Experimenters cannot manipulate variables to produce suicides, abuse, or rapes for obvious ethical reasons. The only choice is to be ready when such events do occur, and then try to answer important questions in retrospect.

Shirley Murphy (1984) used an ex-post-facto design when she studied victims of the Mount St. Helens volcano eruption. She collected data on a variety of physical and emotional symptoms. Door-to-door surveys with pre-set questions or face-to-face interviews can provide clues to alterations in physical and mental health status. Catastrophe research also might use **archival data** from hospitals or social and governmental agencies. A descriptive analysis may be possible that summarizes the traumas reported by the group. With careful planning and execution, it is sometimes possible to test hypotheses about likely changes following such an event. It would still be impossible to directly test hypotheses about what precipitated an event such as suicide or abuse.

ECOLOGICAL MOMENTARY ASSESSMENT: REMOTE OBSERVERS

Technology has made it possible, though costly, to observe a variety of events in the natural environment with much more precision than has ever existed. The technique is called **Ecological Momentary Assessment** or simply EMA (Stone & Shiffman, 1994). It typically depends on electronic monitoring, signaling, and recording apparatus. The forerunner of this approach was biotelemetry, recording signals from organisms moving about their natural environment. We are probably all familiar with a "Wild Kingdom" scenario that captures, collars, and releases an animal with a radio transmitter around its neck. In more recent years, technological advances have allowed medical facilities to monitor a variety of health risk signals (for example, heartbeat, blood pressure, or blood sugar) while patients go about their daily routines.

The primary intent of EMA, in Stone and Shiffman's words, is to "assess phenomena at the moment they occur in natural settings, thus maximizing ecological validity while avoiding retrospective recall" (1994, p. 199). There are four core features of EMA.

1. EMA occurs at the time a behavior or event occurs.
2. EMA requires careful planning and timing of assessments.
3. EMA typically involves numerous repeated observations.
4. EMA is typically done in the subject's own environment.

This procedure allows the investigator to study many stress and health variables in the natural environment that could not be readily studied before. For example, Saul Shiffman and his colleagues (1994) wanted to learn more about the cue properties of drinking and smoking since there are notable synergistic effects of drinking and smoking on mouth and throat cancers. A synergistic effect means that the two behaviors combine to produce a different, and in this case, more powerful, effect than would be predicted from simply adding the two separate effects together. Also, self-report survey data suggested that drinking cues smoking. The researchers used palm-top computers to sample more than 4000 events during a week in the lives of 57 subjects. They concluded that earlier survey data were wrong, that there is more to the link between drinking and smoking than just a situational cueing effect. Although alternative hypotheses were suggested, the researchers' data remain only suggestive of new leads that need to be pursued to better understand this set of high-risk behaviors.

CORRELATIONAL DESIGNS: WHAT IS THE RELATIONSHIP?

Correlational research is not experimental in the strict sense of the term. Nonetheless, this type of research can be very useful in tracking down variables that are potentially relevant for more extensive experimental investigations. Correlation is a statistical procedure that assesses the relationship between two or more variables. More precisely, the correlation coefficient is a quantitative index of the extent to which individuals occupy the same relative position on two scales. Correlation coefficients, expressed as r, range from $+1.00$, a perfect positive association, through 0.00, showing no association, to -1.00, a perfect inverse association. A strong negative relationship is just as informative as a strong positive relationship.

A study by Sorbi and Tellegen (1988) illustrates the correlational approach in stress research. Survey studies suggested that stress events frequently precede the onset of migraine headaches. Since no one had tested the strength of this relationship previously, Sorbi and Tellegen decided to do so. They treated stress as cause (also called the **predictor variable**) and migraine as effect (also called the **criterion variable**).

A group of 29 migraine patients responded weekly to an event-specific coping list. This list contained a stress scale based on the notion that everyday life events are stressful. Stress events could be objectively categorized into threat and challenge. Patients used a diary to record migraine attacks hourly. Sorbi and Tellegen found that threat events preceded migraine but challenge events did not. The reported correlation was $r = +0.50$. This was significantly beyond the .01 level, a result that would be expected to occur by chance less than 1 time in 100.

There are several caveats that apply to correlational research. First, correlation does not imply causation. Associations may be produced by the operation of another hidden variable, or the association may be simply a matter of coincidence. The other side of the logic is often overlooked: *without correlation there can be no causation.* Thus, correlational research can be very useful to identify patterns of association that may be subjected later to closer scrutiny with experimental techniques.

Second, even when the observed correlation is high, the explained variance (technically r^2) is smaller. Explained variance, a technical term, can be understood without going into the statistics behind the term. Even if we assume that there is a tendency for stress to cause migraine headaches, we would not expect stress to be the only cause of migraine. Migraines may occur because of biomedical factors (for example, cardiovascular processes) or some combination of biomedical and psychosocial factors. The correlation observed in the Sorbi and Tellegen study suggests that stress explains no more than 25% ($r^2 = .50^2 = .25$) of the variability in migraine headaches. About 75% of the variability is unexplained by this relationship and must be due to the operation of other, possibly biomedical, factors.

Scientists still regard the laboratory experiment as the pinnacle of research procedure. Nonetheless, designs implemented in the natural environment or with small groups of clients in a clinical setting are known for their great heuristic value. That is, they are a rich source of new hypotheses that may be tested later in more optimal controlled conditions.

CLINICAL RESEARCH: PRE-POST INTERVENTION DESIGNS

Clinical research usually works with clients who seek help for distressing or painful symptoms. Researchers try to find the best treatment to use with a specific type of client presenting a distinct set of symptoms. They are rarely satisfied with the knowledge that a treatment works. They also want to know how it works. This means that they want to identify the effective agent of change that is crucial to treatment success.

It is probably better to think of current clinical research as a give-and-take between lab, clinic, and field settings. Hypotheses generated in applied settings may eventually be tested in more controlled settings. Conversely, insights gained from controlled studies may become the rationale for even more effective clinical interventions.

Single-Subject Research: Baseline Reversal Designs

The simplest clinical study is the **single-subject** design. While many variations are possible, the most general is the so-called **baseline-reversal design,** or *AB* design, in which *A* is the baseline and *B* is the treatment phase. During baseline, the clinician obtains data that indicate how frequent or intense the behavior is before treatment. Then, the clinician selects a therapy that presumably should improve the symptoms and begins treatment. Later, the clinician compares treatment data to baseline data. If the symptoms are gone or reduced, there is reason to believe that the treatment can be used effectively in the future. To be sure that the treatment produced the improvement and not some coincidental outside factor, baseline conditions may be restored. If the symptoms reappear, we have even more confidence that the treatment was the effective agent. This is an *ABA* design.

Mark Hegel and his colleagues worked with three women who displayed hyperventilation syndrome (Hegel et al., 1989). They taught each patient to use controlled diaphragmatic breathing plus the relaxation response. As Figure 2-2 shows, for one patient, chest pain and shortness of breath episodes declined systematically after introducing this treatment. The treatment gains were still evident 12 months later. Results were similar for the other two patients.

An interesting example of an *ABAB* baseline-reversal design comes from the work of Roque and Roberts (1989). As we noted in the use of this design for a case study, the *ABAB* baseline-reversal design tracks behavior for a specified period of time prior to treatment. Then, the investigator begins the intervention and continues to collect data during treatment. Later, treatment is terminated and the conditions that existed in baseline are reinstated as much as possible. Finally, treatment conditions are repeated to ensure that the client is released with maximum therapeutic benefit.

Roque and Roberts carried out their study in the natural environment with a group of unsuspecting subjects, drivers on the public streets of Tuscaloosa, Alabama. Subjects never gave consent for participation, but they were observed anonymously and without disclosure of their behavior to any authority.

Roque and Roberts were concerned about high-risk driving behaviors such as speeding and refusal to wear seat belts. They wanted to find out if public posting of speed-limit compliance would help to control speeding. Their subject population consisted of drivers on a defined stretch of urban highway. Speed was measured through inductive loop detectors. Feedback on the rate of compliance with the speed limit was provided daily by a roadside sign that read "DRIVERS NOT SPEEDING YESTERDAY, *nn%*" on top and "BEST RECORD, *nn%*" below it (see Figure 2-3).

Roque and Roberts monitored speed for 10 days, 24 hours a day, to establish their baseline. The percentage of drivers complying with the speed limit was calculated and used for the subsequent phase of the experiment. As a control, the road sign that would display the percentages was erected so that it was in place during the baseline, but it was covered so that no information was conveyed to the drivers. In the treatment phase, the sign was uncovered and the percentage of drivers who were in compliance with the speed limit was posted. The daily posted rates were accurate reflections of the prior data.

FIGURE 2-2

Frequency of chest pain episodes and average frequency of shortness of breath episodes for patient G. A. for baseline, treatment, and follow-up.

SOURCE: Hegel et al. (1989).

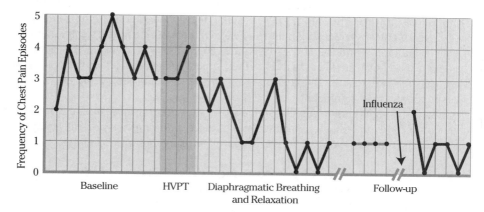

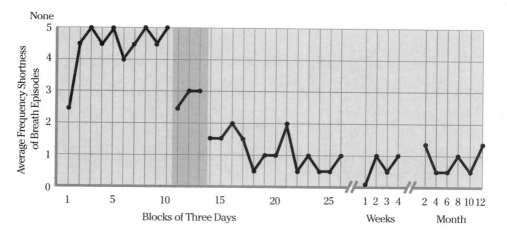

FIGURE 2-3

An environmental sign of the type used by Roque and Roberts to reduce speeding.

SOURCE: Based on Van Houten, Nau, & Marini, 1980.

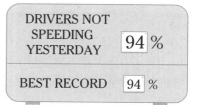

DRIVERS NOT
SPEEDING   94 %
YESTERDAY

BEST RECORD   94 %

The results showed that posting compliance rates led to even more compliance among low- and middle-range speeders. Unfortunately, high speeders did not seem to reduce their speed at all during this intervention.

After the posting period was finished, another baseline was conducted. This second baseline showed an increased speeding level in all groups of drivers, almost like a rebound effect. However, this return to the baseline level yielded convincing data that the posting treatment was effective. Finally, the research team used a fourth treatment period in which inaccurate and inflated compliance rates were posted. When this occurred, more high speeders were likely to reduce their speed. In fact, the higher the posted rate of compliance, the greater the effect on the high speeder. Still, the overall effect on the high speeder was not significant.

Reversal designs can be very helpful, but they lack control, and generality is limited when conducted with a single subject. However, there is nothing that prevents using multiple subjects in baseline-reversal designs, as well as using multiple baselines.

Pre-Post Designs: The Workhorse of Therapy Research

In a **pre-post design,** a group of clients with common symptoms responds (pretesting) to a standard scale (or set of scales). This shows how severe the symptoms are before treatment. Then all clients receive treatment for a set time. In a posttest, clients respond to the same scale (usually an equivalent form of the same scale). The clinician then compares scores on the pretest to scores on the posttest to find out whether the treatment was effective or not.

This design seems elegantly simple on the surface, but it is also subject to problems of control. It is possible that factors external to the intervention really produced the change. Clients may obtain helpful informal therapy from family, friends, or clergy. Clients with acute stress reactions may improve because the stressor retreats as quickly as it entered. In the absence of a control group, we cannot tell.

PRE-POST DESIGN WITH UNTREATED CONTROL To solve this problem, the clinician may use an untreated control group having the same clinical symptoms as the treatment group. One way of managing this is the **wait-list control,** diagrammed in Table 2-2. Volunteers may be solicited through local advertising. After the pretest, the clinician randomly assigns about half the volunteers to a wait-list. To facilitate this process, volunteers are given a convincing cover story, that the clinic can provide treatment to only a few people at a time, and treatment will be provided as soon as space is available.

When the treatment group completes therapy, the clinician treats the wait-list group. Before beginning treatment, though, the group again fills out the scales that were used in pretesting. The logic is straightforward. If the treatment group improved

---

TABLE 2-2
A pre-post design with wait-list control group

NONFACTORIAL DESIGN WITH WAIT-LIST (UNTREATED) CONTROLS			
Treatment Group	Pretest (T1)	Treatment Phase	Posttest (T2)
Wait-List Control	Pretest (T1)	Waiting Period	Posttest (T2)

while the wait-list group did not, then the treatment must be responsible, not external factors. This design is superior to both the baseline-reversal and the pre-post designs, but it still has flaws. For example, we know that if clients simply believe in a therapy, there is greater chance for cure. This is the **placebo effect.** To solve this problem, we use an attention-placebo control group.

PRE-POST DESIGN WITH ATTENTION-PLACEBO CONTROL A study at the Sloan-Kettering Cancer center led by Sharon Manne illustrates this approach[3] (Manne et al., 1990). Manne and her associates were concerned about the extreme distress experienced by children undergoing invasive and painful chemotherapy. Children often must be physically restrained for venipuncture procedures. Manne cited evidence that these children receive as many as 300 venipunctures in the course of treatment. The procedure usually becomes more aversive as the veins become less accessible.

Manne's team designed a behavioral-cognitive treatment program with four components. First, children could divert attention by using a party whistle during venipuncture. Second, paced breathing substituted for undesirable behaviors such as struggle and refusal to sit still. Third, children could earn cartoon or celebrity stickers as positive reinforcement for cooperation. Finally, parents received instruction to encourage use of the party whistle and paced breathing.

Of the 23 children who participated, 13 were in the treatment group and 10 in the attention-placebo group. All subjects provided baseline data during a scheduled venipuncture procedure plus three data sets following intervention. Parents in the attention-placebo group received instructions to use whatever procedures had been successful in previous sessions. For both treatment and control dyads (parent-child pairs), psychologists were present during venipuncture sessions. One flaw existed in the design: the researchers could not use blind control. The treatment team, including medical personnel, knew whether the dyads belonged to the treatment group or the attention group.

Manne's team rated a child's distress over three trials. The results of the experiment were clear. The behavioral-cognitive treatment significantly reduced the amount of observed child distress. Children in the treatment group required less physical restraint after intervention than before and significantly less than the control group. The control group did improve, but not as much. This illustrates the role of attention that would be obscured by an untreated control design. (See Figure 2-4.) Parents also rated their child's pain as much lower following intervention. The intervention was just as successful with young children (three years old) as with older children (nine years old), and with both boys and girls. However, children in the treatment group did not report lower subjective pain. This suggests that behavioral control under distress and subjective experience of distress are not necessarily linked.

Factorial Designs: Combining Independent Variables

The previous designs manipulated only one independent variable. They are easy to interpret, but of doubtful generality. Events in the real world are rarely if ever determined by just one factor. **Factorial designs** combine two or more independent vari-

---

[3]The procedures and analysis are simplified to highlight the main design features and outcomes. Also, the researchers used sophisticated statistical analyses that are beyond the scope of this text.

FIGURE 2-4
Mean frequency of use of restraint across baseline and three intervention trials
(percentage of children).
SOURCE: Manne et al. (1990).

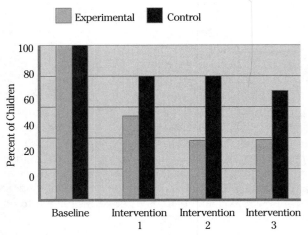

ables in a single experiment. We gain significant information with this strategy. Each
independent variable can be tested as though a single-variable experiment is under
way. At the same time, interactions can be tested. Interactions reflect the way multiple
factors combine to produce outcomes not predicted by the operation of variables
studied in isolation. It is important to note that no single-variable experiment, no matter how well designed, can ever provide information about interactions. Neither can
we link a group of single-variable experiments to obtain information about interactions. The only way to study interactions is to combine the influence of suspect variables in one experiment.

A study conducted by Kenneth Allred and Timothy Smith (1989) illustrates the factorial design. Allred and Smith were following a line of inquiry begun by Suzanne Kobasa
(1979a, 1979b) on the hardy personality. Numerous studies suggested that people who
display a hardy personality are resistant to stress-induced illness. Investigators usually
credited this to an adaptive cognitive style and reduced physiological arousal. To test this
idea, Allred and Smith assessed both cognitive and physiological responses of males of
both high and low hardiness under conditions of a laboratory-manipulated threat.

This study used two independent variables, personality hardiness and threat, as a
stressor. First, Allred and Smith used the Abridged Hardiness Scale and the Revised Hardiness Scale. They divided subjects into high- and low-hardiness groups by taking the
combined median split of the two scales.[4]

---

[4]A median split divides the group into two equal halves. If subjects scored in the same half on each median
split, they stayed in the study. Otherwise, they were dropped from the study.

TABLE 2-3
A schematic representation of the 2 × 2 factorial design used by Allred and Smith (1989) and the expected outcome for the dependent variables

	HIGH THREAT	LOW THREAT
High Hardiness	Low arousal (physiological) Positive thoughts (cognitive)	No change compared to low hardiness
Low Hardiness	High arousal (physiological) Negative thoughts (cognitive)	No change compared to high hardiness

Second, Allred and Smith randomly assigned subjects to receive either a high evaluative threat condition or a low-threat condition. Subjects in the high-threat condition believed that they would take a test that could predict academic and vocational success. Subjects in the low-threat condition believed that they would provide physiological measures while doing a cognitive task where the answers were unimportant. Each independent variable had two levels, resulting in a typical 2 × 2 factorial design, shown in Table 2-3. The dependent variables were systolic and diastolic blood pressure plus a self-statement inventory to assess positive and negative thoughts.

Analysis of the data showed that subjects with high hardiness had only marginally lower arousal when they were waiting for the task to begin. High-hardiness subjects had higher systolic blood pressure perhaps because of more active coping efforts. High hardiness subjects in the high-threat condition also had more positive thoughts than low hardiness subjects in the same condition. The results supported the hardy cognitive style on the one hand, but suggested that the physiological links between hardiness and health status are by no means simple.

Indeed, Dienstbier (1989) has shown that organisms subjected to intermittent stressors develop a type of physiological toughness and resilience that allows for a more efficent response to stress. The base rate for sympathetic operations is reduced, which translates to a lower level of chronic arousal. At the same time, the sympathetic-adrenal-medullary complex can react more swiftly and strongly to challenge or threat. Further, important brain neurotransmitters (catecholamines) are not depleted as rapidly as when sympathetic nervous system activity is high. This is significant because depletion of catecholamines undermines mental and physical performances. The resulting deficits could be critical to successful coping with stress. Finally, experience with intermittent stressors suppresses the pituitary adrenal-cortical response, which appears to translate as enhanced immune system function.

Mixed Designs: Comparing Between Groups Across Time

Quite often, clinical research and field trials require that the investigator compare the effectiveness of a treatment across time. Typically, the dependent measures are taken pre- and posttreatment, but other measures may be taken at different times during treatment and at several follow-up times. It is not uncommon for such work to collect observations years after the original intervention. In the parlance of experimental design, these are repeated measures on the same subjects.

In addition, there may be differences in client traits that are considered theoretically important, or different potentially useful treatments that are still unproved. Indeed, it may be that one treatment is most useful with one type of client while another treatment is most useful with a different type of client. To test hypotheses of this nature, the investigator must use separate groups. The first approach, repeated observations on the same subjects, is a **within-subjects design.** The second approach, assigning different subjects to different treatments, is a classic **between-groups design.** When the project requires both within-subjects and between-groups designs, it is a **mixed design.**

Friedman, Bliwise, Yesavage, & Salom (1991) used a mixed design to compare two different treatments, sleep restriction therapy (SRT) and relaxation training (RLT), for insomnia in adults. Sleep restriction therapy limits the time in bed when sleep is disturbed and increases time in bed as sleep becomes more efficient (Spielman, Saskin, & Thorpy, 1987). Subjects were obtained from the community, carefully screened for inclusion in the study, and assigned to either SRT (n=10) or RLT (n=12).

Multiple dependent measures were used, including total sleep time, time in bed, sleep efficiency (defined as the ratio of total sleep time to time in bed multiplied by 100), and time to the onset of sleep, among others. Each measure was obtained for two-week observation periods and converted to three period means: the first was for a two-week baseline; the second mean was for the last two weeks (weeks 3 and 4) of treatment; and the third mean was for a two-week follow-up scheduled three months after treatment. Total sleep time did not improve for either group during therapy, but it rose significantly in both groups at follow-up. RLT subjects were spending more time in bed after treatment, but were significantly less efficient than SRT subjects. By this criteria, SRT seemed to have the more salutary effect on sleep. The authors note, however, that there were subjects in both groups for whom the treatment did not seem to be effective. This suggests that it is necessary to know more about how client traits interact with the qualities of specific treatments before better matches can be made.

Quasi-Experimental Designs: Comparing Assessed or Static Groups

As noted earlier, a quasi-experimental design is a study that has a family resemblance to a true experiment but is still different in crucial ways. The primary difference in a quasi-experimental design is that the investigator cannot assign subjects completely at random to the different treatments. This may occur because a trait being used for grouping cannot be directly manipulated by the investigator. For example, sex of subjects is used very often as a grouping variable, but the investigator must use the presence of the variable as it already exists in the subjects. Trait anxiety, depression, coping style, and pre-existing medical condition are just a few examples of subject traits that must be assessed by inventory or selected for based on documented diagnosis. In each case, the degree of a trait or the presence versus absence of a trait determines group membership, not random assignment. Many of the so-called experimental designs technically may be quasi-experimental designs by this criteria. For example, the Allred and Smith (1989) study described earlier technically is a quasi-experimental design because the researchers used an assessment procedure to establish groups with subjects of high and low hardiness.

FIGURE 2-5

A comparison of sleep restriction therapy to a relaxation procedure with three months' follow-up.

SOURCE:Friedman et al., 1991.

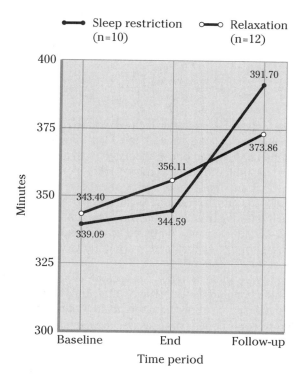

EPIDEMIOLOGY: THE SCIENCE OF EPIDEMICS

Epidemiology, the science of epidemics, seeks to understand the distribution and eti-ology of disease (Lilienfeld & Lilienfeld, 1980). The historical origins of this science are ancient and venerable, but the modern era of epidemiology may be traced to the work of John Snow around 1850. Snow, a founding member of the London Epidemiological Society, noted that death rates were from eight to nine times higher in a London district south of the Thames. Snow discovered that one particular company supplied water to this region and that this was the only company to draw its water from a highly polluted area of the Thames. Snow inferred from this that cholera comes from "poison" transmit-ted by the polluted water.

Epidemiologists use many dependent measures not typically encountered in psy-chosocial research. The most common are mortality, morbidity, incidence, prevalence, and relative risk. **Mortality** is a period death rate per base of the population. For example, the annual death rate from cardiovascular disease is approximately 326 cases per 100,000 peo-ple. **Morbidity** measures the presence of disabling symptoms in a population. Heart pa-tients may experience severe fatigue, require corrective surgery, or suffer nonfatal strokes.

The rate at which new cases of a disease appear in a given period is **incidence.** **Prevalence** is the number of cases of a disease that exist at a given time. Thus prevalence is total cases, whether old or new. The rapid change in AIDS during the middle-1980s illustrates these two measures. Early in 1986, the total number of cases—prevalence—was about 18,907. At that time, new cases began to appear at an alarming rate—incidence. In this case, the incidence statistic was much more important than the prevalence statistic. Finally, **relative risk** (RR) is the measure of association between a marker trait and a disease. It is expressed as a ratio:

$$RR = \frac{Incidence_{exposed}}{Incidence_{unexposed}}$$

Grobbee and his colleagues used this measure in their report on caffeine and cardiovascular disease in men (Grobbee et al., 1990). Men who drank four or more cups of coffee per day (whether caffeinated or decaffeinated) had a relative risk of 1.04. In concrete numbers, 589 non-coffee drinkers suffered some cardiovascular disorder compared to 613 men who drank four or more cups of coffee per day ($613 \div 589 = 1.04$). This difference was so small that it could be explained by sampling differences or measurement error. One interesting result was that men who drank decaffeinated coffee had a relative risk of 1.67 (572 unexposed compared to 1002 exposed). This was statistically significant. The authors concluded that there is no support for the notion that coffee consumption increases risk for coronary.[5]

The logic of epidemiology follows the usual scientific progression from description to explanation to prediction and control (Kleinbaum, Kupper, & Morgenstern, 1982). In general, epidemiology first tries to describe the health status of a population. It counts current cases of illness (prevalence) or measures the rate at which new cases of an illness appear in a given period (incidence). Using these measures, comparisons can be made between subgroups of the population, as Snow did for people living below the Thames as opposed to those living above. Differences between subgroups may lead to a useful and testable hypothesis (pollution of the water caused the illness).

The second step is to explain the **etiology,** or origins, of a disease. Etiology constructs a coherent picture of the factors that contribute to an illness. Numerous markers may be identified, including demographic characteristics (sex, age, ethnic group), biological and genetic factors, environmental variables, socioeconomic variables, and personal health habits and lifestyle (such as coffee consumption). The emphasis is on groups at risk. There is no attempt to predict illness in individuals (Cockerham, 1982).

Epidemiology may test models developed in stage two by trying to predict prevalence and distribution of diseases. If predictions are accurate, there is increased confidence that the etiological model is correct. Finally, they may use the knowledge gained in prior studies to control diseases. This could include preventive steps, eradication, prolongation of life, or improving health status of afflicted persons.

There are many variations to epidemiological studies, more than we can discuss here. I will use a very common procedure, the clinical trial, to illustrate. A **clinical trial** is a field experiment to verify that a therapeutic agent is effective. The study presented next also illustrates a **prospective design:** That is, it followed subjects through the nat-

---

[5]We should note, however, that the results across many studies are mixed, so the jury is still out on the exact role of caffeine in coronary risk.

ural history of a disorder. In contrast, a **retrospective design** attempts to reconstruct probable causes by looking back on a disorder after it has already occurred.

Recently, medical nutrition research suggested that beta carotene may act as a dietary anticarcinogen. Animal models (see below for more detail) suggested that carotenoids slow down development of tumors but do not reduce the number of tumors (Krinsky, 1989). Case-control studies showed that increased consumption of fruits and vegetables with high amounts of beta carotene reduced the risk for cancer. Unfortunately, case-control studies do not allow us to eliminate competing explanations since we cannot control for many other variables.

Greenberg's group reported the results of a large-scale, randomized, double-blind clinical trial in people with a prior history of nonmelanoma skin cancer (Greenberg et al., 1990). They randomly assigned 1805 patients to one of two groups. The treatment (exposed) group (913 patients) received 50 mg of beta carotene daily. The placebo (nonexposed) group (892 patients) received capsules identical in appearance to the carotene capsules.

The team monitored compliance with the therapy through regularly scheduled questionnaires. If subjects did not take the pills, or there was a substantial difference in compliance between the groups, no firm conclusions could be made. Greenberg's group anticipated another potential problem: that the nonexposed group might obtain black-market supplies of beta carotene. As a check on compliance, subjects provided blood samples, which were tested for level of beta carotene. This is a **manipulation check.** Patients in the exposed group had an eight-fold increase in beta carotene while patients in the placebo group showed no change from prestudy levels.

Patients received routine medical examinations at yearly intervals over a five-year study period. There were two dependent measures: time to the occurrence of new skin cancer, and number of new skin cancers. The results clearly conflicted with earlier case-control studies: beta carotene did not protect the exposed group against recurrence of skin cancer. The exposed group had an average of .29 new cancers per study year while the placebo group had an average of .25 new cancers. The rates also did not differ at checkpoints during the five-year study time. The authors point out that their study used subjects with a particular type of cancer. From this sample, then, it would be unwise to conclude that beta carotene offers no protection for all cancers.

META-ANALYSIS: ANALYZING THE ANALYSES

Meta-analysis is the new kid on the block when it comes to analysis of experiments. Richard Light, a Harvard statistician, and David Pillemer, a Wellesley College psychologist, developed the technique in the early 1970s (Light & Pillemer, 1984), but it was Gene Glass (1976) who coined the term. Meta-analysis is observational, not experimental. It generates new data, but only through use of old data, not through manipulation of causal variables. It is a statistical technique that sums up the results of studies concerned with similar hypotheses.

Historically, science has progressed by contributing a volume of studies that probe the breadth and depth of an issue. In the process, a group of studies might seem to converge to a common solution only to be upset by another group of studies showing discrepant results. When a critical mass accumulated, some undaunted soul would pore through the results and try to pull order from the jaws of chaos. The written record of this effort was a **qualitative literature review** (or a narrative review). Entire journals are devoted to these reviews (*Psychological Bulletin* and *Psychological Review*), and they play an invaluable role in helping interested parties keep up with a research topic.

Still, qualitative reviews suffer from the bias of expert opinion. No matter how expert the reviewer is, review still involves subjective judgment. Further, qualitative reviews lack methodological rigor, and they place undue emphasis on the level of significance of studies under review (Johnson, 1989).

In contrast, meta-analysis provides an objective tool to conduct a **quantitative literature review.** Presumably, the results of a meta-analysis can be placed in the public domain for scrutiny, whereas expert opinion cannot. Also, the process is subject to replication and should lead to the same outcomes and interpretations.

In brief, meta-analysis accounts for the magnitude of effect, which is defined as the absolute size of the difference between experimental and control conditions. It is not based solely on statistical significance. In the pooling of the results of many studies, the effect of certain stimulus variables can be more clearly seen. In several situations, meta-analysis led to much different conclusions than those obtained from a narrative review.

An example of this approach is found in the work of Fernandez and Turk (1989). Their research revolves around issues of pain management and the efficacy of behavioral and cognitive therapies to reduce pain. Fernandez and Turk used a pool of 46 articles with a composite sample of 2000 subjects. They showed that previous qualitative and quasi-statistical studies led to confusion about the potency of cognitive coping strategies. Earlier reviews suggested that acknowledging pain was the most effective method of altering pain perception, while neutral imagery was the least effective. Meta-analysis showed the opposite results. On one matter, though, all the analyses agreed: cognitive strategies produce substantive improvement over untreated or placebo controls.

Although meta-analysis has had remarkable success, it is not a panacea. It has its pitfalls and critics. The investigator must make many decisions about studies to include and exclude, how to group studies where definitions vary, how to treat missing data, and so on. Also, studies with significant effects are overrepresented in the published literature, while studies with nonsignificant findings are much less likely to be published. In their meta-analysis of the disease-prone personality, Friedman and Booth-Kewley (1987) found fault with the excessive speculation that has often been the result of meta-analysis. They pointed out that the most valuable product of meta-analysis should be more refined empirical work to resolve discrepancies. Finally, there is concern that meta-analysis distances us even further from the client whose well-being is the primary concern of much of the research.

ANIMALS IN STRESS AND HEALTH RESEARCH

Most of the previous research designs used human subjects, but this does not mean that animal studies are irrelevant to research on stress and health. In fact, a substantial amount of stress research and related health variables began with animal models before moving on to human populations.

Several arguments have been made in support of animal research (Johnson, 1990). First, the need to provide therapeutic assistance to the physically and mentally ill has always seemed a compelling reason to pursue research with animals. This need is based on the demand, indeed the public clamor, for treatments to meet catastrophic health needs. Second, animal research has proven historically to be nearly invaluable in providing information about numerous crucial issues, including brain-behavior relations; genetic substrates of stress, addictions, obesity, or aging; and development of treatments (both behavioral and pharmacologic) for depression and anxiety, to name just a few. Third, animal models enable researchers to control and manipulate certain factors that could not be so easily overseen with human subjects. Fourth, although animal-rights activists recommend simulations and culture experiments instead of outright animal research, these techniques cannot begin to provide the information that is needed where the complexities of human behavior and health needs are concerned. Fifth, the evolution of the comparative sciences (comparative psychology, for example) has produced more detailed knowledge of parallels between animals and humans in biological and psychological systems. When a scientist selects a particular animal subject, the selection is typically directed by that same knowledge of parallels. In turn, generalizations to humans can be made with increased confidence, although final confirmation with a human population is still important. Finally, though not an argument for animal research, it has been noted that the number of animals used in psychological research is in actuality relatively small, and that experiments inflicting severe pain are rare even though their frequency has been highly exaggerated (Coile & Miller, 1984; Miller, 1985).

I will touch on just a few of the more noteworthy examples of animal research. At the biological end of the continuum, psychological research has used animals for a wide range of neuroanatomy, neurophysiology, and neurotransmitter studies. This work has been important to understanding brain-behavior connections, many of which are important to stress-health links. As one example, understanding the role of the hypothalamus in regulating food intake depends largely on animal models. Overall regulation of hunger and food intake is now known to be a complex system that involves brain centers and feedback of information (both neural and chemical) from the digestive system. Further, knowledge of obesity and fat-storage mechanisms has benefited greatly by animal research. In turn, all this knowledge has led to more focused research and better understanding of eating disorders in general, including obesity, anorexia nervosa, and bulimia.

A second important research area involving animals attempts to answer questions about the genetic basis of high-risk behaviors. For example, the past 25 years have seen a great thrust of work on the genetic basis of drug addiction (George, 1988, 1990) and alcoholism (George, 1987; Geer, McKechnie, Heinstra, & Pyka, 1991). Among the more important issues explored via the genetic animal model are (1) sensitivity to drug effects, (2) tolerance, dependence, and withdrawal, (3) and the rewarding (or aversive) effects of drug use. (See the review by Crabbe, Belknap, & Buck, 1995.) Animal models of genetic influence enable an investigator to look at the transmission of a trait over several generations (5 to 7 generations is not uncommon) in a matter of just a few years, when the same research with humans would require approximately 100 to 120 years. Animals from the lowly fly to rodents to primates have served for this type of work.

Hans Selye's research on stress was conducted largely with rats as subjects (1956, 1976). Thus, much of what we know about the body's emergency response system (the physiology of stress) comes from this type of work. Over the past 20 years, we have seen the emergence of the field of psychoneuroimmunology (Ader, Cohen, & Felten, 1987). The basic notions of immunology and of the connections between the immune system and the brain and endocrine system have been based on animal models. Investigators also have provided evidence that the immune system can be classically conditioned. Finally, dose-response links in newly designed medicines or in high-risk toxins like side-stream smoke and carcinogens are based largely on animal research.

There are, of course, sensitive ethical issues beyond the scope of this chapter that have sparked lively debates on both sides of the issue. Perhaps the most intense debates ensued following revelations from Edward Taub's laboratory that involved neglect, if not abuse, of animal subjects. Despite the negative press surrounding this situation, the research program itself is a valuable example of the analogue approach applied to closed-head injury and rehabilitation methods (Pons et al., 1991).

SUMMARY

In this chapter, we have discussed conceptual issues plus several methodologies used to study psychosocial factors related to health and illness. The coverage has been selective to provide a background for studies introduced later in the text. The major points are listed below.

- Thinking about stress and health relationships requires that we use contextual and organistic thinking as opposed to singly-determined mechanistic thinking. The processes that are at work in linking stress to disease are most often multiply determined.
- The logic of scientific discovery is to manipulate an independent variable and to measure its effect on a dependent variable. At the same time, the scientist tries to control or eliminate other variables that might confound interpretation of the results.
- In stress and health research, there are few absolute independent or dependent variables. In other words, the role a variable plays depends largely on where the researcher cuts into the causal chain. An independent variable in one experiment, such as differences in personality types, might actually be a dependent variable in another experiment.
- Case studies look in great depth at a single individual but do not establish cause-effect relations. Case studies can be of heuristic value in generating hypotheses for further clinical testing.
- Assessment instruments must meet the criteria of both reliability and validity. Reliability means that the test measures the same way every time. Validity means that the test measures what it is supposed to measure.
- Using human subjects in research requires that the investigator consider many ethical issues before conducting the research. All research must now be reviewed by an ethics committee (such as the Institutional Research Board) to ensure that subjects are treated ethically.
- Inferential statistics allow an investigator to decide whether an outcome was likely or unlikely to have occurred by chance. If the result is judged significant, it means that the outcome would occur only very rarely by chance. Therefore, it is more likely that the result occurred due to the investigators' manipulation of the independent variable.
- Field studies allow investigators to observe many behaviors that occur in natural settings. Most do not control for extraneous variables and thus cannot provide information about cause and effect. Yet they have ecological validity, and like the case study, they are of heuristic value.

- Ex-post-facto research is research conducted after an event has already taken place. For example, natural catastrophes, such as hurricanes and earthquakes, call for this type of design.
- Ecological Momentary Assessment is an effort to carry out observations in the natural environment as a behavior or event occurs.
- Correlational research assesses the extent to which variables are related to each other. While correlations do not establish causation, without correlation, there can be no causation.
- Simple clinical experiments use single-subject designs and compare baseline data to data following treatment. Extensions of this basic design include the single-group pre-post design, the pre-post design with untreated control group, and the pre-post design with an attention-placebo control group. Each design improves on the preceding by increasing control that eliminates alternative explanations for the success of the treatment.
- Factorial designs are the first step to multicausal hypotheses. They combine two or more independent variables and allow us to test how these variables interact to produce outcomes not predicted from study of the variables in isolation.
- Epidemiological research assesses the distribution of diseases in a population. It also seeks to discover the etiology or causes of disease. When changes in mortality (deaths) and morbidity (disabling symptoms) occur with different rates in subgroups of a population, important clues may appear to guide further research.
- A common research design in epidemiology is the clinical trial. This method randomly assigns subjects to different therapies and then tests the success of the therapy for a certain disease. Psychosocial epidemiology is now extending these methods to study relations between psychosocial factors and health status.
- Meta-analysis is a newcomer to the quantitative analysis of data. It works on data from already completed studies. The technique analyzes effect size, the size of the difference between the experimental and the control group. This enables investigators to evaluate the consistency of findings, assess the importance of either demographic or situational variables used by previous investigators, and resolve contradictions between existing studies.
- Animals are used in various projects to obtain information on disease and health processes that may not be as readily obtained with human subjects. Genetic processes, for example, can be much more easily observed in a rodent sample than in a human sample.

CRITICAL THINKING AND STUDY QUESTIONS

1. What is the significance of the distinction between unicausal and multicausal models for health psychology?
2. How might single-subject case studies be useful to the health psychologist?
3. What are the strengths and weaknesses of the correlational design?
4. When an investigator decides to use a control group, what factors must be considered?

5. What is epidemiological research, and how does it differ from classical laboratory research?
6. What is meta-analysis? How is it being used today to add to our knowledge base in health psychology?

KEY TERMS

alternate-forms reliability
archival data
attention-placebo group
baseline measures
baseline-reversal design
between-groups design
case-study method
clinical trial
confidence level
construct validity
content validity
contextual thinking
control group
control, double-blind
control, single-blind
correlational design
criterion variable
criterion-related validity
debriefing
dependent variable
distal cause
Ecological Momentary
   Assessment
epidemiology
etiology

ex-post-facto design
experimental group
face validity
factorial designs
formistic thinking
hypothesis
incidence
independent variable
inferential statistics
informed consent
Institutional Research
   Board
manipulation check
mechanistic thinking
meta-analysis
mixed design
morbidity
mortality
operational definitions
organistic thinking
placebo effect
precipitating factors
pre-post design
predictor variable
predisposing factors

prevalence
prospective design
proximal cause
qualitative literature
   review
quantitative literature
   review
quasi-experimental
   design
random assignment
relative risk (RR)
reliability
retrospective design
single-subject design
split-half reliability
standardized test
survey research
test-retest reliability
Type I error
Type II error
validity
wait-list control
within-subjects design

WEBSITES research and methods in health behavior

URL ADDRESS	SITE NAME & DESCRIPTION
http://www.socsciresearch.com	Research Engines for the Social Sciences
http://www.cdc.gov	☆Center for Disease Control, provides latest data on epidemiology of disease
http://www.essex.ac.uk/social-science-methodology-school	Social Science Methodology School Home Page—Data Analysis and Collection
http://www.apa.org/science/lib.html	☆American Psychological Association's Introduction to Library Research, for students and nonpsychologists

COMMENTS ON SELF-STUDY EXERCISE 2-1

The following is a brief, non-exhaustive guide to possible responses to the claims in the exercise.

1. Many of the claims for melatonin-improved sleep are based on experiences of aged groups where sleep disturbances are common due to changes in melatonin. In most younger individuals, sleep disturbances are due to factors other than problems in melatonin production. Also, even when the sleep problem is due to distubances in melatonin production, the dosage supplied for relief is up to 10 times the amount medically necessary to restore balance. Finally, many people suffer negative side-effects from taking melatonin, including intense dreams (some enjoyable, some not so enjoyable) and changes in sexuality (some enjoyable, some not so enjoyable).

2. The claims that many food and snack products have low fat and low cholesterol do not point out their other food additives or sodium content. Certain products with low cholesterol may still have unacceptably high levels of sodium. If you have any familial or personal history of heart or blood pressure problems, the high sodium content may be as or more important than the fat and cholesterol.

3. The fat-reduction claim is a favorite, but the level of fat even after the reduction may still be unacceptably high.

4. Testimonials are also a favorite advertising ploy. However, we can never be sure what personally unique variables contributed to the success of the therapy, or for that matter, whether it was actually the hypnosis or some other overlooked factor (for example, a religious conversion experience during the intervention period, or informal therapy from some other source) that actually produced the change. Also, we seldom know where a person giving testimony is in the course of the intervention. If the addiction returns in a few months or the weight is back on, the previous success is really not that meaningful.

5. The fen-phen debacle may be considered an outcome of an unhealthy tradition in medical practice. Many drugs, including the combination of fenfluramine and phenter-mine, are used for purposes not approved by the FDA (Connolly et al., 1997). Even when the effects of an individual drug may have been well-researched, that drug may be combined with another drug while the interaction of the two has never been stud-ied. At the same time, when a drug once considered a great hope (in this case, for those wanting to lose weight) is dropped from use, the consuming public often makes a mass exodus to any new substitute product that offers hope. Now, St. John's Wort is being advertised as a suitable substitute for fen-phen. One problem with many so-called natural vitamins and herbal medicines is that evidence of efficacy may be largely anectodal, whereas scientific data is either incomplete, lacking for the adver-tised use, or completely absent. You may find it interesting to follow up on both ends of this issue by looking briefly at information on FDA approval for fen-phen as well as scientific evidence for use of St. John's Wort. The Connolly study cited above deals specifically with the fen-phen case.

ANSWERS FOR SELF-STUDY EXERCISE 2-2

For the listed hypotheses, the actual independent and dependent variable(s) are shown.
1. IV—levels of exercise in the three groups
   DV_1—good cholesterol (HDLs)
   DV_2—bad cholesterol (LDLs)
2. IV_1—type of coping strategy (problem-focused versus emotion-focused)
   IV_2—type of stress (interpersonal versus disaster)
   DV—current levels of stress
3. IV—behavior pattern (Type A versus Type B)
   DV—risk for coronary disease
4. IV—level of vitamin E use (three groups)
   DV—incidence of cancer
5. IV_1—type of social support
   IV_2—type of surgery (mastectomy or lumpectomy)
   DV—levels of stress

Biopsychological Foundations of Stress

CHAPTER 3

The Cognitive Stress System:

Attitudes, Beliefs, and Expectations

If pleasures are greatest in anticipation, just remember that this is also true of trouble.

ELBERT HUBBARD

Your clinic appointment ends with arrangements made for admission to the hospital. "We have to run some tests," the doctor says. You reply, "Tests? What tests? What do I have? Tell me what's going on. I need to know."

Your supervisor stops by to summon you to a meeting with management in one hour. "We have to discuss the production record of your group" is the only clue. Your response is to the point. "What's wrong with our work?" "I can't say anything more until the meeting. See you then," your supervisor replies.

Your teenager calls to say, "I don't know how to tell you this, but, ah, I just wrecked the car." "You did what? Were you hurt? Was anyone with you? How did it happen? Where are you now?"

These very different events share a common problem: each is ripe for many different interpretations. You may welcome the hospital diagnostics for the prospect of rest, discovery, and the end of uncertainty. On the other hand, you may dread the tests because of what might be found or because you expect the procedures to be uncomfortable, if not painful. The production record may be good or bad; the supervisor's comments do not provide any clues.

The youngster who has to relay the unwelcome news to his parents also faces a variety of uncertainties. He cannot be sure how his parents will react, and he might lose future use of the family car. Also, the parents can only imagine what their car might look like. At one extreme is the image of a scratched car, at the other, the image of a demolished car.

LABELS, GUESSES, AND GAPS

The most common cognitive response to uncertainty is **labeling,** assigning meaning to the event. Hospital tests mean a serious health problem. A meeting with management spells trouble, reprimands, probably a diminished chance for promotion, and so forth. Labeling will occur very early in cognitive processing, even prior to one's having all the relevant information. The process is private and goes unnoticed for the most part. Still, it plays a vital role in transactions with the people we meet daily. It sets the stage for a distress reaction or a positive encounter (Brewin, 1988).

A second process occurs simultaneously. That is, people tend to fill gaps in available information with *guesses,* or inferences about the unknown. "What's wrong with our work?" not only labels the supervisor's summons as a threat, it also shows that the person has already guessed the likely script for the meeting. The inference is that the news is bad, that management will scold the group for poor production.

The true purpose of the meeting might be much different, though. Management may want to use the group for a special project that needs the group's production ability. Instead of reprimanding, management intends to honor. The pessimistic guess about what is going on nudges the process to the negative side of stress. Our knowledge of the **literal brain**[1] suggests that physical arousal will occur. Blood pressure may increase, and adrenaline may flood the system. Metabolic rate quickens, and sweating could occur. Based on their extensive studies of **pessimistic explanatory styles,** Chris Peterson and Martin Seligman (1984, 1987) came to believe that this pessimistic style is a major problem in transactions that lead to stress, depression, and illness.

---

[1]See pages 75 and 131 for more details on the literal brain.

Most events hold some uncertainty because only a small amount of information is available at any given time. We actively seek data to fill these gaps. Information seeking can be an important coping strategy, but obtaining information is also time dependent. The doctor does not know what to expect or what will be found. It may be several days before test results are available. The supervisor could disclose nothing until the meeting. That gives you at least an hour to worry and fret. The teenager can verbally relay only bits and pieces of the total picture. Meanwhile, the mind works overtime drawing its own pictures of what happened or what will happen. These three processes—assigning meaning, filling in gaps, and seeking information—continue in cycles. Only when the mind has achieved a satisfactory evaluation and integration will it cease its struggle to give meaning.

ANTICIPATIONS: HOPE AND DESPAIR

Herbert Lefcourt (1976) related one of the most dramatic examples of the powerful effect of labeling. A woman had been mute and socially withdrawn for nearly ten years. She was in a psychiatric hospital, confined to a ward known to patients as the "chronic hopeless" ward. Then hospital management decided to redecorate. To simplify the work, hospital staff moved these patients to a new location with a special meaning. Patients recognized the new ward as the exit ward—the last step before going home. Shortly after being moved, the mute woman started talking and seemed very happy with her new social

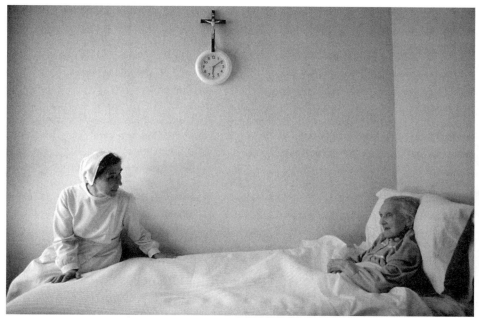

People in chronically ill wards of hospitals and nursing homes often have feelings of hopelessness that can work against their health.

life. Workers soon finished redecorating the chronic hopeless ward, and the residents had to move back. In Lefcourt's words, "Within a week after she had been returned to the 'hopeless' unit, the patient . . . collapsed and died. The subsequent autopsy revealed no pathology of note, and it was whimsically suggested at the time that the patient had died of despair" (1976, p. 10).

COGNITIVE SCIENCE: PROBING THE MYSTERIES OF MIND

Several years ago when my second daughter was about four years old, we visited my parents for a short vacation. It was a hot, humid summer day in Kansas, so my mother thought it would be nice to take the grandchildren to Dairy Queen for a treat. Soon, we were seated enjoying our ice cream, and my high-energy daughter was bouncing from seat to floor and back with ice cream in hand, taking in everything there was to see. We were engaged in "adult" conversation, catching up on the family events of the past year. It soon became clear that my mother was getting increasingly nervous. Finally she said, "Michelle, could you sit down for a minute? Just watching you bounce around is driving me up a wall." To this my daughter perkily replied, while never missing a bounce: "Well, you don't have to watch." In an instant, she had defined the gist of the problem of many stressors: Stress is in the eye of the beholder, a mental construction of the external event that could be quickly defused by relabelling.

On the more negative end of the continuum, observations of voodoo deaths and placebos provide strong supporting evidence that thoughts, labels, and expectations powerfully influence stress reactions and health processes. A great many slings and arrows of modern living might never be suffered were it not for the way we think about our daily transactions.

Stress is not so much a physical property of a situation as it is a transaction between person and environment (Lazarus & Launier, 1978). It is more a product of our cognitive processes, the way in which we think about and evaluate a situation. In much the same way, how we cope and how effective our coping is depends largely on how we think about our resources, how we select coping strategies, and what coping skills we have nurtured.

Labels, thinking, and expectations are the province of the mind. They fall within the domain of **cognitive science.** This new science of the mind is concerned with all the ways in which humans know, think, reason, and decide. Considered private and inaccessible for decades, the mysteries contained in the hidden recesses of the mind are now the subject of intense discussion and investigation. These mysteries are opening up gradually to the probing eyes of cognitive scientists in laboratories around the world. The discoveries of these scientists may hold the key to understanding why one person's distress is another's challenge.

Cognitive scientists first tried to construct general theories about the basic processes in cognition. Now, they also think about the cognitive processes involved in stress and health. In addition, cognitive therapists have begun to develop ways to help people alter self-defeating thoughts and build a sense of control. This chapter concerns cognitive processes such as **perception, attention, appraisal,** and **information seeking.** Later in this chapter, we will discuss a highly regarded model of cognitive processing. Finally, we will look at research on pessimistic explanatory styles and health beliefs as they influence health status.

A MODEL OF MIND: INFORMATION PROCESSING

Cognition is defined as all the ways of knowing, thinking, reasoning, and deciding. It includes attention, perception, memory, problem solving, and creativity. In short, cognition is everything we have come to associate with intelligence. To describe how the mind works, cognitive scientists borrowed a computer model from the fields of language and communication. This is the **information processing model.**[2] It states that the person's transactions with the environment can be likened to an elaborate computer data-processing task. For any task, there are at least three stages: input, throughput, and output. A feedback system also is present to correct errors and to modify output based on internal decision rules.

Our sensory systems serve as input channels. After sensory input comes throughput processes such as memory, reasoning, planning, and problem solving. These mental functions require some internal organization and rules for managing the flow of information. For computers, an outside programmer must write the program and provide the rules. We write our own programs using organizational schemes and rules assembled through experience. Speaking is an output process, as is behaving.

Cognitive scientists hope to discover what goes on at each stage. They also try to find connections between brain structures and cognitive processes. They look for feedback circuits that allow for error correction and flexible processing.

SCHEMATA AND PERSONAL CONSTRUCTS

As experiences accumulate, some ideas about how the world operates become functional parts of long-term memory. We group these ideas in mind files that contain as much information about a certain event or class of events as we have. In addition, we organize the information within a file in a meaningful, coherent way. This allows us to predict with some accuracy what the outcome of personal action should be. We cannot say with certainty how this is done, but two theories propose similar solutions. First is George Kelly's (1955) **personal constructs** theory, a model that evolved from personality research. Second is the **schema theory** from the developmental research of Jean Piaget.[3]

Both personal constructs and schemata are subjective constructions of reality. Both can influence perceptions and reactions. According to Kelly, constructs are not part of reality. Instead, we impose constructs on reality to give it meaning. Constructs are predictive guesses that are tested in reality: The world is just or unjust. Bosses, spouses, and acquaintances are bad or good, happy or sad, friendly or hostile, warm or aloof, charitable or uncaring. Any construct that refers to others also can refer to self. Some constructs become rigid and impermeable to new information, and other constructs remain flexible and permit a wide range of new information.

A key idea in Kelly's (1955) thinking is that people become mentally channeled by the way they anticipate events. Anticipations are similar to putting blinders on a horse—they restrict the view to a very narrow range of the track. Different interpretations simply do not exist because they are outside the restricted channel set by expectations.

[2]Currently, a new model, the neural network model, is challenging the information processing model. Still, the work relevant to stress and health is rooted in the information processing model.
[3]For a comprehensive, readable introduction to Piaget's theory, see Ginsburg and Opper (1979).

A clinical anecdote tells of a couple who came close to a divorce because the husband thought the wife had become unfaithful. She had begun to engage in mysterious, secretive behavior. As it turned out, she had concocted an elaborate ruse to surprise her husband with a special gift. His construct of reality allowed him to see only one interpretation—that she was having an affair with someone else—a construction of reality that proved to be erroneous but placed enormous strain on the relationship.

In Piaget's theory, the mind alters sensory input so it will fit with a previously developed schema. This is called **assimilation.** As new information becomes available, the schema becomes more elaborate. This is **accommodation** to meet external demands. We have schemata for cars: what they are like, how they operate, and how we can operate them. Our schema for bosses probably carries a much different meaning from our schema for colleagues or for lovers. Our schema for mothers differs from our schema for fathers. A schema for situations, also called a *script,* contains the rules for situationally appropriate behavior (Schank & Abelson, 1977). Self-concept is an important personal schema. Negative self-schemata may increase vulnerability to depression in the presence of stressful life events (Hammen, Marks, Mayol, & deMayo, 1985). On the other hand, anticipatory schemata of success or failure can influence the way people approach a situation (Bandura, 1989). In this way, schemata act as the primary *meaning systems* in cognition.

PERCEPTION: STRESS IS IN THE EYE OF THE BEHOLDER

If schemata are the central organizing files of the mind, perception is the selective and organizing gateway to the mind. Ulric Neisser (1976), dean of cognitive scientists, stated that perception is the most fundamental cognitive act. This is appropriate in the case of stress and health as well. One review of work stress noted that employee perceptions of stressful situations influenced employee health and well-being (Beehr & Newman, 1978).

Perception is defined as the interpretation and organization of information provided to the brain by the senses. *Interpretation* suggests that we attach meaning and make value judgments about the information. One basic judgment is whether the event is pleasant and valuable or unpleasant, if not painful. *Organization* implies that we make links to experiences stored in long-term memory. We classify new information; that is, we put it in the same memory bin with similar information. This adds to our store of experiences. In the future, this stored experience will, in turn, add color to the perceptual process.

Even from the first breath of life, these positive and negative evaluations are orderly, not random. Research in behavioral genetics showed that inherited emotional sets and the cumulative effect of experience influence **perceptual biases** (Buss & Plomin, 1975; Thomas, Chess, & Birch, 1970). These emotional sets lead some people to see things negatively and to react accordingly. Other people seem to view most events, even catastrophic events, as positive (Hamilton, 1979).

Misperceptions and Stress

One basic problem is that perception is not perfectly veridical. In other words, mental representations are not always congruent with external reality. Perception falls prey to numerous distortions or subtle alterations in the message. Two of the best known and most severe forms of **perceptual distortions** are delusions and hallucinations. A **delusion** is a mistaken belief, such as "I am Jesus" or "Everyone is out to get me." **Hallucinations**

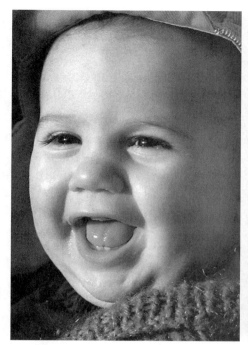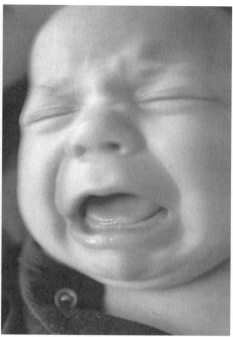

Research on temperament suggests that a genetic factor sets people on a path to a sunny disposition or an irritable disposition.

are tricks the brain plays on some people. These people firmly believe they have seen or heard something that does not really exist.

What about something less extreme, like an imagined threat or the thought that a doctor's examination could be negative? An interesting research project sheds some light on this issue. John (1967) designed an experiment to answer basic questions about how the brain responds to a real physical object. The crucial point in the experiment came when John stopped presenting the geometric forms that subjects saw earlier. At this time, he simply asked the subjects to *imagine* the forms were on the blank screen in front of them. The results were unexpected—there were no differences in the recorded brain waves from the real forms and the imagined forms! In other words, the brain could not distinguish between the perception of the object and its own thought of the object. This led Kenneth Pelletier (1977) to call the brain the *literal brain.*

Such observations help explain how people can become upset when they recall an emotionally distressing event. It also explains why people may panic when merely thinking about surgery or an upcoming major exam. The thought is as real to the mind as the actual event, and the effect on the body is just the same.

Perceptual Vigilance and Attention

The perceptual system appears to have some elaborate processes built in to ensure continued alertness or attention to changes in the environment. As defined by cognitive scientists, attention is the process by which we choose what stimuli are important and where to focus our mental energy. "Choosing" may be involuntary, impulsive, and automatic; or voluntary, deliberate, and selective.

A car crash in front of the house, a firecracker placed under your chair by a mischievous friend, or the cry of "fire!" in a theater will almost always lead to automatic attending. Features of physical stimuli that demand our attention include size, intensity, and motion. In addition, surprise, novelty, and complexity shift the process in the direction of involuntary attention.

A process called **selective attention** protects against overload; helps focus on relevant information, thus improving efficiency; and blocks out unimportant stimuli. Selective attention combined with voluntary sustained attention is **perceptual vigilance.** This requires extreme concentration and deliberate control over competing irrelevant information. Vigilance is vital to certain jobs, such as air traffic control and medical practice. Several serious accidents and near-misses have occurred because of the intense pressure on air traffic controllers, especially in high-density airports such as Boston, New York, and Chicago. In hospitals, medical staff often monitor patient life signs over long periods. Anesthesiologists must be alert every instant to signs of change in vital functions during prolonged surgery.

Sustained attention can produce a variety of problems. For example, vigilance suffers greatly even over short intervals. Within a few hours, an air traffic controller may begin to lose the high level of concentration required for peak accuracy. In addition, the level of arousal required to sustain vigilance appears to take a toll physically and psy-

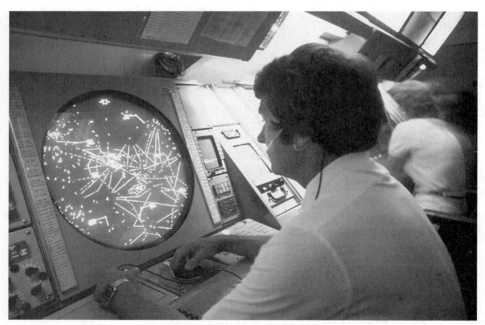

Air traffic controllers work under conditions of high strain because their jobs require them to maintain periods of high vigilance while guiding several planes safely into and out of the terminals airspace.

chologically. Controllers working in congested airports have a much higher rate of physical illness (compared to overall population morbidity), such as high blood pressure and gastric difficulties. They also report more migraines and subjective stress.

Another vigilance problem occurs when patients receive disturbing news of a serious disease or treatment that will affect their future. Some people prefer the path of least resistance, using denial to protect themselves. Some become aroused and vigilant and actively seek any information they can find about their disease and prognosis. They seem to prefer being active and participating in their treatment to sitting back passively. Others become vigilant to the extreme. Janis (1982) called this state **hypervigilance,** when people are on guard constantly as though they must detect the smallest signal to keep on top of the disease. In the long run, hypervigilance usually interferes with decision making. It results in chronic physical and emotional arousal, which may then hinder healing processes.

PERCEPTION, DEPRIVATION, AND OVERLOAD

A large body of research built up over nearly 50 years shows that stimulation levels influence stress. We all have our preferred levels of stimulation and try to avoid the extremes of **deprivation** and **overload.** In the preferred middle ground, the emphasis is on novelty and quality. Sameness and sheer quantity are less desirable. Excessive stimulation aggravates existing stress or is a source of stress itself.

Stimulus Deprivation: Boredom and Stress

Bexton's study of stimulus deprivation at McGill University is almost legendary (Bexton, Heron, & Scott, 1954). Volunteers received $20 per day to lie in bed and sleep. To most students, this seemed like an easy buck. They could quit when they wanted to, and until that time, their basic needs were satisfied. There was only one catch. They had to lie in a cubicle with hands and arms padded and with translucent goggles on their eyes. The subjects could not even hear external sounds because of a masking noise presented through a speaker system.

Bexton's group did not predict what happened. Most of the volunteers quit in the first 24 to 36 hours, and no one went beyond 72 hours. The volunteers slept for the first few hours and enjoyed the relaxation. Soon, though, most of them experienced boredom, restlessness, and increasing anxiety. They tried to generate stimulation by singing, whistling, and talking to themselves. Nonetheless, they experienced a gradual deterioration of intellectual efficiency, followed by unsettling, if not terrifying, experiences. That is, many began to have hallucinations. Some hallucinations were mild, but they seemed to increase in bizarreness and intensity with time. Most were simple geometric forms, but some were more grotesque. One subject saw eyeglasses that turned into deformed, long-legged people walking on the horizon of a small world. To most of the students, the experience was emotionally disturbing and unpleasant. It was too much time with too little input.

How can we explain this result? One possible explanation has to do with the reticular formation, a structure that lies in the brain stem. The reticular formation is the brain's arousal center. It keeps activity going even in the absence of external stimulation. Contact with the outside world, though, is necessary for reality testing. Without it, the brain improvises. It generates its own activity and makes up its own images. As these internal forms stray farther and farther from the norm, they take on the appearance of hallucinations. To use a metaphor, there are no quality controls to ensure that the internal production matches the external blueprint.

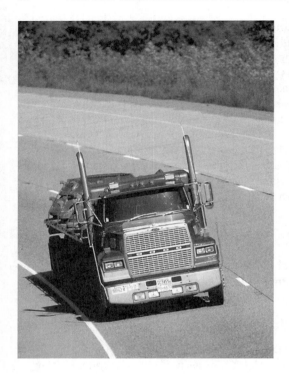

In contrast to air traffic controllers, long-haul truckers often experience sensory deprivation.

This suggests that we need a minimum level of input to keep the cognitive system operating smoothly. It also shows that reduction of input below a minimum level produces stress. Reports from people who function in stimulus-deprived environments such as underwater exploration, polar expeditions, radar operation, and long-distance truck driving confirm these conclusions. Formal research on this issue has helped people prepare to work in such conditions.

Stimulus Overload: Too Much Equals Chaos

Too much stimulation may translate to psychological overload. The expression "this place is a zoo" implies that too much is going on at a pace too fast for the individual's preferred stimulation level. The simple solution, of course, is to get away, be alone, reduce the rate of stimulation even for a short time. When feasible, this coping strategy may be all that is necessary. When this strategy is not feasible, other measures may be called for, such as family problem solving (see Chapter 6), more effective management of space and reduction of noise (Chapter 9), and cognitive coping strategies (Chapters 10 and 12).

MEMORY: I DON'T REMEMBER IT THAT WAY

How often have you heard statements such as these? "I don't remember it happening that way." "No, you were the one who said. . . ." "Your memory is going. It was nothing like that." These comments reflect a fundamental vagary of human existence, the fragility of human memory. Perhaps it would be fairer to say "the vulnerability of human memory." This is not to dispute research over the past century that suggests human memory is both powerful and long-lasting. It is only to note that memory is also subject to numerous forces that selectively discard, suppress, or creatively reconstruct memory to fit personal motives and needs.

Two important memory processes are redintegration and reconstruction. **Redintegration** means reuniting or restoring to a new condition. We recall a set of related bits of information as a unit when we recall one item. For example, during a trial, an attorney prompts a witness to recall some detail from a murder. At that moment, a flood of data related to the prompted recollection may arise. For the most part, redintegration is valuable. However, there is just one problem: Some of the facts recalled never happened. They are inferences or guesses about what must have occurred. Redintegration fills in gaps through a logical fabrication to make complete what is otherwise incomplete. In the heat of battle, it is all the more difficult to distinguish fact from fiction because the recollection makes sense.

In **reconstruction,** we shape memory to fit expectations, beliefs, knowledge, or schemata. This process was shown in a classic study by an English psychologist, Frederic Bartlett (1932). Bartlett used a story from the oral tradition of west coast Canadian Indians of a century ago. Subjects recalling the story anywhere from several hours to several years later showed evidence of distortions in recall. They omitted details and changed facts. Each time they recalled the story, it was shorter, a process called *leveling.* In addition, some details became more prominent, a process called *sharpening.* Subjects changed the story to make it more consistent with English culture. "Hunting seals" became "fishing" and "canoe" became "boat." Elements of the story that were unintelligible without knowledge of the Indian culture were simply discarded or completely changed. This shows that memory can change selectively to fit personal schemata. Errors that lead to interpersonal conflict (marital disputes, for example) may result from inferential, redintegrative, and reconstructive processes.

Very important insights into the influence of stress on memory come from studies of people suffering from posttraumatic stress disorder (PTSD). It appears that we are equipped with two memory systems (Metcalfe & Jacobs, 1996). One is the so-called "cool" system that processes information in a calm, objective fashion. The second system, called the "hot" system, processes information from emotional-fear situations. The first system, under the control of the hippocampus,[4] provides a detailed record of autobiographical events with clear connection to a well-demarcated time-line and context. The second system, under control of the amygdala, tends to be narrowly focused and fragmentary with direct encoding of the fear-inducing cues from the traumatic event.

The implications of this system are numerous and significant. Metcalfe and Jacobs (1996) point out that this system helps to explain the weapon-focus effect that occurs in street assaults or robberies. When an assailant flashes a gun, the victim will often focus so exclusively on the weapon that other details, including significant identifying information about the robber or a getaway car, may be lost in the flood of fear-ladened impressions.

Additional information from the work of de Kloet, Oitzl, and Joëls (1993) suggests that the hot and cool systems respond differently to increasing levels of stress. In this view, both systems increase active responding with stronger storage codes at low levels of stress. However, at high or traumatic levels of stress, the cool system becomes

---

[4]The brain memory system, including the hippocampus, is explored in more detail in Chapter 5.

dysfunctional while the hot system becomes hyperresponsive. This may explain why people who have gone through extreme trauma (collecting bodies of buddies killed in action) are not able to provide a coherent recollection of traumatic events, but they may still relive the fear when certain cues evoke the episode.

APPRAISAL PROCESSES IN STRESS

Probably the most influential cognitive model of stress comes from the work of Richard Lazarus and his group (Lazarus & Launier, 1978). We discussed the basic tenets of this model in Chapter 1. Lazarus defined stress as a mismatch between demands and coping resources. Two cognitive processes, appraisal and coping, are important to the person/environment transaction. *Appraisal* means literally setting a value on or judging the quality of something. **Coping** means engaging in behavioral and cognitive efforts to deal with environmental and internal demands and with conflicts between the two (Coyne & Holroyd, 1982).

Lazarus suggested three appraisals that provide meaning and influence the coping process. These are primary appraisal, secondary appraisal, and reappraisal. **Primary appraisal** yields the initial evaluation about a type of situation. Lazarus (1991) said that primary appraisal "concerns the stakes one has in the outcome of an encounter" (p. 827). **Secondary appraisal** judges the match between coping skills and situational demands. Primary appraisal answers the question "Am I in trouble or not?" Secondary appraisal answers the question "What can I do about it?" **Reappraisal** is based on feedback from transactions that occur after the first two appraisals. This may lead to a change in primary appraisal, which may in turn influence the perception of the skills available to deal with the situation.

There are three types of primary appraisal. Some events are simply **irrelevant** to the person involved. They contain no threat and require no response. A loud, unnerving shout on the street may be recognized immediately as a driver who is irate with another driver for taking a coveted parking space. The shout can be discarded as irrelevant to your well-being as long as you are not the other driver. Other events are **benign-positive.** They are desirable or, at worst, neutral. They make no serious demands on personal skills.

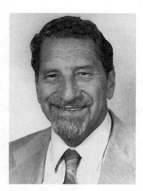

Richard Lazarus, proponent of the cognitive-transactional view of stress.

Events evaluated as **stressful** vary in at least two ways. First, they vary in the nature of the threat to the person. Second, they vary in the nature of the demand placed on personal coping resources and skills. Stress begins when we perceive (primary appraisal) that a situation presents some physical or psychological harm, either real or imagined, for which we have no effective response (secondary appraisal). Stress may end because we alter the meaning of the event so that threat is no longer present. Stress may also end because we use a coping method that removes or neutralizes the threat.

Lazarus proposed three stressful appraisals. The first type of stressful appraisal is **harm-loss.** Events of this nature usually involve real or anticipated loss of something that has great personal significance, such as the death of or separation from a spouse or a child. Loss of a job, prestige, or money is another example. Damage to self-esteem is a psychological loss. The sudden loss of a friend or lover is both loss of support and loss to ego. Wills and Langner (1980) noted "there is no self-esteem threat more powerful than rejection by an intimate partner" (p. 163). Diagnosis of a long-term or terminal illness, mastectomy for breast cancer, and loss of eyesight or hearing are physical harm-losses.

Appraisal of **threat** occurs when a situation demands more coping capacity than is available. The emotional tone of the evaluation is negative. Appraisal of **challenge** refers to a situation we evaluate as demanding and potentially risky, but the emotional tone is one of excitement and anticipation. In addition, we believe the demands can be met whatever they are. The distinction between threat and challenge is still somewhat muddy and not resolved to everyone's satisfaction (Coyne & Lazarus, 1980), but an example might help to clarify the difference. A novice climber climbs small mountains but becomes incapacitated by fear if asked to climb a sheer rock face. For the novice, this extreme demand is a threat. An experienced climber, on the other hand, not only relishes the thought of tackling the dangerous climb but feels honored to be involved.

FACTORS CONTRIBUTING TO STRESSFUL APPRAISALS

What determines whether we appraise an event as stressful or not stressful? At least three factors are critical. These are emotionality associated with the event; uncertainty, because we lack the information needed to evaluate the situation or because we cannot cope with ambiguity; and evaluation of meaning.

Emotionality

The connection between emotions and cognitions has been a controversial issue for decades. One camp adopts the view that emotions are primary and influence the form and focus of cognitions. Another camp takes the view that cognitions are primary and give rise to emotions. Consistent with a transactional view, Lazarus suggested that cognitions and emotions are linked in an ongoing flow of negotiations related to environmental stimuli (Folkman, Schaefer, & Lazarus, 1979; Lazarus, 1991). Cognitions and emotions are thus interdependent. In this view, emotions can influence adaptive transactions and coping processes in four ways.

First, emotions serve as an early warning signal that something is wrong. These emotional reactions are related to biologically primitive survival themes. As transactions with the environment turn out positively or negatively, our memory system stores emotional impressions along with details about an event (Anderson, 1990). Later, when the same event (or a similar event) occurs, it is likely that our perception of the event will be colored by the stored emotional tone. As noted earlier, however, the emotional content (hot—amygdala system) may be more direct and fragmentary compared to the cognitive component (cool—hippocampal system).

Second, emotions interrupt ongoing behavior. In this sense, emotional evaluations are attention-getters. They redirect our focus to something that is more important because of the danger or threat involved. If the situation is powerful enough to "demand" our attention, we are likely to evaluate the event as stressful.

Third, emotions can interrupt cognitive tasks in process and start tasks that are necessary to meet new demands. This is why concentration on practical affairs can be difficult after a highly emotional incident. For example, the death of a loved one may disrupt or intrude on thought processes for months or years. In the extreme, some bereaved people become so obsessed with thoughts of their deceased loved one that they cannot carry on day-to-day activities.

Finally, emotions can be motivators. Some emotions are pleasant; we will engage in a variety of behaviors to maintain those emotions or put ourselves in situations where there is hope that they will be recreated. Marvin Zuckerman (1971) believes that this is even true of the intense emotions aroused in activities such as mountain climbing, sky-diving, hang gliding, or bunge-cord jumping. Zuckerman called those who seek out these intense thrills **sensation seekers.** Once they have experienced the intense high provided by their chosen sport, they feel compelled to repeat the activity to reinstate the high. On the other hand, some emotions are unpleasant; we will do whatever we can to get rid of them. Stress usually results from unpleasant emotional events. In either case, pleasant or unpleasant, emotions can increase behaviors that will control, preserve, eliminate, or reduce internal tension.

Uncertainty, Predictability, and Stress

The second factor contributing to a stress appraisal is uncertainty. We may experience uncertainty in several ways. First, an event may be unpredictable, such as a bombing raid or a tornado. Second, an event may require more knowledge than we have available. We

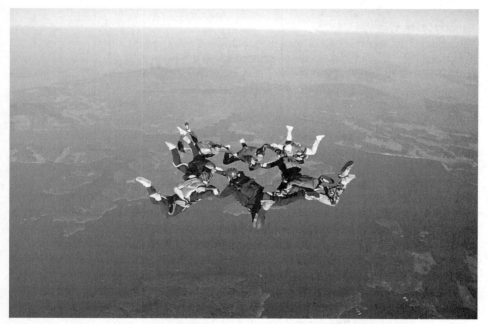

High flyers: While falling at a comfortable 120 mph, skydivers maneuver into formation thousands of feet above the ground. The sport parachutists will break off from the formation and open their parachutes more than 2000 feet above ground.

can call this a quantitative deficit. Third, an event may be more complex than our schemata can accommodate. We can call this a qualitative deficit.

Mishel (1984) studied a group of 100 patients in a Veterans Administration hospital. He found that scheduled medical events alone did not produce stressful appraisals. It was lack of clarity and lack of information about the medical procedures that accounted for the patients' reports of stress. Thus, a strong relationship existed between uncertainty and stress.

The Lazarus group thinks uncertainty is confusion over meaning (Folkman, Schaefer, & Lazarus, 1979). They suggested that we do not have readily available schemata to interpret each and every situation. This makes the event unpredictable, and thus a person does not know what behavior is appropriate. Given this **unpredictability,** a feeling of helplessness or futility may overwhelm the person and lead to a stress reaction.

We know from numerous studies that unpredictability is both psychologically and physically debilitating. When we have no way of predicting an event, we experience chronic arousal. Both subjective tension and bodily strain occur. Chronic physical arousal results in ulcers in laboratory animals (Brady, Porter, Conrad, & Mason, 1958; Weiss, 1968, 1971).

An event preceded by a signal is predictable. Rosenhan and Seligman (1989) noted that when a signal precedes an aversive event (for example, an impending SCUD attack in Tel Aviv), a person will be terrified during the signal but can relax when the signal is off. Also, if the person can do something when the signal occurs to offset the impending doom (for example, get to a shelter), then the person will not experience the same ill effects as when he or she can do nothing.

Research from the Gulf War and the SCUD attacks on Israel showed an interesting example of the powerful influence of uncertainty (Wolfe & Proctor, 1996). Early in the war, the first missile attacks were greeted with large numbers of hospitalizations—psychological causalities, as they were called—due to traumatic stress. It was hypothesized that much of this was due to the widespread rumors that Iraq was using chemical weapons. Later in the war, however, when it became clear that the SCUDs were armed with conventional warheads, there was also a significant decline in the number of psychological causalities.

Two personal traits govern whether uncertainty will result in a stress reaction or not. The first is **tolerance for ambiguity.** The second concerns information-seeking skills. We say an event is ambiguous when it is susceptible to different interpretations, when it is vague or obscure. Tolerance means the ability to withstand or endure.

When uncertainty occurs, we can search for new data that will remove the uncertainty. Several investigators conclude that **information seeking** is one of the most important coping strategies a person can develop. When we search for relevant information, it is assumed that we can tolerate ambiguity until we obtain the necessary information. Uncertainty seems to result in stress only if we do not have the ability to prevail while we check out possible meanings. If we do persevere, new facts may enable us to transform an unpredictable event into a predictable event.

In addition, successful coping depends on our ability to predict what will happen and on our ability to engage in controlling behaviors. A prerequisite to the ability to control is belief in that ability. One study obtained an interesting result in this regard. Jerry Suls and Brian Mullen (1981) wanted to know if perceptions of control and desirability of life events would have any effect on subsequent health in a college sample. They found that undesirability of life change by itself did not produce change in later illness. Lack of control over life change also did not produce change in illness. If undesirable and uncontrollable events occurred together, though, or unwelcome events of uncertain control occurred, there was a significant impact on illness in the following month. The results suggest that information may be important to the extent that it both reduces uncertainty and increases the perception of personal control.

Meichenbaum and Jaremko (1983) proposed that we should engage in **perspective taking** when unalterable stress occurs. This coping strategy involves remembering that most problems are limited in duration, that other areas of life still provide many rewards, and that bad outcomes can still be bearable.

Evaluation of Meaning

The final factor influencing stress appraisal is evaluation of meaning. We have shown several ways that appraisals contribute to meaning. Primary perceptual processes combined with self-schemata and event-schemata contribute to meaning. As an event unfolds, new information may lead to a change in our perception of the event; this change calls up a new schema or event script. Then we may change the meaning of the event from stressful to irrelevant or benign-positive.

SECONDARY APPRAISAL, SELF-EFFICACY, AND MASTERY

As defined earlier, secondary appraisal is concerned with whether we have the skills needed to meet the demands of the situation. Albert Bandura (1977, 1989) proposed a related notion, **self-efficacy.** Self-efficacy is the perception of capability, the belief that we possess the personal skills and performance abilities that will enable us to act correctly and successfully in given situations. It is a self-schema about personal competency and mastery.

Bandura's theory distinguishes between efficacy expectations and outcome expectations. Each time we engage in a behavior, it has some good or bad consequence. These consequences are rewards for appropriate acts or punishments for inappropriate acts. As we mature, we develop **outcome expectations.** That is, we learn to anticipate which behaviors are most likely to lead to which outcomes. An **efficacy expectation** is the belief that we can successfully perform the behavior that will produce the outcome. In Bandura's words, "expectations of personal mastery affect both initiation and persistence of coping behavior. The strength of people's convictions in their own effectiveness is likely to affect whether they will even try to cope with given situations" (1977, p. 193).

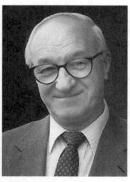

Belief that one's skills are poor (low self-efficacy) would lead to the secondary appraisal that an event is unmanageable and thus stressful. Belief in one's ability to deal with anything that comes along is more likely to lead to the appraisal that the event is irrelevant or benign. Numerous studies show that self-efficacy increases with coping success (Bandura, Reese, & Adams, 1982).

Albert Bandura, author of self-efficacy theory.

Stress Reappraisals

According to the transactional model, every stress situation is a series of negotiations that continues until we control the stress through coping efforts or until the stressor ends spontaneously. Feedback related to coping actions and from people who are involved provide information on both our coping success and the meaning of the event itself. As feedback goes on, we reevaluate the situation, possibly adjusting both coping strategies and meanings in the process.

There are at least three ways in which we deal with stressful events during reappraisal. These are rationalizing, changing the meaning of the event, and reducing the significance of the event. In rationalizing, we attach a personally desirable meaning to an event, although an unbiased analysis would show that the meaning is not appropriate. Consider, for example, someone who has just been fired. After the first shock, he or she might suggest that dismissal is the long-awaited sign to go into private business. Everyone else, though, would consider the chances of this person's becoming a successful business entrepreneur nonexistent.

As noted earlier, changing the meaning of an event may be warranted if new information provides some basis for it. For example, a manager receives word of reassignment to an office in a different region of the country. At first, the manager feels hurt, rejected, and shuffled aside. Later, discussions with management clarifies responsibility, projects, pay, and locale. It becomes obvious that the new arrangement will mean a freer hand, more creative opportunities, a larger work force, and a more relaxed lifestyle for the family in a less overwhelming city. This new data may lead to a significant change in the meaning of the new assignment. In fact, the manager may reinterpret the new post with positive meanings of challenge and opportunity instead of threat and loss.

Another process that occurs in reappraisal is reduction of the meaning of the event. Imagine a union negotiating a new contract where initial talks hint at a sizable pay increase. Employees begin planning for new investments, perhaps even luxury purchases that have been postponed a long time. Then union and management reach settlement on the contract, but the anticipated large pay raise is little more than a token increase. Initially, employees feel frustrated. They may direct anger toward both union and management. Soon the planned investments and purchases are gradually and quietly reduced in significance. "Well, we really didn't need that anyway." "We got along without it all this time, we can make it a while longer." This type of cognitive process seems to operate most frequently in cases where outcomes are essentially out of personal control.

Before proceeding to the next section, take a few minutes to work through Self-Study Exercise 3-1. The activity is designed to help you integrate the information in this chapter in a more personally relevant way.

ATTRIBUTIONS, BELIEFS, AND HEALTH

A major concern in cognitive models of stress is the extent to which attributions and beliefs contribute to high-risk behaviors. Two theories deal with these cognitive processes. First, Christopher Peterson and Martin Seligman (1984) developed a theory of pessimistic explanatory style to explain how cognitions influence health. Second, Irwin Rosenstock (1966) and his associates proposed the **Health Belief Model** to describe how perceptions of vulnerability and beliefs about illness influence health behavior. We will discuss briefly the major tenets of these two models.

SELF-STUDY EXERCISE 3-1

Attributions About Positive and Negative Events

The following statements represent life-event scenarios that happen often enough to college students. Suppose that each one has happened to you, and you must now explain why. Write a brief statement (a phrase or at most a few sentences) that is your most likely way of explaining the outcome of these events. After you have written a response to each one, read the next section of the text and then read the brief explanation for this exercise at the end of the chapter.

Statements about life events	Your explanation for the event
1. Tried out for the college choir and was accepted.	
2. Failed an important test in my major.	
3. Went for a job interview that is related to my major, but did not get the job.	
4. Slipped on the steps outside the dormitory and crashed as my friends watched.	
5. Made a speech in class that was a hit with both my classmates and the teacher.	
6. Went out with some friends, got in a heated argument, and they have shut me out since.	
7. Got several calls this week because of bills that are overdue.	

Pessimistic Attributional Style

The notion of pessimistic explanatory style is an outgrowth of Martin Seligman's work on learned helplessness. Seligman defined learned helplessness as a cognitive-motivational deficit that results from inconsistent but inescapable punishment. Most organisms learn very quickly to escape from aversive stimulation. If punishment occurs on an unpredictable schedule with no hope for escape, the organism will quit trying to escape. Then, even if escape is possible, the organism will fail to get away; it has learned to be helpless. Learned helplessness has been used as a major explanatory construct for depression, and it may be related to deficits displayed by individuals with histories of abuse (Rosenhan & Seligman, 1989).

Seligman's group observed significant differences in people's responses to uncontrollable events. They modified the learned helplessness model in an effort to better account for these differences (Abramson, Seligman, & Teasdale, 1978). This resulted in a general theory of explanatory style that has been applied to numerous outcomes, including failure, depression, illness, and even presidential behavior (Zullow, Oettingen, Peterson, & Seligman, 1988). Explanatory style is the habitual way we explain bad events. In other words, it is how we attribute cause. This theory suggests that causal attributions vary on three dimensions: internal or external; stable or unstable; and global or specific. Table 3-1 provides an example of these dimensions.

TABLE 3-1
Possible causal attributions by a person driving a car that caused a fatal accident

| | INTERNAL | | EXTERNAL | |
	STABLE	UNSTABLE	STABLE	UNSTABLE
GLOBAL	I've never been good with mechanical things.	I can't do anything right when I'm tired.	There are too many jerks on the road today.	The [zodiac] signs were not good for today.
SPECIFIC	I'm just a very poor driver.	I'm not a good driver when I'm tired.	That corner causes a lot of accidents.	A truck blocked my view.

To illustrate these dimensions, consider the plight of a rape victim. She may say, "It's my fault. I shouldn't have been out that late alone." This is an internal attribution. On the other hand, she might conclude that poor lighting and lack of visible police protection were at fault. This is an external attribution. Internal attributions generally lead to more passivity and lowered self-esteem following adversity than do external attributions (Peterson, Seligman, & Vaillant, 1988).

Second, she might believe the conditions that led to her attack are permanent, unchanging. This is a stable attribution. If she thought the conditions were temporary, however, this would be an unstable attribution. A stable attribution would probably lead to a chronic feeling of vulnerability, whereas an unstable attribution might lead to a quicker resumption of normal lifestyle.

Finally, the victim might have a pervasive feeling of vulnerability, a feeling that she might not be safe at any time or any place (Janoff-Bulman, 1988). This is a global attribution. On the other hand, she might recognize that the factors contributing to this incident were limited, a specific attribution. A pessimistic explanatory style exists when we consistently use internal, stable, and global explanations for adverse events. The outcomes of this explanatory style are thought to be passivity, poor achievement, and signs of depression.

One study tried to evaluate the connection between attributional style and personal hardiness (Hull, van Treuren, & Propsom, 1988). Personal hardiness, a trait that will be discussed in Chapter 4, is thought to result in resilience to stress and positive health. The authors of the study provided strong evidence that attributional style plays a mediating role in the hardy personality. Specifically, hardy persons tend to give internal, stable, and global attributions for positive events, and external, unstable, and specific attributions for negative events. Persons low in hardiness are the opposite, giving internal, stable, and global explanations for negative events. As noted, this generally results in poor outcomes.

A longitudinal study examined the connection between pessimistic explanatory style and physical health (Peterson, Seligman, & Vaillant, 1988). Chris Peterson's team used a sample of male Harvard University graduates from the classes of 1942 to 1944. These people agreed to participate in a long-term project on adult development. They provided extensive data on both psychological and physical health, including factual medical records to verify health status. Also, in 1946 they responded to an open-ended questionnaire.

Peterson's group used a technique called CAVE (Content Analysis of Verbatim Explanations) to analyze statements the subjects made. These statements provided scores that allowed the team to classify subjects on the basis of pessimistic versus optimistic styles. Peterson's group wanted to test the hypothesis that men who used internal, stable, and global explanations for bad events would show worse health outcomes than men who used external, unstable, and specific explanations. The results supported the hypothesis. The strongest relationship between pessimistic explanations and health status occurred 20 years later when most of the men were about 45 years old. Results were also significant at 50, 55, and 60 years of age, but the correlations were smaller than those observed at 45.

Although the theory of explanatory style is appealing, it has its critics. Brewin (1988) noted, for example, that the theory is persuasive when dealing with accidents and illness. On the other hand, the presumed link to depression following stressful events is far from clear. Carver (1989) also pointed to flaws in the theory and scaling techniques used. He noted that the model is a multicomponent model (three attributions, presumably with different contributions), yet most research has not bothered to test the specific contribution of the individual components. In this case, he argued, we might see premature closure similar to what occurred with the Type A behavior pattern.

The Health Belief Model

Irwin Rosenstock (1966) developed the Health Belief Model (HBM) from field theory and value expectancy theory. Early surveys of health beliefs provided descriptive support without testing the model's predictive power (Kirscht, Haefner, Kegeles, & Rosenstock, 1966). Since then, many investigators have elaborated and tested the model with different populations (Calnan & Moss, 1984), in varied settings, and with various health/illness behaviors (Cockerham, 1982). The model probably is most applicable to higher socioeconomic groups with above-average education. Notably absent, though, is research on children's beliefs about health, although this lack may be short-lived (Peterson & Harbeck, 1988). The model continues to enjoy popularity, perhaps because it assumes that beliefs are subject to modification. Thus, educational or clinical interventions may be expected to bring changes that could have a positive impact on health status.

Figure 3-1 shows the basic components of the Health Belief Model. The model is multicausal in one sense. It proposes that health behavior results from the joint influence of psychosocial factors, including demographic and social cues aimed at changing risk behaviors. At the core of the cognitive system is a set of personal beliefs about illness. These beliefs mediate the perception of threat and thus affect the likelihood of taking action against illness.

First, the model assumes that people hold beliefs about the *seriousness of disease.* This is a motivating factor that makes health issues important. Someone who believes that death from lung cancer is a likely outcome of smoking probably will be motivated to quit. Support for this motivational part of the model is not as strong as for the rest of the model. Still, David McClelland (1989) has argued that motivational factors have a more important connection to health status than first believed.

Further, each person has a **perception of vulnerability** or susceptibility to disease. This is a personal estimate of the chance of contracting a disease. Some people worry constantly about getting sick. Others think of themselves as the "Rock of Gibraltar,"

FIGURE 3-1
The Health Belief Model.
SOURCE: Becker (1974).

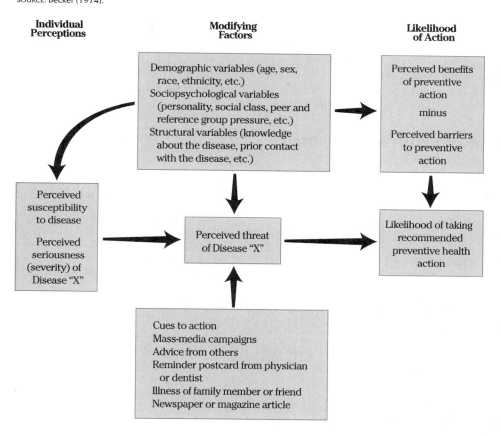

immune to illness. This usually leads to reduced efforts to avoid risks. Even if such smokers believe that lung cancer could occur, they might also believe it will never happen to them.

Finally, each person has a set of beliefs about the *benefits of taking action* to prevent or combat disease. These include perceptions of costs and barriers to action. People might feel that the risk of lung cancer warrants quitting and that they are personally at risk. Still, they might not be willing to endure the side effects that accompany withdrawal from smoking. They might calculate that quitting will lead to a weight increase, which they regard as negative. They might also fear loss of companionship with smoking friends. These would be barriers to quitting.

Rosenstock, Strecher, and Becker (1988) provided a revised explanatory model that incorporates Bandura's (1977) self-efficacy concept. They noted that the early Health Belief Model ignored efficacy expectations because the researchers focused on acute medical distress and simple preventive actions such as inoculations or dental care. Chronic illness, however, did not fit as well with the Health Belief Model.

Long-term health behaviors such as diet and exercise also were not as well predicted by the model. Complying with strict medical regimens or making significant long-term lifestyle changes requires belief in personal competency (self-efficacy) to undertake the change.

At the same time, Rosenstock and his colleagues warned against uncritical acceptance of self-efficacy theory as a "patent medicine" cure. They noted that self-efficacy theory often incorrectly assumes that a client has adequate incentives to change, feels threatened by environmental events, believes outcomes can be influenced by behavior, and does not face barriers to taking actions. These assumptions are contradicted by data collected with the Health Belief Model.

SELF-STUDY EXERCISE 3-2

Health Beliefs and AIDS

Respond to the following statements either true or false. After responding, look for information on the issues addressed as you continue reading. Answers and information about the quiz are given at the end of the chapter.

1. You can tell a person has AIDS because they look sick.   T or F
2. A person having oral sex takes a risk for contracting the AIDS virus.   T or F
3. Using condoms is a foolproof way to avoid the AIDS virus.   T or F
4. Sharing needles for drug injections is a risk factor for AIDS.   T or F
5. Using alcohol prior to sexual activity does not increase risk for AIDS.   T or F
6. To get AIDS, you have to have sex with multiple partners.   T or F
7. Heterosexual intercourse does not carry risk for AIDS.   T or F
8. Effects of the AIDS virus appear quickly, making them easy to detect.   T or F
9. Family members sharing kitchenware and bathrooms
     are not at risk for AIDS.
10. Staying in a monogamous relationship is the only way to prevent AIDS.   T or F

SUMMARY

In principle, the cognitive system encompasses everything that has to do with mental activity from the simplest to the most complex. Of necessity this discussion was selective instead of exhaustive, and it focused on those parts of the cognitive system that are influential in stress and health. The following summarizes the major points made in this discussion.

- A basic cognitive process is labeling, that is, assigning meaning to events. This process begins very early in the flow of information through the brain.
- Cognitive science is the science of the mind. It is a systematic study of all the ways people come to know, think, reason, and decide.
- The information processing model of mind was patterned after the way a high-speed computer works: that is, *input* of information is followed by program operations on the information as *throughput*, which leads in turn to appropriate *output*.
- The theory of personal constructs suggests that we create a subjective reality as we try to anticipate how certain people might respond to us. Our view may be channeled (restricted) because of these biases that precede the actual interactions.

- A related notion is that cognitive schemata serve to organize information from our myriad transactions with our environment. These schemata in turn enable us to assign meaning during new transactions.
- Perception is the interpretation and organization of information given to us by the senses. Unfortunately, perception is subject to bias and distortion.
- An important aspect of information processing is attention. At the simplest level, attention refers to the process by which we choose what stimuli are important and where to focus our mental energy.
- Voluntary sustained attention is called perceptual vigilance. In the short haul, perceptual vigilance can yield more accurate detection of important information, but over the long haul, it can produce stress and lead to higher rates of illness.
- Stimulus deprivation, when we are cut off from adequate and varied stimuli, may lead to distortions in perception.
- Memory is the core storage and retrieval system of the mind. As strong as we may think memory can be, it is nonetheless subject to distortions and breakdowns. In all likelihood, our memory systems work to store themes rather than literal point-by-point detail. When we try to retrieve a memory that seems to be incomplete, we may logically reconstruct or unwittingly use external sources to fill in the gaps.
- Posttraumatic stress disorder includes weak memory for detail of traumatic episodes. This may be due to the hot memory system, which stores primarily emotional tones, at work during extreme crises. The cool memory system at work during normal states stores the themes of experience.
- The cognitive-transactional model of stress suggests stress is a relation between the person and the context. Primary appraisal first evaluates the likelihood of harm-loss, or the presence of threat or challenge. Secondary appraisal then evaluates the coping resources (skills) available to meet demands. When the person has adequate resources to meet demand, there is no stress.
- The important factors that contribute to stressful appraisals include emotionality, uncertainty, and unpredictability. Events that are unpredictable (like SCUD attacks during the Gulf War) can lead to severe stress reactions.
- The personal trait of self-efficacy is important to the secondary appraisal process. People who feel competent to act correctly and successfully in certain situations (such as administering CPR in an emergency) are less likely to experience stress.
- Reappraisal occurs after our first efforts to confront a stressor. We may reinterpret (change the meaning) in a way that effectively eliminates the stressor, or realize that we have skills not previously recognized that will deal with the situation effectively.
- One important issue is the connection between specific cognitive processes and health behaviors or health outcomes. When people habitually attribute bad outcomes to internal, stable, and global causes, they display a pessimistic explanatory style. This cognitive set predicts poor health outcomes.
- The Health Belief Model assumes that perceptions of seriousness of disease combine with perceptions of vulnerability and cost benefits to influence health behaviors. The authors of this model revised it recently to incorporate the notion of self-efficacy to better explain long-term coping behaviors.

CRITICAL THINKING AND STUDY QUESTIONS

1. How does the process of labeling influence the perception of stress?
2. What is the theory of personal constructs, and how does it relate to the notion of constructs of reality? Try to think of a recent experience that exemplifies the personal constructs idea.
3. What are some of the ways in which perceptions may not be accurate?
4. What is attention? Perceptual vigilance? Hypervigilance? What are the good and bad (or undesirable) aspects of each?
5. What is the difference between the hot and cold memory systems?
6. What are the core concepts and terms from the cognitive-transactional theory of stress? Be able to describe the theory in some detail, and also be able to give examples of the different appraisal processes.
7. What is the Health Belief Model? What are its basic terms? How does it connect cognitive evaluations to health risks?
8. What is the pessimistic explanatory style? How may it relate to undesirable mental and physical health outcomes?

KEY TERMS

accommodation
appraisal
assimilation
attention
challenge appraisal
cognition
cognitive science
coping, transactional
    model
delusion
efficacy expectation
hallucinations
harm-loss appraisal
Health Belief Model
hypervigilance
information processing
    model
information seeking

labeling
literal brain
outcome expectation
perception
perception of
    vulnerability
perceptual biases
perceptual distortions
perceptual vigilance
personal constructs
perspective taking
pessimistic explanatory
    style
primary appraisal
    benign-positive
    irrelevant
    stressful
reappraisal

reconstruction
redintegration
schema theory
secondary appraisal
selective attention
self-efficacy
sensation seeker
stimulus deprivation
stimulus overload
threat appraisal
tolerance for ambiguity
unpredictability

WEBSITES the cognitive stress system: attitudes, beliefs, and expectations

URL ADDRESS	SITE NAME & DESCRIPTION
http://www.apa.org/science/lib.html	☆APA's Introduction to Library Research, for students and nonpsychologists
http://www.rbet.org/faq.html	Albert Ellis Institute
http://www.grohol.com/web.htm	☆Psychology Web Pointer. Excellent starting point for general support and psychology resources
http://ideanurse.com/aath/	American Association for Therapeutic Humor
http://cctr.umkc.edu/user/dmartin/pscyh2.html	CyberPsychLink. Very useful for information in psychology and behavioral medicine
http://www.lycaeum.org/drugs/other/brain/	Devoted to epistemology, consciousness, and the mind, with links to institutes, news groups, journals, and the Neuroscience-Net

ANALYSIS AND COMMENTS ON SELF-STUDY EXERCISE 3-1

These statements are roughly similar to those used in attribution research that tries to find out how people explain both the good and bad things that happen to them. Look back through your written explanations and identify your causal attributions: "I failed the test because _____"; or "I did not get the job because _____ ." In each causal statement, try to identify whether you have attributed the cause to something within your control or outside of your control. Also, try to identify whether the cause is something that is short-term and is likely to pass quickly or is something that will go on for a long time. Finally, try to identify whether your explanation is related to a specific skill (for example, "I'm not good at interviewing"), or to a more global self-view ("I cannot seem to make a good impression on anyone").

Attribution theory suggests that there are a few common ways that we explain these events. The list presented in Exercise 3-1 contained two positive events and five negative events. Although researchers will analyze both positive and negative events, the primary focus has been on how we explain bad events. Seligman's group suggested that if we habitually attribute bad outcomes to internal, stable, and global factors, we are likely to be at more risk for helplessness, depression, and possibly adverse health outcomes. Finally, the pessimistic explanatory style is not inescapable; it is a style that can be changed through cognitive interventions.

ANSWERS AND COMMENTS ON SELF-STUDY EXERCISE 3-2

1. False—AIDS carriers may appear to be healthy for quite some time.
2. True—The fluids involved in sexual activity, no matter how transmitted, are primary carriers of the AIDS virus.
3. False—While condoms remain a very important defense against transmitting the AIDS virus, they do fail.
4. True—A needle often aspirates blood from a previous user into the tip. When the next user injects, blood from the previous user is shot directly into the blood stream.
5. False—Although the connection between alcohol and risk for AIDS is still a subject of controversy, it is clear that using alcohol prior to sexual activity tends to reduce the chances that the person will take safety precautions.
6. False—All it takes is one partner with an unknown sex history for someone to contract the virus. Given the high rate of failure among AIDS patients to disclose their condition, there is always some risk even with one partner.
7. False—Heterosexual intercourse accounts for nearly 10% of all AIDS cases. Intercourse with broken genital skin or sores increases the likelihood of transmitting the virus.
8. False—There is a long latency period before appearance of AIDS symptoms, with a median of 10 years. This long time-frame is a sinister window of opportunity for the carrier and contacts to be part of the spread of AIDS.
9. True—The virus is actually very fragile outside the body, and easily killed with standard detergents.
10. False—This statement could be true, but only if both partners have a known sex history, or the partners have been in the monogamous relationship for a period that exceeds the latency of AIDS.

The Health Belief Model proposes that how people think about their personal vulnerability, the severity of the disease, and the cost-benefits ratio of taking protective action influences how they will actually behave. If you responded accurately to most of the items above, it indicates that your awareness of crucial issues in AIDS transmission is good. Presumably then, you will be more likely to engage in self-protective behaviors. At the same time, knowledge alone is not sufficient to motivate people to take the necessary precautions. On the other hand, if your answers were largely inaccurate, it suggests that you might be at risk because you are less likely to know when you are exposed.

CHAPTER 4

Personality and Stress:

Traits, Types, and Biotypes

Bodily traits are not merely physical, nor mental traits merely psychic. Nature knows nothing of those distinctions.

C. G. JUNG [PARAPHRASED]

QUESTIONS

- How do psychologists define personality?
- What is the difference between a typology personality theory and a trait theory?
- What are the so-called five robust personality traits?
- What are the four major health behaviors?
- What are the possible ways in which personality may be linked to health outcomes?
- Is the Type A behavior pattern reliably linked to coronary risk, and if so, how is it linked?
- What is the toxic core of the Type A behavior pattern?
- What are the various links between depression and health?
- Is there evidence that a particular personality profile may be linked to risk for cancer?
- What is the link, if any, between personality and smoking?
- What links exist between personality and alcohol addiction?
- It is preferable to speak of the disease-prone personality?
- How do locus of control, hardiness, and self-esteem relate to stress and health?

The notion that personality is somehow related to coping and health is a recurrent, almost obsessive thought in Western society. It is so ingrained in Western philosophy, medicine, and psychology that many people probably would believe a link exists even if scientific evidence disputed it. Research has shown that personality does correlate with both the type and intensity of the stress response (Bolger & Zuckerman, 1995). It is related to certain types of health problems. In addition, personality may be related to a variety of sick-role behaviors that affect the time course and prognosis for recovery from illness.

Before delving into these issues, however, it is necessary to understand how the term **personality** is used by those who study it most. We all have some idea of what it means to have a pleasant personality. We may also feel quite confident that we know what we are talking about when we describe someone as having a rotten disposition. However, if pressed to define personality precisely and then to measure differences in personality accurately, we would find the job much tougher. That is the problem investigators face in trying to pin down the relationship between personality and stress or health. In the next few pages, we will examine the concept of personality and the major theories of personality that relate to stress and health. Evidence will then be presented linking personality types to a variety of stress reactions and health problems. In some cases, the evidence seems quite strong and indisputable. In other cases, however, the claims are still on shaky ground and should be accepted only with healthy skepticism. Later in this chapter, we will discuss positive personality traits that seem to increase resilience to stress.

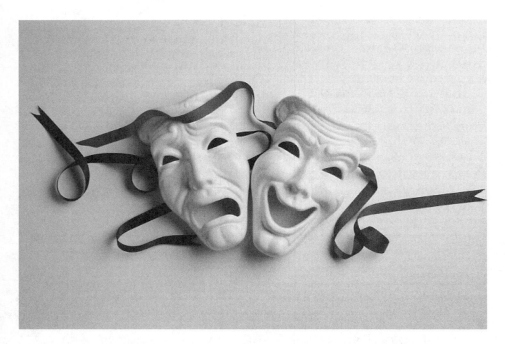

Just as a theater dramatist may put on a mask to present a different persona to the audience, personality is thought of as the outward expression of individual uniqueness.

PERSONA: WHAT LIES BEHIND THE MASK

The concept of personality has changed many times. As originally used by the ancient Greeks, the term *persona* meant a mask such as an actor would wear on stage for theatrical plays of that time. Later, *persona* came to mean the roles individuals played in different aspects of their lives.

More recently, *persona* has come to mean some characteristic or set of characteristics within a person. In figurative terms, personality is the essence of the person behind the mask. It makes the person both real and unique. Personality is also stable and enduring, providing a private reference point in the midst of constant flux and change. Presumably, this durability also allows an outsider to look inside and predict with some accuracy how the person typically behaves.

CLASSIC AND CONTEMPORARY DEFINITIONS OF PERSONALITY

Definitions of personality are relatively easy to come by, but agreement on what personality really refers to is more difficult to find. Liebert and Spiegler (1994) believe that adopting any definition of personality implicitly adopts a particular theory of personality as well. Nonetheless, we will use for our purposes a commonly encountered definition provided by Gordon Allport (1961), who said that personality is "the dynamic organization within the individual of those psychophysical systems that determine his characteristic behavior and thought" (p. 28). Personality so defined is the hub or meeting point for all the biological and psychosocial forces that come to bear on the individual during the course of development.

In spite of disagreement on what personality is, most definitions share common themes such as *uniqueness, organization,* and *style of adapting or coping.* The perceptions, thoughts, feelings, and behaviors of each individual are organized in different patterns. This difference in patterns makes each person in some ways different from every other person and determines the characteristic style of responding.

Theodore Millon (1982) is a theorist concerned about personality in relationship to stress and health. His view is roughly consistent with the psychodynamic view, which is that personality summarizes the person's style of defending against anxiety, resolving interpersonal stress, and dealing with psychological conflicts. Similarly, Millon views personality as the coping style the individual uses to deal with stressful situations.

VARIETIES OF PERSONALITY THEORY

Different types of personality theories have been popular at one time or another. These include (1) the **psychoanalytic,** (2) the **dispositional,** (3) the phenomenological, and (4) the behavioral-cognitive. The psychoanalytic and dispositional theories have received the most attention, especially in regard to stress-health connections. One dispositional model based on the *five robust factors* has received increasing attention in the last ten years, and has already begun to generate research on personality and health behaviors (Booth-Kewley & Vickers, 1994; McCrae & Costa, 1987). Phenomeno-logical theory has not been systematically developed to deal with the stress-health is-sue. Further, although behavioral-cognitive components are included in several mod-els of stress and health, there is not a unified behavioral-cognitive theory of stress and health as such. Because of this, I will summarize only the psychoanalytical and dispo-sitional approaches and discuss the relevance of each to current concerns in stress and health research.

Psychoanalytic Theory in Stress and Health

Psychoanalytic theory, epitomized by the work of Sigmund Freud, describes personality by reference to intrapsychic conflict. The nature of the conflict and the developmental stage during which the conflict first occurs are presumably important in determining the formation of a person's personality.

During the Golden Age of psychoanalysis, many attempts were made to interpret stress responses and health problems in terms of psychoanalytic theory. Most of these attempts were part of the early work in **psychosomatics.** A psychosomatic disorder is one in which a real physical ailment (such as ulcers, asthma, colitis, or cardiac ar-rhythmia) is caused by or influenced by a psychological process, such as ongoing stress or anxiety.

A prominent psychoanalyst, Franz Alexander (1950), was a leading proponent of this view. He proposed that the asthmatic person is a victim of three correlated events. First, a genetically determined weakness in one organ of the body makes it likely that the organ will break down when stress occurs. This can be likened to a "weak link" theory. Second, a specific psychological conflict weakens the person's defense system if and when stress occurs. Third, some threatening situation arises. Presumably, life stress (the threat) arouses the unresolved conflict (the psychological risk), and the person is not able to defend against it. As a result, the weakest link in the body, in this case the lungs, expresses the stress in asthmatic attacks. Although many investigators have looked for ev-idence in support of this idea in the context of a variety of disorders, little evidence has been found in favor of the psychoanalytic view.

Dispositions, Personality Types, and Traits

The second type of theory, dispositional theory, generally proposes that there are "en-during, stable personality characteristic[s]" (Liebert & Spiegler, 1994, p. 156). The two most commonly encountered dispositional theories are the typology approach and the trait approach. A **typology** looks for a small number of dispositional clusters that occur with some frequency. A **trait theory** looks for a large number of dispositions and allows description of an individual based on each of the dispositions. Presumably, people may have many traits but fit only one type.

JUNG'S TYPOLOGY Perhaps the best-known typology is the approach proposed by the Swiss psychiatrist Carl Jung. According to Jung, there were two primary types of peo-ple, the **introvert** and the **extravert.** The introvert is described as socially withdrawn, reflective, not given to displays of emotion, and somewhat closed off from the external world. The extravert is characterized as outgoing, socially active, free in the expression of emotions, and rather open.

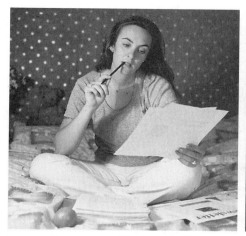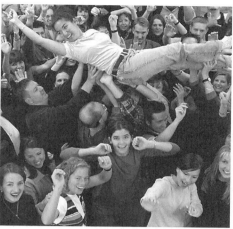

One of the most stable personality traits appears to be the introvert-extravert distinction. The introvert tends to be more reclusive, while the extravert tends to be more social.

BIOTYPES In contemporary stress and health research, attempts have been made to relate certain personality traits to particular diseases. As the reasoning goes, genetic mechanisms determine constitution, temperament, and intellect in each person. The interplay of these factors in turn leads to the emergence of a unique personality, which may be as strong and resilient as genetic endowment can provide—or it may be a personality given to weakness or excess. In the latter case, the nature of the genetics-personality link may produce risks for stress- and health-related problems. One personality type might be more prone to coronary attacks, while another personality type might be more prone to ulcers, and so on.

One major difficulty in trying to establish the personality-illness connection is the proverbial chicken-and-egg problem—that is, do health problems change personality, or do personality disorders contribute to health problems? Another difficulty is that biotype theories tend to convey either the impression that genetics is destiny or a very closely related misperception that personality types are irreversible. Both these notions are unfortunate. Personality, as described earlier, is the hub of all the influences—whether biological, psychological, or social—that weave their way into its fabric from conception. Thus, genetic factors may be pushed or pulled in different directions, to more extreme or less extreme expressions, depending on the forces that come into play after birth. In addition, while the stability of personality is often emphasized, there are indications that changes in personality function can and do occur throughout life.

Trait Anxiety and State Anxiety

Charles Spielberger (1966) believes there is a basic difference between **trait anxiety** and **state anxiety.** Trait anxiety tends to be relatively stable across time and place. People who are high in trait anxiety have a much greater tendency to be anxious whatever the situation and relatively more anxious all the time compared to those low in trait anxiety. For the high trait-anxious person, it takes relatively less external stress to trigger a stress reaction. On the other hand, people who are low in trait anxiety are more relaxed all the time, regardless of the situation. It takes relatively higher levels of stress to trigger an anxiety response in them.

In contrast to trait anxiety, state anxiety is specific to a situation. Job interviews, driving tests, and solo music performances are situations that can produce high anxiety. Students experience a form of state anxiety called **test anxiety.** People in a variety of professions take certifying exams that can make or break a career. A person high in trait anxiety, when faced with high test anxiety, might be overwhelmed or panicked by the test. On the other hand, someone with low trait anxiety might manage with no difficulty as long as test anxiety did not become extreme. State anxiety can vary a great deal within a person.

SELF-STUDY EXERCISE 4-1

Identifying Anxiety-Provoking Events

In the first column of the space provided, identify situations in which you experience the strongest symptoms of anxiety. Try to be as concrete as possible. Instead of saying, "I get anxious when I go out," be specific: "I get anxious when I have to meet new people at important social functions." In the second column, estimate how intense the anxiety is on a scale of 1 to 10, where 10 is the most intense anxiety. Finally, in the last column, note what you typically do when you feel anxiety coming over you. Chapters 11 to 13 will describe some methods to deal with anxieties and fears.

Situations	Intensity of Anxiety	Coping Strategy

A person might be low in trait anxiety, but experience extreme state anxiety when confronted with a robber. The same person caught in a dangerous winter storm might handle the situation very calmly. The concept of state-trait anxiety is important to stress research because of the belief that stress reactions, especially chronic stress, may be related to trait anxiety.

The Five Robust Personality Traits: Looking for a Common Ground

After many years of research, there is an emerging consensus that most personality differences can be captured by five dominant traits. These traits are given as *neuroticism, extraversion, openness, agreeableness,* and *conscientiousness.* However, each of these terms actually begins a continuum that is anchored on the other end with the opposite characteristic, as Table 4-1 shows.

A quick study of the descriptors for these traits suggests that some might be more relevant to stress and health than others. The neuroticism dimension, for example, is described in terms of negative emotions such as worry and nervousness, but also includes

TABLE 4-1
The five robust factors, or the Big Five, appear to describe the most important dimensions of personality differences.

THE FIVE ROBUST FACTORS	DESCRIPTORS OF THE FACTORS
Neuroticism/Stability	Worrying/calm; nervous/at ease; high-strung/relaxed; insecure/secure; vulnerable/hardy
Extraversion/Introversion	Sociable/retiring; fun-loving/sober; affectionate/reserved; talkative/quiet; joiner/loner
Openness to Experience	Original/conventional; creative/uncreative; independent/conforming; untraditional/traditional; daring/unadventurous
Agreeableness/Antagonism	Good-natured/irritable; courteous/rude; lenient/critical; flexible/stubborn; sympathetic/callous
Conscientiousness/ Undirectedness	Reliable/undependable; careful/careless; hardworking/lazy; punctual/late; perservering/quitting

TABLE 4-2
Four major health factors may be useful in describing what people are doing to promote health and prevent illness.

FOUR HEALTH BEHAVIORS	DESCRIPTORS OF THE HEALTH BEHAVIORS
Wellness behaviors	Exercise; proper diet; medical screening
Accident control	Fixing home hazards; knowing first aid
Traffic risk taking	Speeding; failure to wear seat belts
Substance risk taking	Use and abuse of drugs such as alcohol and tobacco

psychological vulnerability. We might expect an individual with a higher degree of neuroticism to be more disposed to interpret events as stressful and to be more reactive to stressor events. We might expect a person who is unconventional and daring to engage in more risk-taking behaviors. Where health behaviors are concerned, we might expect the reliable and careful person to take more precautions and to follow more self-protective guidelines.

Just this type of speculation was the basis of work by Stephanie Booth-Kewley and Ross Vickers (1994). However, they added another critical dimension based on the work of Vickers and Hervig (1984). These investigators found that health behaviors also cluster in a few robust categories—four categories, to be exact. These categories are called *wellness behaviors, accident control, traffic risk taking,* and *substance risk taking.* These are shown in Table 4-2 with their associated descriptors.

As a prelude to their own study, Booth-Kewley and Vickers (1994) summarize information showing that neuroticism is associated with the presence of negative health habits and the absence of positive health habits. Further, extraversion has been linked to substance risk taking, but also to health-promoting behaviors such as regular exercise. The remaining three personality traits have not been studied much in the context of positive health habits. Their study, however, confirmed the previous findings on neuroticism and extraversion, but added detail in regard to conscientiousness and agreeableness. They found that both conscientiousness and agreeableness were positively correlated with wellness behavior, accident control, and traffic risk taking. Openness to experience was only related to substance risk taking. Of the five factors, conscientiousness was most strongly connected to positive health behaviors.

GENERAL MODELS: THE PERSONALITY-HEALTH CONNECTION

Before discussing research on personality and disease, it may be helpful to conceptualize plausible models. As Friedman and Booth-Kewley (1987) point out, "it is silly to postulate a psychological model of disease causation that is physiologically impossible" (p. 541). Four possible models are presented in Figure 4-1. First, it is possible that a given personality profile causes a disease to appear. The Type A-coronary heart disease connection in its most primitive form is an example. This is the typical psychosomatic model that argues for the influence of a psychological variable on a somatic process.

Second, a personality profile may result from a disease process. Depression may be a natural outcome of being diagnosed with cancer (McDaniel, Musselman, Porter, Reed, & Nemeroff, 1995). Anger and hostility may mount when the disease is terminal. In this view, disease is caused by a biological agent. The personality pattern occurs after the fact and plays no role at all in the etiology of the disorder. This **somatopsychic model** argues for the influence of the physiological system on psychological process.

Third, personality may be a perceptual filter through which the disease is viewed and a characteristic response to the disease is organized. In this model, the cause of the disease is still viewed as a biological insult, but the course of the disease is tempered by how the person responds to it. Someone with a preexisting tendency to depression may view the diagnosis of cancer more fatalistically than someone with a positive personality profile. This person also may respond more passively, which may exacerbate the health problem and lead to an overall faster deterioration and poorer prognosis for recovery.

Fourth, personality may be a filter, but it may act through some subtle feedback loop to influence the biological mechanisms that are involved in the disease process itself. In this view, called a *differential reactivity model* (Bolger & Zuckerman, 1995), a personality trait may lead to increased autonomic arousal, hormonal flooding, or some combination of both. If maintained over long periods of time, these altered body functions could lead to physiological changes and further biological insult.

CORONARIES, TYPE A, AND HYPERTENSION

Are there coronary-prone, depression-prone, and cancer-prone personalities? Are there special dispositions that predispose a person to drug dependency or to smoking? If so, what special traits make people vulnerable to their own brand of illness or addiction? What hope is there, if any, that the risks can be reduced? If there are no specific biotypes, might there still be a general set of personality traits that disposes people to increased

FIGURE 4-1
Possible models of personality/health relations.

Model 1: Psychosomatic Model

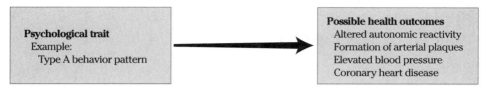

Psychological trait
Example:
   Type A behavior pattern

Possible health outcomes
Altered autonomic reactivity
Formation of arterial plaques
Elevated blood pressure
Coronary heart disease

Model 2: Somatopsychic Model

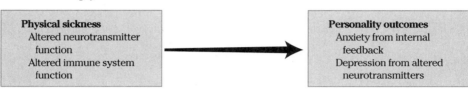

Physical sickness
Altered neurotransmitter
   function
Altered immune system
   function

Personality outcomes
Anxiety from internal
   feedback
Depression from altered
   neurotransmitters

Model 3: Perceptual-Filter Model

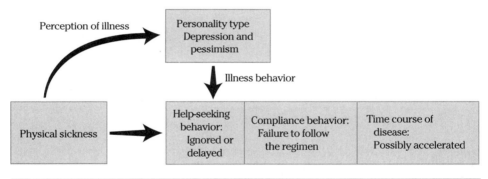
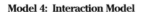

Perception of illness

Personality type
Depression and
pessimism

Illness behavior

Physical sickness

Help-seeking
behavior:
Ignored or
delayed

Compliance behavior:
Failure to follow
the regimen

Time course of
disease:
Possibly accelerated

Model 4: Interaction Model

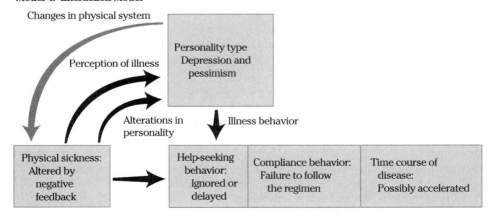

Changes in physical system

Personality type
Depression and
pessimism

Perception of illness

Alterations in
personality

Illness behavior

Physical sickness:
Altered by
negative
feedback

Help-seeking
behavior:
Ignored or
delayed

Compliance behavior:
Failure to follow
the regimen

Time course of
disease:
Possibly accelerated

TABLE 4-3
Comparison of the most prominent theories of personality-disease connections

BIOTYPE	ASSUMED TOXIC CORE	ASSUMED DISEASE LINK	EMPIRICAL STATUS
Type A behavior pattern	Anger directed in; task-oriented anger with chronic activation	Increased risk for coronary artery disease	Converging data from laboratory and epidemiological studies provide the most convincing evidence
Cancer-prone personality	Internalized anger and aggression with abnormal release of emotions	Increased risk for cancer	Methodologically and empirically weak
Smoking and personality	High tension and anxiety	Physical addiction with increased risk for lung cancer and coronary disease	Weak evidence
Alcoholic personality	Genetically set psychological vulnerability; ineffective psychosocial skills; chronic stress	Physical addiction; possible risk for breast cancer	Inconsistent and weak evidence at best
Disease-prone personality	Primary depression; anger and anxiety	Any one of several diseases, including heart disease, arthritis, asthma, ulcers, and headaches	Based on meta-analysis of 101 studies; inconclusive as yet

vulnerability? These are some of the questions to be addressed in the next few pages. Table 4-3 summarizes the variety of personality-illness theories that will be discussed throughout the chapter.

The Type A Behavior Pattern

Perhaps the most widely publicized and popularly discussed biotype is the **Type A behavior pattern** (TABP). The idea of a Type A behavior pattern was first described by two doctors, Meyer Friedman and Ray Rosenman (1974). There are several popular tales of how Friedman and Rosenman came to discover the connection between Type A behavior and **risk of coronary thrombosis** attacks. According to their own story, however, they were led to the discovery by an upholsterer who came to their office to repair furniture. He commented that the doctors must treat a lot of worried people. When they questioned the basis of his opinion, he pointed out the excessive wear on the leading edges of the couches and chairs. This was a sign to him that many of the doctors' clients were literally "on edge." Following this bit of serendipity, Friedman and Rosenman launched the line of research that produced a veritable Type A industry.

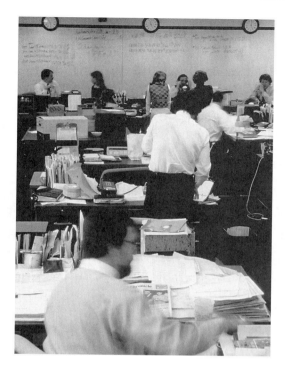

People with a Type-A personality always seem to be working against a clock and tend to feel highly competitive and hostile.

The Type A person is described as one who is time driven, impatient, insecure of status, highly competitive and aggressive, generally hostile, and incapable of relaxing. Time urgency is always prominent in the list of symptoms, but as we shall see later, it is not the core problem. Type A people seem to run with a faster internal clock and perceive time differently than do Type B people (Mueser, Yarnold, & Bryant, 1987). Type A people tend to work rapidly, pushing themselves to complete things at a rapid pace (Yarnold & Grimm, 1982b), and they set higher performance standards (Grimm & Yarnold, 1984). Type A people report more stress symptoms than Type B people do. They are more dominant in interpersonal relationships with Type B people (Yarnold & Grimm, 1982a) and impatient in competitive situations (van Egeren, Fabrega, & Thornton, 1983). They also smoke more and exercise less (Howard, Cunningham, & Rechnitzer, 1976).

Rosenman and Friedman (1974) refer to this pattern as the *hurry sickness*. They listed 13 important trademarks for Type A behavior. These criteria have been translated into a question format in Self-Study Exercise 4-3. It may be instructive to answer these questions before going on. In doing so, stick with your first impressions of how you behave most of the time. Try not to edit answers or to answer based on what you think a Type A person should or should not be. You will find an approximate scoring method at the end of this chapter.

Type A and Coronary Risk

Is Type A behavior related to increased risk for coronary disease, as Friedman and Rosenman suggested? There are two distinct phases of research that attempted to answer this question. A large body of literature provided early evidence that people with the Type A behavior pattern have a much greater risk for heart attacks than people who do not display the hurry sickness. Recent research, however, challenges that simple notion but shows that there is a core of Type A that may be lethal. We begin by reviewing the structure of early arguments. Later, we will discuss current views of Type A and coronary risk.

Biomedical research identified several **coronary risk factors** that were reliably associated with risk for coronary heart disease (CHD). These include (1) age, (2) sex, (3) high cholesterol levels, (4) hypertension, (5) smoking, (6) inactivity, (7) diabetes mellitus, (8) parental history of heart disease, and (9) obesity (Rosenman et al., 1970). In the normal population, approximately 1 of every 162 Americans will suffer a heart attack, although that rate has been dropping for 30 years (Sytkowski, Kannel, & D'Agostino, 1990). The most recent data indicates that more than 737,500 people died from heart disease in 1995, or 281 deaths per 100,000 (Anderson, Kochanek, & Murphy, 1997).

SELF-STUDY EXERCISE 4-2

Coronary Risk Assessment
For an interactive physical risk assessment from the American Heart Association's Webpage, use this URL address and follow the instructions:

http://207.211.141.25/risk/index.html

David Glass (1977) suggested that no matter what combination of physical risk factors was used, they still failed to detect most new cases of coronary heart disease. Presumably, the presence of the Type A behavior pattern could predict CHD better than could all the other risk factors put together. Numerous studies, including the classic longitudinal research project, the **Western Collaborative Group Study** (Rosenman et al., 1964), showed a connection between TABP and significantly higher incidence of CHD (see Rosenman, 1993, for a recent review). The statistics cited revealed up to nearly six times the incidence of CHD for TABP people compared to controls. Although there have been some failures to replicate this finding, most notably the Multiple Risk Factor Intervention Trial (MRFIT), there is still strong evidence that TABP is connected through some means to increased risk for coronary disease (Kuller, Neaton, Caggiula, & Falvo-Gerard, 1980).

The search for the so-called toxic core has led in a number of directions. Some believe that there is a coronary-prone personality with a core of impatience and overactivity (Lloyd & Cawley, 1983). Several teams observed this sympathetic reactivity and suggested that Type A people had an increased risk for several stress-related illnesses, not just for coronary (Goldband, 1980; Irvine, Lyle, & Allon, 1982; van Doornen, 1980). Lovallo and Pishkin (1980) also observed more blood clotting, higher cholesterol levels, and increased triglyceride levels under stress in Type A people. All of this led some investigators to believe that coronary-disease victims experience no more stressful events than healthy subjects but that they translate emotional upsets into bodily symptoms more frequently.

The Changing Face of the Type A Behavior Pattern
In spite of these early promising leads, the alleged relationship between Type A and coronary disease began to evaporate after about 1977. There were failures to replicate

SELF-STUDY EXERCISE 4-3

Criteria Used to Identify Type A Behavior Pattern

1. Do you overemphasize some words in speech and hurry the last words in your sentences?	Yes	No
2. Do you always move, eat, and walk rapidly?	Yes	No
3. Are you generally impatient and get irritated when things do not move fast enough for you?	Yes	No
4. Do you frequently try to do more than one thing at a time?	Yes	No
5. Do you generally try to move the topic of conversation to your own interests?	Yes	No
6. Do you feel some sense of guilt when you are relaxing?	Yes	No
7. Do you frequently fail to take note of new things in your environment?	Yes	No
8. Are you more concerned with getting than becoming?	Yes	No
9. Do you constantly try to schedule more activities in less time?	Yes	No
10. Do you find yourself competing with other people who are also time driven?	Yes	No
11. Do you engage in expressive gestures, clenching a fist or pounding the table to emphasize a point, while engaged in conversation?	Yes	No
12. Do you believe that your fast pace is essential to your success?	Yes	No
13. Do you score success in life in terms of numbers—numbers of sales, cars, and so on?	Yes	No

SOURCE: Adapted from Friedman & Rosenman (1974).

See footnote on page 126 for scoring guide.

early findings of a link between TABP and CHD as well as disturbing negative findings. For example, one study revealed a completely unexpected finding that Type A's had lower mortality after a first coronary event than did Type B patients (Dimsdale, 1988). Ragland and Brand's data also were especially surprising because they showed that Type B's had twice the mortality rate of Type A's after a first coronary attack (1988).

The Toxic Core of Type A Behavior

These unexpected reversals posed a challenge that had to be answered. This required that both the theory and the method be subjected to more intense scrutiny. One major effort in this direction tried to dissect Type A behavior into its component parts. TABP is usually measured by the Structured Interview (SI) or the Jenkins Activity Survey (JAS), an objective paper-and-pencil test of Type A behavior (Jenkins, Zyzanski, & Rosenman, 1965). Research on the properties of these scales showed that they tap a complex pattern with several behavior and affect factors, including strong hostility and anger. Wright (1988) and others (Matthews, Glass, Rosenman, & Bortner, 1977) suggested that these measures are largely measures of **Type A anger.** Must all Type A components be present at some threshold level to increase risk for CHD, or is some subset of TABP factors more toxic than others? Why is CHD absent in some people who nonetheless demonstrate strong time urgency and hostility? Further, why do some people not classified as Type A still experience CHD (Contrada, 1989)? Could there be a common toxic agent, a component of TABP, that is highly related to CHD in both the Type A and non-Type A?

Researchers amassed evidence during the 1980s suggesting that the toxic ingredient was hostility/anger (Blumenthal, Barefoot, Burg, & Williams, 1987; Dembroski & Costa, 1987). The Western Electric Study showed that high-hostility men had five times the incidence of CHD compared to low-hostility men (Shekelle, Gale, Ostfeld, & Paul, 1983). A recent meta-analysis of 83 studies points to negative affect as the most important ingredient, although depression also emerged as a strong component (Booth-Kewley & Friedman, 1987).

One group headed by Logan Wright set out to determine more precisely the importance of several TABP components (Wright, 1988). First, they identified a cluster, a triad of factors that was more strongly connected to TABP and coronary risk than either global measures or single components. This triad included *time urgency, chronic activation,* and *multiphasia.* Time urgency has already been described. Chronic activation is a tendency to be "wired" on a long-term basis, to stay aroused and keyed up from sunup to sundown, day in and day out. Chronic activation is more than just high energy and fast-paced activities. It is also muscular tension and hormonal flooding. Research suggests that the hormones associated with anger may be metabolized differently depending on whether one can respond with a large-muscle response or one bottles up the response.

Multiphasia is the tendency to engage in multiple activities at the same time, a type of double-timing to crowd more and more into less and less time. Examples include the person who reads a technical article while exercising on a stationary bike, the business manager who must take work along on vacations, or the student who works on a term paper while attending a recital. The emergence of this triad of factors provided support for the argument that a subset of TABP would provide a better prediction of CHD than would global Type A measures.

To get at the hostility/anger issue, Wright's group broke anger down into smaller components. In this view, we may experience anger related to tasks or situations, such as dirty or demeaning jobs that have to be done. We may be angry with people in certain situations, such as when they stand in the way of personal achievements. In such cases interpersonal relations may be tainted with aggression. We can also be angry with ourselves. Whatever type of anger is present, it might be contained and bottled up, or it might be expressed outwardly, thereby ventilating emotional energy. This led Wright to use measures that tap "anger-in" and "anger-out." Anger-in proved to be the strongest element predicting risk for CHD. It is noteworthy that anger-out proved to be a combination of time urgency and chronic activation, suggesting that time urgency and activation are really task-oriented anger. This is consistent with Rosenman's view as explained later.

In the end, Wright's program pointed to the multicausal nature of coronary artery disease. Wright's group identified five separate paths to coronary artery disease: inherited risk based on family history, risks that accrue from personal lifestyle choices such as overeating and lack of exercise, anger directed inward, anger directed outward—in other words, time urgency and chronic activation—and finally, the traditional global TABP identified by Rosenman and Friedman.

Rosenman (1993) criticized arguments for the hostility-CHD link based on the fact that hostility scales are weak and the concept itself is subject to shifting definitions. He argued that enhanced, inappropriate competitiveness is the toxic core. However, this core is a multifaceted construct composed of aggressive drive, accelerated pace (Wright's chronic activation), impatience, and hostility/anger. Thus, Rosenman's position is not incompatible with the anger-out and multiple paths suggested by Wright. Further, a recent large-scale meta-analysis showed that, although hostility accounts for a relatively small amount of variance in heart disease, it is nonetheless a significant independent risk factor for CHD (Miller, Smith, Turner, Guijarro, & Hallet, 1996).

Rosenman goes on, though, to present a forceful argument that any proposed psychological construct must be sensibly linked to physical pathology that explains increased coronary risk. He reviews evidence that chronic activation and competiveness lead to heightened noradrenergic activity, which can produce negative outcomes (vasoconstriction and arterial plaques) in the cardiovascular system. More will be said about this in Chapter 5.

Intervening in Type A Behavior

The techniques used to change Type A behavior run the gamut from Rosenman and Friedman's philosophical reeducation to detailed behavior management programs focused on narrowly defined aspects of the Type A pattern (Rosenman & Friedman, 1977). Many individuals identified as Type A have made dramatic changes to a more temperate lifestyle.

Probably the most extensive investigation of such change has come in the **Recurrent Coronary Prevention Project.** In this project, over 1000 patients who had survived a heart attack were studied over a 4.5-year period (Friedman et al., 1994). From this group, 270 people went through a conventional cardiac counseling (CC) program that provided advice on diet, exercise, medication, and other medical information on the heart and surgical interventions. Another 592 people received the same cardiac counseling, but they also received a Type A behavioral counseling package (TAC) that included relaxation training, methods to alter Type A behaviors, reformulating Type A belief systems, and restructuring the environment. At the end of the 4.5-year period, more than 35% of the TAC group, but less than 10% of the CC group, showed marked reductions in Type A behavior. Most significantly, just 12.9% of the TAC group suffered a recurrent cardiac event while 21.2% of the CC group had one. Also, there was a significantly lower death rate among the TAC group compared to the CC group after the first year, a difference that continued through the remaining 3.5 years of the study.

One reason for caution in interpreting results from Type A intervention studies is that they often use people who have suffered a coronary attack. In many cases, the attack was life threatening. The intrinsic motivation in such a scare may be all that is necessary to get people to change their lifestyles. Thus, how much the treatments contributed to change is not clear. It may be that the motivation to change and the information on what to change are more important than the specific means of change.

The Hypertensive Personality

A concept related to the Type A behavior pattern is that of the **hypertensive personality.** Franz Alexander (1939) believed hypertensive patients fight an internal struggle between two strong but incompatible feelings. On one hand, the person feels passive and dependent. On the other hand, the person has strong aggressive and hostile impulses. Because expression of hostility is threatening, the person must fight continuously to keep it under control. Theoretically, this internal conflict should produce long-term autonomic arousal, constriction of blood vessels, and increased blood pressure. Over a period of time, permanent arterial changes occur, and hypertension results.

Alexander's theory was largely speculative and was based on clinical observations of patients, as opposed to carefully thought out, controlled studies. Early efforts to identify a specific pattern of traits common to hypertensives yielded inconsistent results (Sparacino et al., 1982). Further, a lengthy review by Iris Goldstein (1981) led to the conclusion that there is no support for the notion that hypertensives are psychologically different from people with normal blood pressure.

Goldstein's conclusion is supported by an extensive meta-analysis of results from more than 25,000 subjects (Jorgensen, Johnson, Kolodziej, & Schreer, 1996). Jorgensen's group found that elevated blood pressure is associated with more negative affect and with lower overall outward expression (consistent with early speculation). However, they also looked very critically at moderator variables, and found that gender, occupation, age, and awareness of blood pressure status influence the nature of the relationship. Based on this, they concluded that traditional simplistic notions of personality causing elevated blood pressure are untenable. Linking their analysis with numerous other reviews, they proposed a biopsychosocial synergistic model, as shown in Figure 4-2. This model suggests that bidirectional influences are at work in regulating blood pressure. This view is consistent with the idea introduced earlier in this chapter that personality and affect may influence biological processes, but maintains that the reverse is equally true—biological processes can influence affect and personality.

THE DEPRESSION-PRONE PERSONALITY

"Depression is the common cold of mental illness" (Rosenhan & Seligman, 1989, p. 307). It afflicts literally hundreds of thousands of people. At any moment, about 1 of every 15 Americans suffers moderate to severe **depression.** The chances are 1 in 3 that sometime in your life you could have a depressive episode severe enough to require clinical treatment. For some, the affliction is barely noticeable, a blue Monday that turns into Tuesday. For others, it is an unhappiness with self and all that life has to offer, an unhappiness that colors all waking perceptions. And for others, depression is the beginning of the end, the bottomless pit of sorrow and despair leading to hospital isolation, attempted suicide, or death.

As this description suggests, depression runs along a continuum of severity. Yet there is also a body of evidence pointing to distinct types of depression. A genetic mechanism may play a major role in distinguishing less severe depression from severe depression. The most severe form, **bipolar depression,** is present in no more than 5% to 10% of cases. It appears to be genetically determined, while most other forms of depression appear to result from daily pressures.

To say that a person is depressed describes the emotional tone, to be sure, but there is much more than that. Depression is a condition so pervasive it changes virtually all the activities normally considered part of daily life. Depression is a disturbance in mood, a prolonged emotional state that colors all mental processes. The most significant mood seems to be a feeling of hopelessness coupled with helplessness. The person may lose weight because of loss of pleasure in eating. Sleep disturbances also occur frequently. Some people sleep a great deal when they become depressed, but at odd hours, so that

FIGURE 4-2

A biophychosocial synergistic model for personality factors, behavior, and high blood pressure.

SOURCE: Jorgensen et al. (1996).

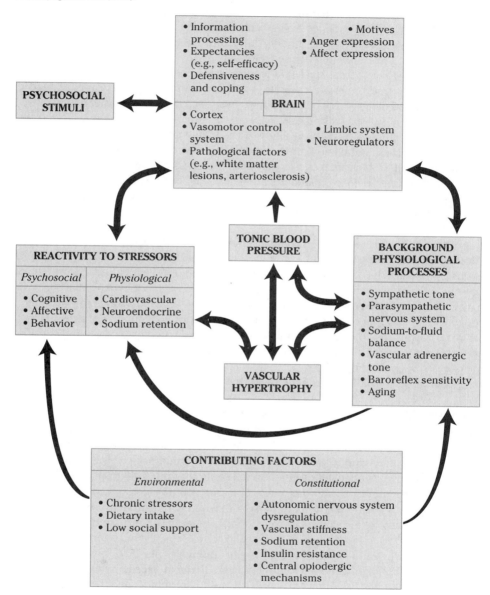

normal activities are disrupted. Others may go to sleep readily but wake up early and not be able to get back to sleep. With both eating and sleeping problems, the person tends to feel fatigued and run down all the time. Normal reserves of energy are depleted, and motivation suffers.

Depression also says something about how the person thinks. It is more than just sluggish thinking. The person feels personal worthlessness to one degree or another. He or she may have vague feelings of being guilty of some type of transgression. In the depressed person's mind, this sin accounts for why people don't care. Concentration suffers, so sticking to any kind of task that requires sustained attention becomes difficult, if not impossible. In some serious cases, thought disturbances may occur, including suicidal thinking and delusions of persecution or of serious illness, such as cancer.

Several observations make the study of depression relevant to the study of stress and health. First, a number of physical illnesses (including coronary heart disease, cancer, asthma, headaches, and ulcers) are commonly associated with depression (Friedman & Booth-Kewley, 1987; McDaniel et al., 1995). Risk for illness may increase because depression tends to increase the circulation of adrenaline and cortisol. These in turn may result in suppression of the immune system. Illnesses may also occur because of the cumulative effect of loss of appetite, poor eating habits, lack of exercise, fatigue, and sleep disturbances.

Second, many illnesses are accompanied by depression because of the sheer strain of dealing with the illness. For example, chronic low-back pain usually results in serious depression when the pain has lasted for more than two years (Garron & Leavitt, 1983). Depression occurs in this case even when there is no evidence of depressive episodes before the back pain.

Third, depression seems to be one major reaction to personal crises or to failure to cope with a crisis. It also seems to be a common reaction to a number of stressors, such as loss of work, loss of savings and investments, and divorce or separation. Finally, depressed people experience more stress in their daily lives, yet they seem to have fewer personal resources and social supports to deal with the stress than do their nondepressive counterparts (Mitchell, Cronkite, & Moos, 1983).

Stress, Depression, and Suicide

Suicide and depression are often linked in folklore. There is good reason to be concerned about the potential for suicide when depression has dragged on for some time. What is often overlooked is that people rarely commit suicide while in a state of depression. This is because both the mental processes required to plan and execute the act and the physical stamina needed to carry out the act are not available. The most dangerous period is when the person is swinging back to a more normal mood state. Unfortunately, this shift tends to make the impact even more devastating for the family.

Suicide is the third leading cause of death among people 15 to 24 years of age (Anderson et al., 1997). In white adolescent males, suicide increased by 64% from 1970 to 1977 (U.S. Department of Commerce, 1979). In a study of gifted high school students, Ferguson (1981) discovered that stress and suicidal thoughts tend to go together. That is, the more stress builds up, the more likely the person is to think about suicide and self-destructive behavior. There does not appear to be any difference in this tendency, however, when gifted adolescents are compared to normally intelligent adolescents.

Knowing the warning signals of suicide and what to do if a friend threatens suicide can be literally a matter of life and death.

THE CANCER-PRONE PERSONALITY

Cancer is one of the most terrifying diseases of our time. Approximately one in four people will be diagnosed with cancer at some time in their lives, while two in three families will have to deal with the disruption, pain, and suffering caused by cancer. The search for a cure has led in all directions—to medicines, surgery, radiation therapy, vitamins, diet, carrot juice, and apricot pits. Many people, desperately seeking to hang on to life and loved ones, grasp at any straw that seems to offer a hope of understanding and beating the dread disease.

But treatment looks beyond just controlling or curing, to eliminating the threat of cancer. In turn, eliminating cancer depends on identifying more precisely the causes of cancer. This is all the more problematic because cancer is not a single disease, but an array of nearly 100 different types. The search for causes has led through many genetic, biochemical, physiological, and environmental studies to a partial understanding. There is new evidence that cancer may be caused by an oncogene, a type of production controller in the cell. **Oncogenes** regulate when and how rapidly new cells are produced. If the oncogene is disturbed—say, through some environmental toxin or carcinogen—production typically goes into an uncontrolled mode, leading to a rapid proliferation of harmful cells. A mutant p-53 oncogene has been linked to certain cancers, and several other oncogenes have been linked to different cancers (Arbeit, 1990).

In spite of the advances in the biomedical arena, there is still speculation about the possible role of psychosocial stressors in cancer risk (Cunningham, 1985; Levy & Wise, 1987). Parallel to the coronary-prone personality (TABP), some have suggested a **cancer-prone personality.**

The personality characteristics most frequently attributed to cancer patients are internalized anger and aggression. Numerous studies reviewed by Morrison and Paffenbarger (1981) showed that cancer patients tend to have higher levels of depression, anxiety, anger, hostility, denial, and repressed emotionality. It should be noted, however, that four of these emotional traits (depression, anxiety, anger, and hostility) are associated with other diseases such as asthma, headaches, ulcers, coronary heart disease, and arthritis (Friedman & Booth-Kewley, 1987). This suggests that the emotional tones may be part of, but not unique to, the cancer-prone personality.

Suggestions abound that these emotional problems are linked to childhood trauma, an unhappy childhood, or family maladjustment. Separation from a parent or death of a parent or sibling has been found in cancer patients' histories more frequently than in those of other patients (Kissen, 1967). One writer even suggested that vulnerability to cancer relates to lack of breast feeding in infancy (Booth, 1969). Family histories of cancer patients reveal more unhappy home lives, domestic strife, and neglect during childhood. This may contribute to the feelings of loneliness, desertion, and denial seen in many cancer patients. Unfortunately, most of the studies that provided evidence for these statements suffered from one or more inadequacies. They lacked control groups, used patients who already knew their diagnosis, and/or analyzed the data improperly.

In spite of improved controls, there is still conflicting information. For example, one team found more repression and less "self-reported" depression relative to a control group (Dattore, Shontz, & Coyne, 1980). Paula Taylor's group used life events, repression-sensitization, and **locus of control** to predict presence of cancer (Taylor, Abrams, & Hewstone, 1988). They found that these variables could explain no more than 8% of the variance. One of the better-controlled studies was carried out using women with breast cancer (Greer & Morris, 1975). The pattern of suppressed anger and abnormal release of emotions was verified in this group. They could find no evidence for the personality traits previously attributed to cancer patients.

Even granted that this difference in anger and release of emotions is the crucial difference between cancer-prone and noncancer-prone people, there is still the issue of how the differences could be physically translated into cancer. Before discussing one model, it should be noted that probably no one would suggest that psychosocial stress could, in and of itself, produce cancer (Levy & Wise, 1987). The assumption is that predisposing factors interacting with host traits trigger the disease with suitable precipitating conditions. One part of the precipitating matrix could be reduced resistance due to psychosocial stress. One general model of this type, proposed by Barofsky (1981), is shown in Figure 4-3.

The hypothesized path from psychological conflict to tumor production may involve any one of several mechanisms. The most frequently suggested path is via elevated adrenocortical production resulting from stress. Certain prolonged stressor situations may produce suppression in the immune surveillance system, which controls the production of Killer-T cells involved in the detection and destruction of cancer cells. As a result of this suppression, tumors could form with little or no resistance.[1]

FIGURE 4-3

A theoretical model of how psychosocial stress and personality may influence the production of tumors.

SOURCE: Adapted from Barofsky (1981)

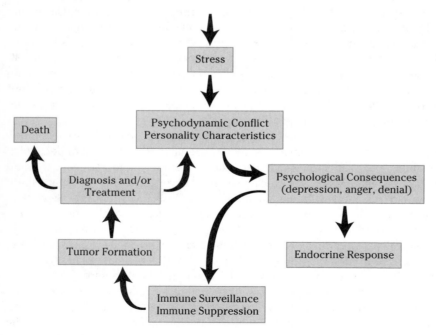

----

[1]More will be said about this in Chapter 5.

As the model shows, diagnosis of cancer and the resulting treatment add to the load of stress. Additional conflict, anger, hostility, denial, and depression generally occur as a result of cancer. The intensity and duration of such conflict may be related to personal coping resources. But even the strongest will go through some period of disruption as they integrate the information about their uncertain future. Many of the early studies are criticized, however, because they used patients with already-diagnosed cancer. It is impossible under such circumstances to separate the psychological characteristics due to the illness from those that have led to the illness. In other words, it would be impossible to distinguish between the somatopsychic hypothesis and the psychosomatic hypothesis in these conditions.

As already noted, defensive coping reactions can significantly influence the course of a disease process. Katz and his colleagues provided some insight on this issue in their study of a group of women hospitalized for breast biopsy (Katz et al., 1970). At the end of the study, they concluded that being in a stress situation alone does not account for arousal of either the emotions or the physical emergency reactions so often expected from a stressor. Rather, both emotional defenses and physical arousal of the adrenal system appear to depend on how the stress is cognitively perceived, interpreted, and defended against. They found that high rates of adrenal reactivity were associated with apprehension, worry, fear, dejection, discouragement, and despair. On the other hand, low adrenal reactivity was associated with hope, faith in God, belief in fate, and pride in one's ability to handle a life-threatening situation.

A final issue concerns the attitudes and emotions that are curative and that enable one to survive the threat of cancer. It is well known, if quietly admitted, that the best medicine may be to no avail when administered to someone who has already given up the struggle for life. Even if no strong relationship exists between the origins of cancer and some personality type, the evidence suggests that the way in which a person responds to the threat may have a lot to do with surviving the physical insult of cancer. The Katz study is one example supporting this. Chronic worry, fear, hopelessness, and despair generally hasten the destructive disease process. On the other hand, hope, faith in a supreme power, and personal courage generally operate to marshal the best body defenses available.

PERSONALITY AND SMOKING

Smoking is considered a high-risk, self-defeating behavior that probably serves to reduce tension for many people. In spite of an overall decline in smoking from a peak around 1955, tobacco use in 1990 still occurred among more than 25% of the population (28% males and 23% females) (Centers for Disease Control, May 22, 1992). A 1991 Youth Risk Behavior Survey of high school students reported that a median 12% reported smoking on 20 of the preceding 30 days (Centers for Disease Control, September 18, 1992). It is estimated that everyday nearly 3,000 adolescents take their first steps to a lifelong habit of smoking (Jason, Ji, Anes, & Birkhead, 1991). Smoking is thus of great significance in considering both health and stress.

There are many theories about what maintains smoking. Strong evidence has accumulated for more than a century that nicotine is addictive. For example, the

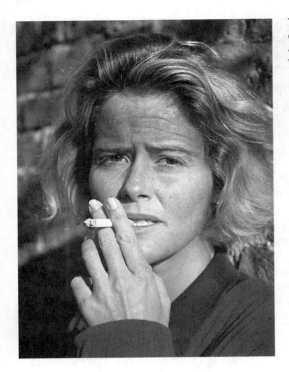

The personality of smokers is described as extraverted, neurotic, and tense with less ability to withstand stress.

dose-response relationship,[2] one of the most reliable signs of physical dependence, was already the subject of study at the turn of the century (Henningfield & Woodson, 1989). Another theory suggests that smoking is primarily a tension release for people who are overly anxious. Support for this notion comes from reports that frequency of smoking increases and decreases with the rise and fall of stress. Theories on what motivates people to start smoking point to peer pressure and peer reinforcement, parental modeling, some set of personal traits, or some combination of all of these.

To this point, little research has been done relating personality traits to smoking. In general, the smoker is described as extraverted, somewhat neurotic, and tense. There is a sex difference, however, in that higher anxiety is found in female smokers than in male smokers. It is noteworthy that these findings relate to the factors that cause people to begin smoking, not to what keeps people smoking (Spielberger & Jacobs, 1982). Heavy smokers show more psychological disturbance than light smokers, and they show less tolerance for stress when not allowed to smoke than when allowed to smoke. In addition, people with psychosocial assets—feelings of self-efficacy, internal control, and good social networks—are able to both resist pressure to begin smoking (Stacy, Sussman, Dent, Burton, & Flay, 1992) and to quit smoking more readily than those lacking such assets.

[2]The dose-response relationship simply states that the larger the dose, the stronger the effect.

Camp, Klesges, and Relyea (1993) summarize six major risk factors for beginning smoking:

1. Presence of smoking friends or family members
2. Overestimation of peer smoking by a factor of 2
3. Perception of maturity, independence, or toughness as a value of smoking
4. Perception that personal support is lacking, or lower expectation for academic success (Ellickson & Hays, 1992)
5. Being a risk taker or being rebellious, and
6. The emotional and/or pharmacological effects of smoking

From the standpoint of stress research, the findings are consistent with an interaction model. They suggest that people with higher levels of tension, anxiety, and psychological disturbance may be more vulnerable to pressures to start smoking. Given stress of the right type and intensity, they are more likely to become trapped in the smoking habit. On the other hand, strong parental models, suitable outlets for tension, guidance for constructive emotional release, and educational programs that enable teenagers to cope with pressure from peers may prevent the habit from starting.

Because of the potential harm of smoking, an increasing number of programs have been designed to help people quit smoking or to reduce the number of people, especially adolescents, who take up smoking for the first time. The first type of treatment deals with the forces that keep people smoking once they have started. The second type of program deals with the factors that induce people to start. Getting people to quit smoking is just as problematic but involves another level of complexity, as noted earlier: the fact that smoking is a physically addictive process constitutes a significant barrier to quitting.

THE ALCOHOLIC PERSONALITY

The concerns that prompted research on personality and smoking also prompted a great deal of research on the **alcoholic personality.** Drinking is related to a variety of stress-reduction and escape behaviors that indicate ineffective coping skills. Drinking also tends to increase and decrease relative to the amount of stress experienced. Alcoholics generally have higher risks for illness, in part due to changes in the gastrointestinal system that lead to increased risk for infectious disorders (Watzl & Watson, 1992). Other examples of risk include the finding that moderate alcohol consumption increases vulnerability to breast cancer by 50 to 100% (Schatzkin et al., 1987). Alcoholism is also related to more rapid mental and physical deterioration (Porjesz & Begleiter, 1982), and an overall higher death rate compared to nonalcoholics. The personal and social costs of drinking are staggering. The road slaughter that occurs each year because of alcohol-related auto accidents is enough to suggest that society must come to grips with this major killer.

It is now generally accepted that alcoholism has a genetic component that may be expressed in a different basal metabolism or some other physical system (Blum, Noble, Sheridan, & Finley, 1991; Le, 1990). Presumably, this makes the person more vulnerable to the addictive properties of alcohol. In addition, there is a pattern of **positive assortative mating** (alcoholics marrying alcoholics) that increases the risk of alcoholism for offspring (Hall, Hesselbrock, & Stabenau, 1983). Still, many factors intervene in the person's development to determine whether the person actually becomes alcoholic or not.

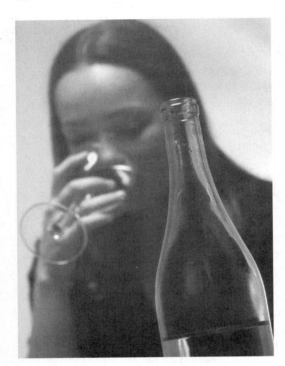

Efforts to portray the alcoholic person suggest that the person may have feelings of personal inadequacy, high levels of fear, chronic levels of stress, and weak psychosocial skills.

The diathesis-stress model may be one of the best theoretical models available to describe the overall mix of factors contributing to alcoholism. This model states that predisposing (risk) factors will be expressed only if a precipitating (stress) event of sufficient intensity is encountered. According to Alterman and Tarter (1983), the predisposing factors include a genetically transmitted psychological vulnerability. These factors include conduct disorders in childhood, hyperactivity, and attentional problems. Stress factors include a disordered family and disturbed family interactions, type of peers with whom one associates, ethnic background, and deprived environment.

The emerging portrait of the alcoholic is of a person with chronic distress, externally controlled (Apao & Damon, 1982), combined with weak or ineffective psychosocial skills (Nerviano & Gross, 1983). Alcoholics also appear to suffer from an alcohol-induced myopia—the inability to process information outside a narrow range—that contributes to the lowered inhibition on impulsive responses and leads to even more difficulty (Steele & Josephs, 1990). Difficulty in psychosocial skills usually revolves around feelings of personal inadequacy, higher levels of fear than normal, and problems with concentration. These traits are revealed in conflict with authority, more frequent and intense expressions of hostility, and aggressiveness. This combination of factors may serve to reduce effectiveness on the job and in a variety of interpersonal relationships from the casual social to the intimate.

When an alcoholic hits the road, some of these characteristics may be intensified. In addition, the tendency for alcoholics to be higher risk-takers increases the likelihood that something bad will happen (Giesbrecht & Dick, 1993). A study from Australia (Federal Office of Road Safety, 1994) covering the decade from 1982 to 1992 revealed that 30% to 40% of drivers and motorcyclists killed had blood alcohol content over the legal limit. Donovan's group proposed a model that integrates personality factors with behavior leading to **"high-risk driving"** (Donovan, Marlatt, & Salzberg, 1983). This model is presented in Figure 4-4.

FIGURE 4-4
Hypothetical model of the effects of social-skill deficits, heavy alcohol use, and hostile-aggressive disposition on high-risk driving.
SOURCE: Donovan, Marlatt, & Salzberg (1983).

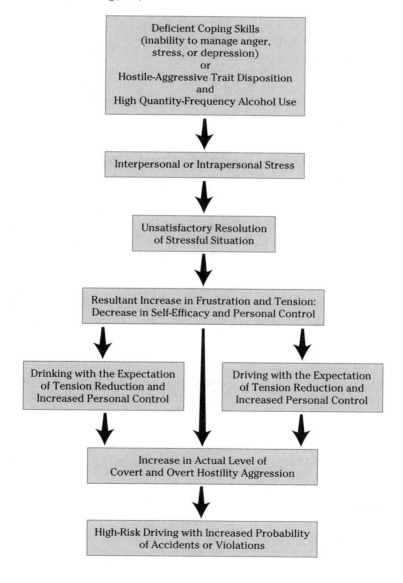

BIOTYPES OR THE DISEASE-PRONE PERSONALITY: THE FINAL SCORE

This extended analysis should make one thing clear: the issues confronted by those working in this arena are very complex. The problems are of great interest and may have important practical outcomes, even though the results seem at times to be weak, inconsistent, and diffuse. On the surface, it may seem that this gives grist to the medical mill's contention that the lingering acceptance of a personality-disease connection is little more than folklore (Angell, 1985).

Friedman and Booth-Kewley (1987) take the view that the issue may not be resolved by looking at specific biotypes but by seeking a **disease-prone personality.** They conducted a meta-analysis of 101 studies that dealt with 5 personality variables and 5 diseases. The personality variables were anxiety, depression, an anger-hostility-aggression complex, an anger-hostility complex, and extraversion. The diseases were asthma, headaches, ulcers, arthritis, and heart disease. Cancer was not included because of the numerous cancers that exist.

The results are instructive. First, Friedman and Booth-Kewley obtained modest support for a personality-disease link. This comes from the fact that each disease is linked to each of the personality factors in a common fashion. In general, a higher level of any of the personality factors (more depression, for example) is related to a greater likelihood of the disease. While the relationships are weak, they are statistically reliable. If there is a dominant trait, it is depression. This led the authors to suggest that depression may have been neglected in favor of the anger trait suggested by Type A research. The analysis provided by Booth-Kewley and Friedman is consistent with the hostility-CHD analysis discussed earlier (Jorgensen et al., 1996).

Second, from this limited sample of personality variables and disease, it is apparent that the notion of biotypes is not supported. This notion would be supported only if one disease reliably connected to a specific trait, while another disease reliably connected to a different trait. On the other hand, the notion of a generic disease-prone personality may be acceptable where negative affect is linked with negative health outcomes. Friedman and Booth-Kewley suggest that, like diet, personality may produce imbalances that can predispose one to disease. It is not so much the specific things you eat, but the lack of balance that presents the problem. The commonality of the traits-diseases relationship also argues against the psychosomatic model (a specific personality causes a specific disease) and against the somatopsychic model (a specific disease causes a specific personality profile).

Finally, the small correlations obtained remind us once again that health status is determined by multiple causes (Wright, 1988). These multiple paths to disease rule out simplistic explanations. The logic of this is based on the small correlations, which indicate that personality accounts for only small amounts of variability in disease. Numerous other factors must be drawn into the equation to explain the origin and progress of a disease. At the same time, as Friedman and Booth-Kewley note, the mere fact that the explained variance is small should not lead us to think it is inconsequential. The number of lives involved even in a small amount of variance can be of great consequence.

CONTROL, HARDINESS, AND SELF-ESTEEM

We have focused much of our attention on traits that seem to have a negative impact on health. At the same time, investigators are very much interested in those that might provide some type of resilience to stress, as well as health protection. Three traits that have been linked in positive ways to stress and health will be discussed here. These are locus of control, **psychological hardiness,** and **self-esteem.**

Locus of Control, Coping, and Mastery

The concept of locus of control comes from the work of Julian Rotter (1966, 1990). Bonnie Strickland (1989), recent president of the American Psychological Association, recognized the concept's importance and reviewed uses of the construct in current research. Rotter (1990) believes that the thousands of studies stimulated by the construct proves its heuristic value. He suggests further that numerous other control concepts, including self-efficacy, are more or less variations on the locus of control construct.

Locus of control refers to the expectancy that personal actions will be effective to control or master the environment. In Rotter's model, people vary on a continuum between the two extremes of **external** and **internal locus of control.** Lefcourt (1976), a protégé of Rotter's, defined external control as the perception that positive or negative events are unrelated to one's own behavior and thus are beyond personal control. External people view most events as dependent on chance or controlled by powers beyond human reach.

The internal person, on the other hand, feels that very few events are outside the realm of human influence. Even cataclysmic events may be altered for good through human action. Lefcourt (1976) defined internal control as the perception that positive or negative events are a consequence of personal actions and thus may potentially be under personal control. If the theme song of the external is "Cast Your Fate to the Wind," the theme of the internal is "I Did It My Way."

Internal people as a group seem to have more efficient cognitive systems. They expend a substantial amount of mental energy obtaining information that will enable them to influence events of personal importance. They expend greater efforts to cope with or achieve mastery over their personal, social, and work environments (Phares, 1976). Internal people also show a greater tendency to implement a specific plan of action. As Phares (1976) noted, "Whether one terms it action taking, confronting, or mastery, internals seem to be more disposed toward behavior that will enhance their personal efficacy, even in the sense of rectifying inadequacies" (p. 66). In this way, a sense of mastery that enables them to cope more successfully with stressful events that may develop. Phares's research also suggests that locus of control is malleable.

A number of investigations have linked locus of control to coping with stress and dealing with family or personal health problems (Donham, Ludenia, Sands, & Holzer, 1983; Ludenia & Donham, 1983). One review (Averill, 1973) outlined three major types of personal control. These are behavioral control, which involves some direct action; cognitive control, which primarily reflects a personal interpretation of events; and decisional control, which means the person has a choice among several different courses of action. The author stated that each type of control is related to stress in a complex fashion, sometimes increasing it, sometimes reducing it, and sometimes having no influence at all. The relationship of personal control to stress is primarily a function of the meaning of control for the individual (p. 286).

Locus of control seems to be important in health behavior. One study of tubercular patients showed that internally oriented patients had much more knowledge about their disease than externally oriented patients did. This is noteworthy because the information they obtained was negative. Results such as this are interpreted as consistent with the idea that internals are knowledge seekers. The results may also relate to the internals' belief that they can do something positive to influence the outcome of the disease process if they have appropriate information (Lefcourt, 1976).

Health service providers face several difficult problems with their clients. These include the facts that people (1) are not highly motivated to engage in effective preventive health care and (2) do not follow prescribed medical programs very carefully when sick. Abella and Heslin (1984) guessed the problem might be related to locus of control—that is, people who are internally oriented might be motivated to control aspects of their environment related to their own health. On the other hand, externally oriented people might not be so motivated, because personal actions are perceived to be unrelated to either positive or negative outcomes. The outcome of the study suggests that the person who both values health and has an internal locus of control is most likely to engage in preventive health behavior.

Psychological Hardiness

Some people seem especially resilient and unflappable. Stress rolls off with little or no apparent disruption to their actions or feelings. Suzanne Kobasa (1979a, 1979b) provided evidence that personality plays a significant role in helping us resist stress-related illnesses. She says resilient people have psychological hardiness. According to Kobasa, three major traits contribute to hardiness: control, commitment, and challenge. *Control* is defined and measured as locus of control, described in the previous section. *Commitment* is a sense of self and purpose. *Challenge* reflects the degree to which safety, stability, and predictability are important. Those with high hardiness are described as having a well-integrated sense of self and purpose. In addition, they see change as stimulating and as providing them with opportunity for growth.

In one study of 137 male business executives, Kobasa and her colleagues looked at both hardiness and exercise as buffers against illness (Kobasa, Maddi, & Puccetti, 1982). They found that stressful life events increased illness, whereas both hardiness and exercise reduced illness. In this sample, the more stress increased, the more exercise and hardiness proved their worth as buffers. Executives who were rated lowest in hardiness and exercised the least had the highest rate of illness. Conversely, those who were rated high in hardiness and exercised the most had the lowest rate of illness. Kobasa (1982) also observed the positive buffering effect of hardiness in a sample of lawyers.

Since then, many studies have focused on the relationship of hardiness to health behaviors. Hannah (1988) observed that hardiness results in more appropriate health behaviors only when it is also combined with high health concern. Nagy and Nix (1989) showed that hardiness is related to both lower stress and preventive health attitudes. Susan Pollock (1989) showed that hardiness is related, directly or indirectly, to physiological and psychological adaptation in chronically ill adults. The direct route is the influence of hardiness on the perception of illness. Pollock suggested that hardiness directly influences the perception of illness. She also believes that coping efforts and social supports indirectly influence adaptation. Hardy people appear to engage in more active coping and draw on more resources than the less hardy do.

Contrada (1989) showed that hardiness is associated with reduced diastolic blood pressure under conditions of laboratory stress. This relates specifically to the challenge component of hardiness. Contrada also assessed TABP using the traditional SI and JAS measures and found that the hardiness construct added significantly to the prediction of diastolic blood pressure (DBP) by the Type A construct. Those who were strongest Type B and strongest on the hardiness measure had the lowest DBP. Allred and Smith (1989) found that hardy subjects gave more positive self-statements under conditions of threat, but they question the presumed organic link of hardiness and health.

Hannah and Morrissey (1987) found that hardiness develops with age in adolescents. Hardiness or resiliency also may explain the extraordinary adaptation of children and adolescents raised in adverse environments (Neiman, 1988; Richmond & Beardslee, 1988). It buffers against burnout in stressful occupations such as intensive-care nursing (Lambert & Lambert, 1987; Rich & Rich, 1987). In the case of intensive-care nursing, commitment appears to be the main hardiness ingredient.

Since Kobasa proposed the hardiness construct, it has been subjected to close and critical scrutiny. There is evidence that hardiness has many faces. The existential constructs of self-actualization and inner-directedness bear more than just surface similarity (Campbell, Amerikaner, Swank, & Vincent, 1989). Another term frequently used is *resilience* (Werner, 1984). Gary Leak and Dale Williams (1989) noted that the commitment component of hardiness is similar to Alfred Adler's notion of social interest.

Frederick Rhodewalt and Joan Zone (1989) conducted one of the more interesting studies of hardiness. They compared adult women who were divided into hardy and nonhardy groups. Their results support the contention that hardiness may be more important when it is absent than when it is present. In this view, nonhardy people tend to appraise more events as undesirable and report that negative events require more adjustment. Thus, higher levels of stress may result more from negative affect combined with poor coping skills, as opposed to the view that hardiness provides special resilience to stress.

Self-Esteem, Stress, and Coping

The term *self-esteem* is frequently used to refer to a sense of positive self-regard. In the simplest possible terms, it is feeling good about yourself. Self-esteem is sometimes confused with **self-concept.** *Self-concept* is a very broad term that includes all the ways in which people compare themselves to others and evaluate themselves physically, mentally, and socially. Self-esteem thus feeds into self-concept. Recent research suggests that self-esteem is made up of three psychosocial factors and two physical factors (Fleming & Courtney, 1984). The three psychosocial factors are self-regard, social confidence, and school ability. The two physical factors are appearance and ability.

The relationship of self-esteem to coping is complex. It includes feedback from many previous successful or unsuccessful attempts at coping. When people feel good about themselves, they are less likely to respond to or interpret an event as emotionally loaded or stressful. In addition, they cope better when stress does occur. This feeds back positive information that further increases self-esteem.

Many investigators have been trying to determine what specific aspects of self-esteem are more closely related to coping failure and success. When people with low-esteem are put in a threat situation, they tend to show both poorer overall coping and lower overall competency. According to Rosen, Terry, and Leventhal (1982) the difficulty with coping in low-esteem people can be traced to two basic negative self-perceptions. First, low-esteem people have higher levels of fear under threat than do high-esteem people. Second, low-esteem people perceive themselves as having inadequate skills to deal with threat. They are less interested in taking preventive steps and seem to have more fatalistic beliefs that they cannot do anything to prevent bad things from happening. They are a step behind at the start because they believe they cannot cope.

SUMMARY

In this chapter, a variety of personality theories specifically related to issues of stress and health have been reviewed. Several biotypes have been shown to have at best weak links to health, while others appear more strongly related to vulnerability to stress or specific health problems. The major points made in the course of this chapter follow.

- Personality is defined as the unique organization of characteristics that determine the person's general style of adapting or coping.
- Personality theories differ in their emphasis on internal versus external characteristics, and whether they believe few or several traits must be used to describe a person. Psychoanalytic theory, for example, described personality by reference to internal psychic conflicts.
- Dispositional theories propose that there are enduring and stable personality traits. A typology looks for a relatively few characteristics to describe personality while a trait theory looks for a relatively large set of characteristics to describe people.
- One typology derived from the work of Jung has proven very durable—that is the distinction between the introvert and the extravert. Introverts tend to be more reclusive and tolerate solitary and reflective pursuits while extraverts tend to be more socially outgoing and prefer being with others.
- A typology of interest to stress researchers is the state-trait anxiety distinction. State anxiety is felt only in certain situations, such as test anxiety. Trait anxiety is a more enduring anxiety that may be present in general regardless of the type of situation.
- Recent research has focused on the Five Robust Personality Traits: neuroticism, extraversion, openness, agreeableness, and conscientiousness. These traits seem to provide a common ground for describing personality.
- Personality traits may be related to health behaviors. Recent research supports the notion that certain core health behaviors are useful in describing what people do to prevent illness and promote health. These behaviors include wellness behaviors, accident control, traffic risk taking, and substance risk taking.
- A psychosomatic model argues that a psychological process influences the physical, whereas a somatopsychic model argues that physical processes influence the psychological. In fact, there may be multiple ways in which the physical and the psychological interact with each other.
- The Type A behavior pattern is an action-emotion complex with a strong toxic core of hostility that more accurately predicts coronary risk than global Type A measures do.
- There is little evidence to support the notion that other diseases (cancer, for example) are related to specific personality types.

- People who become addicted to smoking may be more extraverted, neurotic, and tense. High anxiety appears in female smokers more than in male smokers.
- People who become addicted to alcohol appear to have chronic distress combined with weak or ineffective psychosocial skills.
- Negative affect appears to be the central ingredient in most studies that look for a link between illness and personality.
- A general illness- or disease-prone personality may exist, but the notion of specific personalities predicting specific diseases does not receive substantive support.
- Research on locus of control looks at whether people feel they do or do not have control over many of the important events around them. Internally controlled people feel they can exercise effective control while externally controlled people feel that most of what happens to them is a result of forces out of their control. Internally controlled people are more likely to seek knowledge about illness and take positive actions to combat illness than are externally controlled people.
- Psychological hardiness is a trait that seems to increase resistance to stress.

CRITICAL THINKING AND STUDY QUESTIONS

1. What is the difference between a typology of personality and a trait view of personality?
2. What are some of the logical problems involved in trying to establish links between personality and illnesses?
3. What are the distinguishing characteristics between state and trait anxiety and how are they related to health and illness behaviors?
4. How is the Type A Behavior Pattern described? What appear to be the major characteristics of TABP that increase risk for coronary?
5. Are there specific personality traits that predict illnesses like hypertension and cancer? Do more than just answer the question in yes/no form. Try to identify the strengths and weaknesses of arguments pro and con on the issue.
6. Is there evidence to suggest that people who become addicted to cigarettes or alcohol have specific personality types? If so, what does the evidence say?
7. What is the disease-prone personality? What is the core trait of the disease-prone personality? Does this construct help resolve issues in regard to a link between personality and illness?

KEY TERMS

alcoholic personality
alcoholism, and high-risk
   driving
biotypes
bipolar depression
cancer-prone personality
coronary risk factors
depression

depression-prone
   personality
disease-prone
   personality
dispositional theory
extraversion
hypertensive personality
introversion

locus of control,
   and health behavior
   external
   internal
oncogenes
personality, definition
positive assortative mating
psychoanalytic theory

psychological hardiness
psychosomatics
Recurrent Coronary
    Prevention Project
self-concept
self-esteem, and stress
smoking, and personality

somatopsychic model
state anxiety
test anxiety
trait anxiety
trait theory
Type A behavior pattern
Type A, and anger

Type A, and coronary
    risk
typology
Western Collaborative
    Group Study

WEBSITES the cognitive stress system: attitudes, beliefs, and expectations

URL ADDRESS	SITE NAME & DESCRIPTION
http://www.cmhc.com/guide/anxiety.htm	☆Mental Health Net. Anxiety reactions including Posttraumatic Stress Disorder
http://www.grohol.com/web.htm	☆Psych Central—Web Pointer. One of the most comprehensive link sites for mental health and personality issues
http://www.unl.edu:80/stress/mgmt/	University of Nebraska Stress Site with Personality section
http://www.psycom.net/depression.central.html	Dr. Ivan's Depression Central. Includes links to many depression-information sites, including Seasonal Affective Disorder
http://207.211.141.25/	☆American Heart Association, Web page with loads of information on heart health

Approximate scoring for the Type A scale used in Self- Study Exercise 4-3:
If you answered most of the questions "yes," you would be described as a Type A person. If you answered "yes" to over half of them, you might still be regarded as Type A but not an extreme Type A.

CHAPTER 5

The Physiology of Stress:

The Brain, Body, and Immune Systems

*It is highly dishonorable for a reasonable soul to live in
so divinely built a mansion as the body she resides in,
altogether unacquainted with the exquisite structure of it.*

ROBERT BOYLE

QUESTIONS

- What is the mind, and how
  does it operate in the stress
  processes?
- What are the immediate
  responses of the brain to a
  stressor event?
- What are the major
  subdivisions of the nervous
  system?
- What is the role of the
  brainstem in life support
  functions and stress reactions?
- What is the visceral brain, and
  what is its role in reacting to
  stress?
- How do the sympathetic and
  parasympathetic systems differ?
- How does the master gland
  function in stress reactions?
- What is the immune system,
  and how may it be helped or
  hindered by stress?
- How does stress influence
  the cardiovascular system?
- What is the effect of stress on
  the digestive system?

The human body is the most beautiful and intricate, yet efficient, machine ever devised. The more we come to understand its design, the more we admire its perfection. Still, the more we understand its intricacies, the more mystery seems to unfold. For every door opened in the labyrinth of the body, research discovers more doors that need to be opened.

The next few pages will provide a tour through the body beautiful, the body functioning at its normative best. We will discuss six systems: the nervous, respiratory, endocrine, immune, cardiovascular, and digestive systems. I selected these systems because (1) stress research suggests they play a prominent role in defensive reactions of the body, (2) these are the systems we most frequently abuse through misbehavior, and (3) we can influence these systems through modest behavioral and/or attitudinal lifestyle changes.

MIND, BRAIN, AND BODY: SOME DEFINITIONS

The terms **mind,** *brain, and body* will be used frequently in this discussion. The issue of how the mind interacts with the body has been a thorn in the flesh of science for a long time.[1] It is necessary, therefore, to make clear how these terms will be used.

In this book, *mind* will be used to mean all the processes of the brain, whether we are aware of these processes as they occur or not. *Mind* describes what is happening when we remember, make decisions, solve problems, reason, reflect, and observe our own reflections. The *mental system* will refer to the interconnected operations of the mind—for example, perceiving, evaluating, reflecting on, and responding to external stimuli. The term *brain* refers to the mass of neural tissue housed in the skull.

There is no dispute that the brain is a physical organ. Yet the way it behaves and our awareness of this behavior makes the brain difficult to talk about without considering its uniqueness. Terms such as *mind* and *mental process* capture that uniqueness adequately. There is little need to become bogged down in a mind/body dispute that is now centuries old. No one has proposed a satisfactory resolution to this conflict yet. Moreover, no empirical data or logic will resolve the issue to everyone's satisfaction. As William Uttal (1978) noted, "in almost all cases, it [the debate] will necessarily be based on softer criteria including ones based on emotion, values, and intuitive and aesthetic judgments of consistency, completeness, or productiveness" (p. 81).

CHARTING THE BACK ROADS OF THE MIND

Tracking the flow of information through a system as complex as the body is not an easy job. The problem is all the more difficult because neural control is maintained through an intricate system of checks and balances, including duplicate pathways and feedback circuits that keep things running smoothly most of the time. Duplication of pathways (called *redundancy*) makes it possible for one part of the brain or body to communicate with other parts even when one pathway is jammed. Feedback circuits allow the brain to *attenuate* (regulate or modify) new input at different stages of processing. In spite of this complexity, scientists have made exciting progress that moves us closer to understanding the body's most complex organ.

---

[1]This is primarily a problem carried over from a philosophical tradition that tried to come to grips with a profound mystery without the benefits of contemporary biomedical and neuroscience research.

Physical Reactions to Anxiety Events

In Self-Study Exercise 4-1, you were asked to identify situations in which you experienced strong symptoms of anxiety. In this self-study, use the anxiety-provoking situations you described earlier, but now expand your analysis. For each of the situations, try to recall as vividly as possible what your typical body reaction was. Most people will experience more than one physical symptom during a stressful event, so feel free to list as many as you can actually recall. Compare your perception of physical arousal with some of the descriptions provided as you continue to read.

SITUATIONS (KEYWORD FROM 4-1)	PHYSICAL SYMPTOMS

THE BRAIN: ITS ROLE IN STRESS AND HEALTH

The brain still conceals many mysteries. It is among the last frontiers of our quest to understand the body. Details of the brain's structure and functions are remarkably intricate. If we waded into this tangled web without some perspective, we could soon lose our bearings. This is the perennial forest-and-trees problem. Before proceeding, then, a brief example may help.

Imagine you are taking a walk late in the evening. You round a corner and a mugger jumps out and demands money. In what may seem like an eternity to you, the brain has already invoked thousands of connections. It has tapped relevant experiences and information about muggings. It quickly calculates such things as the size of the mugger; the type of weapon, if any; and even something as subtle as the robber's disposition and seriousness of intent. Meanwhile, your body mobilizes its energy for the emergency. You may feel your heart racing, palms sweating, knees knocking. In a flash, you may consider several possible plans of action. Should I run? Scream? Fight? Talk? Give in without resistance? Just as quickly you may estimate the risk of these various plans.

It would be nice if we could all be cool under fire, as was one man featured in a recent Ann Landers column. He and his station manager were confronted with a husband-and-wife armed robbery team. While the husband took the manager to the back to get the money, the man coolly asked the woman if she would like to register for the current sweepstakes. The woman liked the idea and promptly filled out a registration sticker while keeping the man under guard. After the robbers left, the man pulled the sweepstakes slip and handed it to the investigating officers! The inept robbery duo were arrested minutes later.

For most of us, the sight of a dangerous felon probably leads to a more distinct stress-type reaction in which, instantly and automatically, most highly controlled processing is suspended and only survival matters. You are not likely, in other words, to

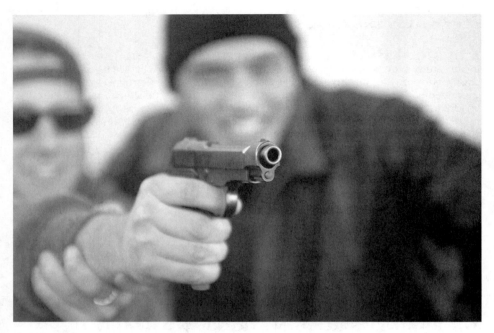

Being confronted by an armed robber usually produces an extreme stress response that suspends controlled mental processing and moves into an automatic survival mode.

continue thinking about a solution to a math or business problem when a gun is aimed at your heart. This does not mean that the cognitive system suspends all rational activity, even though it may not be as rational as that of the cool station attendant. The brain matches the event to existing schemata, including event scripts that may guide behavior—perhaps based on things that have been read or seen on TV—for self-protection in emergencies. Personality traits probably also interact with event data to bias the interpretation and the action plans.

At the biologic level, the brain activates descending pathways of neural and hormonal control. The result may be increased output from the pituitary, elevated adrenal flow, and increased blood pressure and heart rate. Normally, the neural-hormonal systems that regulate this adaptive reflex operate as negative feedback loops. That is, they feed back data to a brain comparator that recognizes when an adequate adaptive response exists. Then the negative feedback loop inhibits or shuts down further activation. After a time, the body returns to normal arousal levels.

There are times, however, when parts of the stress system operate as a positive feedback loop—that is, the loop actually increases activity in the circuit and takes the stress reaction to yet a higher level, a process that is called amplification. Whether the system works to soften or intensify the blow seems to depend on a number of factors, including the type, severity, and duration of the stressor. Under conditions of prolonged stress, the biological system may flood itself with its own chemicals. The body's defenses then work continuously at high speed. This can lead to changes in several biologic systems, including the immune system. In the early stages, these bodily changes may go undetected because they are so subtle. Still, the long-term effects can include changes that affect structural integrity of body organs (for example, stomach ulcers or accelerated hardening of the arteries) and result in serious physical illness. Later, the body loses its ability to resist added stressors and shows signs of exhaustion. This, of course, is a restatement of the General Adaptation Syndrome, which we discussed in Chapter 1.

The Literal Brain

Earlier in this book, the notion of the literal brain (Pelletier, 1977) was introduced. Simply stated, the brain makes no distinction between actual threat and imagined threat. A thought is just as important to the mind as an external event. To the brain, perceived threat is simply threat. When threat is present, the brain sounds the alert, and the body begins mobilizing defensive reactions. In this way, the brain induces change in life-sustaining functions even when only perceived threat is present. In the next few pages, we will look at the components of this literal brain. In the process, we will detail the ways in which these various components function in stress reactions.

Functional Neuroanatomy: A Primer

The nervous system consists of two divisions, the **central nervous system (CNS)** and the **peripheral nervous system (PNS).** The central nervous system contains the brain and spinal cord. The peripheral nervous system is comprised of two subsystems, the **autonomic nervous system (ANS)** and the **somatic nervous system (SNS).** Finally, the autonomic nervous system has two major parts, the **parasympathetic** and the **sympathetic nervous systems.** Figure 5-1 summarizes these divisions. For this discussion we will confine our attention to the brain and autonomic nervous system, since these systems play the major role in the stress response.

Neuroanatomists, scientists who specialize in mapping the structure of the brain, now recognize several layers of tissue in the brain. Each layer represents a distinct stage in the brain's development. From old to new, these layers are the brain stem; the visceral brain (comprised of many different parts); and the new brain (neocortex), or cerebral cortex.

The Brain Stem

The **brain stem** is a bulb-like outgrowth at the top of the spinal column. It houses control centers that involuntarily regulate vital life functions. The brain stem centers that we are concerned with include the **medulla** and the **reticular formation (RF).** Figure 5-2 shows these structures.

The medulla is like a neural Grand Central Station. It contains nerve fibers arriving from the body and departing the brain through the spinal cord. Two types of nerve fibers leave the brain through this concourse: the autonomic nerves, which control many visceral activities, and the motor nerves (corticospinal tract), which govern muscle control (Liebman, 1979).

The most important brain stem centers, the *autonomic nuclei,* carry on life-support processes such as respiration, heart action, and digestion. For example, the

FIGURE 5-1
Major divisions of the nervous system.

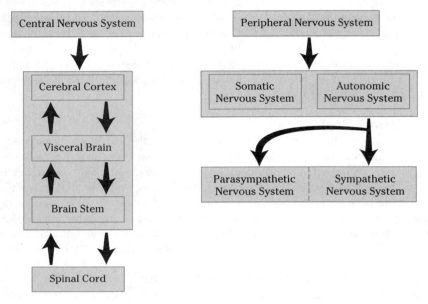

FIGURE 5-2
Brain stem, reticular
formation, and locus
coeruleus system, with
cardiovascular and
respiratory control centers
shown.

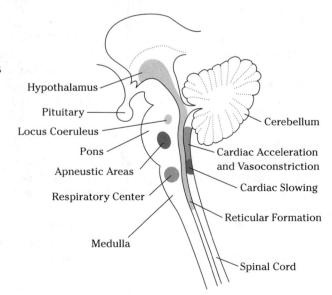

brain stem respiratory center regulates the rhythmic nature of breathing. In normal states, breathing occurs at an even pace (about 12 breaths per minute) and with good balance between inspiration and exhalation—about 2 seconds and 3 seconds, respectively (Guyton, 1977).

Stress can alter this balance, as some everyday situations illustrate. Anxiety over public speaking can result in a person's appearing to be out of breath. If someone runs a red light in front of you, your breathing might stop momentarily; then you would breathe rapidly for a short while. During such stressful events, the cerebral cortex signals the autonomic respiratory nuclei, which in turn signals the respiratory system. Then, the balance of inhalation and exhalation is tipped in the direction of more inhalation, or very deep breathing. This puts more oxygen in the blood than normal. Probably the most common reaction to a stressor is an increase in the rate of breathing.

Anxiety Hyperventilation

A condition called **anxiety hyperventilation** shows what can happen under extreme stress. In hyperventilation, excessive ventilation of the blood supply occurs as it tries to release carbon dioxide. When this happens, the person feels dizzy, perhaps even to the point of blacking out. Shortness of breath occurs, and the heart pounds. The person may experience *parathesia,* a numbness or tingling in parts of the body. This heightens anxiety because people typically perceive these symptoms as an impending heart attack. This is not only uncomfortable; it can be very frightening.

Clinicians regard hyperventilation as a psychogenic reaction. In other words, it is a condition that comes from psychological traits and social circumstances, not from physical pathology. The condition can be relieved in one of two ways. One is to breathe voluntarily at a measured slow pace or to hold the breath for short periods. The other is to breathe into a paper bag and rebreathe the same air. One research group showed that practiced breathing and relaxation is an effective treatment for hyperventilation and resulting chest pain (Hegel et al., 1989).

Control over the activity of the heart also comes from autonomic nuclei in the brain stem. Both the sympathetic and parasympathetic sides of the autonomic system operate to keep the heart pumping smoothly. The sympathetic system drives the heart to higher rates when necessary. Sometimes it can drive the heart to beat as many as 250 beats per minute (normal heart rate is 70 beats per minute). The action of the sympathetic system also increases the strength of the heartbeat. The parasympathetic system moderates the strength of the beat and decreases the rate.

The Reticular Formation

The reticular formation (RF) is a bundle of fibers that runs upward like a great rope through the middle of the brain stem into the hypothalamus and thalamus. Although we speak of it as a single structure, it is actually a very complex system in its own right, comprised of approximately 90 separate nuclei. It may be viewed as the great sentry system of the brain, but one of its nuclei, the *locus coeruleus,* is also extremely important in the stress response. The work of the RF is threefold: two-way communication between brain and body, selection (gating) of sensory information for processing by the cerebral cortex, and vigilance or arousal.

BRAIN-BODY COMMUNICATION   The reticular formation is a major two-way path for communication between the brain and the rest of the body.[2] The descending pathway relays signals from the hypothalamus to several organs controlled by the autonomic system. It also relays involuntary motor impulses to voluntary muscles.

The brain signals the presence of psychosocial stressors via the descending pathway and the hypothalamic-pituitary adrenal cortex pathway, or the HPA complex as it is most commonly known. (Figure 5-3 shows these connections.) In this way, nonphysical stressors can lead to major changes in physical systems. The most important changes occur in the cardiovascular, glandular, and immune systems. With prolonged stress, these changes may produce undesirable effects.

FIGURE 5-3
Effects of prolonged stress in the hypothalamic–pituitry–adrenal (HPA) complex and autonomic systems.

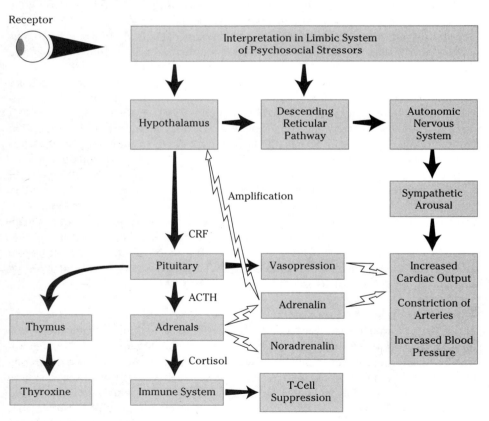

The second pathway, the ascending RF, signals the brain that physical stressors, such as extreme temperatures and injury to the body, exist. These stressors may be translated into a variety of emotional states that produce psychological discomfort and tension. The reticular formation, combined with thalamic centers, controls the awareness of pain. Because pain usually produces negative emotions, an amplification effect may occur that increases sensitivity to the pain itself. Still, this signal system leads to activation of normal healing processes. The body can even produce its own analgesic-like substances, opiates, to reduce the level of pain experienced while healing is in process. More will be said about this later in this chapter.

GATING The RF receives input either directly or indirectly from each sensory system. In turn, it can influence receptor sensitivity and alter the state (open or closed) of sensory relay stations. The general outcome of this changing sensitivity is to help the flow of information through one sensory channel while restricting the flow in another. Because of this, a great amount of information initially sent to the brain is lost or distorted. This may not seem like an efficient way of doing business, but it ensures that vital information gets to its destination.

To borrow some terms from communication theory, the RF works to increase the ratio of signal to noise. If every bit of sensory data entered the brain, the brain would simply be overwhelmed. Think of what it would be like to have every radio and TV in your home running full blast while every member of your family talks at once. That is noise! When you turn the radios and TVs down to background level, the sound of only one person talking is signal. By being selective in what gets through—enhancing signal while reducing noise—the brain can operate more efficiently.

One important question is "How does the RF know what information is important and what is not?" Only the most general answer can be given. The RF receives input from almost every part of the brain, including centers responsible for motivation, emotion, attention, and associative processes. Changes in any of these internal states bias the way in which the RF selects information. An example may help illustrate this point.

Imagine a parent who puts his or her baby down for a nap and then takes a brief nap also. The TV is on, and there is moderate street noise. In spite of this, the parent rests comfortably, somehow effectively blocking out the noise. Then the baby whimpers softly. Its cry is not as loud as the other sounds, but the parent gets up and immediately attends to the child's needs. Since the baby's cry typically has higher motivational strength than street noise or TV talk, the RF permits this signal to get through and awaken the sleeping parent.

VIGILANCE AND AROUSAL: THE LOCUS COERULEUS The third function of the RF, vigilance or arousal, is very important to the way in which the higher brain centers work. This function is part of the work carried out by the locus coeruleus (LC), which is located in the brain stem region at about the mid-pons level, as shown in Figure 5-2. The LC looks for important information reaching the senses. Then it provides an alerting signal to higher centers of the brain: "Get ready, I have something important for you." Evidence for this notion comes from surgical procedures that isolate the cortex from the RF and from clinical observations of patients with damage to the RF. When damage occurs in the LC region, the result is depressed cortical activity, and in extreme cases, coma.

The LC is the central nervous system site for production of norepinephrine, one of the major stress hormones. The LC works with the HPA complex to form a positive feedback loop (Michelson, Licinio, & Gold, 1995). When stimulated by **corticotropin-releasing factor (CRF),** the LC increases its firing rate, and when norepinephrine is released from the LC, it stimulates the hypothalamus to release CRF. When the LC is active, activity in target cells is enhanced, or stated in other terms, signal-to-noise ratio is improved (Valentino, Drolet, & Aston-Jones, 1995). Further, when the LC is active, it is accompanied by another part of the stress response, autonomic arousal.

The Visceral Brain

The **visceral brain** is a complex set of structures in the center of the brain. The name comes from its extensive connections with the **hypothalamus,** which controls visceral systems involved in fight-or-flight reactions. Because this group of structures plays a primary role in interpreting potentially emotional stimuli, it is crucial to any explanation of how the brain responds to stress. The most important structures of the visceral brain are the **thalamus,** the hypothalamus-pituitary complex, and other centers associated with the **limbic system.** These structures are illustrated in Figure 5-4.

THE THALAMUS The thalamus contains several nuclei that are the major relay centers for every sensory system except the sense of smell. It is in an excellent position to evaluate

FIGURE 5-4
Cross section of the cerebral cortex showing the major motivational and emotional control centers associated with the "visceral brain."
SOURCE: Goldstein (1994).

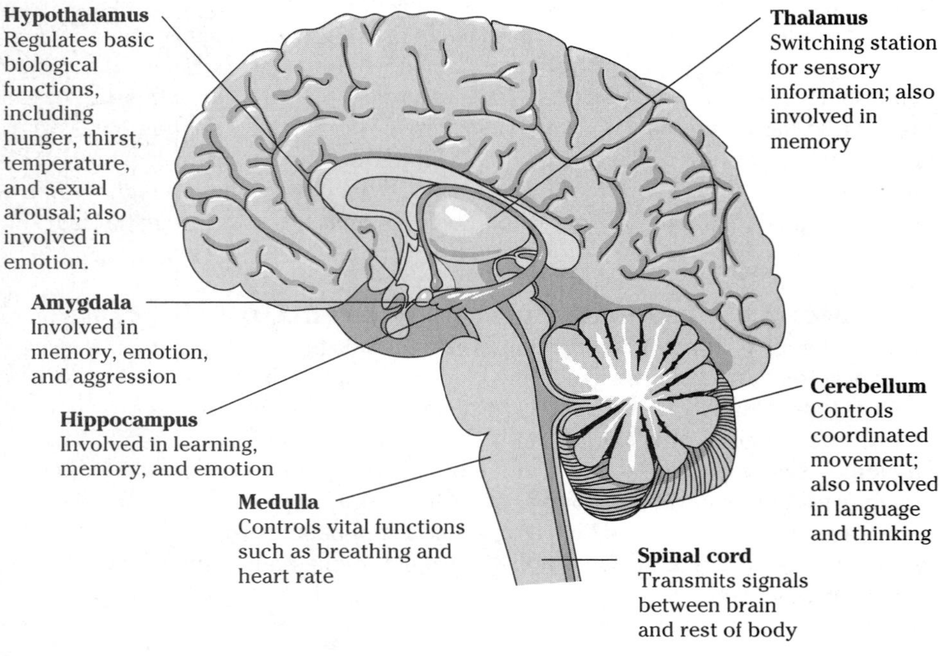

Hypothalamus
Regulates basic biological functions, including hunger, thirst, temperature, and sexual arousal; also involved in emotion.

Amygdala
Involved in memory, emotion, and aggression

Hippocampus
Involved in learning, memory, and emotion

Medulla
Controls vital functions such as breathing and heart rate

Thalamus
Switching station for sensory information; also involved in memory

Cerebellum
Controls coordinated movement; also involved in language and thinking

Spinal cord
Transmits signals between brain and rest of body

the emotional content of information the senses provide. The first clinical observations supporting this view came from observing patients who had physical damage to the thalamus. Such people overreact to emotional stimuli. Some patients also showed uncontrollable weeping or laughing without any accompanying subjective experience (Grossman, 1973).

One interesting recent discovery is the role the thalamus plays in the perception of pain. Pain researchers commonly identify three types of pain. Pricking pain comes from a knife cut or a needle, for example. Burning pain is the second type, and aching pain is a deep muscle or bone pain (Guyton, 1977). Each specialized pain pathway terminates in the thalamus. Burning and aching pain also have connections to the RF.

There is some evidence that we can exercise cognitive control over the perception of pain. This might occur by shutting neural gates that are part of the pain pathway (Melzack & Wall, 1965). Another possibility is that cognitive processes might increase the level of **endorphins** (literally the "morphine within") in the pain region. Scientists do not understand these mechanisms well enough to say exactly how pain can be cognitively mediated. Still, they have taken promising steps to provide therapies for people with chronic pain. For example, stimulation techniques act on pain gateways; these techniques have enabled terminally ill patients to control pain levels without drugs.

THE LIMBIC SYSTEM The limbic system is the part of the primitive brain concerned with survival. It includes the thalamus, hypothalamus, **amygdala, hippocampus,** and septum. Again, you can refer to Figure 5-4 for details. The functions most often associated with the limbic system include anger, aggression, punishment, reward, sexual arousal, and pain.

For example, damage to the amygdala typically results in greatly increased appetite. Damage to the septum may result in extreme irritability or even rage responses with unprovoked aggression. The amygdala produces the opposite type of reaction, suggesting that these two centers balance aggressive tendencies: the amygdala starting, and the septum moderating, aggressive tendencies. The septum and the hypothalamus also may serve as major reward or pleasure centers in the brain.

Damage to the hippocampus can disturb formation of new memories, and may slow down or block several types of learning. Most often, these are learning processes that require some kind of avoidance or discrimination response. The hippocampus has extensive connections with the emotional-motivational complex, but it still seems to function as the "cool," more objective and analytic memory system (Metcalfe & Jacobs, 1996).

THE HYPOTHALAMUS The general location of the hypothalamus is just above the roof of the mouth, toward the back. It connects directly to the **pituitary gland,** the **master gland** of the body. Through this connection, the hypothalamus powerfully affects nearly every visceral system in the body. Another measure of the hypothalamus' significance is that nearly every area of the brain interacts with the hypothalamus in some fashion. For example, the hypothalamus has elaborate connections with the RF and the limbic system. Sexual behavior originates in the limbic region but depends on the hypothalamus for control.

Because of this intricate linkage system, the hypothalamus is sensitive to psychosocial and emotional stimuli. It responds to cognitive stressors that originate from associative thinking or obsessional ruminations. The limbic system can also influence the operation of the autonomic system through this linkage. For example, sleep is cocontrolled by centers in the hypothalamus and the RF. Finally, the hypothalamus is very richly supplied with blood, and it monitors the level of nutrients in the blood and body-fluid volume. The hypothalamus also monitors concentrations of hormones originating in other parts of the body. As part of a complex feedback loop system, it is crucial to mediating stress reactions.

The role of the hypothalamus in stress is most clearly revealed in five functions. These are (1) initiating activity in the autonomic nervous system; (2) via **CRF,** stimulating the secretion of **adrenocorticotrophic hormone (ACTH)** from the anterior pituitary; (3) also via **CRF,** acting on the locus coeruleus, which increases CNS noradrenaline; (4) producing antidiuretic hormone **(ADH),** or **vasopressin,** and (5) stimulating the thyroid glands to produce **thyroxine.** To perform these tasks, the hypothalamus has two dedicated centers. One center stimulates sympathetic activity and the production of pituitary stress hormones.[3] The other center slows down sympathetic activity[4] and inhibits the production of pituitary stress hormones. Understanding these five functions is central to understanding how the stress response begins.

The Autonomic Nervous System

The autonomic nervous system (ANS) is the primary control system for three different types of tissues: cardiac muscle tissue, most glandular tissue, and all smooth muscle tissue (Pinel, 1993). The ANS controls heart activity, blood pressure, digestion, urinary and bowel elimination, and many other bodily functions. Control of the ANS comes from the brain stem, the hypothalamus, and the spinal cord.

The ANS is comprised of two parts, the parasympathetic nervous system and the sympathetic nervous system. These two systems exist in a state of dynamic but antagonistic tension. When one is active, the other is relatively quiet or passive. There are times, however, when both systems must be coactivated for certain processes to work (Berntson, Cacioppo, & Quigley, 1991). For example, extreme fear responses typically combine increases in heart rate and blood pressure (sympathetic control) with emptying bowels and bladder (parasympathetic control). Second, the male sexual response requires parasympathetic control for the erectile response, and sympathetic control for the ejaculatory response

The parasympathetic nervous system is in control when we are quiet and relaxed. Most of the positive reconstructive processes occur with parasympathetic dominance. Blood concentrates in central organs for such important work as digestion and storage of energy reserves. Breathing is typically slow and balanced. Heart rate slows, and blood pressure drops. Body temperature also drops, and muscle tension decreases.

The sympathetic nervous system is the fight-or-flight system. It springs into action during emergencies or during states of heightened emotionality. The alarm signal itself originates within the hypothalamus. Guyton (1977) identified eight effects of sympathetic arousal. Paraphrased, these are as follows:

1. Increased blood pressure
2. Increased blood flow to support large active muscles, coupled with decreased blood flow to internal (for example, digestive) organs not needed for rapid activity
3. Increased total energy consumption

---

[3]This center is called the posterior medial center, which means "toward the back and middle of the hypothalamus."

[4]This center is called the anterior lateral center, which means "to the front and side of the hypothalamus."

4. Increased blood glucose concentration
5. Increased energy release in muscles
6. Increased muscle strength
7. Increased mental activity
8. Increased rate of blood coagulation (pp. 600-601)

When the emergency is past, the hypothalamus recalls the parasympathetic system to dominance. Thus, the body begins to repair destructive effects from the emergency period.

You may have heard that you should not eat while angry and should engage only in pleasant conversation while eating. This is because anger changes salivary and digestive processes. Indigestion can occur because the body diverts blood from the stomach to support muscle tension during aroused emotional states. Other undesirable effects of prolonged sympathetic arousal include elevated blood pressure and ulcers.

The Master Gland

The master gland, or pituitary gland, secretes six important hormones (among numerous hormones) from its anterior region and two from its posterior section. The hypothalamus controls these hormonal secretions through its own secretions. One hormone, the **corticotropin-releasing factor (CRF),**[5] tells the anterior pituitary to release ACTH. Release of ACTH activates the adrenal glands. Almost any kind of stress, physical or psychosocial, will lead to a swift rise in the level of ACTH. One psychosocial stressor that typically triggers ACTH release is the death of a spouse or other loved one.

Shortly after ACTH release, the adrenals secrete several hormones, including **cortisol (hydrocortisone), epinephrine,** and **norepinephrine.** Cortisol provides more energy to the body through conversion of body stores into glucose and is a necessary part of the body's stress reaction. However, some stress conditions can lead to hypersecretions of cortisol, a process that can have negative consequences because of the **immune suppression** effect. Immune suppression reduces the number and effectiveness of lymphocytes (Dantzer & Kelley, 1989), which generally translates to less resistance to infections and disease. Further, immune suppression typically reduces the number of natural killer cells, cells that are specialized for tracking down cancer cells (Herbert & Cohen, 1993). These issues will be discussed in detail later. Figure 5-5 shows interactions within this system.

The other two hormones, epinephrine (also called **adrenaline**) and norepinephrine (also called **noradrenaline**), have the same general effect as the sympathetic nervous system. Output from the adrenal glands thus amplifies actions of the sympathetic nervous system. Epinephrine and norepinephrine levels vary with intensity of stimulation. Under conditions of severe stress, the body can be flooded with epinephrine and norepinephrine.

Epinephrine has a powerful effect on the heart. It increases both the rate and strength of the heart's contractions and raises blood pressure. By a feedback loop to the hypothalamus, epinephrine can increase secretions of ACTH and other hormones to even higher levels. This amplifies the effect of changes in other visceral systems and increases the level of activity in its own loop. This is why activation of the hypothalamic-pituitary-adrenal complex can have such powerful effects under conditions of prolonged stress.

---

[5]This is called corticotropin-releasing hormone (CRH) in some sources.

FIGURE 5-5
Stress excitation and adrenal inhibition in the hypothalamic-pituitary-adrenal complex.
SOURCE: Guyton (1977).

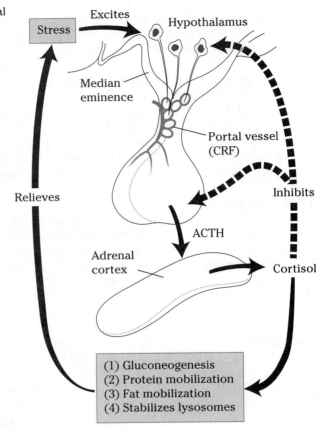

The brain is also extremely sensitive to the presence of another group of hormones called *adrenocorticosteroids*. These hormones can produce alterations in mental function, which in turn raise adrenocorticosteroid levels even higher. Under these conditions, people become more vulnerable to stress because they cannot deal effectively with daily problems (Riscalla, 1983).

For a short time, some psychologists believed they could link specific emotions to specific physical processes. In this view, love might be a specific neural-hormonal pattern that is the same for any person feeling love. Another emotion—for example, happiness—might be associated with a different neural-hormonal pattern. Up to now, the only consistent evidence of an association between a neural-hormonal pattern and a specific emotion involves epinephrine and norepinephrine. Epinephrine is present in greater amounts when fear occurs, whereas norepinephrine is present in greater amounts when anger occurs (Ax, 1953).

Recent research clarifies the roles of epinephrine and norepinephrine in stress reactions. Early work led researchers to believe that psychological stressors, such as mental arithmetic, continued vigilance, and public speaking, were all associated with increased levels of epinephrine in the bloodstream. Further, researchers suspected that norepinephrine increases with physical stressors such as physical restraint or immobilization (Tanaka et al., 1983), submersion in ice water (Aslan, Nelson, Carruthers, & Lader, 1981), isometric stress, and physical exercise. However, the evidence supporting this distinction—epinephrine-psychological stress, norepinephrine-physical stress—was often inconclusive, if not contradictory. More recent research has confirmed that this distinction is correct.

Ward and his team of Stanford researchers (1983) used a very sophisticated, continuous blood-sampling technique and a high-power statistical procedure called *time-series analysis* to do this. They also discovered the reason for the early confusing results. The researchers concluded that the two hormones behave very differently in their speed of reaction and the speed at which they clear out of the bloodstream. Epinephrine is fast-acting and leaves the bloodstream quickly. Norepinephrine clears out of the bloodstream much more slowly. When investigators mixed mental and physical tasks in testing procedures, norepinephrine was still present, especially when mental tasks came later. Thus, norepinephrine logically seemed related to mental stressors. But if the mental and physical stressors are tested at different times, it is clear that epinephrine increases with mental stressors and norepinephrine increases with physical stressors.

Research by Richard Dienstbier (1989) showed that exposure to intermittent stressors leads to a host of interrelated changes in the arousal complex. Dienstbier called these changes, which have positive effects for the organism, **physiological toughness,** a term adapted from Neal Miller's work. The first positive effect of these changes is to reduce the base rate for sympathetic operations. Remember that the usual outcome of stress is to activate or increase the level of the sympathetic system's operation. Dientsbier's research suggests that, after experience with intermittent stress, the body does not work as hard as before because of the reduced base rate for sympathetic nervous system activity. A second positive effect is that the sympathetic-adrenal-medullary complex can react more swiftly and strongly to challenge or threat. Third, brain catecholamines are not depleted as rapidly as when sympathetic nervous system activity is high. This is significant because depletion of catecholamines undermines mental and physical performances. The resulting deficits could be critical to successfully coping with stress. Further, catecholamine depletion may be one of the mechanisms involved in depression, and depression may complicate coping efforts in numerous ways. Finally, experience with intermittent stressors suppresses the pituitary-adrenal-cortical response. This can enhance immune-system function because an active pituitary-adrenal-cortical response typically increases cortisol levels and suppresses immune function.

Gold and his colleagues argue, however, that the catecholamine-depletion notion is too simplistic (Gold, Goodwin, & Chrousos, 1988a, 1988b). They showed that stressors can produce a long-term kindling and sensitization of neuronal response, thus impairing the normal feedback restraint on CRF. In their view, this lack of restraint on CRF leads to hypercortisolism, which leads to increased anxiety and other mood/behavioral disturbances commonly associated with depression. Taylor and Fishman (1988) concur with this position. They showed that CRF is a "central integrating signal" in the stress response.

Vasopressin

Vasopressin (ADH) is one of two major hormones produced in the hypothalamus but released by the posterior section of the pituitary gland. It regulates fluid loss through the urinary system. Most significantly, vasopressin influences heart activity and blood pressure. Receptors that feed information to the hypothalamus monitor both the volume and pressure of blood in the venous cavities of the heart. With low volume and pressure, vasopressin production increases. With high volume and pressure, vasopressin production decreases. In this way, the hypothalamic-pituitary system regulates the heart's output. Further, when blood pressure is low, vasopressin constricts arteries, thus causing blood pressure to increase. Traumatic injury is a severe biologic stressor that includes loss of blood volume. When traumatic injury occurs, ADH production increases immediately and dramatically to preserve pressure and restore volume. In addition, vasopressin can directly affect vasoconstriction. During severe stress, ADH can elevate already high blood pressure caused by other neural and hormonal processes (Blessing, Sved, & Reis, 1982).

Thyroid Glands and Thyroxine

Physical and psychological stress can have powerful effects on the rate of metabolism, the rate at which the body burns fuel. Changes in the metabolic rate influence mood, energy, nervous irritability, and mental alertness. Regulation of these changes is a three-step sequence. First, when psychosocial stress or strenuous physical exercise places a demand on the system, the hypothalamus releases a neural hormone called **thyrotropin-releasing factor (TRF).** Release of TRF stimulates the pituitary gland; then the pituitary signals the thyroid, which releases the hormone thyroxine. Second, as demand increases, TRF output increases, thus accelerating metabolic rate. Third, through a negative feedback circuit, the hypothalamus is able to adjust the level of TRF. When demand is past, TRF output decreases and metabolism reverts to normal.

A side effect of this sequence is that high levels of thyroxine make the system more responsive to adrenaline. Thus, another amplification effect occurs. The prevailing notion is that adrenaline is a short-term stress hormone, whereas thyroxine is a long-term stress hormone.

Other behavioral effects stem from high thyroxine levels. Mental activity heightens, and the person typically feels more nervous and anxious, always tired, yet achieving sleep only with great difficulty. Blood flow increases greatly, resulting in higher blood pressure. Usually, respiratory rate and intensity also increase. Finally, elevated secretions of gastric juices and stomach motility occur, with resulting diarrhea. These may be recognized as symptoms that occur during periods of stress.

NATURAL DEFENSES: THE IMMUNE SYSTEM

The immune system is second only to the CNS in sophistication and complexity (Heninger, 1995). Its one basic function is to help the body resist disease. *Immunity* is "the power of an individual to resist or overcome the effects of a particular disease or other harmful agent" (Memmler & Wood, 1977, p. 281). **Immunocompetence** is the degree to which the immune system is active and effective. When foreign agents (for example, poisons, germs, or toxic substances) invade the body, it defends itself by producing **antibodies** to attack and destroy the invaders. The body may also use its inherited immunity to fight battles against other agents, such as bacteria, viral infections, and blood poisons.

The immune system produces two types of cells, the **T-cell** and the **B-cell.** The thymus gland, sometimes called the "master organ" of the immune system, produces T-cells. T-cells provide **cellular immunity.** They fight bacterial infections (such as tuberculosis) as well as some viral infections. T-cells also attack cancer cells, fungi, and cells from transplanted organs. B-cells derive from bone marrow and provide **humoral immunity.**[6] They are responsible for antibody formation and can neutralize foreign agents (Nossal, 1987). Cellular immunity is often called the cell-mediated immune response, while humoral immunity is often called antibody-mediated response. Cell-mediated immune reactions are apparently more sensitive to stress than antibody-mediated reactions (Heninger, 1995).

Scientists generally regard the immune system as an autoregulated system working with minimal input from the CNS. The immune system's sole purpose is to recognize what is self and what is not-self, and then attack and kill not-self. Some changes in this view began to occur in the early 1980s. Robert Ader (1983) noted that "the immune system is integrated with other physiological systems and, like all such systems operating in the interests of homeostasis, is sensitive to regulation or modulation by the brain" (p. 251). Ader provided convincing evidence for (1) the influence of conditioning on the immune function; (2) the relation between psychosocial factors, such as life stress and immunocompetence; and (3) the relationship between use of psychoactive drugs and immunocompetence.

A new scientific discipline, **psychoneuroimmunology,** reflects the importance of this view. Psychoneuroimmunology seeks to uncover the intricate relations between psychosocial stressors and neural-immunologic systems that govern adaptive biologic response to stress (Jemmott, 1985).

Stress and the Immune System

Uncovering the processes that link stress and immunity has not been easy for scientific sleuths. Still, the work over the last 15 years has led to remarkable advances in understanding how stress can influence the immune system. Initially, researchers concluded that stress lowers the body's resistance to disease by suppressing the number of disease-fighting cells available. The net outcome for the person presumably would be an increase in the frequency or intensity of afflictions. Lowered resistance could also slow down recovery from existing disease. There are elements of truth in this representation, but more detail is required to understand the complex connections.

To begin, animal research showed that numerous stressors suppressed T cell circulation (Irwin & Livnat, 1987; Keller et al., 1981). One research team also showed that genetic factors influence immune response to stress (Irwin & Livnat, 1987). Abrupt changes in social contact increased tumor growth in laboratory mice (Sklar & Anisman, 1980). Observations of human reactions to stress generally confirm this result (Locke, Hurst, Heisel et al., 1978). Plaut and Friedman (1981), for example, showed that stress increased risk for contracting infectious diseases, allergic reactions, and autoimmune disease in humans. Stone's research team showed that antibody response is lower on days with high negative mood and higher on days with high positive mood (Stone et al., 1987). Other researchers showed

---

[6]A useful mnemonic is to simply remember that the connection is T-cell—thymus, and B-cell—bone marrow.

that grief after the death of a spouse (Bartrop et al., 1977) and after an abortion (Assael et al., 1981) can lower the number of lymphocytes available to fight disease. In sum, these results present a substantive argument for a stress-immune response interaction.

Research concerned with grief and immune suppression especially began to call into question the more simplistic views of stress and immune function. For example, a large-scale epidemiologic study looked at mortality in a group of parents whose sons died in war or in auto accidents (Levav, Friedlander, Kark, & Peritz, 1988). Death rates of this group of bereaved parents were no different from those of the general population. In fact, fathers who lost sons in war had lower mortality rates than those who lost sons in accidents. This suggests that the social context of stress can lead to very different outcomes.

Recent work has begun to focus on more careful examinations of specific stressors and specific immune illnesses. After an extensive review of viral infection studies and stress, Heninger (1995) found evidence that stress from negative life events is associated with impairment of immune function across seven different types of viruses.

One of the better controlled studies in this tradition was carried out by Sheldon Cohen's laboratory (Cohen, Tyrrell, & Smith, 1991). This project focused on stress, colds (rhinovirus), and the immune system. The project is exemplary for three reasons. First, it was a true experimental design that used a controlled virus challenge. Second, it collected medical and serological data on infections and colds over time using a prospective method while subjects were under direct control of the investigators. Third, it used meticulous controls to eliminate alternative explanations for the relationship between stress and immune response to cold viruses. Among the variables controlled were individual differences in immune system reactivity, recent prior exposure to a virus, recent negative changes in dietary behavior, loss of sleep and increased fatigue, and increased reliance on smoking to allay anxiety. It is possible that these health behavior changes could predict an immune illness better than stress.

Cohen's group used multiple measures of life stress, coping, and negative affect. Recall that negative affect is considered an important correlate of negative health outcomes. After participants completed all the psychosocial and biomedical tests, Cohen's team exposed the 420 subjects to one of five respiratory viruses, and quarantined them for seven days either singly or in pairs.

The outcome of Cohen's study (Figure 5-6) showed that the rates of infection and clinical colds increased in a dose-response manner: that is, the higher the stress-index score, the higher the rate of colds. However, stress levels were not related to increases in clinical colds among the previously infected. Thus, in Cohen's view, the link between stress and colds is primarily due to increased rates of infection among subjects with higher stress-index scores, not to increased frequency of cold symptoms following infection. This is an important distinction since it indicates that the alteration in the immune system occurs in response to stress even when the full-blown symptoms of a cold do not appear.

Robert Dantzer and Keith Kelley (1989) have cautioned against a simplistic view of immunosuppression. They believe that immune-system interactions with stressors are part of a long-loop regulatory feedback system that includes reciprocal influences. Dantzer and Kelley see this as a "true mechanism for communication between physiologic systems," as opposed to a fortuitous indirect effect. Because stress also can enhance immune function, it is important to understand the conditions under which either suppression or facilitation may occur. Dantzer and Kelley pointed out that the influence of stressors on the immune system depends on the nature, duration, and frequency of stressor events.

FIGURE 5-6

Exposure to cold virus challenge showed a relationship between stress and the rate of colds.

SOURCE: Cohen et al. (1991).

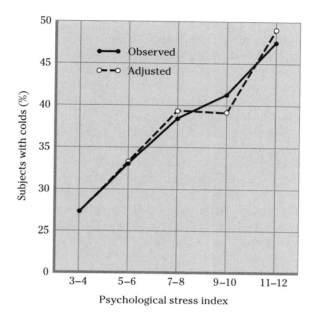

The Brain and Immune System

As evidence continues to accumulate, one major neural-hormonal axis emerges as crucial to CNS regulation of the immune system, and it also provides important clues in regard to the conditions related to immune activation versus suppression. This is the hypothalamic-pituitary-adrenal (HPA) complex. As shown earlier in Figure 5-5, when psychosocial stressors occur, a sequence of events called a neural cascade begins. First, higher cortical and limbic system analysis defines the stressor internally as a threat that requires a response. Signals sent to the hypothalamus initiate release of CRF, which directs the anterior pituitary to release ACTH. In response, the adrenal cortex secretes **glucocorticoids,** which are steroid hormones (cortisol, aldosterone, and desoxycorticosterone) that mobilize energy resources (raising blood glucose), combat inflammation, and promote healing by stimulating the immune system (Pinel, 1993).

One of these hormones—cortisol—has been the subject of intense study to determine its role in the stress response. Originally, cortisol was the designated bad guy, the hormone that seemed to produce negative effects in the immune system. In normal conditions and in a first response to mild stressors, the HPA complex seems to operate in what is called a permissive mode. Here, cortisol seems to have only a positive effect (Michelson et al., 1995). In this condition of lower activation, cortisol actually redirects energy and works through a negative feedback loop to restrain CNS stress reactions. Thus, a primary function of the glucocorticoid system is to contain the stress response so that it does not damage itself by extremes. In response to higher-level stressors, however, the HPA complex seems to operate in what is called a suppressive mode. Here, the glucocorticoids, including cortisol, begin to have a generally suppressive effect on the immune system that can increase vulnerability to illness.

A laboratory model using rats suggests another CNS mechanism that may explain how different types of stress may alter a part of the immune system. In this study at the University of California, Los Angeles (UCLA), investigators manipulated the predictability of the shock stressor (Shavit et al., 1984). They wanted to learn more about the role of **opioid peptides** in stress-related immune deficiency, especially as it related to **natural killer cells.** Opioid peptides are the brain's natural pain killers. Natural killer cells are a type of lymphocyte specialized to recognize and kill tumor cells and other foreign bodies.

In the UCLA study, two groups of rats received two different stress conditions. The crucial difference was that one group received shock on an unpredictable schedule (UPS) while the other group received shock continuously (CS). Both groups showed the expected analgesic-pain blocking response, but the UPS group blocked pain through activation of the natural opioid mechanism in the brain, a stress-induced analgesia. The UPS group also showed suppression of natural killer-cell activity in the opioid-analgesia group, but this did not occur in the CS group. The investigators concluded that the production of opioid peptides is one mechanism that mediates the relation between certain types of stress and suppression of natural killer cells.

Two critical factors in the relation of stress to immunity are chronicity and intensity (Ader, 1983). *Chronicity* refers to a condition that goes on seemingly without end. Under conditions of prolonged stress, the health-promoting response may become fatigued. The body could then exhaust the vital supply of adrenal hormones, and an impaired immune response may follow. This is a replay of Selye's (1956) stage concept of alarm, reaction, and exhaustion.

Intensity is the strength or power of a stressful condition, which admittedly depends in part on personal appraisal processes. The evidence now suggests that acute stressors imposed on top of a background of chronic high stress has the most detrimental effect on immune function (Heninger, 1995). Still, the effects vary by type of stress, and even the component of the immune system affected can be different.

Using a meta-analytic technique to review stress and immunity literature, Herbert and Cohen (1993) came to the following conclusions:

1. Objective stress events produce larger immune changes than self-reported stress.
2. The immune response varies with the duration of the stressor, with acute stressors generally increasing immunocompetence and chronic stressors generally impairing immunocompetence.
3. Interpersonal stressors result in different immune outcomes than nonsocial events. Although there is some conflicting evidence, it appears that interpersonal stressors, especially those that are chronic, produce a greater negative change in immune function than nonsocial stressors.

The Body at War with Itself

One side effect of the way the immune system works is the development of allergies. **Allergies** may be described as wars between special antibodies and external agents called **allergens.** The warfare results in the rupture of two different white blood cells and the release of toxic materials into the bloodstream. One of these materials is the substance histamine.

HIVES AND HAYFEVER The most common allergies are anaphylaxis, urticaria, **asthma,** and **hay fever.** Anaphylaxis, though rare, is extremely serious because it can lead to circulatory shock and death within a few minutes of onset. Urticaria is a type of anaphylaxis localized in the skin. The skin becomes inflamed and swollen, a condition most commonly called "hives." Hay fever occurs when the allergic reaction occurs in the nasal area, leading to increased capillary pressure and rapid fluid leakage into the nose. Physicians commonly prescribe **antihistamines** for both urticaria and hay fever because histamine is the primary cause of the difficulty. Antihistamines are not used for asthma because other products of the allergic reaction are involved.

In Japan, one research group provided evidence for the relation of stress to skin diseases (Teshima et al., 1982). Using a clinical sample, the investigators found that lifestyle changes and substantial daily stress preceded the appearance of urticaria. Lifestyle changes occurred most frequently in schools, residence, type of work, marriage, promotion, and so forth. The stressors most frequently experienced were overwork, interpersonal difficulties, or family difficulties. Autogenic training, a relaxation-imagery method described in Chapter 12, was effective in reducing the levels of histamine in the blood.

ASTHMA Asthma is "an intermittent, variable, and reversible obstruction of bronchial airways" (Pinkerton, Hughes, & Wenrich, 1982, p. 234). Asthma has received more attention than other allergies, probably because of the sheer number of asthma patients and the cost of treatment. Asthma afflicts possibly 12 million Americans and handicaps about 9 million of these. Annual costs in 1985 dollars reached about $4.5 billion (Weiss, Gergen, & Hodgson, 1992).

Many clinicians have speculated that psychological factors contribute to the etiology of allergic reactions such as urticaria and asthma. We discussed evidence on this issue in Chapter 4. Clinical studies suggested that hypnosis is useful in relieving these conditions, which supports the psychogenic argument (Hall, 1982-1983). There is still no convincing evidence, though, that either family stress or personality is important in the origin of asthma. Psychosocial factors might play a role in the day-to-day intensity of reaction. Evidence also shows that conditioning can affect the immune system. This might, then, produce an asthmatic attack. Again, there is no proof that such a mechanism exists. More importantly, behavioral treatment programs have had little or no success in treating asthma. Perhaps the most important observation is that lifestyle serves to intensify symptoms and/or defeat medical treatment. This suggests that psychological factors are mediators, not precipitators of asthma.

ACQUIRED IMMUNE DEFICIENCY SYNDROME No health issue of the recent past has demanded more attention than **acquired immune deficiency syndrome (AIDS).** Batchelor (1984) called AIDS "a modern-day black plague." **AIDS** is the name for a disease that does not itself kill but is nonetheless deadly. AIDS kills indirectly by threatening integrity of the immune system, the body's primary defense against bacterial, viral, and malignant diseases. Early in medicine's struggle to get control over AIDS, the Centers for Disease Control (CDC) referred to AIDS as a syndrome "characterized by opportunistic infections and malignant diseases in patients without a known cause for immunodeficiency" (cited in Seligman et al., 1984, p. 1286). Intensive research in the early 1980s uncovered the cause, a virus dubbed the HTLV-III/LAV. Later, an international committee christened it the **human immunodeficiency virus** or HIV (Coffin et al., 1986).

Just as the HIV does not kill directly, it does not destroy the immune system as one unfortunate early myth suggested. What it does is selectively attack the T_4 lymphocyte (CD4 T-cell), a white blood cell that is key to immune response (Burny, 1986). In simplified form, it works like this. The HIV is a **retrovirus** containing an enzyme that allows it to make a DNA copy of its own genetic material (Lee, 1989). It grabs on to host cells at vulnerable points and then takes over the cell by replicating its own code.

The T_4 lymphocyte cell has a large number of so-called CD4 receptors on the surface. These receptors are the Achilles heel of the T_4 cells. They are like handles the HIV can hold on to. Once attached to the cell, the HIV replicates itself and destroys the cell's function. As the HIV continues to infiltrate, it produces several abnormalities in the immune system. Probably the most notable change is impaired cellular immunity through reduction of helper T-cells. The complete story of how the HIV brings about destruction in the CD4 T-cells is not known, but biomedical research is looking at several mechanisms (Greene, 1991).

SELF-STUDY EXERCISE 5-2

Internet Multimedia Tour of AIDS and HIV
For a multimedia tour of the body with information on AIDS and HIV, log on this Webpage and follow the instructions:

http://www.thebody.com/cgi-bin/body.cgi

In the body, the effects may be seen in opportunistic infections such as PCP, pulmonary tuberculosis, meningitis, and cancers such as Kaposi's sarcoma and cervical cancer. Further, the infected lymphocyte cells migrate to the brain where the HIV has a specific affinity for CNS cells (Bridge, 1988). There, it can lead to CNS abnormalities that produce the AIDS dementia complex.

AIDS presents several serious problems for diagnosis, tracking progression, and treatment. It is a disease with a long latency, a large number of possible symptoms, and a period when the person is asymptomatic. Although the rate at which AIDS advances shows wide variability among people, there is nonetheless a typical steady progression toward more severe symptoms. The progression and prototypical time course has been mapped by Fauci, Pantaleo, Stanley, and Weissman (1996), as shown in Figure 5-7. Two markers are plotted, the gradual decline in CD4 T-cells and the presence of detectable virus in the blood. Immediately after the primary infection, CD4 T-cells drop by almost half and may be associated with acute HIV infections, the first signs that the AIDS virus is present. The fact that these first infections are acute (short in duration) may mislead people into believing the illness is just another common ailment. This is a sinister window of opportunity when the victim can unwittingly pass the HIV to others.

In the next stage, the immune system does mobilize a credible though weak response, and CD4 T-cells rebound against the HIV infection. Still, the presence of the virus is almost undetectable during this clinical latency period. The CD4 T-cell count then begins an irreversible decline and sooner or later reaches a threshold level below which the body can no longer resist the appearance of symptoms. The median length of this latency period is 10 years. From this point on, physical symptoms and opportunistic infections appear largely unchecked, and the time course to death is typically about two years.

FIGURE 5-7

Typical course of HIV infection showing the gradual decline in CD4 T-cells (dark circles) and the detectable presence of the virus in the blood (viremia).

SOURCE: Fauci et al. (1996).

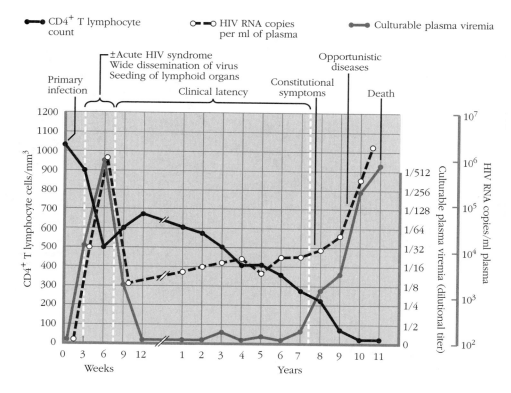

AIDS was unknown in the United States prior to 1977. It presumably entered with infected persons from Africa through Haiti (Bridge, 1988). Today, the disease has become more than an epidemic: it is **pandemic,** a disease that has spread throughout the world. Thus AIDS has earned the dubious distinction of being the first disease to engulf the entire globe. At first, there were few signs that AIDS could be controlled, but developments since about 1995 give renewed hope that control may be possible.

Some indication of the rapid growth in AIDS cases, but also encouraging signs of a reversal in trend, can be seen in Figure 5-8. At the end of 1981, there were only 398 total cases reported, but by the end of 1986, 41,518 adult U.S. cases had been reported. By the end of 1991, a total of 254, 826 AIDS cases and 155,899 deaths had been reported in the United States since the epidemic began in 1981. As of June 1997, there had been 604,176 cases and 374,656 deaths (Centers for Disease Control, 1997a).[7]

---

[7]This 16 years, from 1981 to 1997, is roughly comparable to the 16+ years of military engagement in Vietnam. During that time, 58,022 military personnel lost their lives. Reported loss of life from AIDS is nearly 6.5 times greater.

FIGURE 5-8

Estimated incidence of AIDS, AIDS-opportunistic illness (AIDS-OI) and deaths in persons with AIDS, adjusted for delays in reporting, by quarter-year of diagnosis/death, United States, 1984–1996.

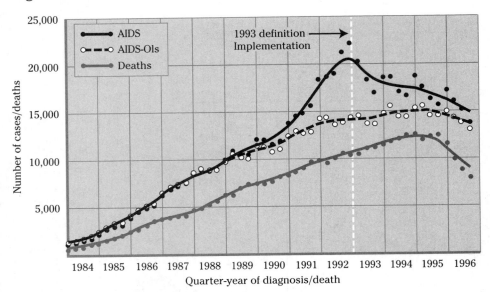

In the United States, AIDS is related to specific at-risk groups, primarily male homosexuals (47% of total AIDS cases) and intravenous drug abusers (21% of total AIDS cases). (See Figure 5-9.) Although these remain the high-risk groups, AIDS can be transmitted through heterosexual contact as well. Based on CDC statistics, heterosexual contact has accounted for 9% of total AIDS cases, but worldwide the figure is much higher (Centers for Disease Control, 1997a).

The common modes of AIDS transmission—high-risk sexual behavior, sharing needles and injecting drugs—suggest that AIDS is a behavioral disease that may respond to behavioral interventions. Various community-based and mass media intervention programs aimed at reducing these high-risk behaviors have shown some measure of success.

One ingredient receiving additional attention is alcohol use. Alcohol may impact AIDS either by altering immune system vulnerability or by increasing high-risk behaviors. (See the review by Dingle & Oei, 1997). Animal models show that alcohol does increase the vulnerability of human cells to risk for HIV infection, but evidence does not exist for a similar pattern in humans. In regard to the second issue, alcohol is thought to contribute to indiscriminate sexual activity that increases the risk of contracting and transmitting the disease. Although there is some data to support this claim, overall the evidence is weak.

At the outset, many fears about AIDS were based largely on ignorance of modes of transmission. Now substantial evidence exists that members of a family with an AIDS patient have little or no risk of infection (Friedland et al., 1986). Further, epidemiological

FIGURE 5-9
Distribution of AIDS cases by reported mode of exposure.

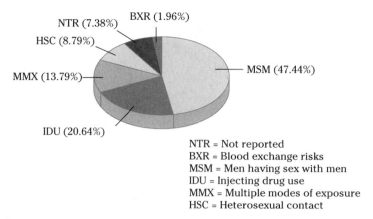

NTR (7.38%)   BXR (1.96%)
HSC (8.79%)
MMX (13.79%)   MSM (47.44%)
IDU (20.64%)

NTR = Not reported
BXR = Blood exchange risks
MSM = Men having sex with men
IDU = Injecting drug use
MMX = Multiple modes of exposure
HSC = Heterosexual contact

and clinical studies show that routine, nonsexual contact in offices, restaurants, or medical facilities does not transmit the virus. The virus is fragile and is easily killed by soaps and bleaches (Batchelor, 1988).

Still, there is what Herek and Glunt (1988) first called "an epidemic of stigma" that surrounds most AIDS patients. Anne Crawford's (1996) meta-analysis of stigma studies showed a greater degree of stigma associated with AIDS than with comparable illnesses. AIDS patients may experience forms of psychosocial stress due to reactions from friends and community. For example, members of the gay community suffered from heightened anxiety, panic attacks, loss of self-esteem, fear of isolation from friends and loved ones, and loss of self-sufficiency (Morin, Charles, & Malyon, 1984). For many, anxiety about the possible course of the disease combined with distress due to social reactions to their condition can be almost as difficult to deal with as the disease itself.

Research on psychosocial processes in immune function is also relevant. Kiecolt-Glaser and Glaser (1988) suggested that positive psychosocial factors may reduce the impact of the virus. Conversely, negative psychosocial factors (for example, the perception of high risk and lack of social support) may intensify the effect of AIDS. In such cases, a type of social victimization may be in process that subjects a person to negative consequences due largely to being part of one of society's less-favored groups.

THE CARDIOVASCULAR SYSTEM

The heart is a miracle organ by any standard. It works day and night, seldom missing a beat as it pumps life-giving blood through the entire body. The pulse rate of a newborn child is around 120 to 140 beats per minute. In the mature adult, the heart beats 60 to 70 times per minute. At this rate, the average heart beats 3900 times per hour, or 93,600 beats each day. During light exercise, the pulse rate can rise to around 100, and in strenuous exercise it can go much higher. Astronauts have pulse rates around 140 beats per minute during the most stressful periods of liftoff and reentry.

Stress and the Heart

Biomedical research has devoted much attention to the physical origins of heart failure. Now, more attention has shifted to psychosocial factors and lifestyle forces that contribute to cardiovascular problems. The major focuses are on stress, personality (TABP), diet, exercise, and abstinence or temperance from the use of addictive drugs. Here we will examine the effect of stress in elevating blood pressure and increasing the pace of atherosclerosis.

Hypertension

Hypertension is an elevation in blood pressure above accepted levels, no matter what produced it. This is the usual diagnosis given when systolic blood pressure exceeds 160 and diastolic exceeds 120. Yet even slight increases in blood pressure over 140/90 predict increased risk of premature death (Taylor & Fortmann, 1983). Serious danger exists when systolic pressure reaches 200.[8] **Essential hypertension** is the term given to hypertension of unknown origins. It may be due to higher peripheral resistance or increased cardiac output (Taylor & Fortman, 1983). Activation of the sympathetic nervous system, as in stress-anxiety reactions, increases cardiac output, resulting in an increase in blood pressure. Under normal circumstances this condition will last only a matter of hours. With continued sympathetic arousal and prolonged constriction of the arteries supplying the kidneys, long-term hypertension may appear.

In addition to sympathetic arousal, control from the HPA complex initiates release of epinephrine and norepinephrine, along with renin from the kidneys. In addition to increasing cardiac output and elevating blood pressure, adrenaline and noradrenaline speed up the rate of damage to the arteries. Renin is a chemical that stimulates production of a peptide called *angiotensin*, "the most potent vasoconstrictor known" (Guyton, 1977, p. 231). The presence of these three hormones duplicates and amplifies the effect of sympathetic arousal. Thus, cardiac output and blood pressure can increase to even higher levels than with sympathetic arousal alone.

Taylor and Fortmann (1983) suggested that hypertension should be viewed in a systems context. This position suggests that single-cause models of hypertension are inadequate, given ample evidence of multiple biologic systems that interact in different ways to produce high blood pressure.

Research also has considered how genetic/constitutional factors influence hypertension and stress reactions. In one study, people with a family history of hypertension showed higher resting systolic and diastolic blood pressure compared with those with no family history of hypertension (Jorgensen & Houston, 1989). These investigators also observed higher systolic blood pressure and diastolic blood pressure under conditions of laboratory stress. The link to life-event stress, though, was different for men and women. Men showed higher resting systolic pressure with more negative stress events. Women showed higher resting systolic pressure with fewer negative events. Catherine Stoney and her colleagues reviewed several studies that point to a sex difference linking physiological reactivity to stress and coronary heart disease (Stoney, Davis, & Matthews, 1987). Greenberg and Shapiro (1987) showed that stressors combined with caffeine had an additive effect in raising blood pressure that was not dose-dependent. Systolic pressures were higher in subjects from families with a history of hypertension, but this did not change in response to caffeine.

---

[8]Blood pressure measured at peak heart output is the *systolic* pressure, and measured at the resting phase of the heart is *diastolic* pressure. In the normal heart, these pressures are 120/80, respectively.

The medical treatment of hypertension typically follows a stepped-care, antihypertensive medication program. Patients also make lifestyle changes that include diet, weight control, and relaxation methods designed to offset stress (Taylor & Fortmann, 1983). McCaffrey and Blanchard (1985) reviewed stress management approaches to the treatment of essential hypertension. They concluded that pharmacotherapy is clearly superior to stress management therapy. Despite the usefulness of stress management therapy, few would ever consider treating essential hypertension in isolation from pharmacological interventions.

Atherosclerosis

In medical terms, **atherosclerosis** is a disease of the large arteries "in which yellowish patches of fat are deposited, forming plaques that decrease the size of the [opening]" (Memmler & Wood, 1977, p. 299). The yellowish patches of fat, called *arterial plaques,* are deposits of cholesterol and other lipids. A variety of factors, including genetic risk, diet, lack of exercise, and stress, can all contribute to the formation of arterial plaques. Rosenman and Friedman (1974) were among the first to note the relation between stressful events and the appearance of cholesterol. They reported that tax accountants in the two weeks before the April 15 income tax deadline had greatly increased serum cholesterol levels compared with levels in either February or March.

Several aspects of the stress response influence risk for atherosclerosis. First, stress activates the HPA complex and arouses the fight-or-flight response under sympathetic control. Further, the system increases circulating catecholamines, or stress hormones that also act to prepare the system for emergency. This arousal elevates heart rate and blood pressure, increases blood volume to peripheral muscles, and raises respiration rate. Prolonged stress hastens damage to the arterial walls. Where atherosclerosis is already present, the system is less resilient to stress.

Behavioral interventions to reduce coronary risk may be effective in both young and old. Heather Walter and her colleagues conducted a five-year school-based intervention with a large sample of children in and around New York City (Walter, Hofman, Vaughan, & Wynder, 1988). They found that changes in dietary intake and health knowledge occurred during the study. The positive effects on blood cholesterol were small but significant in one school system, and favorable but not significant in the other school system. Further research suggested there is some benefit to lowering cholesterol even after myocardial infarction (Rossouw, 1990). Patients with symptoms of coronary disease have a relative risk five to seven times higher than those without signs of coronary disease. Although prevention of coronary disease in the normal population is important, this research program suggested that risk factors are equally modifiable before and after myocardial infarction.

Another effect of stress and sympathetic arousal is the increase of the tendency for blood to coagulate. Even when no injury has occurred, the effect in the bloodstream is the same. There is a buildup of blood platelets (also called *thrombocytes*), which become part of the arterial plaques. Because plaques reduce the physical space that blood has to pass through, pressure increases. Plaques also cause a breakdown in the wall of the artery itself. The body then tries to repair this breakdown. The platelets, rather than helping in this process, contribute to the problem by making the plaques even thicker. At this point, it is mostly irrelevant how the plaques got there. Stress only adds to the problem.

In the later stages of atherosclerosis, fibrous cells also infiltrate the plaques and add to the scar tissue on the artery wall. Calcium deposits further harden the cell walls and narrow the corridor. Blood must be squeezed through a much smaller space than normal, and the heart must work even harder to produce blood flow. Just as a weight lifter develops larger muscles with increasing workouts, heart muscle also grows as it works harder. Unfortunately, heart muscle grows faster than the supply network that keeps blood flowing to the heart. The muscle that pumps blood to the rest of the body does not have enough of its own resource to stay healthy, a condition called *myocardial ischemia*. Rozanski's (1988) research group observed irregular ventricular-wall motion during mental-stress tasks. They concluded that personally relevant stress may precipitate myocardial ischemia in coronary-artery–disease patients.

THE DIGESTIVE SYSTEM AND ULCERS

One of the early conclusions of Selye's research was that stress can have disastrous effects on the digestive system, including perforated ulcers and death. The executive-monkey study convincingly showed this. Many other observations support the notion that psychosocial factors contribute to the origin of ulcers. Urban populations have a higher prevalence of ulcers than rural populations; for example, the prevalence of ulcers increases in wartime. Certain occupational groups with higher levels of psychological stress, such as air-traffic controllers, are also more prone to ulcers (Pinkerton, Hughes, & Wenrich, 1982).

There are several different types of ulcers. **Peptic ulcers** occur when excess amounts of gastric juices are used to digest food. Figure 5-10 shows how a peptic ulcer originates and develops. In the absence of neutralizing secretions, these juices attack the stomach lining. The result is irritation, bleeding, and in severe cases, a break in the stomach wall itself. In sum, peptic ulcers result when acidity and peptic activity overpower mucosal defense (Soll, 1990).

Peptic ulcers may be of three types: the acute, the chronic, or the so-called stress ulcer. There are probably several physical causes for the stress ulcer. The most likely include excess production of hydrochloric acid and pepsin under control of the parasympathetic system, and excess secretion of adrenal hormones under the control of the HPA

FIGURE 5-10
Model of the pathogenesis of peptic ulcer.
SOURCE: Soll (1990).

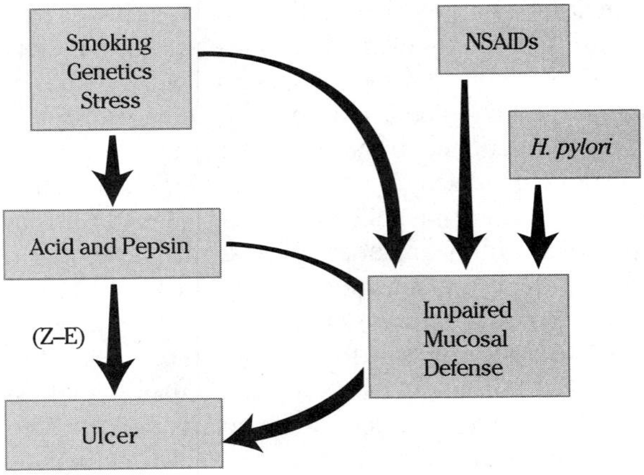

complex. Nonsteroidal anti-inflammatory drugs (NSAIDs) irritate the stomach lining; but aspirin is probably the worst barrier breaker (Soll, 1990).

Gastric ulcers are deeper erosions in the stomach lining. They occur most frequently on the bottom curved surface of the stomach, just below the outlet to the intestines. They can be caused by excessive use of aspirin and alcohol. They may also result from chronic anxiety and depression (Stephens, 1980).

SUMMARY

In this chapter, we have seen how the brain translates emotional or stressful stimuli into specific physical processes. Most of the time, these processes work to our benefit, but under prolonged stress, they may prove to be detrimental to our health. The major points made in the course of the chapter are summarized below.

- Mind and body must work together to produce the kind of outcomes that occur under stress. This suggests that mind is nothing more than the brain at work when we are thinking, feeling, and responding.
- When confronted by a stressor event, the brain swings into action quickly. It uses interpretive processes to assign meaning to the event and begins to marshall energy reserves to meet the challenge.
- The brain is divided into two major subdivisions, the peripheral nervous system (PNS) and the central nervous system (CNS). The PNS is subdivided into the autonomic nervous system and the somatic nervous system.
- The autonomic nervous system works to maintain homestasis, or a balance between energy conserving (parasympatheic) and energy expending (sympathetic). When emergencies occur, the sympathetic system springs into action to help in the fight-or-flight response.
- The brainstem contains most of the life support systems such as respiration and cardiovascular activity. It can force these systems to higher activity under stressful conditions, such as anxiety hyperventilation.
- One core system in the stress response is the hypothalamic-pituitary-adrenal (HPA) complex, which mobilizes the body's natural defenses to fight the stress.
- A second core system is the sympathetic-adrenal medullary (SAM) system. The SAM system duplicates or mimics some of the activities of the HPA system including increasing heart rate, cardiac volume, increased blood pressure, respiration, and so forth.
- One possible negative consequence of prolonged stress is flooding with cortisol, one of the stress glucocorticoids. This may suppress the immune system and increase vulnerability to illnesses.
- Immunocompetence is the ability of the system to ward off disease through its production of T-cells and B-cells.
- Prolonged stress may also accelerate wear and tear on the heart through increased blood pressure and increased plaque formation.
- Continued stress may alter the operations of the digestive system leading to a breakdown in the stomach or intestinal lining. If not treated properly, ulcers can occur.

CRITICAL THINKING AND STUDY QUESTIONS

1. Describe the overall sequence of events from a first encounter with a stimulus (one that may or may not be stressful) through the brain's neurochemical response leading to an external behavior.
2. What are the primary functions of the sympathetic and parasympathetic systems, and how do they operate in relation to each other?
3. How does the HPA complex respond to a stressful event?
4. How does the SAM complex respond to a stressful event?
5. Describe the effects of stress on the (1) immune system; (2) cardiovascular system; and (3) digestive system.

KEY TERMS

acquired immune
   deficiency
   syndrome (AIDS)
adrenocorticotrophic
   hormone (ACTH)
allergens
allergies
amygdala
antibodies
antihistamines
anxiety hyperventilation
asthma
atherosclerosis
autonomic nervous
   system (ANS)
B-cell
brain stem
cellular immunity
central nervous system
   (CNS)
corticotropin-releasing
   factor (CRF)
cortisol (hydrocortisone)
endorphins

epinephrine
   (adrenaline)
essential hypertension
gastric ulcers
glucocorticoids
hay fever
hippocampus
humoral immunity
hypertension
hypothalamus
immune suppresion
immune system
immunocompetence
limbic system
medulla
mind
natural killer cells
neuroanatomists
norepinephrine
   (noradrenaline)
opioid peptides
parasympathetic nervous
   system
nervous system

pandemic
peptic ulcers
peripheral nervous
   system (PNS)
physiological toughness
pituitary gland (master
   gland)
psychoneuroimmunology
reticular formation (RF)
retrovirus
somatic nervous system
   (SNS)
sympathetic nervous
   system
T-cell
thalamus
thyrotropin-releasing
   factor (TRF)
thyroxine
vasopressin (ADH)
visceral brain

WEBSITES the physiology of stress: the brain, body, and immune systems

URL ADDRESS	SITE NAME & DESCRIPTION
http://www.med.harvard.edu/AANLIB/home.html	☆Whole Brain Atlas, from the Harvard Medical School
http://www.mic.ki.se/Diseases/index.html	A top site for AIDS information
http://www.teachhealth.com	Medical basis of stress
http://www.thebody.com/cgi-bin/body.cgi	☆The Body: A Multimedia AIDS and HIV Information Resource
http://www.healthseek.com	Searchable database with a huge selection of stress materials
http://www.psy.aau.dk/bobby/pni.htm	Resources for psychoneuroimmunology

PART THREE

Social Systems and Stress

CHAPTERS

CHAPTER 6

Stress in the Family:

Adjustment, Conflict, and Disruption

Most of the complaints about the institution of holy matrimony arise not because it is worse than the rest of life, but because it is not incomparably better.

JOHN LEVY AND RUTH MUNROE

<table>
<tr>
<td>

OUTLINE

</td>
<td>

QUESTIONS

</td>
</tr>
<tr>
<td>

Focus on the Family

SELF-STUDY EXERCISE 6-1

A Case Study in Family Stress

Family Stress: Problems in Definition

A Transactional Theory of Family Stress

Transitional Stress

Separation and Divorce

The Single-Parent Family

Violence in the Family

Battered Wives

Sexual Abuse of Children

Positive Coping in the Family

</td>
<td>

• How do individual stress reactions differ from a family stress reaction?

• How should we define family stress?

• Is a transactional theory applicable to family stress?

• What are the unique stressors that occur in family transitions?

• What specific stressors occur for those going through separation and divorce?

• What stressors do single parents typically encounter?

• What are the contributing factors to violence, abuse, and neglect in families?

• What are the physical and psychological signs of sexual abuse?

• How can families deal with stressors in more positive ways?

</td>
</tr>
</table>

The winter of 1996–97 was a harsh one on the great northern plains. Blizzards rolled like waves, one after another, over the Dakotas, dumping nearly 120 inches of snow. Some homes looked like snow cocoons as they were literally wrapped—along with the people in them—in drifts as high as the rooftops. If this were a ski resort in the Colorado Rockies or Utah's Wasatch range, it would be a winter paradise. Instead it was just a prelude to a flood of near biblical proportions. The water rose to nearly 54 feet, more than 25 feet above flood stage, and when the levee system protecting Grand Forks, North Dakota, gave way on April 17, it was the beginning of a period of great loss and instability for many families. Nearly 75% of the city (about 40,000 people) had to be evacuated, many never to return to their homes, their neighbors, and neighborhoods as they were before.

Sheryl Adams and her husband faced enough difficulty even before the flood. Sheryl was near the end of her term with a difficult pregnancy that required regular medical supervision. They were expecting triplets and knew that the time of delivery could be especially risky for her and the babies. However, the Grand Forks flooding closed down the local hospitals, and any patients who needed continued care were relocated to other hospitals in the region. Doctors were unable to provide specialized and high-tech care to many people, like Sheryl, who could require it at a moment's notice.

The only reasonable solution for Sheryl was to relocate to Fargo, nearly 80 miles away, where medical services continued in spite of record flood levels. There she could wait, guaranteed not only continuing medical supervision of the pregnancy, but also quick access to the hospital when the time for the babies' delivery arrived. There was just one problem: they did not have the funds to afford rental for an uncertain time. Her story was told on television newscasts up and down the Red River valley, and within an hour, Sheryl had received hundreds of calls and offers of places to stay or support to arrange for accommodations. The happy ending of the story was the delivery of three healthy babies and the beginning of the road to a more normal family life.

Family stress does not always come in large doses as it did for Sheryl. Still, family stress is a problem of substantial proportions. This chapter provides a perspective on what we know about stress in the family, about family coping strategies, and about how networks of support can help the family survive. First, some working definitions will be presented, followed by the description of a comprehensive theory of family stress. Later, stress from marital disruption, child abuse, and sexual abuse will be discussed. Finally, this chapter will present some coping and problem-solving strategies for the family.

FOCUS ON THE FAMILY

Most research on stress and health has focused on the variety and quality of *individual* reactions to stressors. It is now apparent that this approach has limits. Stress is seldom, if ever, an isolated event affecting only one person in one remote situation. Stress often envelops the family in both destructive and constructive ways. Stress spills over from the job, children bring it home from the classroom, and social events originate stress that ends up at home.

A search for the sources of stress in the family is a search for the interplay of forces between the family unit and its members. The appearance of stress in any family member is likely to alter a family's functioning during the time stress is present. On the other hand, the way a family unit responds to stress affects the burden each family member carries. Consider a family that has suffered severe economic loss. Ideally, family leaders keep their emotions in check and use rational problem-solving behavior. Some leaders, though, may display hysterical, irrational, and "catastrophizing" behavior (Ellis, 1962). The rest of the family may then interpret the situation as much worse than it really is. More vulnerable family members, such as very young children, may develop feelings of anxiety and insecurity. Worse yet, they may learn that this behavior is the "adult" way to respond to stressors and then carry that style with them into adult life.

The family is a fertile ground for the emergence of stress as well as for stress-spillover effects. The family cycle has distinct phases—mate selection, marital adjustment, family planning, childbearing, child rearing, career decline, and retirement. Each phase has its unique joys and sorrows, harmony and stress, from the first breath of commitment to the dying breath of a spouse. Later in this chapter, I will outline some of these stage stressors. For the interested reader, I have included references that provide coverage of stress in marriage and the family (Aldwin, 1994; Boss, 1988; Curran, 1987; Elkind, 1994; Menaghan, 1982).

Finally, attempts to resolve stress normally occur first at home. People usually do not seek outside help until after personal resources fail and the home no longer provides solace and solution. It is more customary for a spouse or parent to serve as confidant to the stressed member. Unfortunately, the person under stress may "unload" problems in an emotional outburst. In other cases, the person cannot open up about the internal conflict, but he or she carries the burden so visibly that it affects other family members.

Involvement in one member's stress may consume so much energy and family resources that the entire family becomes distressed and maladjusted. When this happens, it is unlikely that anyone can obtain the support needed to bear the strain and resolve feelings of helplessness, guilt, loneliness, neglect, or anger. The long-term effects of stress in the family are exemplified by what has been happening recently in farm families (Conger & Elder, 1994).

SELF-STUDY EXERCISE 6-1

Identifying Family Stress

Respond to the following statements about family situations as either true or false. If you are in a committed relationship, respond in terms of that relationship. If you are not in a committed relationship, respond as you best remember your family life as you were growing up. After responding, look at the end of the chapter for information on the issues addressed.

1. We always seem to be fighting about money and budget matters.	T or F
2. The children always seem to be fighting about something.	T or F
3. Overall management of the household is pretty evenly divided among family members, and everyone shares in chores.	T or F
4. I never seem to have enough time for myself.	T or F
5. There is not enough time for all the different duties that have to be attended to.	T or F
6. My significant other and I never seem to have time for each other.	T or F
7. We both seem to be pretty tired by the time the work day is done and necessary household chores are finished.	T or F
8. Although I work and work, I don't seem to be accomplishing the things I really wanted to accomplish.	T or F
9. We typically lay out everything we need for ourselves and the children before we go to bed.	T or F
10. There seems to be difficulty communicating with each other on important matters.	T or F
11. Instead of not having enough to do, we seem to be on the go all the time.	T or F
12. The children pretty much set their own bedtime schedule.	T or F

A CASE STUDY IN FAMILY STRESS

For many American farmers, the past two decades have seen frustration, unsteady prices for commodities, increasing production costs, staggering indebtedness, foreclosures, and the death of the family farm. Projections in one state suggested that 40% of its farmers could lose their farms. While the economic load carried by the head of the family in these cases is immense, the emotional load apparently can be unbearable. The prospect of loss is more than just economic. It is psychological and social, a personal failure witnessed by the entire extended family. Many farms have been "in the family" for years. Loss of the farm signifies a separation, an enforced detachment, from all that has carried family pride and tradition for years. In one Iowa community of 8000, three farmers committed suicide within 18 months because of despair over the prospect of losing their farms (Turkington, 1985).

Family members suffer emotionally as well. Some members, especially the children, have little or no direct control over the situation and no responsibility for the origins of the difficulty. They become victims of the family disruption. The incidence of depression, poor schoolwork, and suicide among children of farm families has increased with pressures on the family. The problems described here, though, are not necessarily confined to the farm family. The types of stressors vary from rural to suburban families, but the general outcome is much the same.

One body of evidence supports the notion that stress in the family increases vulnerability of individual members to physical and emotional distress (Bloom, Asher, & White, 1978). On the other hand, numerous factors unique to the family increase resistance to distress. One benefit found in a family's support for its members is the **social buffer** it provides against the storms and stresses of daily life (Cobb, 1976). Early theory suggested that the presence of social buffers might have a direct, positive effect on coping. More recent analyses suggest that lack of social support is the key factor because its absence interferes with adjustment (Walker, 1985). Whichever occurs—vulnerability or resistance—depends on the psychosocial traits of family members, the dynamics of family interactions and communications, and the problem-solving strategies established by the family.

FAMILY STRESS: PROBLEMS IN DEFINITION

To this point, I have not used the term **family stress** as some authors have used it (McCubbin et al., 1980), because the previous definition of stress is not wholly appropriate when referring to groups. A group of people cannot experience stress the same way an individual does. Qualitative differences exist that require different levels of analysis and different intervention strategies.

Personal Versus Family Stress

First, it seems intuitively acceptable to say that a family is under stress. Everyday language frequently uses just this type of expression. One example came from the 17-day ordeal following the hijacking of TWA Flight 847 from Athens, Greece. Televised interviews with families who had husbands or brothers still held hostage amply documented the fear, torment, frustration, and anger many of the families felt. In a similar vein, studies of families who lost loved ones, homes, or investments through natural catastrophes (Hurricane Andrew) or disasters caused by humans (the Oklahoma City bombing) show the terrible stress families sometimes have to endure. Few would quibble with the notion that families in any of these situations are families under stress.

Still, a problem exists when we use the concept of stress this way. Simply put, we speak of families under stress, but individuals are the ones who really grieve and become depressed, frustrated, or angry. Family-stress theory thus straddles a fence between "the hazard of blatant reductionism to the level of individual behavior" and "the hazard of assuming that groups have the properties of individuals" (Klein, 1983, p. 93). We need to shift our focus, then, from the personal system to the **family as system**—a set of connected elements that function as a whole, yet a unit that can be disrupted.

Family is a descriptive term that refers to a unique social cluster of persons who enjoy a special relationship through love, mutual commitment, and reciprocal dependence. Traditionally, a family has formed through marriage and extended itself through procreation, but nontraditional families share many features of traditional families. Families share common goals and values. They work cooperatively to realize their goals and usually become more closely united when threats to family integrity appear.

To meet family needs, the system has adult leaders and child followers. There is a parallel division of teachers and learners. Usually, some division of labor exists for productive earning and household management. Stress on the family may cause the system to malfunction, disrupting harmony and destroying the organization of the family. Family leaders may experience more difficulty managing family resources. Earning

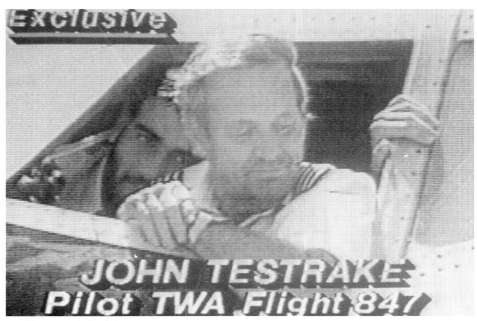

Captain John Testrake under the gun of a hijacker, while the world, including families of the crew and passengers, watched.

productivity may decrease, and the child's socialization may stop. When this happens, the family is a maladaptive system. On the other hand, a family that functions as an organized, coherent, and integrated unit is an adaptive system.

To summarize, family and personal stress are qualitatively different. Individuals experience emotional distress, but families suffer a loss of harmony. Individuals suffer from lack of concentration and loss of fluid thinking, but families experience reduced resources for collective problem solving. Individuals suffer from ulcers or migraines, but families break up through separation or divorce. For individuals, stress is an insult to a biopsychological system. For families, stress is an insult to a social system.

Stressors, Stress, and Crises

Several authors use stress definitions that recognize differences between personal and family stress. McCubbin and Patterson (1983, p. 8) defined **stressor** as "a life event or transition impacting upon the family unit which produces, or has the potential of producing, change in the family social system." The death of a parent, long-term hospitalization of a family member, loss of income, departure of a family member to military service, or imprisonment of a family member all qualify as stressors in this view.

The same authors define stress in terms of the family's response to an event. That response depends on how the family interprets or assigns meaning to the event and on the seriousness of the threat. Finally, McCubbin and Patterson define a **crisis** or **distress** as the disorganization or incapacity that results from the family's lack of resources and problem-solving skills to manage the stress.

A TRANSACTIONAL THEORY OF FAMILY STRESS

Although numerous family-stress theories exist, Reuben Hill (1949) provided one of the most comprehensive. To its credit, the model is still highly respected and continues to evolve (Patterson & Garwick, 1994). The theory's sterile title—**ABCX Model**—obscures its basic message: Some *event* (**A**) interacts with the family's *resources* for meeting crises (**B**), and with the family's *definition* of the event (**C**), to produce a *crisis* (**X**). Later, the ABCX model became the double ABCX model when it was extended to include the family's perception of other stressors and family resources (McCubbin & Patterson, 1983). More recently, Patterson (1989) dubbed it The **F**amily **A**djustment and **A**daptation **R**esponse (FAAR) Model with an emphasis on positive adaptation processes within the family.

It is noteworthy that the FAAR model parallels the cognitive-transactional model of personal stress proposed by Lazarus (1993). In the family, a stressor exists only if the family has appraised (defined) the event as threatening and the family's resources (secondary appraisal) are inadequate to meet the demands. Table 6-1 lists the essential features of this theory and compares it to theories introduced later, a systems theory and a cognitive-contextual theory.

Components of Family Stress and Coping

The original ABCX model had three core notions: *amount of change, family vulnerability,* and *family appraisal*. Figure 6-1 shows the general model. **Amount of change** is the degree of adaptive change in the family required to meet the demands of the stressor event.

TABLE 6-1
Summary of three theories of family stress

STRESS MODEL	DEFINITION OF STRESS	SOURCE(S) OF STRESS	MODEL'S STRENGTHS	MODEL'S WEAKNESSES
FAAR model	An event that interacts with resources and appraisals to produce a crisis	Various events that require family adjustment	Parallels the interactional model Some empirical support Potential to be a comprehensive theory	Still largely theoretical/speculative Difficult to give terms operational reference Concept of family appraisal is problematic as are levels of meaning
Systems theory	No definition given	Family violence and marital conflict	Indirect but large body of supporting evidence Compatible with other, more comprehensive theories	Primarily developed to explain family violence Limited in scope Difficult to give terms operational reference
Cognitive-contextual theory	No definition given	Parental conflict	Parallels and complements the interactional model	Primarily developed for one type of family stress Limited in scope

Death of the major wage earner produces a substantial change in the family structure, as does divorce. Less dramatic but still powerful is the change produced when the major wage earner takes an assignment that involves relocating the family to a new city. Conversely, imprisonment of a family member might be *welcomed* (and require little if any change), if it removes a child molester or spouse beater from the home. Thus, the influence of change is still dependent on how the family appraises or defines the change.

Charles Figley (1993) studied stress in military families during the Persian Gulf War. He noted that military mobilization often gives families very little notice of activation and precious little time to set personal and family affairs in order beforehand. Single parents may have to quickly arrange for child care, while a parent left behind may have to do likewise—as well as look for temporary work. There is also an assortment of legal matters necessary to these situations, which most civilians are unaware of. The departing family member typically has to make sure that a will and power of attorney are complete or up-to-date so that important matters can be dealt with correctly in the event of death or incapacity. Young children typically do not understand the urgency of national needs

FIGURE 6–1
FAAR model of family stress.
SOURCE: Adapted from McCubben & Patterson (1983).

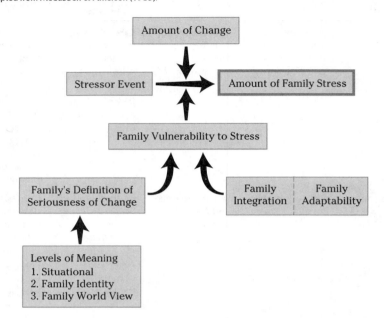

when weighed against their own perception of the tension in the adults around them and their feelings of being abandoned. In so many ways, then, the family subject to military call-up can be under tremendous pressure for change. On a positive note, stress from family disruption tends to subside quickly upon return to normal (Rosen, 1995), although the returning member may still bring emotional baggage home that continues to produce problems in the family.

FAMILY VULNERABILITY The second factor, **family vulnerability,** is the degree to which the family is defenseless or open to insult, injury, and disruption. Families in the path of the Red River flood were at risk in a variety of ways, but those with little insurance and few financial resources were more vulnerable. Sheryl's family was even more vulnerable at this particular time because of a difficult pregnancy, loss of medical support, and few financial resources. It is easy to see, then, that stressors interact with family vulnerability to produce a crisis. Assuming that vulnerability is constant, the more threatening an event is, the more likely the family will have a crisis on its hands. Similarly, holding threat constant, the more vulnerable the family, the more likely the family will experience stress. This relationship holds true when the event produces short-term or acute stress. Still, small stressors can pile up, or one milder stressor can become chronic. This may be likened to the proverbial "straw that broke the camel's back." Then, the effect is the same as that of a severe short-term stressor.

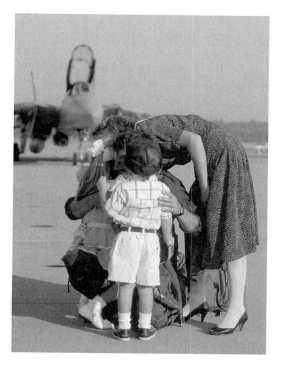

The Gulf War split up families for varying periods of time and required substantial adjustments. In many cases, the adjustments are just as significant after a military operation as they are during the operation.

FAMILY APPRAISALS Numerous factors contribute to family vulnerability. As Figure 6-1 shows, the family's definition, or **appraisal,** of the seriousness of the change, combined with family integration and adaptability, lead to vulnerability. The family's definition of seriousness combines personal assessments (what the change means to each person individually) and group assessments (what the change means to the family as a social unit). The actual stress felt by any member probably depends on his or her personal awareness of the implications of the change. In addition, individual stress may depend on the extent to which the person can influence or help alter the course of the stressor event or reduce the impact of the change.

Continuing refinement of the FAAR model, Patterson and Garwick (1994) break down the family's definition of a stressor into three levels of meaning: situational, family identity, and family world view. In their words, "family meanings are the interpretations, images, and views that have been collectively constructed by family members as they interact with each other" (p. 288). In the context of coping with a chronically ill child, Patterson and Garwick report that it is not uncommon for parents to focus on positive aspects of their child while minimizing the difficulties or limitations imposed by the illness. They see the child's tenacity and the family's resilience in the face of overwhelming odds. They see growth in their own coping skills, and strengths in siblings that might not otherwise have bloomed. This is the family's situational meaning, their social construction of reality related to the pressure of caring for their child.

At the second level of meaning, family identity, the family carries out rituals that define who the family is as a unit. These rituals, though not always deliberately acted out and even in some cases occurring below the level of subjective awareness, set boundaries for who is included and who is not, what structure is important, and what activities are valued or devalued. Patterson and Garwick cite marriage and death as two events involving boundary rituals. When a premature birth occurs, the infant may spend weeks or months in intensive neonatal care, physically absent from the family but psychologically present. This is an example of a boundary ambiguity that can place great pressure on family identity.

Finally, the most abstract dimension is the family world view, which represents a collective sense of value, purpose, and commitment. It also includes certain assumptions about the world and one's relationship to it. The birth of a child with a serious defect or illness may challenge the family's view of a just world or a kind and benevolent god. It may lead to types of marginal existence because the family must restructure its routines and redirect so many of its resources to caring for the child. In the face of this type of stress, many families seek some type of professional help, which may be provided in the form of a support group, education, or help in reformulating goals and redirecting emotional energies.

FAMILY RESOURCES Another factor contributing to family vulnerability is the family's resources for meeting the demands of the stress event. Family resources are a combination of **personal resources** possessed by the individual family members and resources that are part of the family system. Family-stress research has focused on four aspects of personal resource. These are financial status or economic well-being, health status or physical well-being, psychological resources (usually assessed as personality variables), and educational level. Educational level is an indirect measure of cognitive skills, which presumably aid realistic appraisals and contribute to problem-solving ability.

FAMILY DECISION MAKING AND PROBLEM SOLVING Perhaps the most significant family resource consists of the family's pattern of decision making and competence in problem solving. David Klein (1983) addressed several issues in family problem solving. One issue is the way the family addresses stress. Another is how the family socializes children to become competent problem solvers and mature adults who can withstand stress. Based on earlier research, Klein noted several problematic areas in family problem solving. Families often are forced to work on problems, for example, when energy levels are low, such as after work or even later in the evening after the younger children are in bed. In this sense, family problem solving is embedded in ongoing family routines instead of being a distinct activity, like a department meeting. Families also tend to defer to power and authority rather than to specific expertise. Moreover, problem solving is complicated by a so-called cascade effect. This occurs when a variety of emotional problems attach to the coattails of the primary problem needing to be solved. If the family cannot find effective ways of staying focused on the problem and identifying working solutions, it is likely that stress will build and family functioning will become more chaotic and dysfunctional.

Coping with Family Stress

McCubbin and his colleagues (McCubbin et al., 1980) specified four general hypotheses of how family coping actions work to ward off stress. The first is the notion that coping behaviors reduce family vulnerability. Consider a family member who is emotionally disturbed or who threatens to leave the family unit after conflict. The family needs to allo-cate time and energy to this issue. Dealing with the issue satisfactorily may remove the threat, thus restoring balance to the family and reducing vulnerability. The second hy-pothesis is that coping actions may strengthen or maintain family cohesiveness and or-ganization. Third, coping may reduce or eliminate stressor events. Fourth, coping may ac-tively operate on the environment to change it.

Investigators acknowledge that faulty coping can produce stress for the family. Some coping strategies are inferior, misguided, or out of touch with reality. According to McCubbin's analysis, faulty coping efforts can damage the family system in at least three ways. First, coping may produce indirect harm to the family unit or members of the family. One example McCubbin gives is when the family compensates for inflation by cutting back on health care. Second, coping efforts may produce direct damage to the family when, for example, a family member abuses alcohol or attempts suicide as a way out of current problems. Third, coping may increase family risks by retarding adaptive behaviors. This is most obvious when the family engages in denial or refuses to accept reality. For example, when a child becomes ill, possibly terminally ill, the fam-ily may reorganize realistically or unrealistically. When the latter is the case, the long-term picture is usually bleak.

Stages in Family Coping

In studies of families with fathers missing in action in Vietnam, the McCubbin group observed three stages in the family's adjustment (McCubbin et al., 1980). These were resistance, restructuring, and consolidation. The initial reaction of most family mem-bers was resistance, as they tried to deny or avoid the reality forced on them. As they began to acknowledge this unalterable reality, members began to reorganize their lives around the notion of a partial family. They redefined family roles. Children as-sumed more of the responsibilities for day-to-day maintenance of the household, and the mother looked for employment. In addition, the mother became more indepen-dent while exercising a stronger authority in the family. One interesting note was that the extended family (for example, in-laws) frequently had difficulty adjusting to this new strength in the mother. They expressed disapproval, which only served to in-crease her stress. Finally, the family consolidated its gains by making the reorganiza-tion permanent, and used this growth as a springboard for more changes in family life. In part, this included assigning new meanings to the crisis and a restructured lifestyle for the entire family.

Based on his study of families under stress during the Persian Gulf War, Figley (1993) identified several effective coping strategies. I have rephrased these strategies below as recommendations for use in a variety of family stress situations.

1. Increase and maintain the network of social support available with family and close friends, as well as social service agencies with professional resources and support groups.

2. Avoid unproductive worry, catastrophizing, and other negative thought patterns. Such thought patterns often occur when we are frustrated, angry, or dealing with major uncertainties. One way to avoid unproductive negative thinking is to get more involved in productive activities, especially helping activities. Flood survivors often found that their problems appeared much less significant when they immersed themselves in helping others.

3. Maintain good personal health habits, since effective coping works best when a sound mind pursues solutions with the support of a sound body. Letting good nutrition habits wane and regular exercise cease in favor of the work of worry is counterproductive in the long run.

Criticism of the FAAR Model

In spite of the continued popularity of the ABCX/FAAR model, it has not escaped criticism. Alexis Walker (1985) noted the tendency for ABCX theorists to identify a stressor at a given point. Yet most stressors result from a cumulative history of forces. In other words, the original model ignored process in favor of a time-anchored event. The updated FAAR version addresses this issue by recognizing that the family's definition of the stressor is itself a result of a dynamic stream of events. Second, Walker contended that family resources are not adequately defined. Third, the family's definition (appraisal) is problematic. Each family member probably has his or her personal representation of the stressor event. According to Walker, it is unlikely that there is a "family mind" that formulates a unitary definition of the event. Patterson and Garwick (1994) might respond that the behaviors of the family nonetheless reveal something about shared definitions and values.

Walker argued that family-stress theory should be contextual and systems oriented. Stress must be viewed in sociohistorical context. This includes understanding the ways external systems (social networks, communities, and agencies) influence the family. It also entails understanding how changes in family support systems alter the family process for better or for worse. Unfortunately, Walker does not provide a testable contextual-systems model.

TRANSITIONAL STRESS

We noted earlier that transitions create stress for family systems. Transitions are normative to some extent—that is, they are part of the natural history of every family. Although some transitions occur frequently, they are not normative according to society's standards; for example, divorce occurs frequently, but it is still not normative. Society generally has accepted the notion that divorce is incompatible with the value of a stable family unit. For this discussion, we will use Fosson's (1988) scheme.

Fosson identified five major family transitions that are likely to produce stress. These are formation of a new family unit, addition of new family members, separation of members from the family unit, loss of a family member, and disintegration of the family unit. Disintegration will be covered in more detail later in this chapter when we discuss separation and divorce. For now, we will discuss only Fosson's first four transitions.

Creation of a New Family Unit

Society customarily creates new family units through legal means or religious ritual or by recognizing reciprocal commitment between two people. In so doing, the unit is distinguished in a special way from other social units. Family members take on roles and responsibilities different from those they had before. The family dyad has an implicit or explicit understanding about sharing emotional support and maintaining exclusive intimacy. They divide obligations in some equitable fashion, and they negotiate patterns of communication and mechanisms for decision making and financial management. When two people share similar histories, values, and patterns of decision making, the transition probably will be smooth. The more pronounced their differences are, the more likely they are to encounter stress.

Adding a New Family Member

The birth of a baby or adoption of a child also requires adjustment in roles and responsibilities. The new roles of father and mother alter the exclusive companionship of husband and wife. The infant demands time and attention, which changes the pattern of interaction for the parents. These interactions are important to the parents' sense of fulfillment or frustration. Husbands may feel deprived of companionship. Wives as primary caregivers may feel that they do not control their own time. The interactions also begin to establish patterns of reciprocity and autonomy in the child. Discord may occur when the couple do not share common child-rearing values. When either parent sees the child as a rival for the spouse's affection or time, or when the child's demands seem to compete with career goals, stress may result. Additional stress occurs when boundaries between parents and grandparents become fluid and the child receives mixed messages about standards and conduct.

Separation of a Family Member

When members leave their nuclear families, alignments among family members also change. Support systems for both parents and children are disrupted. Siblings may be left without their best friend. Parents may lose a sense of closeness to their child. When the child leaves for college, family resources may be taxed. When children are unprepared for college life, they may turn pressure back onto the family by introducing emotionality and uncertainty into family interactions.

The effect of separation may be even more traumatic when it comes under duress. Teenagers may leave because of conflict with family values. Some may engage in antisocial behavior that leads to jail, or they may volunteer for military duty. The family may go through a type of grieving process under these circumstances.

A common separation stress is the "empty nest" syndrome, when the last child leaves and the parents are again a dyad. Parents may miss the excitement and structure that revolved around helping their children reach maturity. At this time, they may find it necessary to reassess mutual and individual goals and establish new ways of interacting.

Loss of a Family Member

Those experiencing separations of the type mentioned in the preceding paragraphs retain the clear hope and expectation that continued interaction is possible. The death of a family member provides no such hope. The loss of a young family member is usually more traumatic than the loss of an older one. A sudden loss is usually more difficult than loss following chronic illness. The grieving process may be difficult, but as Fosson (1988) noted, the family system does not change greatly and stress is usually not insurmountable. Events of this nature may draw family units together, making them even stronger.

SEPARATION AND DIVORCE

Living in a family unit where everything goes smoothly engenders enough day-to-day tensions. No matter how devoted two people are to each other, there will be disagreements at times. Even the most loving of brothers and sisters fight occasionally. Family members also have many different needs and wants that can put pressure on the family budget. A study based on a large Chicago sample (Pearlin & Schooler, 1978) found that the one family stressor most consistently identified was financial pressure. Returning veterans from the Persian Gulf War likewise were most concerned about money—but also about family adjustment and employment (Figley, 1993).

If life is this way in families that are presumably close-knit, think what it must be like in families where quarreling and fighting are the rule rather than the exception, where alternating periods of separation and reconciliation keep everyone off guard; where one never knows when Dad will walk out the door next or whether it will be the last time before divorce breaks the family up for good. Starting with the work of Holmes and Rahe (1967) on life-change, the three events commonly identified as the most potent family stressors are death of a spouse, divorce, and marital separation. Children and adolescents are no different in their perceptions: divorce for them is the most stressful event, second only to the death of a parent or close friend. These events can produce both emotional and physical health problems in the family, including adjustment problems for the children (Grych & Fincham, 1990).

Demographic statistics compiled in Europe, Canada, and the United States all point to a rapidly changing face of the typical family. In Great Britain, there are 16 divorces for every 30 marriages, while in the U.S., the figure is about 12 divorces for every 23 marriages (Facts on File, August 31, 1995). In the U.S., 27% of children live in a single-parent home (Facts on File, October 20, 1994), a rate that is virtually duplicated (26%) in Canada (Maclean's, July 1, 1996). In Great Britain, divorce increased sixfold between 1961 and 1991 (Wilkinson, 1996), but divorce rates in the U.S. actually dropped about 6% between 1979 and 1984 (Heatherington, Stanley-Hagan, & Anderson, 1989). In spite of this drop, 40% of the children born in the 1970s and 1980s are still likely to experience divorce (Grych & Fincham, 1990).

The decline in divorce rates might be related in part to changing ideas about marriage itself: More people establish homes now without the legal sanction of marriage. Still, alarm exists about the trend to end marriages frequently, even casually, making little effort to salvage the relationship. Many social scientists are now trying to discover the factors that contribute to marital conflict and divorce (Amato & Keith, 1991; Grych & Fincham, 1990). The hope is not just to stop the rush to divorce but to reduce the toll on survivors of divorce.

Personal Traits and Divorce

Bernard Bloom and his colleagues carried out a comprehensive review of stress and **marital conflict** (Bloom, Asher, & White, 1978). They reported that divorced and separated people contribute disproportionately to the numbers of psychiatric patients, whereas married people are underrepresented in psychiatric populations. Divorced and separated groups also are 4.5 times more likely to become alcohol dependent than married persons. One obvious question is whether the reported difficulties follow marital disruption or cause marital disruption. The evidence suggests that the problems were present before marriage and contributed to marital disruption; marital disruption probably intensified the problems.

The Aftermath of Marital Disruption

Disruption in marital relations produces numerous additional problems. Divorced people more frequently commit suicide and homicide. Divorced, separated, or widowed persons generally have substantially higher rates of illness and disability than married or never-married persons (DiIulio, 1997). As one example, divorced men who smoke one pack of cigarettes per day have about a 71% greater risk of premature death from cancer than married men who smoke the same amount. Given the already high risks that exist with smoking, this is a significant jump in overall risk. Divorced people are involved in motor vehicle accidents more frequently, and they average about three times the death rate from auto accidents as married people. Table 6-2 summarizes divorce as a family stressor along with two other stressors, single parenting and violence in the family.

THE SINGLE-PARENT FAMILY

When marital conflict ends in divorce or separation, the troubles are often only beginning, especially for the partner who retains custody of the children. In an early study of single parents, 90% of whom were women, the parents reported a set of common problems in their struggles to keep the family intact (Schlesinger, 1969). These included difficulty in managing the children, the necessity to go to work, financial problems, difficulties with sexual expression, and feelings of failure and shame. Most often, mothers and children could stay in the original home, retaining some sense of continuity and stability. On the other hand, fathers most often had to abandon those same homes, homes they had worked hard to provide. This appeared to contribute to fathers' feelings of isolation and rootlessness immediately after divorce.

Nancy Colletta (1983) compared low-income families with moderate-income families and found that low income presented the major problem. Low-income mothers had more difficulty related to child-rearing practices, baby-sitters, and health crises. These problems did not occur in moderate-income families, where stress was lower for both mother and child. Unfortunately, Colletta did not assess the families' educational levels; this could also have influenced the reported stress levels.

Single-parent families tend to be more disorganized, which increases stress on individual members (Heatherington, Cox, & Cox 1976). Divorced parents felt more anxious, angry, rejected, and depressed than did married parents (Heatherington, Cox, & Cox, 1977). Kessler and Essex (1982) advanced the theory that married people show less depression than single people because they are less emotionally damaged by stressful experiences. Single parents may be both psychologically and physically vulnerable. Kiecolt-Glaser and her colleagues found evidence that marital disruption suppresses the immune system, which increases vulnerability to illness and even death (Kiecolt-Glaser, Fisher, et al., 1985).

TABLE 6-2
Summary of major family stressors

FAMILY STRESSORS	CONTRIBUTING FACTORS	POSSIBLE CONSEQUENCES
Separation and divorce	Physical illness or disability	Increased physical illness
	Mental illness or emotional instability	Increased anxiety, tension, and/or mental illness
	Alcoholism	Suicide
		Homicide
		Increased motor vehicle accidents and deaths
Single parenting	Family disorganization	Increased feelings of guilt, shame, and failure
	Postdivorce conflict	
	Time management and work	Increased anxiety
	Financial pressures	Child's frustrated expectations
	Child care	
	Interpersonal conflict with extended family and ex-spouse	
	Intrapsychic conflict	
	Adult responsiblilty placed on children	
Family violence and abuse	*Historical variables:*	Damaged self-image and self-esteem
	Developmental history of family violence and abuse	Poorer long-term emotional stability and adjustment
	Parental rejection	Feelings of failure and incompetence
	Modeled aggression	
	Failure to learn how to parent effectively	Feelings of helplessness and hopelessness
	Current variables:	Failure to thrive
	Family disorganization	Instrumental but maladaptive acts to restore balance
	Life-change stress	
	Traumatic bonding or co-dependencies	
	Premature, difficult, or unhealthy baby	
	Child misbehavior	
	Tacit or explicit support for sibling abuse	

Children in the Single-Parent Family

Just as divorced parents experience great stress while adjusting to the single-parent reality, so do children. As noted earlier, the number of children living in single-parent homes has increased dramatically. Probably 40% to 50% of children born in the 1970s and 1980s will spend about five years in a single-parent home (Heatherington, Stanley-Hagan, & Anderson, 1989). Many children must take on adult responsibility at the expense of enjoying their childhood. Avis Brenner (1984) noted that children may enjoy the signs of adult status, but they still miss the privileges of being children. Several behavioral changes are noted in children of divorce, including withdrawal, dependency, inattention, and unhappiness. They are more likely to commit suicide and to be involved in violent criminal acts. Finally, children of divorce tend to perform lower overall on mental health status measures (Zinsmeister, 1997).

Another problem in the single-parent family is that children of divorce and separation may create as much stress as they suffer. Single mothers tend to have more difficulty with their sons, whereas single fathers tend to have more difficulty with their daughters (Heatherington, Stanley-Hagan, & Anderson, 1989). Because women head roughly 90% of the single-parent families, the difficulties encountered more frequently result from problems in dealing with a son. This appears to increase the mother's anxiety and feelings of helplessness and incompetence. The long-term cycle may be one of escalating tensions between the two, eroding the relationship and resulting in the mother's loss of self-confidence.

One of the most frequent problems for children is the continued hopes and dreams that their mother and father will get back together again. It appears that this dream is especially unshakable, lasting for years in some children (Heatherington, Stanley-Hagan, & Anderson, 1989). It takes a gentle but persistent effort to help children of divorce accept reality without adding greatly to their inner turmoil.

This problem can carry over into postdivorce and remarriage as well. All too often, adults expect children to accept remarriage as a blessing. What many adults do not realize is that remarriage shatters their child's dreams of reconciliation. In addition, the child has little time to mourn the death of the dream when the parent remarries. Single parents intending to remarry would do well to consider this source of stress for their children. One solution is to include children as much as possible in the decision process. This might also help them put to rest any hopes that still exist for the dissolved marriage.

Postdivorce Conflict and Stress

Even after divorce, many factors force the separate families to interact, beginning with visitation rights and schedules. In joint custody arrangements, parents must arrange for moving the children from one home to another. Both partners usually share continued interest in the children's development. There are the father's financial obligations and the mother's concern when payments are inconsistent. These continued contacts may represent new opportunities for predivorce conflicts to resurface (Amato, 1996).

One research team (Cline & Westman, 1971) identified five patterns that seem to mark postdivorce conflict. These are listed with explanatory comments.

1. *Hostilities over parenting.* Fathers' parenting styles tend to change more than mothers' parenting styles, an alteration that may contribute to conflict.
2. *Hostilities over matters unrelated to the children.* Parents may carry over bitterness and acrimony about the cause of the divorce, or they harbor anger over perceived injustices in the divorce settlement.
3. *Pressure from the children to maintain contact between mother and father.*
4. *Tugs-of-war, choosing sides, and shifting alliances.* One parent may use a child as a pawn to wage a war of nerves against the other parent. This pattern can be especially destructive to everyone. More often than not, the children are the real losers. Children of divorce fare best where the parents maintain an

amicable relationship (Rofes, 1982), share the children with warmth and regard for each other's rights (Wallerstein & Kelly, 1980), and help the children understand that the love of both parents is not dependent on a marriage contract alone.

5. *Continued interaction caused by grandparents and the extended family.* One forgotten aspect of divorce is that divorce does not just shatter the dreams of the nuclear family; it shatters the dreams of members of the extended family as well. Parents of the divorced couple may perceive their child's divorce as their own parenting failure. In addition, they have vested interest in their grandchildren and frequently want to retain some contact, which can become another source of stress to both the mother and father.

VIOLENCE IN THE FAMILY

Of the family stressors receiving attention today, none rate higher than **spouse abuse** and **child abuse.** Crime statistics reveal that family quarrels or ongoing patterns of family violence lead directly to many physical injuries and deaths (Centers for Disease Control, September 6, 1996). Unfortunately, counting just the physical scars ignores the real toll: the lifelong emotional scars that abused people carry wherever they go. At the least, abused children tend to suffer a damaged self-image; poorer emotional adjustment, if not mental disturbance; more disturbed family relationships; lower impulse control; and inferior coping skills (McCauley et al., 1997). They tend to display more antisocial and criminal behaviors, more addiction-risk behaviors, and more suicidal behaviors (Garneski & Deikstra, 1997). Adult female survivors of childhood sexual abuse also reveal clinical signs of posttraumatic stress syndrome, suggesting that childhood sexual abuse is an etiological factor in PTSD (Rodriquez, Ryan, Vande Kemp, & Foy, 1997). Finally, a history of childhood abuse often is associated with numerous physical conditions, such as gastrointestinal tract symptoms, headaches, pelvic or genital pain, and nonepileptic seizures (McCauley et al., 1997).

Violence in the family is not a modern problem, and it certainly is not as rare as some like to think. Gelles and Straus (1979) took the position that violence is *normal.* They based this judgment on the sheer frequency of violence in the family. They also suggested that conflict is inevitable in social relationships, although physical violence is not (Gelles, 1985). Police records do not help dispel this notion, as nearly 20% of homicides are a direct result of family violence (Emery, 1989).

Defining Child Abuse and Neglect

Congress reauthorized the **Child Abuse Prevention and Treatment Act** (CAPTA) in 1996 (Public Law 104-235, Section 111; 42 U.S.C. 5106g), which defines child abuse as:

- Any recent act or failure to act resulting in imminent risk of serious harm, death, serious physical or emotional harm, sexual abuse, or exploitation
- Of a child (a person under the age of 18, unless the child-protection law of the State in which the child resides specifies a younger age for cases not involving sexual abuse)
- By a parent or caretaker (including any employee of a residential facility or any staff person providing out-of-home care) who is responsible for the child's welfare

CAPTA defines sexual abuse as:
- Employment, use, persuasion, inducement, enticement, or coercion of any child to engage in, or assist any other person to engage in, any sexually explicit conduct or any simulation of such conduct for the purpose of producing any visual depiction of such conduct; or
- rape, and in cases of caretaker or interfamilial relationships, statutory rape, molestation, prostitution, or other form of sexual exploitation of children, or incest with children

Current national data indicate that over 1 million children were victims of substantiated child abuse and **neglect** in 1995 (U. S. Department of Health and Human Services, 1997). About 52% of the cases involved neglect, 25% involved physical abuse, 13% sexual abuse, 5% emotional maltreatment, 3% medical neglect, and 14% other forms of maltreatment. In 1995, data from 45 reporting states indicated 996 deaths from abuse or neglect. Among the cases of abuse and neglect, more than half of the children were under the age of 7 years, and overall, about 52% were female and 47% were male. As bleak as these numbers may seem, there is evidence that the statistics substantially underestimate the true rate of abuse and neglect. The true rate may be closer to 1.5 million children.

The National Clearinghouse on Child Abuse and Neglect (1997) says that child neglect is simply failure to provide for the child's basic needs. Still, Brenner (1984) may have described it best when he said that neglect occurs when "children live with caretakers who are unwilling or unable to become involved with them and who are emotionally and sometimes physically absent" (p. 115). Brenner's description of the neglected child is almost nauseating, but it reveals the silent and insidious tragedy of neglect:

> Households . . . cluttered with garbage, piles of clothing, excrement, dirty dishes, and stained mattresses lacking sheets and blankets. Drugs, liquor, poisons, and matches are discarded wherever they have been used last. It is not unusual to find a baby lying naked in a crib covered with feces and next to it a bottle of soured milk. (p. 117)

Having witnessed some of these conditions and more (for example, chickens perched on a baby's crib, adding animal excrement to baby feces), I can only say that mere words cannot convey the magnitude of the horror.

Attempts to identify the factors that contribute to abuse and neglect have turned up some leads. There are also some constructive plans emerging for preventing child and spouse abuse, but these plans have opened the door for yet other forms of abuse.

Abuse and Developmental History

First, parents who maltreat their children often have a developmental history that predisposes them to do so. Both retrospective and prospective studies confirm this conclusion. This does not mean that all abusive parents were themselves abused as children. Suffering personal abuse or neglect as a child is only one factor that sets the stage for becoming an abusive parent.

Another factor is the powerful influence of observing aggression. Albert Bandura's classic work on modeled aggression supports the idea that parents' reciprocal aggression may contribute to children becoming abusive in adult life (1973). Further, being rewarded for aggressive actions within the family contributes to becoming abusive in adult relationships.

Parental rejection also may be a key factor that contributes to becoming an abusive parent. Abusive parents may be looking for the love and acceptance from their children that they did not receive from their parents (Rohner, 1975). In effect, abusive parents create a role reversal in which the parents are the "cared-for" and the children are the longed-for "care-givers." When the parents do not receive the care they expect from their children, they may turn to abuse.

Lack of developmental experiences that enable children to pass into adulthood with suitable parenting values and skills is equally important. These include learning experiences with child care during childhood and adolescence. Blumberg's research suggests that parents who abuse their children are woefully ignorant of the most rudimentary information about the sequence and timing of a child's growth and maturation (1974). Without this knowledge, it may be difficult for parents to comprehend that the way a child thinks and behaves is natural and is not contrived expressly to irritate. Theodore Dix (1991) believes that emotional expression and control are at the core of parental competence. On the one hand, emotional sensitivity to the child's needs contributes to effective parenting. On the other, inappropriate emotional expression or control in the parent serves to undermine effective parenting.

Life-Change, Stress, and Abuse

Many adults who were abused as children, however, raise their own children with love, sensitivity, and regard. This shows that developmental history alone cannot account for one's being abusive as an adult. Other forces must interact with developmental influences. One suspect in this equation is family stress. Abuse of a spouse or child creates extreme stress, especially when the attack is unexpected. This may suggest that stress is only an outcome of maltreatment.

Is it possible, though, that stress may also cause abuse? Several investigators have addressed this issue. Life changes such as a spouse's death, divorce, loss of a job, and economic hardships correlate strongly with child abuse and neglect *when the developmental history described earlier is also present* (Conger, Burgess, & Barrett, 1979; Smith, 1984). Stress as a cause of maltreatment may begin a vicious cycle in which abuse creates more stress, which then perpetuates abuse.

One of the most powerful family stressors is marital conflict. Conflict appears to run high in families where child abuse occurs (Smith & Hanson, 1975). Unfortunately, it is not always clear whether the conflict preceded or followed the child abuse. Steinmetz (1977) showed that spouses who use physical and verbal aggression in resolving marital conflict also use the same tactics in disciplining their children. Finally, the transition to parenthood may create stress. For some parents, the birth of a child is a disruption. In addition, they lack preparation for the responsibilities of parenting, and this may be enough to tip some over the edge into child abuse. This is especially true when the first child is premature or abnormal (Lowenthal, 1987).

Finally, family disorganization may be related to a pattern of abuse. Disorganization disables family coping capacity, which usually leads to increased stress. Among the most powerful disorganizing influences are unemployment and economic privation. Research in the United States and Great Britain showed that unemployment is probably the most important factor related to abuse and neglect (Light, 1973).

Children as Causes of Stress and Abuse

Another factor that has received attention is the role the child plays in raising levels of tension and stress in the family (Smith, 1984). According to this view, infants are still innocent, unwitting provocateurs. Older children may be both less than innocent and at least partially aware of what they are doing. Based on this notion, investigators looked for patterns of physical and/or psychological traits of children that might be linked to aggression in adults.

First, evidence exists that many maltreated children are premature babies (Klein & Stern, 1971). Premature and maltreated infants often lack social responsiveness (Egeland & Brunquell, 1979). Parents may see this as a source of mild irritation at first. Should this pattern continue, parents may feel rejected and begin to question their competence as parents. Soon, a parent may feel a strong sense of frustration followed by anger and ultimately aggression. Another line of evidence shows that some parents find their premature babies' crying and appearance aversive and disagreeable (Lowenthal, 1987). As Jay Belsky (1980) noted, "child maltreatment must be considered an interactive process; although children may play a role in their own abuse or neglect, they cannot cause it by themselves" (p. 324). In Belsky's view, the interaction is between the parent's traits and the child's characteristics.

Older children may prompt abuse through misbehavior. Studies of family interactions reveal that when parents punish or discipline a child, the child probably will react with more coercive actions toward the parent (Patterson, 1977). The interaction may deteriorate into "a war of wills" as each combatant seeks to control or resist control with escalating punitiveness and counteraggression. This may end only when the more powerful adult physically attacks the less powerful child.

Sibling Abuse

An overlooked aspect of child abuse concerns physical injuries caused by siblings. We now recognize that sibling rivalry can take on sinister twists, producing traumas equaling those that parents inflict. Tooley (1977) described children abused by siblings as "weaponless and without safe refuge" in their homes (p. 26). One study found that sibling abuse had occurred in over half the families studied (Straus, Gelles, & Steinmetz, 1980).

One sinister aspect of sibling abuse is that it can occur in the presence of parents. Tooley described three different parental patterns enabling sibling abuse to occur. First, some parents simply choose to ignore or deny that abuse is going on. Second, some parents apparently are unable to manage a violent child, or the child intimidates an inadequate parent. The parent, then, may indulge the child, allowing attacks on the other children to occur without interference. Third, some parents may encourage sibling aggression to act out their own violent impulses.

A Systems Model of Family Violence

In a thoughtful review of family violence, Robert Emery (1989) noted both conceptual and methodological problems in family violence research. He also advanced a theory of the child's reaction to parental conflict. Emery suggested that current definitions of abuse are social value judgments rather than operational definitions. This makes it difficult to assess the true incidence and severity of abusive acts. Further, it is difficult to construct credible theories of process and outcome. This in turn undermines efforts to design effective interventions to prevent abuse and to offset the effects of abuse.

The theory Emery advances is brief. First, he points out that even one-year-old children show distress in response to displays of anger between their parents. They show negative emotions such as crying and aggression even when the anger does not include them. Second, distress motivates instrumental acts by a child to reduce or offset the distress. These acts may include diverting attention to other problems or directly intervening to protect a parent. Third, the function of the child's instrumental act is crucial. In Emery's view, the child acts to preserve order, homeostasis, in the family system. To do this, the child may act as a scapegoat—a personally maladaptive response, but a response that is adaptive for the family system. Emery noted that this theory is very new but has a substantial body of evidence to support it.

After an extensive literature review of marital conflict and child adjustment, John Grych and Frank Fincham (1990) proposed a **cognitive-contextual theory** for understanding children's reactions to marital conflict. (See Figure 6-2 and also compare this theory to other theories summarized in Table 6-1.) In this model, parental conflict is a stressor that places adaptive demands on children. Children try to make sense of conflict through an appraisal process that combines cognitive and affective elements. Qualities

FIGURE 6-2
A cognitive-contextual analysis of children's reactions to and appraisals of marital conflict.
SOURCE: Grych & Fincham (1990).

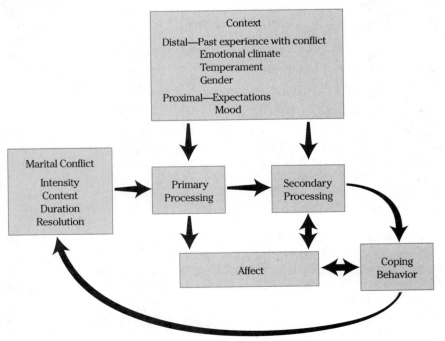

of the conflict, such as intensity, directly affect the child's first appraisal. In the second stage, the child assigns causal attributions for the events. The child may assign blame to a parent. Worse yet, the child may assume personal responsibility for the conflict. Coping efforts, if successful, reduce tension and negative emotions. On the other hand, failures in coping may both add to family tension and increase the child's distress. Historical factors relating to the child's experiences in the family and to the family system itself will influence the child's appraisal.

BATTERED WIVES

Spouse abuse involves man[...] ample, abusive men and battered [...] of violence already established. [...]ld, the more likely she was to be f[...] In a recent study, 50% of women [...] adults (McCauley et al., 1997).

One issue of concern [...]ut will also keep coming back fo[...]nes because they are dependent [...]y exists for most adults. Adults pre[...] again, adults stay in abusive relat[...]

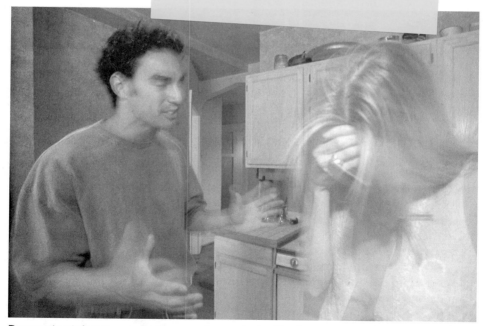

Domestic violence comes in many forms, but wife abuse is one of the most commonly reported. Many community agencies provide shelter and housing for abused women.

Traumatic Bonding and Battered Women

Don Dutton and Susan Painter (1981) believe the answer to this paradox is **traumatic bonding.** There is no simple definition of traumatic bonding; it is a complex process in which personal, familial, and social forces operate in consort and collusion to lock the woman into the abusive union. In the interest of brevity, only an outline of the process appears here.

First, as Dutton and Painter noted, domestic violence is more often than not a series of events in which periods of quarreling and abuse alternate with almost equally passionate attempts by the abusive male to make amends. This pattern may beguile women to think the abuse is an exceptional part of the relationship or to ignore it altogether (Rounsaville, 1978). Many clinical and laboratory studies with both human and animal subjects support the argument that alternating abuse and passion increases the chance of traumatic bonding. Rajecki's group reviewed emotional bonding in infants. They concluded that inconsistent treatment by the source of affection (punishment by a parent who also bestows love) intensifies the child's attempts to become closer to the parent (Rajecki, Lamb, & Obmascher, 1978).

A second factor involved in traumatic bonding is the power imbalance between the abuser and the abused. This imbalance may mask mutual dependency needs in which the abused identifies with the abuser and gains some sense of power. At the same time, the abuser needs the partner's submission to his needs.

SEXUAL ABUSE OF CHILDREN

Sexual abuse of a child may be the most despicable violation of the trust given to parents. About 29% of childhood sexual abuse (CSA) events were instigated by the birth parent; about 25% were instigated by a non-birth parent or parent-substitute; and the remaining 46% were instigated by someone outside the family (U. S. Department of Health and Human Services, 1997). Offenders appear to operate from one of three motives: they are seeking tenderness, they are exercising power not available in other aspects of their life, or they are venting sadistic rage (Groth & Burgess, 1977).

Physical and Psychological Symptoms of Sexual Abuse

Investigators report numerous physical and psychological problems in sexually abused children. These include sleep disturbances with nightmares; general restlessness, sometimes hyperactivity; eating problems that may include stomach aches and vomiting; and a **failure-to-thrive syndrome.**[1] The child may experience genital irritation, painful discharge of urine, or bed-wetting and soiling.

Preventing Childhood Sexual Abuse

Prevention occurs through public awareness programs, parent education programs, skills-based curricula and awareness education (for example, the "Red Flag/Green Flag" for appropriate touching) for children, and home visitation programs, often through some type of child protection agency. A wide range of information is available via the

---

[1]Failure-to-thrive syndrome generally refers to a state in which the child is listless, disinteresed, and lacks energy and initiative, and also shows signs of despondency and lack of joy in living.

Internet[2] to guide people in understanding CSA and to help them locate regional and local support services. A first step to preventing CSA is to know the warning signs. The following is a composite of behaviors that children may display after sexual abuse.

- Appearance of new and strong fears, such as fear of the dark, of being alone, of sleeping alone, of strangers, or of men.
- Insistence on having mother nearby and refusal to go to formerly favored places.
- Changes in emotionality such as increased irritability, worry about staying clean, withdrawal from normal activities and circle of friends, crying, and sleep disturbances.
- Changes in habitual behaviors, such as occurrence of bed-wetting, loss of appetite, and excessive bathing.
- Appearance of more "adult-like" behaviors, including overt interest in and expressions of sexuality, seductive talk and actions, and so on. This may include intense acting-out behaviors, including sexual acting-out such as promiscuity or prostitution.
- Sudden changes in school performance, inability to concentrate, failing grades, and indirect attempts to divulge sexual actions and fears.
- Major changes in children's relationships with parents, wherein parents (or the perpetrator) become overprotective and jealous of other friends, and show inordinate attention and control. Such changes may be a clue to the offender's identity.
- Appearance of clandestine contacts between the perpetrator and the child, such as contriving to be alone and being secretive.

These signs do not all appear in any given child. The most important and easily detected signs are physical injury—irritation, bruises, and swelling and bleeding in the genital region. Signs of venereal disease reveal sexual contact. Beyond these physical signs, the most important clues include marked changes, usually for the worse, in behaviors or performances that children normally display.

Effects on the Family

Repercussions in the family are countless. The most basic include strains in familial relationships, changes in natural family roles, and distortion in patterns of affection (Muldoon, 1979). Unhealthy alliances frequently shift the balance of power to the abused daughter, especially when she is old enough to recognize the power she wields. Mary de Young (1982) pointed out that the daughter holds power over the offender because his security depends on her silence. The offender also may resort to a variety of forms of bribery or threat to keep the victim silent. This may include increased attempts to buy the child's loyalty and silence through gifts of money and clothes, trips, and favors. The perpetrator may try to interpret morality and reality for the child to prevent the child from developing a sense that the sexual activities are wrong. The child usually lacks mature cognitive structures to interpret the meaning of the interaction; this only aids the deceit (Orzek, 1985). The cognitive deficit also may contribute to the child's self-blame and feelings of guilt and shame.

[2]See the Websites listing at the end of the chapter for more information.

As noted earlier, the child's psychological problems typically carry over into the adult years. Survivors of child sexual abuse often experience later disturbances in marital relationships, and continue to harbor negative—at best, confused—feelings toward their family. They feel a mixture of hate, sympathy, understanding, and faint affection mixed with strong ambivalence for the father. Surprisingly, 38 (79%) of the victims in de Young's study felt more strongly negative toward their mothers than toward their fathers. de Young (1982) concluded that this negative feeling arose from the daughters' perceptions that the mother was in a position to stop the abuse but chose not to do so. Therefore, feelings of anger toward the offending father or stepfather ("How could he do this to me?") are easily transferred to the nonparticipating mother ("How could she *let* him do this to me?") (p. 58).

POSITIVE COPING IN THE FAMILY

There are positive and constructive aspects of coping in the family. Because the family is a social system, it provides a variety of intimate contacts and supports not routinely available in society. In this sense, the family serves as a major source of **social support.**

The Family as a Social Support System

A major moderator of stress is the extent of social support available. Social support may be defined as help given by spouses, parents, and friends. Pearlin's group suggested that social support is "access to and use of individuals, groups, or organizations in dealing with life's vicissitudes" (Pearlin, Lieberman, Menaghan, & Mullan, 1981, p. 340). Gerald Caplan's team looked at social support as attachments to individuals and groups that reduce vulnerability to stress and improve the person's ability to cope with "short-term challenges, stresses, and privations" (Caplan & Killilea, 1976, p. 41).

Social support functions at two levels in the family. First, the family is a social support network for its members. Second, families are embedded in a community. The extent to which that community provides a social support network for the family is important in moderating stress. Unfortunately, some communities function as sources of stress instead of as support networks.

Sidney Cobb (1976) provided a systematic theory of social support. According to Cobb's analysis, social support conveys three types of information to a person. First, social support leads a person to a sense of being cared for and loved. Second, social support leads a person to a sense of being esteemed and valued by other people. Third, it leads a person to a sense of belonging to a communication network with mutual obligations.

Cobb's analysis can be extended to the gamut of social systems. Social support groups exist at every stage of the life cycle. They wax and wane in importance as personal needs shift. There is a time, for example, when the teenage peer group is the teenager's most important, perhaps only, support network. As the young adult looks for employment and seeks to become a respected member of the community, the social network will consist of bosses, work associates, and community leaders. Thus, many different social groups may provide support to moderate the effects of stress.

Research shows that social support is important to early development, recovery from surgical procedures, and to health. For example, Forssman and Thuwe (1966) conducted a study of children born after their mothers had requested an abortion. The researchers showed that unwanted children were more likely to have trouble with the law. Also, these children were more likely to require psychiatric treatment in their youth than were matched control children who were presumably "wanted" by their parents.

There are health implications of social support as well. Children experience less stress from hospital procedures when parents and staff can provide a warm, supportive environment. This is why many hospitals now allow parents to stay with their children. Parents now have the legal right to stay with their infant or young child (Brenner, 1984).

In addition to social support, a child's acceptance of hospital procedures may depend on cognitive expectations. Children can be prepared for their hospitalization through presurgical visits in which they meet their hospital care-givers. They can view films in which similar-aged and same-sex children model the hospital procedure (Melamed & Siegel, 1975). When this occurs at the child's level of cognitive development, he or she can deal more adequately with the anxiety of hospitalization or outpatient surgical procedures. However, this may depend on other psychological characteristics of the child (Saile, Burgmeier, & Schmidt, 1988). Some children may be sensitized by modeling procedures. In addition, prior experience with hospitals and medical procedures influences children's response to modeling.

An extensive study of 10,000 men with angina pectoris showed the importance of support in the marital relationship. Men with a satisfying love relationship were significantly less likely to present symptoms of angina, even when physical risk factors were present (Medalie & Goldbourt, 1976). Social support is also important in compliance with medical prescriptions and treatment programs. One review (Baekeland & Lundwall, 1975) looked at 19 projects that studied social support. All 19 studies observed that social isolation and/or lack of affiliation related strongly to dropping out of treatment. Other research shows that social support is crucial to minimizing the impact of stress from job loss (Cobb, 1974), long-term illness and recovery, grief after the loss of a loved one, and retirement (Shapiro, 1983). Finally, social support may moderate the effects of essential hypertension, increase the chances of surviving a heart attack, and increase the expected length of survival in cancer patients (Turner, 1983).

SUMMARY

Family stress differs from stress at the personal level. That is, family stress disrupts a system, an organization, whereas personal stress has consequences for the psychological and physical well-being of the individual. The major points made in the course of this chapter are summarized below.

- A family is descriptive of a social cluster of persons who enjoy a special relationship through love, mutual commitment, and reciprocal dependence.
- Family stress is defined as pressure that disrupts or changes the family system. It reduces harmony and resources for collective problem solving.
- The family stress model, dubbed the ABCX model, was originally proposed by Reuben Hill. This model proposed that family stressors occur as a result of an event interacting with a family's resources for meeting crises and the family's definition of the event.
- Later, Hill's colleagues modified the model to the **F**amily **A**djustment and **A**daptation **R**esponse (FAAR) Model. This model added details on how a family assigns meaning to events.

- Many family stressors are connected to transitions that occur as the family is formed, changed with the addition of children, and transformed by children leaving or the family breaking up.
- Separation and divorce fragments the family system, but typically produces serious personal stressors for individual family members, especially children who may feel powerless or, worse yet, feel that they are in some way guilty of contributing to the breakup of the marriage.
- Single-parent families tend to be more disorganized, and children in such families tend to be placed in a position of conflict in which they are neither truly child nor adult. These children also tend to maintain hopes that their parents will reunite, a hope that is dashed when one parent remarries.
- Abuse occurs most in families where the parents have a developmental history that predisposes them to neglect or abuse. The parents may have been abused themselves, or they may have witnessed abuse.
- Family stress only increases the likelihood that abuse will occur.
- When the wife is the target of abuse, there may be a traumatic bonding that serves to keep the abused person in the family in spite of the suffering.
- Children can contribute to stress through a variety of misbehaviors, but they can also instigate abuse of siblings. This source of abuse is often overlooked, but it may be partially supported by parents for various reasons.
- Signs of sexual abuse include both physical and psychosocial symptoms. Preventing sexual abuse is important to the child's long-term well-being, but involves more than just knowledge. It requires the will to act to stop something that is terribly wrong.
- When the family functions as a sensitive social support system, many outside stressors may be minimized. Families can structure problem solving to avoid common pitfalls and increase the chances of finding useful solutions.

CRITICAL THINKING AND STUDY QUESTIONS

1. How does family stress differ from personal stress? What are the core features of family that require us to adjust our thinking about stress in the family compared to personal stress?
2. What are the basic terms and propositions of the FAAR model of family stress? Try to give examples from your own experience that invoke each of the major components.
3. How do transitions contribute to stress in the family? What transitions have occurred in your family? Did these transitions create stress for only some of the family members or for the family as a unit or both?
4. What are some of the factors that work against smooth and effective problem solving in the family? Are there ways to improve family problem solving so that the effects of these factors are reduced?
5. What are some of the contributing factors to family violence and abuse? Does knowing about these factors help in some way to prevent the appearance of abuse?

KEY TERMS

ABCX model
  amount of change
  family appraisal
  family vulnerability
child abuse
Child Abuse Prevention
  and Treatment Act
child neglect
cognitive-contextual
  theory

crisis
distress
failure-to-thrive
  syndrome
family as system
family resources
family stress
life-change and abuse
marital conflict
personal resources

social buffer
social support and family
  stress
spouse abuse
stressor
systems model
  (Emery's) of
  family violence
traumatic bonding

WEBSITES stress in the family: adjustment, conflict, and disruption

URL ADDRESS	SITE NAME & DESCRIPTION
http://www.healthtouch.com/level1. leaflets/101810/102031.htm	Women's Mental Health & Physical Addictions. Impressive set of links for career, family, and domestic violence information
http://www.tezcat.com/~tina/psychdir/ main.shtml	☆Abuse Survivors' Resources
http://hammock.ifas.ufl.edu/txt/fairs/he/ 30922.html	Stress Management: Strategies for Families, from the University of Florida Extension Service
http://education.indiana.edu/cas/adol/ mental.html	Mental Health Risk Factors for Adolescents. A comprehensive site including links for abuse, stress, and suicide
http://www.sidran.org	☆The Sidran Foundation's site for survivors of abuse, trauma, and PTSD
http://www.pitt.edu./HOME/GHNet/ GHWomen.html	University of Pittsburgh site devoted to women's health issues

ANSWERS AND COMMENTS ON SELF-STUDY EXERCISE 6-1

The "correct" answers are not really correct in the absolute sense of that term, but rather are based on observations by family specialists about the kinds of things that produce more stress for the family. Thus, if you respond the same way as the designated answer, you are carrying on in your family life the kinds of things that tend to increase stress. The suggestions nested in the comments, then, are intended to guide in the direction of reducing stress in the family.

1. True—Money matters are routinely among the top two or three stressors for families. Rule number one is to let expertise prevail: that is, the one who is the best money manager should be in charge of the checkbook and accounts. If you cannot agree or continue to have financial problems in spite of your best efforts, then seek guidance from a financial advisor.

2. True—Constant squabbling among children is usually a sign of inadequate or non-existent rules and parental discipline. Children need boundaries set in order to develop a clear sense of self. In the absence of discipline, they will set their own, often overly fluid boundaries. If this is a major problem in the household, look for library and community resources on parenting or, in more serious situations, seek out professional help for the family.

3. False—The most stressed families typically have very uneven division of labor. When both adult members are working, it is even more important to share equally in the household work load. If children are present, they should have some responsibility within the limits of their age and mental ability.

4. True—Down time for self is one of the most important methods of reducing stress. If you have trouble managing it, work on setting well-defined boundaries of time that are consistent from day to day so the rest of the family gets used to it.

5. True—Time constraints define another one of the major stressors. The solution is to do a time audit—in other words, find out how you spend your time on a daily basis. More will be said on this topic in Chapters 10 and 14.

6. True—Partners in the relationship need regular time together to keep the relationship flourishing and healthy. If too many other activities are encroaching on this time together, the solution is to set priorities and eliminate the activities that are less essential in favor of the ones that are vitally important.

7. True—Physical fatigue has a spreading—often insidious—effect on other aspects of home life. It tends to lower overall efficiency in household management, and it generally increases irritability. Proper sleep, exercise, and judicious use of time without overcrowding can usually correct this problem.

8. True—A feeling of failure or simply lack of success can have an undermining effect in family relationships. This problem is magnified when the member who feels this way begins to blame the other member(s) for the shortcomings. Setting priorities and then setting goals that can be accomplished in attainable chunks can go a long way to correcting this situation.

9. False—Families under stress often are lacking in organization, so that every action seems to be a crisis that is magnified by a clock that is relentless. A few minutes of preparation in the evening can greatly reduce the chaos that often besets busy families in the morning.

10. True—Mere talking is not communicating. Communicating is sharing feelings and needs, reasons, and intentions, all the while retaining sensitivity to what the other family member is trying to communicate. If communication is stifled or garbled, some of the other aspects of family stress may be getting in the way. Getting them solved can in some cases help to reopen lines of communication. If the problems are more deep-seated, then personal and/or family counseling may be called for.

11. True—A constantly crowded schedule is one of the major stressors among modern families. As noted earlier, setting priorities about what is essential can help to keep the schedule from dominating the family life.
12. True—This is related again to parenting skills and discipline. The more children are allowed to set their own rules, the more chaotic family life can be, and the less time there is for some of the other important matters that maintain the vitality of the committed relationship and the routine of operating a household.

CHAPTER 7

Job Stress:

Dissatisfaction, Burnout, and Obsolescence

Many ... have reached the top of the success ladder but are beginning to suspect it may be leaning against the wrong wall.

SAM KEEN

QUESTIONS

- What are the unique features of job stress?
- How should job stress be defined?
- What are the economic costs of job stress?
- What are the physical and psychological symptoms of job stress?
- What are the major sources of work stress?
- Are boredom and monotony really stressors?
- How is technological change related to job stress?
- What are the symptoms of job burnout?
- Does job stress differ across occupational groups?
- Is telecommuting more or less stressful than working in a central site?
- What are some coping techniques to reduce job stress and burnout?

S unday, May 19, 1985: A headline in *The New York Times* business section read "War-ren Anderson: A Public Crisis, a Personal Ordeal." This headline introduced the inside story of a corporation and its chief executive officer struggling to deal with a tragedy of immense proportions (Diamond, 1985). For both Union Carbide and Warren Anderson, it was a period of intense, unyielding stress. Half the story described the pub-lic, legal, and corporate pressure on Union Carbide Corporation following the Bhopal tragedy. The accident tarnished the company's image worldwide, contributed to plum-meting stock, slowed the pace of company expansion, and produced multibillion-dollar lawsuits.

The rest of the story, more intimate and personal, concerned Anderson's dramatic changes in lifestyle. Though Anderson was not directly involved in the events that led to spilling toxic gases, he had to take ultimate responsibility as the company's chief execu-tive officer. Immediately after news reports revealed the immensity of the tragedy, he as-sembled technical and medical experts to help at Bhopal. In Bombay, he met two of Union Carbide's Indian officials. Upon arrival in Bhopal, police arrested and jailed all three. Anderson spent several hours in jail before flying to New Delhi, but his Indian col-leagues spent nine days in jail. Anderson's wife, Lillian, said the few days he was in India were filled with more terror for her than she had known during her entire life.

When Anderson returned to his Connecticut office, he devoted attention only to matters related to Bhopal. He left day-to-day operations to junior officers. Anderson said that he felt "like I'm taking tests all the time. You know there is going to be a grade on everything you do and say" (p. 8F).

Meanwhile, Lillian kept a doctor on call for fear that her husband might collapse from the stress. All the while, she kept her worries secret lest she add to the load he car-ried. The Andersons felt they were prisoners of Bhopal, a private jail they carried wher-ever they went. Reading the paper, watching the news, or going out for an evening din-ner might bring unwelcome reminders of what had happened. They lay down at night with "lumps in [their] chests," and both experienced difficulty sleeping. Always regarded as a low-profile couple, their lifestyle became almost reclusive.

DIMENSIONS OF JOB STRESS

This case study highlights important aspects of **job stress.** First, work stress generally involves both the organization and its employees. Job stress is not a private matter for the employee to deal with alone and in isolation. Employees may transport personal and family problems to the job, but work problems also spill over to the home (Rousseau, 1978).

Second, job stress produces negative effects for both the organization and the em-ployee. For the organization, the results are disorganization, disruption in normal opera-tions, lowered performance and productivity, and lower margins of profit. For the em-ployee, the effects are threefold: increased physical health problems, psychological distress, and behavioral changes. Problems with health may not be so much related to the onset of a specific disease but to the quiet and gradual loss of health. Psychological distress usually comes with loss of job satisfaction and several related negative emotions. The resulting changes in behavior tend to affect both productivity within the company and lifestyle outside the workplace.

Third, job stress requires both organizational and personal solutions (Ivancevich, Matteson, Freedman, & Phillips, 1990). Employee assistance programs that focus solely on the employee perpetuate the myth that job stress is the worker's problem and the worker's fault. Removing job stress also requires some intervention and change in the organization. Until this happens, personal coping strategies are little more than Band-Aids that help the employee survive from one crisis to the next. We will discuss several organizational and personal intervention strategies later in this chapter.

DEFINING JOB STRESS

One definition of job stress focuses on job features that pose a threat to the worker (Lee & Ashforth, 1996). Threat may be due to excessive job demands, insufficient supplies to meet workers' needs, or the possibility of loss. When the job requires too much work in too short a time, job overload exists. Supply deficits concern things employees expect from their jobs: adequate salary, job satisfaction, and promotion or growth in the job. A threat of loss may include demotions, unattractive relocations, or outright severance from the job (Latack, Kinicki, & Prussia, 1995).

The transactional view of stress applied to the work environment says that *job stress* is work demands that exceed the worker's coping ability. At a broader level, job stress involves interactions of work conditions with worker traits that change normal psychological or physiological functions or both (Beehr & Newman, 1978; Edwards, 1992). While some forms of stress may actually increase worker productivity, we are generally concerned with finding solutions to distress in the work setting that impairs job performance.

THE COSTS OF WORK STRESS

A preeminent concern is the immense personal and economic loss from job stress and from unsafe conditions on the job. The federal government reported that 6,220 job fatalities occurred in 1995, an incidence that represents some decline since 1980 (Department of Labor, 1997; Stout, Jenkins, & Pizatella, 1996). During 1992, in addition to the more than 6000 fatalities, 60,300 deaths occurred due to occupational illnesses—for example, lung diseases and lead poisoning (Leigh, Markowitz, & Landrigan, 1997). Among the total of 6.8 million job-related illnesses and injuries, there were about 865,000 occupational illnesses (U.S. Department of Labor, 1997).

Beyond the incalculable costs of loss of life, occupational illnesses and injuries represent great loss of productivity for the industry, loss of wages for the worker, and distress for many who must now contemplate a future without meaningful work and wages, and a future that has been compromised with failing health. The direct costs of injuries and illnesses totaled $65 billion in 1992 (Leigh et al., 1997). Indirect costs including lost wages add another $106 billion loss. The total cost—$171 billion annually—calculates at $468 million dollars lost each business day. As Leigh and his colleagues pointed out, these annual losses are as great as losses from cardiovascular disease ($164 billion), or from cancer ($171 billion), and 6 times the loss from AIDS-related illnesses ($30 billion).

Although data are hard to come by, it is widely believed that acute reactive stress contributes to many job-related accidents and fatalities (Green, 1985). The Bureau of Labor Statistics estimates that American workers lose 3.5 % of their total work hours through absenteeism (Veniga & Spradley, 1981). Probably one in every three workers, on any given day, calls in sick because of stress-related problems. One recent estimate suggests that stress-related claims cost nearly 10% of a company's annual earnings (Gibson, 1993).

SYMPTOMS OF WORK STRESS

Mere monetary computation of losses overlooks the most important outcomes of work stress. Adults spend roughly half their waking life on the job. Because more wage earners now work overtime or hold two jobs simultaneously, that figure may be an underestimate. Conditions at work thus contribute significantly to lifestyle and health. The effects may spread, either positively or negatively, to all facets of life.

Terry Beehr and John Newman (1978) reviewed many job stress studies and concluded that three negative personal outcomes result from work stress: mental health symptoms, physical health symptoms, and behavioral symptoms. The following sections summarize some of these symptoms, but the list will probably change in the future as we increase our knowledge of work stress.

Psychological Symptoms of Work Stress

Psychological distress and mental disturbance bear an important relation to work conditions. This is evident from the inclusion of an occupational-stress category in the *Diagnostic and Statistical Manual of Mental Disorders*, Fourth Edition (DSM-IV—American Psychiatric Association, 1994; Sauter, Murphy, & Hurrell, 1990). The following symptoms occur in various occupational settings as a result of work stress.
- Anxiety, tension, confusion, and irritability
- Feelings of frustration, anger, and resentment
- Emotional hypersensitivity and hyperreactivity
- Suppression of feelings, withdrawal, and depression
- Reduced effectiveness in communication
- Feelings of isolation and alienation
- Boredom and job dissatisfaction
- Mental fatigue, lower intellectual functioning, and loss of concentration
- Loss of spontaneity and creativity
- Lowered self-esteem

Perhaps the most predictable consequence of job stress is job dissatisfaction. The employee feels little motivation to go to work, to do a good job while at work, or to stay on the job. Other symptoms occur at different stages on the road to job dissatisfaction and vary from one person to another. Current research on workplace motivation is beginning to integrate systems variables with human factors to obtain a better balance between job demands and job satisfaction (Katzell & Thompson, 1990).

Anxiety, tension, anger, and resentment are among the more commonly reported symptoms. Some people find job pressure so great they increase their psychological distance and gradually become depressed. This may occur after the employee tried but failed to correct the stress situation. When this occurs often, the outcome may be *learned helplessness,* which prevents the employee from making changes even when it is within his or her power to do so. On the other hand, some employees probably never try because they bring a load of learned helplessness to the job.

Physical Symptoms of Work Stress

One of the alleged outcomes of unmanaged stress is a gradual deterioration in physical health. Before clinical pathology appears, however, several physical symptoms give warning of something wrong. A few of the identified physical symptoms are listed here (Cordes & Dougherty, 1993; Latack & Kinicki, 1995).

- Increased heart rate, blood pressure, and potential cardiovascular disease
- Increased secretions of stress hormones (for example, adrenaline and noradrenaline)
- Gastrointestinal disorders such as irritable bowel syndrome, colitis, and ulcers
- Increased frequency of bodily injuries and accidents
- Physical fatigue, and possible chronic fatigue syndrome
- Respiratory problems, including aggravation of existing conditions
- Skin disorders
- Headaches, low back pain, and muscular tension
- Sleep disturbances
- Impaired immune function, including possible increased risk for cancer

Adequate research exists to verify the effects of work stress on the cardiovascular and gastrointestinal systems. Links to physical fatigue, bodily injuries, and sleep disturbances are also well verified. The remaining disorders are not as reliably established as resulting from work stress.

Stress also comes from unsafe work environments. The National Institute for Occupational Safety and Health (NIOSH) lists the ten leading work-related diseases or injuries as follows: occupational lung diseases; musculoskeletal injuries; occupational cancers; severe occupational traumatic injuries; cardiovascular disease; disorders of reproduction; neurotoxic disorders; noise-induced loss of hearing; dermatologic conditions; and psychological disorders (Levi, 1990). Among the psychological outcomes of working in unsafe, hazardous, or dangerous occupations is a general increase in stress, depression, and smoking, as well as lower trust of management (Roberts, 1993).

Obvious examples of unsafe work environments are plants that produce toxic chemicals or materials using unsafe methods. Asbestos, the most common toxic chemical (Cullen, Cherniack, & Rosenstock, 1990a), causes white-lung disease and cancer. Benzene causes leukemia and aplastic anemia. Coal dust causes black-lung disease. Radiation causes cancer, leukemia, and genetic damage. Lead causes kidney disorders, anemia, central nervous system damage, sterility, and birth defects. NIOSH estimates that 1 million of the 16 million working women of childbearing years work in jobs with the potential for exposure to hazards that could produce birth defects or miscarriages. In addition, workplace toxins have a detrimental effect on the male reproductive system, leading to lower or no production of sperm, lowered sex drive, and possible damage to sperm chromosomes (U.S. Department of Health and Human Services [NIOSH], 1997). Behavioral methods may be effective in reducing exposure (Hopkins et al., 1986), but the need to alter unsafe production environments is still evident.

One problem in making the work-stress-health connection clear-cut is that employees bring physical health problems to the job. These problems may be related to high-risk behaviors in the social environment. Work conditions may intensify a health problem and make it visible, but then the job may get the blame. James House (1987) argues that current research does not provide a strong and convincing picture of the relationship between stress and disease, because research fails to consider the etiology of chronic disease. Further, as we have noted earlier, many affective variables, especially negative affect, are most important to stress and health. However, these negative affective variables have not been adequately reflected in job stress research.

Paul Spector and his colleagues also argue that current research uses simple, linear, cause-effect models that do not do justice to complex stress-health relationships (Spector, Dwyer, & Jex, 1988). They suggest that three hypotheses must be entertained when investigating stress-health relationships. First, performance indicators might alter workers' perceptions of stress, a *reverse causality model*. Another is the *reciprocal causation* notion that both outside events and performance outcomes cause perceptions of stress; this in turn feeds back negatively to performance. Finally, there is the *external cause* model, which suggests that some individual dispositional variable is responsible for both performance outcomes and perceptions of stress. Spector's group found little evidence for the dispositional approach. They did, however, find evidence for the reciprocal causation model without ruling out the reverse causality model.

Behavioral Symptoms of Work Stress

Several behavioral symptoms reveal job stress. These include the following:

- Procrastination, work avoidance, and absenteeism
- Lowered performance and productivity
- Increased alcohol and drug use and abuse
- Outright sabotage on the job
- Overeating as escape, leading to obesity
- Undereating as a withdrawal and sudden weight loss, probably combined with signs of depression
- Increased risk-taking behavior, including reckless driving and gambling
- Aggression, vandalism, and stealing
- Deteriorating relationships with family and friends
- Suicide or attempted suicide

Procrastination is often disguised as busywork. The comment "just getting organized" may be a mere coverup to avoid doing something bothersome. Work stress frequently combines with other problems such as alcoholism and drug abuse. There is evidence that alcohol dependence and abuse are more frequently linked with certain occupations—for example, construction and transportation (Mandell, Eaton, Anthony, & Garrison, 1992). Further, it is clear that mixing alcohol and the job increases the risk for occupational injury by as much as 35% (Dawson, 1994).

Behavioral Symptoms with Organizational Impact

Work stress has a major impact on employee mental and physical health, but it also affects the organization. Stress is associated with poor job performance, absenteeism, and accident proneness. The employee experiences low job involvement and loses a sense of responsibility to the job. The employee also displays a lack of concern for the organization and for colleagues. The final outcome may be the employee's leaving the job. A cautionary note about absenteeism is necessary. Dan Farrell and Carol Stamm (1988) conducted a meta-analysis of 72 studies on absenteeism to resolve inconsistencies reported in previous studies. They found that the only significant correlates of absenteeism were work environment and organizational variables, including control policies (warnings, incentives, dismissals, and so forth). Demographic and psychological factors did not predict absenteeism.

SOURCES OF WORK STRESS

Attempts to identify the sources of stress on the job disclose many culprits. First, stress is an interaction between the objective work conditions and the perception that skills match job demands. Thus, the sources of job stress noted here are not solely responsible for job stress. Instead, they add potential for stress in combination with worker traits and perceptions. The most commonly identified sources of work stress are summarized in Table 7-1 with both contributing factors and possible consequences (Cooper, 1983; Cordes & Dougherty, 1993). These are job-specific stress, role stress, interpersonal stress, career development, organizational structure and development, and the home-work interface. We will use this list to structure the discussion that follows. Before reading further, it may be instructive to fill out the Work Stress Profile (Self-Study Exercise 7-1) on page 200.

Stress Related to Job Conditions

Specific work conditions that contribute to stress include job complexity, work overload or underload, unsafe physical conditions, and shift work. *Job complexity* is the inherent difficulty of the work to be done. Several factors contribute to job complexity. They may include the amount and sophistication of information required to function in the job, as well as expansion or addition of methods for performing the job.

WORK OVERLOAD Work overload can be divided into **quantitative** and **qualitative overload.** Quantitative overload results when the physical demands of the job exceed the worker's capacity. This occurs when the employee must do too much work in too short a time. Some jobs may require physical strength beyond the worker's capacity or set unreasonably high quotas. The assembly line may keep moving no matter how strained or fatigued the worker is. The day may be heavily scheduled, with no downtime. Qualitative overload results when work is too complex or difficult. This occurs when the job taxes either the technical or mental skills of the worker.

ASSEMBLY-LINE HYSTERIA Work underload means that the job is not challenging or fails to maintain the worker's interest and attention. George Everly and Daniel Girdano (1980) called this **deprivational stress.** They suggest that understimulation is most frequently found in assembly-line workers and in large bureaucracies. NIOSH described an **assembly-line hysteria** in which victims display symptoms of nausea, muscle weakness, severe headaches, and blurred vision, where no physical basis for these symptoms exists. Instead, the symptoms may be a psychological response to a job that is boring, repetitive, lacking in social interaction, and low in satisfaction.

TABLE 7-1
Summary of major job stressors

JOB STRESSORS	CONTRIBUTING FACTORS	POSSIBLE CONSEQUENCES
Job conditions	Quantitative work overload Qualitative work overload Assembly-line hysteria People decisions Physical dangers Shift work Technostress	Physical and/or mental fatigue Job burnout Increased irritability and tension
Role stress	Role ambiguity Sex bias and sex-role stereotypes Sexual harassment	Increased anxiety and tension Lowered job performance
Interpersonal factors	Poor work and social support systems Political rivalry, jealousy, or anger Lack of management concern for worker	Increased tension Elevated blood pressure Job dissatisfaction
Career development	Underpromotion Overpromotion Job security Frustrated ambitions	Lowered productivity Loss of self-esteem Increased irritability and anger Job dissatisfaction
Organizational Structure	Rigid and impersonal structure Political battles Inadequate supervision or training Nonparticipative decision making	Lowered motivation and productivity Job dissatisfaction
Home-work interface	Spillover Lack of support from spouse Marital conflict Dual-career stress	Increased mental conflict and fatigue Lowered motivation and productivity Increased marital conflict

DECISION-MAKING RESPONSIBILITY AND STRESS Qualitative overload may occur when a manager must make decisions that affect company production and employees' futures. Managers may have to plan production schedules, procure materials, evaluate staff, and make recommendations for hiring, firing, and layoffs. When decisions merely involve *things,* as opposed to people, managers may function effectively. When the manager's decision involves responsibility for others, stress is more likely.

SELF-STUDY EXERCISE 7-1

Work Stress Profile

This scale provides some information on work stress. Instructions for scoring and interpreting the scale appear at the end of the questionnaire.

The following statements describe work conditions, job environments, or personal feelings that workers encounter in their jobs. After reading each statement, circle the answer that best reflects the working conditions at your place of employment. If the statement is about a personal feeling, indicate the extent to which you have that feeling about your job. The scale markers ask you to judge, to the best of your knowledge, the approximate percentage of time the condition or feeling is true.

NEVER = not at all true of your work conditions or feelings
RARELY = the condition or feeling exists about 25% of the time
SOMETIMES = the condition or feeling exists about 50% of the time
OFTEN = the condition or feeling exists about 75% of the time
MOST TIMES = the condition or feeling is virtually always present

	NEVER	RARELY	SOMETIMES	OFTEN	MOST TIMES
1. Support personnel are incompetent or inefficient.	1	2	3	4	5
2. My job is not very well defined.	1	2	3	4	5
3. I am not sure about what is expected of me.	1	2	3	4	5
4. I am not sure what will be expected of me in the future.	1	2	3	4	5
5. I cannot seem to satisfy my superiors.	1	2	3	4	5
6. I seem to be able to talk with my superiors.	1	2	3	4	5
7. My superiors strike me as incompetent, yet I have to take orders from them.	1	2	3	4	5
8. My superiors seem to care about me as a person.	1	2	3	4	5
9. There are feelings of trust, respect, and friendliness between me and my superiors.	1	2	3	4	5
10. There seems to be tension between administrative personnel and staff personnel.	1	2	3	4	5
11. I have autonomy in carrying out my job duties.	1	2	3	4	5
12. I feel as though I can shape my own destiny in this job.	1	2	3	4	5
13. There are too many bosses in my area.	1	2	3	4	5

	NEVER	RARELY	SOMETIMES	OFTEN	MOST TIMES
14. It appears that my boss has "retired on the job."	1	2	3	4	5
15. My superiors give me adequate feedback about my job performance.	1	2	3	4	5
16. My abilities are not appreciated by my superiors.	1	2	3	4	5
17. There is little prospect of personal or professional growth in this job.	1	2	3	4	5
18. The level of participation in planning and decision making at my place of work is satisfactory.	1	2	3	4	5
19. I feel that I am over-educated for this job.	1	2	3	4	5
20. I feel that my educational background is just right for this job.	1	2	3	4	5
21. I fear that I will be laid off or fired.	1	2	3	4	5
22. Inservice training for my job is inadequate.	1	2	3	4	5
23. Most of my colleagues are unfriendly or seem uninterested in me as a person.	1	2	3	4	5
24. I feel uneasy about going to work.	1	2	3	4	5
25. There is no release time for personal affairs or business.	1	2	3	4	5
26. There is obvious sex/race/age discrimination in this job.	1	2	3	4	5

> **NOTE:** Complete the entire questionnaire first! Then add all the values circled for questions 1–26 and enter here.   Total 1–26 [ ]

	NEVER	RARELY	SOMETIMES	OFTEN	MOST TIMES
27. The physical work environment is crowded, noisy, or dreary.	1	2	3	4	5
28. Physical demands of the job are unreasonable (heavy lifting, extraordinary periods of concentration required, etc.).	1	2	3	4	5
29. My work load is never-ending.	1	2	3	4	5
30. The pace of work is too fast.	1	2	3	4	5
31. My job seems to consist of responding to emergencies.	1	2	3	4	5
32. There is no time for relaxation, coffee breaks, or lunch breaks on the job.	1	2	3	4	5
33. Job deadlines are constant and unreasonable.	1	2	3	4	5

	NEVER	RARELY	SOMETIMES	OFTEN	MOST TIMES
34. Job requirements are beyond the range of my ability.	1	2	3	4	5
35. At the end of the day, I am physically exhausted from work.	1	2	3	4	5
36. I can't even enjoy my leisure because of the toll my job takes on my energy.	1	2	3	4	5
37. I have to take work home to keep up.	1	2	3	4	5
38. I have responsibility for too many people.	1	2	3	4	5
39. Support personnel are too few.	1	2	3	4	5
40. Support personnel are incompetent or inefficient.	1	2	3	4	5
41. I am not sure about what is expected of me.	1	2	3	4	5
42. I am not sure what will be expected of me in the future.	1	2	3	4	5
43. I leave work feeling burned out.	1	2	3	4	5
44. There is little prospect for personal or professional growth in this job.	1	2	3	4	5
45. In-service training for my job is inadequate.	1	2	3	4	5
46. There is little contact with colleagues on the job.	1	2	3	4	5
47. Most of my colleagues are unfriendly or seem uninterested in me as a person.	1	2	3	4	5
48. I feel uneasy about going to work.	1	2	3	4	5

> **NOTE:** Complete the entire questionnaire first! Then add all the values circled for questions 27–48 and enter here.
>
> Total 27–48 [ ]

	NEVER	RARELY	SOMETIMES	OFTEN	MOST TIMES
49. The complexity of my job is enough to keep me interested.	1	2	3	4	5
50. My job is very exciting.	1	2	3	4	5
51. My job is varied enough to prevent boredom.	1	2	3	4	5
52. I seem to have lost interest in my work.	1	2	3	4	5
53. I feel as though I can shape my own destiny in this job.	1	2	3	4	5
54. I leave work feeling burned out.	1	2	3	4	5
55. I would continue to work at my job even if I did not need the money.	1	2	3	4	5

	NEVER	RARELY	SOMETIMES	OFTEN	MOST TIMES
56. I am trapped in this job.	1	2	3	4	5
57. If I had it to do all over again, I would still choose this job.	1	2	3	4	5

> **NOTE:** Now go back and add the values for questions 1–26. Do the same for questions 27–48. Enter the values where indicated. Then add all the values circled for questions 49–57.
>
> Total 49–57 [   ]

Last, enter those sums for each of the following groups of questions and add them all together to get a cumulative total.

QUESTIONS:	1–26 Inter- personal	27–48 Physical Condition	49–57 Job Interest	TOTAL 1–57
TOTALS:	[ ] +	[ ] +	[ ] =	[ ]

The first scale measures stress due to problems in interpersonal relationships and to job satisfaction or dissatisfaction, as the case may be. The second scale measures the physical demands of work that wear on the person daily. The third scale measures job interest and involvement. For each of the scales, you can gain some sense of how much job stress you live with relative to the original test group by locating your scores on the scale provided below. On each scale, a high score means more job-related stress. If you are high in one of the areas, say interpersonal stress, it could be of some help to pay attention to the interpersonal aspects of your job.

	← Low Stress →			← Normal Stress →			← High Stress →		
Interpersonal	.. 39	43	46	51	54	57	62	68	75 ..
Physical	.. 35	40	44	48	52	55	58	62	67 ..
Interest	.. 13	15	17	18	19	21	23	25	27 ..
Total	.. 91	101	111	117	123	134	141	151	167 ..
Percentile	.. 10	20	30	40	50	60	70	80	90 ..

The work stress profile has been tested in a sample of 275 school psychologists. The three scales are virtually identical to those identified in other work stress scales. The reliability of this scale is quite high. For the total scale, the reliability is .921. Reliabilities for the three subscales are .898, .883, and .816, respectively. A reliability of 1.00 indicates perfect reliability. The high reliability shown by this scale may be due in part to the fact that it was tested on a single occupational group. Additional studies with other occupational groups will be needed to determine if the scales are stable across a variety of occupations.

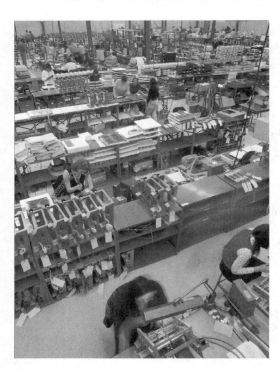

Assembly line workers may encounter boredom because of the monotonous, repetitive nature of their work.

Stress also increases as managers assume more responsibility for their decisions. Conversely, stress declines when management spreads out the responsibility for decisions—say, within a committee. A decision that must be made by some deadline can be highly stressful. Some people even try to avoid making deadline decisions. In many jobs, though, there is no time to waste. People working in life-and-death situations, such as emergency service crews, cannot take their ideas to a board room or request a computer simulation showing the likelihood of success for a plan of action. Presidents, military leaders, and pilots of stricken aircraft also fit in this category.

PHYSICAL DANGER Physical danger is a potential source of job stress, especially when the worker confronts the threat of injury. People in emergency service jobs, such as police officers, miners, fire fighters, soldiers, and bomb disposal squad members, confront this type of stress. Successful coping is closely related to one critical factor: whether the employees feel adequately trained to handle the emergencies. This is consistent with the cognitive view that stress results when demands exceed capacity.

SHIFT WORK Shift work requires that workers rotate schedules. This can produce disturbances in sleep patterns, neurophysiological rhythms, metabolic rate, and mental efficiency. These reactions occur because of disturbances in the **circadian rhythm,** a type of internal body clock. Jet lag is one example of this type of disturbance.

The primary pacemaker for the circadian rhythm is the hypothalamus (Czeisler et al., 1990). This may account for several body processes that change with disturbances in

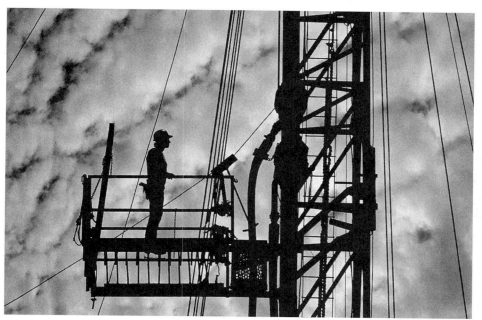

The constant rotation of working time against the natural rhythms of the body may produce a number of undesirable health consequences for shift workers, such as those who work in the mining and oil industry.

the body clock. For example, in the morning the body secretes only small amounts of the stress hormones, adrenaline and noradrenaline. These secretions increase as the day progresses. Also, some people describe themselves as "morning people." They feel most alert and work most efficiently in the morning. Then they fizzle out by mid- to late afternoon. Other people are "night owls." They never seem to get going until midday and do not hit full stride until even later. They may work late into the night but struggle to get out of bed in the morning.

One circadian rhythm is the 24-hour sleep-waking cycle, with the norm of nighttime sleep and daytime work. Shift-work schedules force people out of this cycle, though. An extreme example is the so-called graveyard shift that runs from around midnight to 8:00 in the morning. The body's clock is temporarily disturbed on this schedule. Physical and psychological effects may occur as described earlier. The person may feel out of sync mentally and physically. Irritability may increase, and typical family interactions may be disrupted. Observations of these difficulties with shift-work have led to closer monitoring of workers, adjustments in shift-work to reduce distress, and expansion of employee assistance to help offset any problems (Koller, 1996).

There is evidence that the 24-hour cycle may not be the best for everyone. Some people might be better off on a 23-hour cycle, while others might function best on a 26-hour cycle. Unfortunately, time-based societies do not take circadian rhythms into account when setting work schedules, so the worker suffers while trying to adjust. Research suggests that people can adjust to shift work, but it is not easy. Fast adapters adjust in about one week. Slow adapters require about three weeks. Overall, shift cycles that work with at least a three-week interval will accommodate the majority of people, but some people feel that they never do adjust. Recent evidence (Czeisler et al., 1990) shows that controlled exposure to bright light and darkness can help night-shift workers adapt in as little as three days.

Role Ambiguity: What Am I Doing Here?

Role ambiguity as a source of work stress is a frequently cited problem, especially in very large and/or ill-structured organizations. The term *role* refers to society's expectations that a person will display certain behaviors when he or she occupies a certain position. Thus, *role ambiguity* occurs when you do not know what management expects you to accomplish. A *Quality of Employment Survey* (Quinn & Staines, 1979) showed that 52% of workers reported conflicting demands. Role conflict is central to the midcareer crisis. In a midcareer crisis, the employee feels stress from such conditions as overpromotion, underpromotion, lack of job security, and thwarted ambition.

The effects of role ambiguity include low performance and low job satisfaction, high anxiety, tension, and motivation to leave the company (Moch, Bartunek, & Brass, 1979). French and his colleagues showed that women perceive more role ambiguity than men (French, Caplan, & Van Harrison, 1982). They also observed that women had higher levels of life stress compared to men. Among the possible reasons for this are sex-role stereotypes and dual-career families that place more pressure on women (Cramer, Keitel, & Rossberg, 1986). However, Martocchio and O'Leary (1989) conducted a meta-analysis of sex differences in occupational stress and discovered no significant sex differences in experienced and perceived work stress. How this inconsistency will be resolved remains to be seen.

Interpersonal Stress: Does Anyone Care?

Personal relationships on the job are very important to job satisfaction. Broad social networks, including support from workers, management, family, and friends, relieve strain (Fisher, 1985). This statement is consistent with Cobb's (1976) findings that social support serves as a buffer against stress. Social support on the job appears to temper physiological stress reactions by reducing the amount of cortisone released, lowering blood pressure, holding down the number of cigarettes smoked, and promoting complete cessation of smoking.

The *Quality of Employment Survey* previously mentioned revealed that 30% of the workers doubted that supervisors cared about their welfare. This concern is often related to leader characteristics and organizational structure. Management style and what the manager believes about employees are also critical.

Career Development: Where Am I Going?

Job stress mirrors the developmental peaks and valleys in the employee's career. According to one national study of work stress, people bring several specific hopes to a job. They hope for rapid, or at least steady, advancement. They hope for some freedom in the job and increased earning power. Employees hope to learn new things and work at new jobs. Finally, they hope to find solutions to certain work problems (Veniga & Spradley, 1981). For some employees, the promotion does not come. The job that once looked so secure may be eliminated. Job loss for many is the ultimate in work stress. In any given year, even during a strong market economy and high employment, nearly 1.5 million people will lose their jobs (Latack, Kinicki, & Prussia, 1995).

When their hopes and dreams only flicker faintly, employees often lose a sense of accomplishment and self-esteem. Minor irritants they would have casually brushed aside when the dream was fresh now irritate and fester inside. Four factors are closely related to stress in career development: underpromotion, overpromotion (also called the **Peter Principle),** lack of job security, and frustrated ambitions. Contrary to what some managers believe, job insecurity—not rising production demands—increases stress and generally lowers productivity.

Organizational Structure: What Are They Doing Up There?

The structure of a business can also produce stress. Most often, employees complain about rigid structure, interoffice or intraoffice political squabbles, and inadequate supervision from management. Employees also dislike lack of involvement in decision making and restrictions on their behavior, including lack of managerial support for individual initiative and creativity. Paul Spector (1986) conducted a meta-analysis of studies dealing with autonomy and participative decision making. He found that when *perception* of control is high, workers experience high levels of job satisfaction and low levels of physical symptoms. The same pattern occurred for actual participation in decision making.

The Home-Work Connection: Sanctuaries and Spillover

Most people think of home as a sanctuary, a place that is private and quiet and where one can be alone. It is a retreat that allows rebuilding and regrouping of inner strengths to meet outside demands. When pressure invades that sanctuary, however, it may magnify the effects of stress at work. Denise Rousseau (1978) provided evidence of a **spillover** from events at work to events at home. Rousseau believes that work experiences are positively related to nonwork experiences. If a person has a job that diminishes self-esteem and produces low satisfaction, that person will have similar experiences in social life. Research has discovered spillover in numerous occupations, including logging, manufacturing, and professional work.

Spillover is only one of five models that seeks to explain the home-work connection. *Compensation theory* suggests that positive events in one area compensate for deficits in the other. *Segmentation theory* considers home and work as two independent arenas that do not influence each other. *Instrumental theory* assumes that we use one area to obtain things for the other. Finally, *conflict theory* states that work and home are incompatible and that sacrifices have to be made in one to fulfill obligations in the other (Burke, 1986; Zedeck & Mosier, 1990). This is a situation in which research may not resolve the issue in favor of one theory. There is support for each model, perhaps because each reflects a valid way to link home and work in cognitive schemata. Personal appraisals of job satisfaction and typical stress reactions appear to influence which process is functioning for a given employee.

One example of stress due to the home-work connection is **dual-career stress.** Zedeck and Mosier (1990) report that the once-traditional nuclear family with a working husband, homemaker wife, and children now makes up only 11% of the nation's families. Nearly 40% of the work force now consists of dual-earner couples, and nearly 45% of married women are working outside the home. Even among those with children under 6 years, 37% of married women are working. These figures show substantial increases from

1960 figures, which were 31% and 19%, respectively (Cooper, 1983). A recent correlational study of dual-career women showed that coping strategies and marital adjustment combine to protect against stress. Dual-career women use more coping strategies when marital adjustment is good. They also report lower levels of stress compared to women whose marital adjustment is poor (McLaughlin, Cormier, & Cormier, 1988). Unfortunately, we cannot judge from this correlational analysis whether the use of coping strategies is responsible for both better marital adjustment and lower stress or whether other variables are responsible for both.

ARE BOREDOM AND MONOTONY REALLY STRESSORS?

For some time, the popular conception of job stress included the idea that monotonous, repetitive jobs (for example, assembly-line work) are stressful. In support of this notion, research showed that blue-collar workers tend to experience high job **boredom,** while professionals tend to experience low boredom (French, Caplan, & Van Harrison, 1982). Three terms often used interchangeably in discussions of job stress are *boredom, monotony,* and *repetition.* It may be more accurate to say that workers perceive repetitive, low-complexity jobs as monotonous. This produces a psychological state of boredom. Using the terms this way keeps job features distinct from subjective feelings.

Boredom does seem to have some bad side effects. For example, monotonous jobs are associated with low self-esteem, job dissatisfaction, and low life satisfaction (Johansson, Aronsson, & Lindstrom, 1976). Stress theory predicts that monotonous jobs should increase physiological arousal, but this does not occur. Physiological arousal depends on other factors, such as the complexity or risks, or both, involved in the job itself. Boredom in itself does not appear to produce stress.

Richard Thackray (1981) strongly disputed the idea that boredom is a stressor. He based his argument on a review of laboratory and field studies. Thackray defined boredom and monotony as highly repetitive and unchanging job conditions. Lack of change normally produces a desire for change or variety. Yet laboratory studies of repetitive work show lowered levels of physiological arousal, not heightened arousal.

In a field study of highly mechanized logging work in Sweden, Johansson's team showed that certain groups of employees were more vulnerable to disturbances such as sleep disorders, gastrointestinal disorders, headaches, and nervous tension. Following these observations, another team examined physiological and psychological differences between a high-risk group and a low-risk control group (Johansson et al., 1976). They found higher levels of urinary adrenaline in the high-risk group. The high-risk group also reported stronger feelings of subjective tension and negative mood when compared with the control group. Physical symptoms of illness were higher in the high-risk group, although this difference was not statistically significant.

In looking at the jobs in the high-risk group, the research team noted several important characteristics that might account for the results. The high-risk workers were in positions that required complex judgments and continuous attention. Most importantly, they worked under a forced tempo. Their production rate was a bottleneck in the plant's flow of production. All employees worked on a piece-rate system. What these men produced determined how much all the men earned. The high-risk group thus bore a great respon-

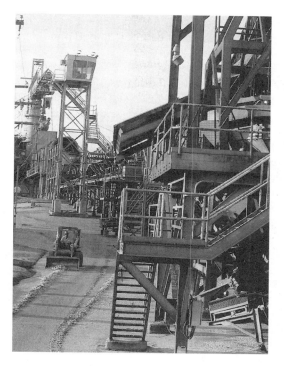

When pay for the work force is dependent on lock-step production, any worker who occupies a strategic position is likely to experience more stress than other workers.

sibility. The objective features of the job—that it was mechanized and repetitive—made no difference. The group worked with a psychosocial pressure that radically changed the meaning of the job from "monotonous" to bearing responsibility for the "livelihood" of their fellow workers.

TECHNOSTRESS: THE CHANGING FACES OF JOBS

Job obsolescence is a major problem confronting workers in technological societies. Changing technology often forces workers to find new work, perhaps several times during their careers. Estimates now indicate that the average skill turnover for many jobs is around 10 to 15 years. In other words, many jobs that existed 10 years ago may have changed to such a degree that they now require substantially different skills. Because an average career may last from 40 to 45 years, many workers may need to retrain or find a new job three to four times during their career. Nowhere is this more evident than in technologically intensive industries.

Craig Brod (1982, 1988) defined **technostress** as "a condition resulting from the inability of an individual or organization to adapt to the introduction and operation of new technology" (1982, p. 754). Thus, technostress refers to the strain felt by workers who must change their skills to keep up with changing jobs or whose jobs may no longer exist because of new technology. As one example, in 1982, Gavriel Salvendy wrote that almost 10 million people were using computers in jobs that did not exist a few years before. It is clear from what has happened in the intervening years that computer technology has invaded business and industry in a way that no one could have imagined at that time.

Technostress often intensifies because employees prefer to stay as comfortable as possible and usually resist change that requires adaptive effort. In addition, employees may view acquiring new skills as a threat to their self-esteem instead of as a positive road to personal growth and advancement. They may only come to accept technological change when management clearly and convincingly communicates the potential benefits and defuses the threats of new technology. As Naisbitt (1982) suggested, high tech must be balanced by high touch, the human side of innovation.

Brod (1982) suggested that technostress can be managed first through education aimed at understanding technostress and the human response to it. Second, the employee may apply several stress-management techniques to technostress, such as cognitive reappraisal and stress inoculation. Finally, self-assessment may help the employee detect negative thoughts and attitudes that stand in the way of change.

JOB BURNOUT: THE END OF WORK STRESS

If the buzzword of the stress-prone personality is "Type A," the buzzword of work stress is **job burnout.** *Job burnout is not a symptom of work stress, it is the result of unmanaged work stress.* Job burnout is now conceptualized as a three-pronged outcome including (1) emotional exhaustion, (2) depersonalization, and (3) reduced personal accomplishment (Cordes & Dougherty, 1993; Lee & Ashforth, 1996). Emotional exhaustion is a feeling of being emotionally used up, that one has given everything that one can and there is nothing more to give. Depersonalization occurs when people (customers, patients, and students, for example) are treated as mere objects. They are viewed with a cold, calculating detachment rather than as people to become engaged with in a humane and caring way. The feeling of reduced personal accomplishment is characterized by a tendency to be harsh on oneself, demeaning one's accomplishments and talents, and viewing one's career as flawed, if not largely unproductive and meaningless.

According to Veniga and Spradley (1981), there are five stages in burnout. In the *honeymoon stage,* youthful ideals motivate the novice, who feels an abundance of energy, enthusiasm, and job satisfaction. The person may continue with energy and satisfaction if early problems are constructively managed. In the second, *fuel shortage* stage, the actual signs of burnout begin to appear and intensify as time goes on. In the third, *chronic* stage, symptoms of exhaustion, illness, anger, and depression are continuously evident. In the *crisis stage,* symptoms are so severe the person may feel as though life is falling apart. In the final stage, *hitting the wall,* the person can no longer function and shows signs of serious deterioration. When this occurs, management or the employee or both must act quickly before stress turns into burnout.

There is a tendency to equate **workaholism** with job burnout. While the association is not perfect, evidence shows that the more hours you work per week, the more likely you are to burn out. Industry now considers the workaholic a liability, not an asset. Many workaholics work 80 hours or more per week. Some have physical systems that allow them to work longer and run on less sleep than others. For most people, such long hours severely strain the physical system, even though the costs may not appear until later. Workaholics may be driven by a fear of failure. This is a negative, stifling motivation rather than a positive, enhancing one. While they work hard, workaholics are not necessarily productive and creative. In fact, the opposite may be closer to the truth—that is, workaholics may work long hours because they are unable to concentrate on one thing at a time and thus need more time to complete a task.

WORK STRESS IN SPECIAL GROUPS

Certain occupational groups apparently experience more stress than others. Space does not permit a lengthy discussion, but some groups merit comment.

Working Women and Job Stress

Women still face blatant discriminatory practices that add stress to their working conditions. Women still are locked into a variety of dead-end, lower paying, and lower prestige jobs compared with men. No more than 2% of senior managers in the private sector, and only 8.6% in government, are women (Morrison & von Glinow, 1990). Although federal and state legislation was designed to protect against discriminatory practices, recent evidence reveals that the earning gap between women and men is still nearly 30%. For example, in 1970, white women earned about 59% of the salary of white men. In 1980, after years of effort and legislative work, women still earned just 59% of the salary of white men. However, by 1990, women's earnings had grown to 69%, and in 1995, they were at 71% of white male earnings.

Employed women often live in a dual-career home that is not yet egalitarian. The woman then works two jobs, one on the outside, the other as a homemaker. Numerous social and economic values continue to support this practice. Women's position in the work force and the stress they bear are not likely to change dramatically unless social attitudes change. Macewen and Barling (1988) showed that conflict between the roles of mother and career woman has a negative effect on marital adjustment. Their research did not indicate support for the reverse notion, that marital adjustment influences interrole conflict. Unfortunately, there is still little research available to help couples deal with dual-career stress (Higgins, 1986; Kater, 1985).

Sexual Harassment: Women's Hazardous Work Conditions

Perhaps the most oppressive form of stress comes from **sexual harassment** on the job. The recent news has been filled with tales of harassment in various settings and occupations, ranging from military drill sergeants to advertising to investment firms to medical professionals. Statistics vary greatly from setting to setting, but one survey revealed that nearly half of the women had been exposed to sexual harrassment in the workplace (Wyatt, 1995). A report in the *New York Times* indicated that nearly 75% of female doctors are harassed by patients in addition to harassment from physicians and interns.

Sexual harassment may be part of some misguided male's gamesmanship to prop up his ego. It is widely regarded as a pervasive power game designed to keep women in their place (Dan, Pinsof, & Riggs, 1995). Still, the effect is the same: exploitation and oppression combined with personal conflict and higher levels of stress.

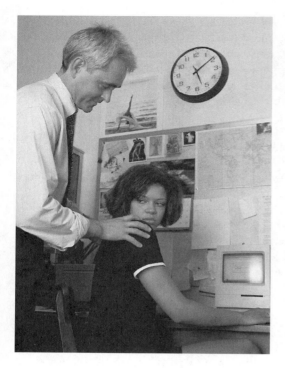

Although some touching in the workplace may be construed as social gestures of support and friendship, touching may be regarded as unwanted and offensive. It may then constitute sexual harassment and be subject to legal sanctions.

More active efforts may be needed to weed out those who harass. Women can use legal remedies that are not always easy to implement, but social changes seem to be working to support more active opposition to harassment. Still, filing a legal suit against a supervisor or colleague may be an act of courage necessary both to protect a highly valued professional career and to advance the position of women in the workforce.

Pletcher (1978) recommended that women keep a detailed diary of contacts, dates, times, incidents, words, and so forth. This may include instances of sexual innuendo, offensive jokes, and, of course, pressure, coercion, or job blackmail. Periodically, the woman should send notes from this diary by registered mail to herself or a trusted friend. The envelope should remain sealed for use in future legal action. Courts generally admit such documents as evidence, and they can prevent a defense attorney's attacks on memory.

Although many have argued that this battle must be waged by women, there may be times when men are valuable, even necessary, allies. More men now recognize that men who engage in harassment are an embarrassment. More men are now ready and willing to help impose sanctions or rid the company of offenders. Finally, involving men may increase pressure for change of sociocultural conditions that reinforce a dual standard of sexuality.

Stress in Air Traffic Controllers

Tragic air accidents often serve to focus attention on the stress in air traffic controllers (ATCs). The collision on February 1, 1991, of a USAir liner and a commuter plane at Los Angeles, probably the result of confusion in the control tower, reminds us again of this problem. In the world's most congested airports, airplanes take off or land every 30 to 45 seconds. ATCs are responsible for the safety of thousands of people each day and for protection of the airlines' multimillion dollar investments. Maintaining strained attention, as is necessary during long hours of radar monitoring, places extreme pressure on ATCs. Early studies of ATCs showed stress effects that included hypertension, peptic ulcers, diabetes, headaches, indigestion, chest pain, and burnout.

Subsequent studies began to question the generality of these early findings. A study of ATCs in low-density airports found none of the stress effects observed earlier (Melton et al., 1977). Another study revealed the mediating effect of air traffic density. Stress effects did not occur away from the most densely populated airports. Further, physical symptoms do not appear until after three years of service. This led John Crump (1979) to conclude that "the stress of ATC work is no greater than could be expected in 'normal' populations" (p. 244). In Europe's largest airport, in Frankfurt, Germany, ATCs indicated they were primarily dissatisfied with the administration, pay, and working conditions, not the stress of managing the airplanes (Singer & Rutenfranz, 1971). Thus, the potential dangers of this job must be considered on a site-by-site basis.

TELECOMMUTING OR THE ELECTRONIC SWEATSHOP?

An interesting, though controversial, development resulted from the personal computer revolution. The futurist Jack Nilles coined the term **telecommuting** to refer to people who work at home on jobs that depend on the computer or who transfer the results of their work to their employers via computers (Nilles, Carlson, Gray, & Honneman, 1976).

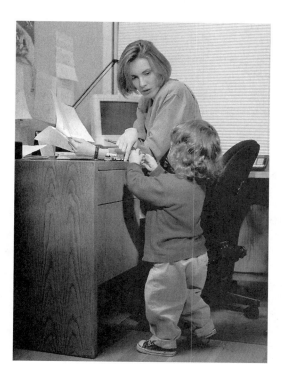

With the advent of the computer and the ability to connect to the world from home, more people are choosing to work in what is called the cottage industry.

The first signs of telecommuting or teleworkers appeared several years ago, primarily in large and specialized industries (Turnage, 1990). In the early 1980s, IBM and other Fortune 500 companies sponsored a study of telecommuting. They found about 100,000 people telecommuting. Recent estimates suggest that as many as 15 million teleworkers may exist in the United States (Turnage, 1990) and around 4 million in Great Britain (Norman, Collins, Conner, Martin, & Rance, 1995).

The expectation was that teleworking would reduce pressures from the traditional workplace. In contrast to a centralized shop and direct supervision, telecommuting could offer solutions to several management/employee problems. Among the expected benefits were distancing from office politics and assembly-line conflicts; decentralized work (flexplace) and reduced energy waste from commuting; flex scheduling and job sharing (between spouses or friends) with personal control over the flow of production; release time for personal business; and reduced difficulties in child care (Keita & Jones, 1990; Zedeck & Mosier, 1990). Businesses also were expected to benefit from lower overhead and higher productivity. On the down side, concerns voiced chiefly by labor suggested that the "romance" with telecommuting would ultimately lure workers into "electronic sweatshops" with more work for less pay, fewer benefits, and less legal protection. It now appears that the so-called second industrial revolution is unlikely to materialize as expected, if at all, because few of the expected benefits have been realized (Norman et al., 1995).

Within business, flextime increases productivity when resources have to be shared (Ralston, Anthony, & Gustafson, 1985). One small study found no difference in reported stress between those who worked in an office, those who telecommute with regular trips to an office setting, and those who work exclusively at home (cottage industry). However, the homebased group reported feeling more isolated and lacking in social support (Trent, Smith, & Wood, 1994).

COPING WITH JOB STRESS AND BURNOUT

Dealing with job stress requires intervention at both the organizational and personal levels. Unfortunately, much of the emphasis in organizations has been solely on teaching workers how to manage or reduce stress. Employee Assistance Programs (EAPs) still seem to assume that stress is a problem within the employee, and consequently, very little emphasis has been placed on sources of stress within the organization (Ivancevich et al., 1990; Murphy, 1984). In the next few pages, I will summarize some positive methods for coping with job stress.

Personal Strategies for Relieving Job Stress

Managing work stress may operate on several levels. It may involve interventions to change attitudes and perceptions, and permit emotional catharsis. Educational and counseling interventions may target problem-solving skills to change negative aspects of the work environment, including organizational features. Finally, tension-reduction strategies can be used to reduce physical arousal.

Cognitive methods usually focus on the distorting perceptions and irrational thought patterns that contribute to stress. People suffering burnout are all too quick to blame others, but blaming does nothing to correct the situation. Blaming also abandons personal control instead of encouraging belief in self-efficacy.

Numerous techniques reported in the literature depend on experimental models of stress management. Others involve active employee assistance programs (EAPs) in major businesses. Many stress management programs teach relaxation training to reduce tension and excess physiological arousal. Other interventions help employees reduce feelings of depression. Unfortunately, much of the research in these settings is still largely pragmatic and atheoretical (Ivancevich et al., 1990), which makes it difficult to know what elements are effective in producing change.

Over the years, several general suggestions for dealing with job stress have emerged. These include the following:

1. Maintain good physical health through a positive program of nutrition and exercise.
2. Accept yourself as you are with all your strengths, weaknesses, successes, and failures. Also, remember that you do not have to be competent in everything to have positive self-esteem.
3. Keep a confidante, a close friend you can talk to with complete candor. If you do not have a strong social support network, take time to develop one. The emphasis should not be on quantity, but on quality.
4. Take positive, constructive action to deal with the sources of stress in your job. This may require devoting time to learning new coping strategies through EAPs, or local university classes.
5. Maintain a social life apart from the people with whom you work. This does not mean you should not have friends from work. It simply means that you should have some part of your social life that does not allow for work problems to intrude.
6. Engage in creative activities outside the workplace. Cultivate hobbies and avocations that allow room for your personal growth.
7. Allow time for yourself. Short periods of quiet isolation should not be regarded as selfish, but personally restorative. Such periods may be used for contemplation, meditation, or problem-solving. Quiet isolation does not even have to occur each and every day to be beneficial.
8. Engage in meaningful work.
9. Apply an analytic (scientific) method to personal stress problems.

Physical exercise is often ignored as a coping strategy for job stress. Physical exercise is an excellent change of pace from the job, especially for desk-bound workers. It provides release for emotional and mental tension. It reduces frustration and allows displacement of anger or aggression that might be self-destructive. Finally, it reduces risk of coronary disease and lowers absenteeism, job injuries, and health-care costs (Gebhardt & Crump, 1990).

Another effective coping technique is to *change gears* through some interesting hobby or creative activity. A hobby that keeps you physically, mentally, and spiritually active is important to maintain a sense of perspective. Social activities can also provide a way of changing pace. However, people often socialize with others from work. This may transport job problems to the home (another spillover effect) and remove opportunities for relaxation.

Accuracy in self-assessment is also important in minimizing job stress. A mismatch between job requirements and job skills may occur because employees do not accurately evaluate their skills for the job demands. It is true that management makes promotion decisions based on assessments of performance in lower-level jobs that are not directly comparable to the higher-level jobs. We often forget, though, that when the mismatch occurred, there was an employee with an inaccurate self-assessment waiting to be promoted. After the promotion, when the employee is unable to keep up with the job, a cycle of frustration and recrimination may take place. The job that looked attractive in prospect may now threaten the employee's future with the company. Peter (1969) described this situation in *The Peter Principle,* which is based on promoting people to their highest level of incompetency.

Using the scientific or analytic method in managing stress means forming hypotheses about what may be the source of a problem. It means that a person collects data from relevant sources, including friends and colleagues, then evaluates a hypothesis in light of the data. The person may use the information to intervene or plan some constructive course of action that will prevent the problem from recurring. In this sense, the scientific method is not for theory building but for application to the real world.

Perhaps the most important way a person can cope with job stress is to work on becoming more aware of the stressors that are unique to his or her position. A person can use a personal inventory or diary, use an objective resource person, or cultivate the art of listening to his or her own body. The body can sound the alarm in early stages of stress and enable a person to prevent it from worsening.

Coping by Taking Legal Action

Employees should be aware of the legal remedies at their disposal. These may be used to settle personal grievances or effect organizational reform. For example, employees have the right to file a complaint with the Occupational Safety and Health Administration (OSHA) regarding unsafe and hazardous work conditions. Federal agencies must then conduct site inspections and evaluations. The agencies may levy fines or recommend other sanctions against companies that do not correct the conditions. Most public organizations (government, schools, universities) have strict laws against sexual harassment, and well-established protocols for filing, hearing, and resolving charges of harassment. The business sector has not been as proactive, but there are still well-defined federal, state, and local policies and procedures to protect and assist those who have been wronged. One method of coping is to learn about these resources when the first signs of difficulty appear. The list of Websites provided at the end of the chapter includes information directed to this end.

Organizational Strategies: Employee Assistance Programs

Many companies now have employee assistance programs. At the beginning of the 1980s, fewer than 300 firms offered such programs. By the early 1990s, over 2400 firms, including several prestigious Fortune 500 companies, provided employee assistance programs.

An employee assistance program offers a variety of services to deal with different facets of employee adjustment to work. Most programs extend to areas beyond the job and include assistance for problems that may have developed outside the job but that affect job performance. These services include personal counseling, classes on stress management and coping (Ivancevich et al., 1990), job retraining, career-change counseling, and support for families of employees in stressful occupations (Hildebrand, 1986). Some programs include a professional staff retained by the company solely to assist its employees. Beyond this, corporations are developing a broad range of services to help employees retain the enthusiasm and freshness of a new employee. Child-care programs, fully-equipped gyms, spas, and exercise and nutrition programs are becoming more common (Gebhardt & Crump, 1990; Ilgen, 1990). These programs address some important needs but do not always directly deal with the issue of reform of the organization itself.

SUMMARY

In this chapter, we have looked at the issues of job stress and burnout. The costs of job stress to both business and the employee reaches into the billions of dollars each year. The psychological costs cannot be calculated in such units of exchange, but the losses are no less real. The following represents the major points discussed.

- Job stress involves negative effects for both the employee and the employer. It is rarely a problem that can be corrected just by focusing on the employee, because it typically involves mismatches between organization and employee.
- A transactional view suggests that job stress results when the demands of work exceed the worker's ability to cope.
- In addition to economic costs, job stress takes its toll in many physical ways including increased accidents and injuries, increased illnesses, and deaths from job-related conditions.
- The symptoms of job stress include physical, psychological, and behavioral disturbances. The most notable psychological symptoms include frustration, anger, hyperreactivity, withdrawal, and depression.
- Some of the more noticeable physical symptoms include increased heart rate and blood pressure, gastrointestinal disorders, chronic fatigue, and sleep disturbances.
- The sources of job stress include physical conditions of the job, work overload, role ambiguity, interpersonal relationships on the job, career development, organizational structure, and the home-work connection.
- One major source of stress depends on the extent to which the job satisfies the employee's long-term goals related to self-esteem, meaningful work, and advancement. When these needs are not met, it increases the likelihood that the employee will hit the slippery slope to job stress and potential burnout.
- Burnout is the end of unmanaged job stress. It includes emotional exhaustion, depersonalization, and reduced personal accomplishment.
- Certain occupational groups, such as women and emergency service providers, are more subject to stress because of job discrimination or because of the dangerous nature of their jobs. When stress occurs because of discriminatory or harassing activities, it is important to know what avenues are available to obtain relief.
- The advent of telecommuting signalled a shift from centralized business to decentralized business including the potential for home-based businesses or cottage industries. Although there are some advantages for many people in this way of working, it is not clear that stress is markedly reduced overall or that one form of stress is replaced by another.
- With early recognition of the onset of stress, effective interventions—including cognitive appraisal, relaxation training, and physical exercise—may be applied to reduce, if not eliminate, the effects of stress. Personal coping skills must be combined with corporate interventions to reduce long-term stress.

CRITICAL THINKING AND STUDY QUESTIONS

1. What are the primary functions of the sympathetic and parasympathetic nervous systems? What are the core features of job stress?
2. What is spillover? How may this feature of job stress contaminate relations both at home and at work?
3. Although several symptoms of job stress are described as behavioral, what are some of the likely psychological processes (inferred) that may be behind the behavioral?
4. Why do you think jobs with personnel responsibility tend to place high stress loads on the people in those jobs?
5. Are there occupations not mentioned in the text that you think might also be subject to high levels of stress? If so, what are they? Is there empirical evidence to support your hypothesis?

KEY TERMS

assembly-line hysteria	job stress	shift work
boredom	Peter Principle	spillover
circadian rhythm	qualitative overload	technostress
deprivational stress	quantitative overload	telecommuting
dual-career stress	role ambiguity	workaholism
job burnout	sexual harassment	

WEBSITES job stress: dissatisfaction, burnout, and obsolescence

URL ADDRESS	SITE NAME & DESCRIPTION
http://www.welltech.com	☆WellTech International. Website for Worksite Health Promotion
http://www.dol.gov	The Department of Labor. Provides latest information on government regulations for the workplace, as well as links to other government agencies
http://www.jobstresshelp.com	The Job Stress Help Page. Links to numerous job-stress sites
http://rhi.hi.is/~agnes/	Mental Health Net. Occupational stress information
http://www.labor.org.au/ library_catalog/0002425.html	Human stress, work and job satisfaction
http://www.feminist.com	This feminist website provides information on job discrimination and legal issues for women in the workplace.
http://www.umanitoba.ca/ student/counselling/cnews/ cnews296.html	Managing job interview stress

CHAPTER 8

Social Sources of Stress:

Social, Technological, and Life-Changes

Our method of dealing with [social] dangers … is likely to be too slow and dangerous for the rate of change that exists today.

AUBREY KAGAN

QUESTIONS

- Do road rage incidents signal frustration with the complexity of modern living?
- What social conditions have been used to explain stress and illness?
- How does rapid social change contribute to stress?
- How can we measure life-change stress?
- Do stressful life events really produce illness?
- Are there weaknesses in the argument that life-change stress produces illness?
- Are there links between race, socioeconomic status and health?
- Do religious beliefs serve in some way to help people cope with stress?
- What is posttraumatic stress disorder?
- What factors predispose some people to become victims of crime?
- How can we avoid becoming victims of crime?
- What attitudes often get in the way of taking safety measures?

W e are reminded often of the complexity of modern society. The explosion of technology and information provides many benefits, but also threatens to overwhelm our senses, perhaps even fatigue our decision processes. Social structure is more regulated through complex legal codes, yet social order seems perilously close to disintegrating into chaos. Laws meant to maintain order are routinely ignored, and we overlook personal responsibility in favor of blaming social conditions, all the while forgetting that we are each helping to create the social condition.

Recent events on our nation's highways seem to provide object lessons in personal frustration that translates into the spread of even more social stress and disorder. The automobile and the freeway have become symbolic of a free society, the freedom to go and come whenever and wherever we please, be it for work or pleasure. Yet, as freeways become more crowded and the pressures of modern commuting pile up, the car has also become a weapon used by modern road warriors to express road rage.

CASE STUDIES IN ROAD RAGE: THE BENIGN AND MALIGNANT

At the relatively benign end of the road-rage continuum, Mr. Cline, a driver's education teacher, apparently became incensed when another driver, Mr. Macklin, cut him and his two female pupils off on the streets of Chapel Hill, North Carolina. Cline instructed his pupil to chase Macklin, a 21-year-old waiter. When they finally intercepted him, Cline punched Macklin, giving him a bloody nose. Still, this confrontation wasn't over. When Macklin drove off, Cline instructed his pupil to take up the chase again. The episode only ended when Cline was arrested for speeding and charged with assault (AP, 16 October 1997).

There are numerous instances from the dangerous end of the road-rage continuum. In Colorado Springs, 55-year-old Vern Smalley managed to get a tail-gating 17-year-old boy to pull over. Instead of apologizing for any discourteous driving behavior, the boy threatened Smalley. Instead of giving the boy a simple scolding, Smalley shot him to death (Vest, Cohen, & Tharp, 1997). In Massachusetts, a driver who wanted to go faster continually flashed his lights at a slower driver. The slower driver pulled to the side with the irate driver right behind. The slower driver then became the aggressor: Bringing a crossbow with him out of the car, he killed the impatient driver (Free, 1997).

Lest you think males are the only ones involved in this, women have added their share of road aggression scenarios as well.[1] At an on-ramp for I-71 in Cincinnati, Ohio, 24-year-old Rene Andrews apparently pulled out and cut off a 29-year-old mother, Trade Alfieri. Enraged, Alfieri passed Andrews and hit the brakes suddenly, causing Andrews to swerve into a parked tractor-trailer. Andrews suffered multiple injuries, but her greater loss was the end of her 6-month pregnancy. Later, Alfieri was sentenced to 18 months for vehicular homicide against the fetus (Adler, 1997).

---

[1] According to one largely unscientific survey covering 585 incidents, 45% of road-rage events were initiated by women and 55% were instigated by men (Free, 1997).

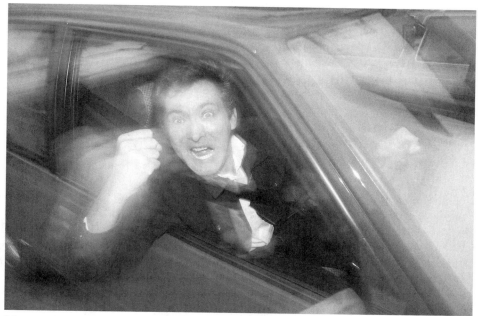

Many people have been confronted with angry, aggressive drivers who seem to feel the slightest inconvenience on the road is a direct affront.

CUTTING TO THE CHASE: POSSIBLE CAUSES FOR ROAD RAGE

According to a report from the National Highway Traffic Safety Administration (Martinez, 1997, July 17), each year approximately 28,000 traffic deaths may be attributed to anger out of control among drivers. Analysts are quick to offer answers. At the statistical level, the length of highways (total miles) has remained essentially constant since 1987, but the number of miles driven has gone up nearly 35%. In 1983, only about 55% of urban freeways were clogged during rush hour, but now nearly 70% are clogged. The number of cars on the road nearly doubled in the last 20 years, a sign of more multi-car families. During the past 10 years, the total number of cars actually grew at a faster rate (17%) than the population (10%) itself (Vest, 1997).

What is going on in the mind of the aggressive driver is always hard to fathom, but there are some suggestions. First, roadrage does not appear to be the isolated behavior of a few half-crazed sociopaths. It is instead a "subculture" of driving exemplified by a significant and growing number of drivers. Like the so-called California "oozing-stop" that is now almost nationally normative, road-rage events have increased by nearly 51% since 1990, and threaten to become a de facto standard of conduct on the road.

Second, the car has become a symbol of power, but it also bestows a certain anonymity for the driver. Thus, it is very tempting for someone struggling to cope with personal stresses to vent frustration as aggression on the road. In this view, the car is a modern answer to the great old-West equalizer, the six-shooter. Large sport-utility vehicles and 4 x 4 trucks especially combine the feeling of power with an aura of invincibility. As roads get more crowded, everyone is more anonymous—the other driver is no longer a person. It is easy, then, to dehumanize, even victimize other drivers, to see the other person as deserving any outrage we feel about even the slightest sign of road misbehavior. This defense seems to work well until we find ourselves looking down the fist of our next-door neighbor (as one driver did) or find out that the person we just cussed out or flipped off was our employer's wife (as another driver did). As soon as the other driver is mentally reconstructed with real human qualities, the rage subsides and the silliness of our own behavior is suddenly all too painfully obvious.

Third, constant time pressures exerted by jobs and busy family schedules make time spent on the road seem even more important. This magnifies the significance of any impediment to our speedy retreat from a pressure-packed day on the job or our ease of access to our conveniences. Finally, economic and market forces, especially the loss of a job or a recession, appear to increase road rage incidents. In this brief excursion into one of society's newest phenomena, we have touched on several themes (crowding, time pressures, power, and anomie) that are considered important in understanding social stress.

STRESS AND ILLNESS: THE ORIGINS OF SOCIAL THEORY

For many years, sociologists, psychologists, and politicians expended tremendous effort to identify pressures imposed by social conditions. Many studies suggested that crime, mental illness, and poor health increase in direct proportion to the degree of (1) financial stress or poverty, (2) urban crowding, and (3) lower socioeconomic status (Brenner, 1973; Faris & Dunham, 1939; Hollingshead & Redlich, 1958; Srole et al., 1962). Obviously, these three factors are closely related.

Still, early social analyses often overlooked the effects of racism that exposes certain groups to discrimination and extreme stress. Stress for several minority groups is further intensified by lower socioeconomic status, crowded living conditions, and "programmed failure" in educational systems that do not readily accommodate to the psychosocial needs of culturally diverse students (Peters & Massey, 1983; Taylor, 1997). Poverty and poor education combine synergistically to produce even worse economic hardships, a fact that is amplified among women (Aneshensel, 1992). Economic stress has a consistent, small but direct effect on physical health. Since unemployment has a negative effect on economic stability, it too has an indirect effect on overall health (Dooley & Catalano, 1984).

The Dodge-Martin Theory

Two social theorists, Dodge and Martin (1970), were among the first to state the relationship between social pressures and personal stress. Although they based their theory on statistics of *death rate* in the population (mortality), they believed that the theory applied to the *frequency of illness* (morbidity) as well. In brief, their theory stated that social factors, including excessive stress, contribute to both chronic (long-term) and acute (short-term) illnesses. However, they believed that different specific social factors account for different types of illness.

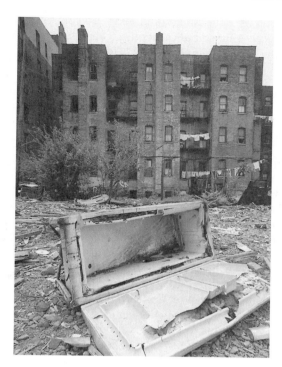

Social theories of stress suggest that low socioeconomic groups experience greater stress because of financial pressures and crowding into inner city slum areas.

Preventive Action or Delayed Reaction

Other writers have noted similar connections between social upheaval, stress, and illness. One life-change researcher, Aubrey Kagan (1974), pointed to the dramatic increase in ill health associated with the Industrial Revolution. This era gained notoriety from its rapid expansion of technology and monstrous pressures on social structures. A similar analysis may be appropriate for the Great Depression. Still, Kagan thought that the greatest danger for modern technological society would turn out to be an inability to respond at a pace that would keep up with the rate of change itself. In the final analysis, this could become modern society's Achilles' heel. Kagan's point makes plain the compelling need to understand the effects of social stressors in contemporary society.

Lifestyle Incongruity: Social Status and Health

William Dressler (1994) proposed that social status is linked to health outcomes through **lifestyle incongruity.** Lifestyle incongruity is a disparity between the desire and the ability to consume market goods. Many people would like to buy fancy cars, large homes, and the latest electronic gadgets. They would like to adopt leisure activities such as jet setting to Acapulco, skiing in Aspen, or hanging out on the Riviera. All of this comes at a very high cost and most people do not have the economic means to support such a lifestyle. This disparity between desire and economic ability is captured in catchy phrases such as "having a Ferrari need but a Volkswagen pocketbook" or "trying to live a Vail lifestyle on a ski bum's income." Dressler provides evidence to support his notion that lifestyle incongruity predicts lower overall family health status.

Social Causation, Social Drift, or Social Selection

Social theory often focuses on differences in outcomes for different social groups. That is, if a particular group shows more evidence of mental or physical illness compared to another group, then it is appropriate to ask if there are unique sets of social and personal traits in the groups that explain the difference. Three views have emerged to explain different outcomes: the *social causation* view, the *social drift* perspective, and the *social selection* viewpoint. The **social causation** view suggests that low-status groups have higher rates of disorder because they encounter more adverse, harsh, even traumatic conditions (Aneshensel, 1992). Here, the stressors normally connected with lower socioeconomic status play a causal role in the emergence of the disorder. The **social drift** notion suggests that disorders create a natural mobility or drift into lower social position. In this case, the stress that usually goes with being in a lower social position is an outcome of a previous disorder, not the cause of the disorder. Similar to the social drift theory, the **social selection** viewpoint suggests that people are selected out of social roles because they can no longer function with their disorders. As a result, they tend to end up working in lower status positions, living in less desirable communities, and pressured because of poorer financial stability. In general, there is more evidence for the social causation point of view than for the social drift or social selection notions.

Criticisms of Early Social Theory

Unfortunately, many early theories took a single-cause, single-effect approach. They looked for the cause of stress only in social structure (sociogenic) or only in the person (psychogenic). Social theories such as those just described focused solely on social structure, largely ignoring the person's contribution to stress reactions. *Relational analyzes* were not yet considered. Taylor (1997) reviewed many factors linking health status to social stressors. She noted that this type of analysis cannot focus exclusively on either the environment or on traits of the person, but must consider how people function in various contexts and subcultures. Her arguments serve to remind us that a contextual relational analysis is as important at the social level as it was at the personal level.

Early theories also ignored contradictory data. For example, many people raised in poverty and ghetto conditions not only survived but seemed immune to stress (Werner, 1984). Many people do not become disabled even when terrible things happen. A good stress theory should explain how people escape the effects of stress as readily as it explains why people succumb to stress.

This chapter and the next will focus on society, life-changes, and environment. The separation of these topics from attitudes and personality is for organizational convenience and thematic coherence only. *The focus is still on the interaction between environmental contexts and personal appraisal.* From a systems perspective, a person is a complex, self-referenced, comparator system that is enmeshed in larger social-cybernetic systems.

A SEARCH FOR SOCIAL STRESSORS

A review of stress literature suggests that there are relatively few but powerful sources of social stress. A major national study (Institute of Medicine, 1979) identified four sources contributing to stress and poor health: (1) uprooting stress, the effect of dislocation and frequent relocations; (2) dehumanizing societal institutions that deliver services mechanically and impersonally; (3) the existence of many obstacles to efficient and effective delivery of human services; and (4) the rapid spread of technology. More recent research suggests that attention also must be given to socioeconomic status (SES) and race as powerful variables that explain a number of negative health outcomes. SES (lower status) and race (African-American) are both connected to higher rates of morbidity and mortality (Taylor, 1997).

For our purposes, we will consider four social factors: (1) rapid sociological and technological change, (2) dehumanizing and victimizing forces, (3) SES and race, and (4) environmental stressors, including overcrowding, pollution, and so forth. The first three topics provide the major themes for this chapter. Environmental stress will be discussed in Chapter 9.

STRESS AND SOCIAL CHANGE

Alvin Toffler created something of a social furor when he named *future shock* the most important contemporary stressor. In his book by the same name, Toffler (1970) discussed the information overload that results from too much change in too short a time. Future shock is a disorder that typifies highly developed technological societies. It occurs when the pace of change is so rapid it exceeds our ability to integrate change. In short, future shock is the premature arrival of the future.

In his later work, *The Third Wave,* Toffler (1980) described the end of *second-wave* civilization. Industrialism, religious idealism, and a representative but centralized democracy formed the core of second-wave society. Second-wave civilization was the society of 300 years past, much of it the society of our immediate past, and still *part of a crumbling present.* Toffler suggested that current changes are not revolutionary in concept only, but also in pace and impact. The old society, with entrenched values and traditions, is being torn down to make way for a new society. The new society frames a new set of values and traditions on the rubble of the old. The transition will produce excitement for some but despair for others.

There is continuing, perhaps even growing evidence that supports Toffler's social commentary. The pace of social and technological change is astounding. Technological changes dramatically alter the way people work, learn, and spend their leisure time. The computer revolution has placed nearly 100 million units in businesses and homes in the United States alone. Since 1978, nearly 43 million jobs have been lost or transformed due to robotics and computers ("Information technology," 1997, January-February). In the mere 14 years since its inception, the Internet has created a cyberspace inhabited nearly 3 hours per day by 15 to 20 million users. Growth is so fast, it is estimated that web users may reach 88 million households by the year 2000 (McGrath, 1997). The TV addiction of the 80s has given way to chat room addictions in the 90s.

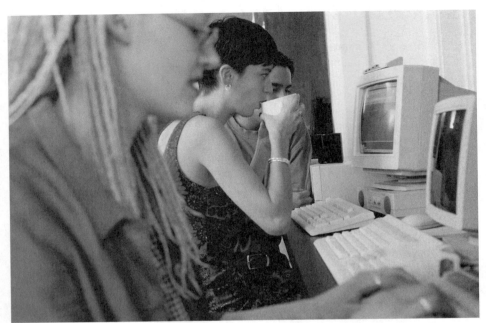

The immense popularity of the World Wide Web is reflected in this new type of coffee shop, called the Cyber Cafe, where people sip gourmet coffee and track down interesting cyberspace connections.

Education changes, and our children ask questions about problems that did not even exist 30 years ago. Science changes the amount and range of information available; *it will change even faster in the future.* Scientists now publish about 7000 articles per day. The amount of scientific and technical information published grows at the rate of 13% per year. At this rate, the volume doubles every 5.5 years. Turnage (1990) noted that information technology has halved in cost and doubled in power every 2 to 4 years. These scientific and technological information resources are increasingly available on the World Wide Web, and are becoming a constant for many educational activities. Technological change, though, only scratches the surface of what lies ahead.

Lifestyle changes mirror social change. Changes in the family challenge old values and religious traditions. Use or misuse of environmental resources leads to competition, if not violent confrontation, between special-interest groups. Organized religion abandons traditions and revises once-unwavering positions, shaking the foundation of personal values in the process. The Internet again plays a newfound role. It has disrupted family relationships, lured young and old alike to distant liaisons with people known only by a cyberspace moniker and whatever line the online romantic felt like spinning at the time. Committing crime, disseminating the literature of hate and racial divisiveness, spreading adult as well as child pornography, and luring the unsuspecting into the world of child prostitution and pornography have all become easier in cypberspace. At the same time, sociopolitical systems, still recoiling from the unexpected pace of growth, are struggling to redefine social values in this new context. Deciding how to police the web must wait while society tries to decipher what values are at stake and what crimes, if any, have been committed.

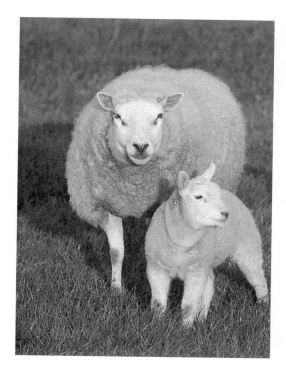

Excitement and fear both went up dramatically in 1997 with the news that a sheep by the name of Dolly had been cloned. At about the same time, another researcher announced plans to clone a human.

The assumptive world, the world order neatly built and packaged in our cognitive schema over the past decades, has changed in a matter of a heartbeat. Personal beliefs and ethical philosophies formed in the crucible of aging ideologies may be incompatible with the new order. For some, adjusting schemata to fit new realities may be easy. For others, it may be that they are not only unprepared for change, they may also be antagonistic to it. Others may simply endure with tension a world they barely recognize and no longer understand.

Personal Stability and Social Change

Confronted with technological developments such as surrogate mothers, test-tube babies, organ transplants, and the real prospect of human cloning, people find their choices are less certain. Personal beliefs and ethical philosophies are more difficult to articulate.

The psychological impact of this revolution is highly visible in three outcomes: anxiety, anomie, and demoralization. Confusion and anxiety tend to increase with rapid social change. Some authors even call this "the age of anxiety." Self-identity becomes less sure as relationships that provided personal security seem more tenuous. To use Durkheim's (1951) term, a feeling of **anomie** may increase. Anomie is a sense of being alone and lost in a huge, impersonal social structure that has no room for individual differences. **Demoralization** is the psychological result that occurs when environmental demands exceed a person's capacity to meet them (Dohrenwend & Dohrenwend, 1982).

These feelings may motivate a desperate, almost spiritual, quest for renewed stability. On one hand, people may cling tenaciously to the structures of the past. On the

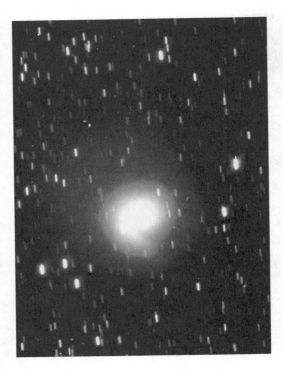

The plausible structure of the Heaven's Gate cult included the notion that the comet Hale-Bopp brought a spaceship that had come to transport them to a world level above the human.

other hand, people may be vulnerable to a variety of new—even seemingly strange—sources of stability. A rapidly fragmenting populace enthusiastically, and financially, supports new "cults" and "isms." Cultural diversity extends to religious pluralism. Each church has its own drive-up, tune-in, advice-column insights into human nature. Churches also have cash-and-carry solutions: buy a pamphlet, a book, an audio or videotape, and carry out the secret of happiness, marital bliss, or effective parenting. Each church captures some part of its followers' imaginations by offering to restore sanity in a world that is no longer comprehensible.

Bernice Martin (1981) noted that myriad cults and religions exploded onto the American cultural scene in the 1960s and 1970s. She used a term from Berger and Luckmann, *plausibility structures*, to describe the attraction:

> [Cults] seem to "prop up the subjective self" in a time of extreme cultural fluidity. [Cults] claim to be liberating while much of their real appeal lies in the latent function of providing firm and definitive conceptions of private individual identity which can be strongly internalized and which are usually backed up by psycho-social support structures. (p. 222)

LIFE-CHANGE, STRESS, AND ILLNESS

Rapid social change appears to function as an important source of stress. Some outcomes of social change may exist as subtle, if not insidious, pressures on personal adaptive reserves. Other effects may be more direct, as well as much more serious. A 1949

Conference on Life Stress and Bodily Disease formally recognized the importance of life stress and illness (Rabkin & Streuning, 1976a). In the 1970s and 1980s, several investigators launched empirical research programs to discover the relationship, if any, between **life-change and illness.** The details and conclusions of this scientific pursuit will occupy our attention for the next few pages.

LIFE-CHANGE UNITS: THE EMPIRICAL STORY

Two separate research groups began the most notable research on life-change and illness. The first team consisted of Thomas Holmes from the University of Washington and Richard Rahe of the U.S. Navy Medical Neuropsychiatric Research Unit. The second team consisted of Barbara and Bruce Dohrenwend (1982) at Columbia University. Because the Dohrenwends' work built on the legacy of Holmes and Rahe, we will treat the two lines of inquiry as a single program. Later, I will summarize the major criticisms of this approach.

Holmes and Rahe (1967) set out to answer two important questions. First, they wanted to know what life-change situations are most stressful. Second, they wanted to know what physical problems, if any, may develop because of stressful life-changes. They reasoned that both constitutional variables and temporal factors in life govern risk for illness. In the words of Richard Rahe (1974):

> Constitutional endowment helps to explain an individual's susceptibilities to particular types of illnesses but does little to explain why an individual develops an illness at a particular point in time. . . . Recent life changes appear to act as "stressors" partially accounting for illness onset. Conversely, when subjects' lives are in a relatively steady state of psychosocial adjustment with few ongoing life changes, little or no illness tends to be reported. (p. 58)

To answer the first question, Holmes and Rahe developed a scaling procedure to assess the degree of stress associated with commonly encountered life events. Taking a direct approach, they asked a large group of people to identify their most stressful events. Then Holmes and Rahe assigned weights to the events based on the group's ratings. They recognized that life events did not have to be extreme (such as war or trauma) in order for stress to be present. Instead, they focused on naturally occurring stressors, or life events such as marriage, divorce, childbirth, and death of a loved one (Dohrenwend & Dohrenwend, 1982).

In regard to the link between stress and illness, Holmes and Rahe followed an old trail. Early laboratory investigators discovered that numerous physical ailments, including ulcers and death, may be related to severe stress. If this finding were also true of people in a natural environment, some important implications for detecting and preventing the sources of illness might emerge.

To begin this phase, Holmes and Rahe asked approximately 5000 clients to write down events they considered most stressful. From this pool of responses, they built a list of 43 life-change events that included the positive (marriage), the negative (going to jail), frequent events (minor traffic violations), and rare ones (death of spouse or child). The common core is that these events require some adaptive struggle or **social readjustment** to manage them effectively. Social readjustment is "the intensity and length of time necessary to accommodate to a life event, *regardless of the desirability of this* *event*" (Holmes & Masuda, 1974, p. 49). Adaptive struggle may reveal itself in psychological conflict and anxiety for a time and may be the motivation for a lifestyle change.

In the next phase, Holmes and Rahe asked 394 people to rate the 43 events based on their experiences with the stressors. Further, they asked the clients to note the relative degree of disruption each event caused. Holmes and Rahe assigned marriage an arbitrary value of 500. Then each person judged whether the remaining events required more or less readjustment than marriage and assigned to each event a value proportionate to the value of 500. For example, if clients judged that death of a spouse required twice as much readjustment effort as marriage, they assigned it a value of 1000. After collecting this data, Holmes and Rahe computed the average severity of life-change produced by each event. Finally, they ranked the events from most intense to least intense.

THE SOCIAL READJUSTMENT RATING SCALE

The outcome of this process was the **Social Readjustment Rating Scale (SRRS)** shown in Self-Study Exercise 8-1. Note that the first item, death of spouse, is assigned a value of 100. The original rating used an arbitrary maximum value of 500, but after computing the final mean ratings, the investigators assigned the most severe stressor a value of 100. They adjusted all the means to this standard so the relative intensity of each event is still reflected accurately. Holmes and Rahe called this adjusted event value a **Life Change Unit (LCU).** Now, presumably, the total amount of stress a person experienced in a given time could be measured by adding together all the LCUs for checked events.

Note that the three items ranked most stressful by this sample (death of spouse, divorce, and separation) involve life-changes in marital status. In fact, eight of the top ten stressors are either family- or work-related. Also, very few items are *high-severity* stressors, whereas a large number are *low-to-moderate-severity* stressors.

In addition, many events are pleasant events. Most people probably think that marriage, pregnancy, completion of school, change in line of work, outstanding personal achievement, vacation, and Christmas are positive events. Still, according to Selye's view, positive events produce stress, some events more than others. As Selye's definition suggests, the body does not distinguish between positive and negative stressors. The excitement of marriage is almost as taxing as the grief suffered with the loss of a close member of the family.

Take a moment to respond to the scale before reading further. Circle the number on the left for any events you have experienced in the past six months. After you have done this, locate the LCU score for the event in the right-hand column and circle it. Then sum the circled LCU scores. Information on interpreting the results will be provided in the following pages.

DO STRESSFUL LIFE EVENTS
REALLY PRODUCE ILLNESS?

After they obtained these severity ratings, Holmes and Rahe wanted to know if life-changes affected personal adjustment and health, and if so, how. Previous research suggested that stressful life-changes could precipitate a variety of harmful effects, including

SELF-STUDY EXERCISE 8-1

Social Readjustment Rating Scale

RANK	LIFE EVENT	LCU
1	Death of spouse	100
2	Divorce	73
3	Marital separation	65
4	Jail term	63
5	Death of close family member	63
6	Personal injury or illness	53
7	Marriage	50
8	Fired at work	47
9	Marital reconciliation	45
10	Retirement	45
11	Change in health of family member	44
12	Pregnancy	40
13	Sexual difficulties	39
14	Gain of new family member	39
15	Business readjustment	39
16	Change in financial state	38
17	Death of close friend	37
18	Change to different lines of work	36
19	Change in number of arguments with spouse	35
20	Mortgage over $10,000	31
21	Foreclosure of mortgage or loan	30
22	Change in responsibilities at work	29
23	Son or daughter leaving home	29
24	Trouble with in-laws	29
25	Outstanding personal achievement	28
26	Wife begins or stops work	26
27	Begin or end school	26
28	Change in living conditions	25
29	Revision of personal habits	24
30	Trouble with boss	23
31	Change in work hours or conditions	20
32	Change in residence	20
33	Change in schools	20
34	Change in recreation	19
35	Change in church activities	19
36	Change in social activities	18
37	Mortgage or loan less than $10,000	17
38	Change in sleeping habits	16
39	Change in number of family get-togethers	15
40	Change in eating habits	13
41	Vacation	13
42	Christmas	12
43	Minor violations of the law	11

SOURCE: Holmes & Rahe (1967).

psychological disturbances and physical illness. Three lines of evidence contributed to the belief that stressful life-changes produce some deterioration in health, if not outright illness. One line of evidence, presented earlier, came from laboratory and clinical research programs based on Selye's theory.[2]

The second line of evidence comes from observations of reactions to natural disasters, such as earthquakes and floods, and observations of individuals under conditions of abnormal stress, such as soldiers in combat. The term **posttraumatic stress disorder** refers to the emotional-behavioral pattern that follows such extreme conditions. Information on stress reactions to catastrophic events will be presented in Chapter 9.

The third line of evidence represents the concerted effort of many investigators working over nearly two decades. Most have used the scaling techniques of Holmes and Rahe; others have adapted their scaling procedure or developed similar techniques. In all cases, the efforts shared a common goal: to assess the relationship between the amount of stress and the amount of illness in populations in the natural environment.

Physicians and Life Crises

Holmes and Rahe asked a group of 200 resident physicians to list all the "major health changes" they had experienced in the previous ten years and to fill out the SRRS. Each responding physician (88 total) received a score based on the sum of LCU values. Of the 96 major health changes reported, 89 occurred with total LCU scores over 150. When the LCU score was under 150, the majority reported good health in the following year. When the LCU score was above 300, over 70% of the physicians reported illness in the following year (Rahe, 1974). This led Holmes and Rahe to use 150 as a preliminary definition of *life crisis*.

Further analysis permitted Holmes and Rahe to establish more precise categories for life crises: 150 to 199 LCUs defined a *mild* life crisis, 200 to 299 LCUs defined a *moderate* life crisis, and anything over 300 LCUs defined a *major* life crisis (Holmes & Masuda, 1974). (If you have already responded to the scale, you can compare your score against this standard.) The working assumption is that the more life crises that accumulate, the more likely the person will incur some illness shortly afterward.

In an extensive review of studies aimed at testing this assumption, Holmes and Masuda found an impressive array of supporting evidence. Retrospective studies found increased life-change associated with myocardial infarction, fractures, diabetes, tuberculosis, pregnancy, and leukemia (Rabkin & Streuning, 1976a; Rahe & Arthur, 1978). Similar outcomes obtained in other cultures established the cross-cultural generality of the life events-illness relationship.[3] Studies of children, of identical twins, and of college students provided similar results. Among adults, the findings appear to hold across various occupational groups.

Hungarian Refugees and Carrier Pilots

Hinkle (1974) and his colleagues were among the first to provide evidence concerning the life events-illness connection. They studied several groups, but two groups in particular are of interest. One group consisted of Chinese-born graduate students, technicians, and professional people living in New York City. The second was a group of refugees who

---

[2]Recall the Brady executive monkey study, which showed development of ulcers in response to chronic stress.

[3]Included in cross-cultural replications were the countries of England, Wales, Norway, Sweden, Denmark, France, Belgium, Switzerland, Japan, Malaysia, San Salvador, and Peru, and the state of Hawaii.

escaped to America following the "Black October" Russian invasion of Hungary. Both groups had undergone severe dislocation, separation from families and stable social support groups, and extreme culture shock. Dislocation and acculturation are both known to be significant stressors (Riad & Norris, 1996; Smart & Smart, 1995).

For the most part, the Chinese group showed little evidence of illness. At first, this result seemed to contradict the expected pattern. Information from the Hungarian group, though, provided a possible explanation. The Hungarian group showed a significant change in illness *during the ten years preceding their flight.* They described their time leading up to the confrontation with the Hungarian regime as one of insecurity and frustration. During the revolution and escape, and in spite of severe disruption in their lives, they actually showed improved health. It appeared that the general excitement and the anticipation of making a fresh start in a new country served as a type of inoculation against sickness. Hinkle concluded that the effect of dramatic social change on a person's health could not be judged solely from the nature of the change itself. Other factors must be important, including a person's psychological characteristics.

Other investigations confirm this conclusion. For example, observations of enlisted sailors showed that only a few men accounted for most of the sick days taken. Sailors who worked in routine, menial jobs that required less skill were sick most frequently. Often their jobs were either hazardous or uncomfortable or both. Further, these sailors were less mature and less capable compared with those who did not report illness (Nelson, 1974).

Rubin (1974) conducted an interesting study in the real-world environment of aircraft carrier pilot trainees. The situation these trainees encountered appears similar in many respects to the Brady "executive monkey" study described in Chapter 1. Here is how Rubin described the training situation and aircraft:

> The F-48 Phantom jet fighter-bomber is a two-man aircraft. The pilot, in the front cockpit, has complete flight control. The radar intercept officer (RIO), in the rear cockpit, monitors the radar and other instruments but has no flight control. He does have excellent visibility. In an emergency both the pilot and the RIO can eject themselves from the aircraft, a procedure not without hazard. The RIO is aware of these hazards and the aircraft's position during the landing attempt, but he must rely completely on the pilot's skill for his own personal safety. (p. 228)

In other words, RIOs are in exactly the same situation as the monkeys who could not control the shock. The RIOs could only put their safety in the hands of the pilots and hope.

Measurements of the physical responses of both the pilots and the RIOs showed an interesting pattern of reactivity. While the RIOs showed higher levels of subjective anxiety on all days tested, the pilots showed the type of stress reaction pattern observed in the laboratory animals. Again, in the words of Rubin (1974):

> These results indicate that aircraft carrier landing practice was considerably more stressful for the pilots than for their RIOs. In the context of the "executive" monkey paradigm, the "executive" naval aviator, who had to perform a highly complex task while avoiding serious potential harm to himself, his partner, and his aircraft, showed an unequivocal adrenal cortical stress response. The passive partner, on the other hand, although completely aware of the risks involved, showed only a slight, statistically insignificant adrenal response. (pp. 231–232)

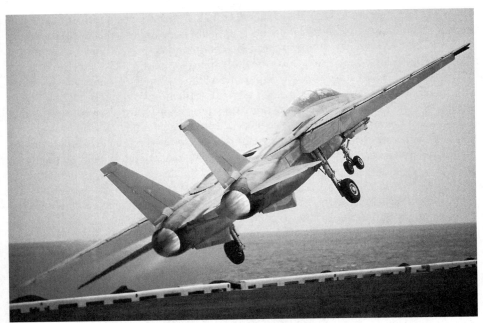

Carrier pilots have a tremendous responsibility, but during landing and takeoff, the RIO has no control and may experience more subjective stress than the pilot.

David Krantz and Shera Raisen (1988) reviewed a growing body of biobehavioral literature concerned with the effects of social stress on ischemic heart disease. They conclude from this review that three environmental variables contribute to increased coronary risk. These are low socioeconomic status, low social support, and occupational settings marked by low control and high demand. Still, Krantz and Raisen point out that the effects are typically small and the relationships complex. Thus, the notion of simple, one-way paths of causation does not fit the data.

THE CASE AGAINST LIFE-CHANGE AND ILLNESS

Research on life-change and illness has been criticized since it began. Lost in the shuffle is the counter-argument that life stress may be growth promoting, or that positive events may promote health, a position that has drawn little empirical attention (Ray, Jefferies, & Weir, 1995; Zautra & Sandler, 1983). The substance of life-change criticism will be examined briefly.

Most of the early studies on life stress and illness used retrospective designs, which contain several weaknesses. First, reliability of retrospective data is suspect because of errors in memory, subjective biases in reporting illness, over-reporting, and intervening distortions that may affect subjects' perceptions of the events (Rabkin & Struening, 1976a). Further, early prospective studies showed the expected relationship, but it was much weaker in the prospective studies than in retrospective studies. This led to a skeptical attitude in the scientific community.

Later, more carefully designed prospective studies caused even more skepticism. David Schroeder and Paul Costa (1984) reported on such a study that found no evidence for the connection. Subjects took a medical examination prior to a year designated as the target year. Later, the subjects reported on life-change using a "56-item Holmes-Rahe-style" checklist. Schroeder and Costa employed physicians' records of illness to assess the number of *new diseases not present at the prestress examination*. They found no correlation between the amount of life-change in the previous 12 months and the incidence of illness.

Still, disconfirming prospective studies such as Schroeder and Costa's must be weighed against positive prospective studies. It may be that moderator variables will be discovered that resolve the discrepancy between outcomes. Additionally, studies have shown that positive events, rather than contributing to more morbidity, actually reduce morbidity (Ray, Jefferies, & Weir, 1995).

One argument against the life stress-illness connection is both simple and powerful. This argument states that illness is often confounded with psychiatric and psychological problems. Psychiatric disability is stressful and causes disruptions in life. Evidence shows that illness occurs with greater prevalence in psychiatric populations. Thus, illness shows a correlation to life stress with no necessary causal connection. Also, it may be that psychiatric disability leads to distorted perceptions of life stress and biased reporting.[4] These arguments cannot be easily discounted.

Another criticism focused on the biased content of life-change scales. Life-stress scales appear to be contaminated with items related to mood and disposition. New evidence reveals that ratings of life stress may reflect a pessimistic style and negative emotional set more than they reflect inherent properties of the event involved. Support for this argument comes from the work of Brett and her colleagues, who use the notion of negative affect (Brett, Brief, Burke, George, & Webster, 1990). Negative affect is a mood-dispositional dimension that reflects pervasive individual differences in negative emotionality and self-concept. When Brett's group used measures of life-change free of negative affect bias, the relationship to physical symptoms mostly disappeared. When they constructed scales with extreme negative affect, the relationship to physical symptoms was even stronger than to total life-events scores. This provided even stronger evidence that the major contributing factor to the life-change–illness connection was negative affect. This finding is all the more interesting when we consider the role negative affect plays in coronary risk.

Finally, Brett's group showed that the negative affect scale correlated even more strongly with depression. Negative affect may be a general mood-dispositional tendency that carries with it the burden of depression and lower quality of health. The stress connection may be incidental or only a reflection of the person's dispositional tendencies. This would argue against life stress as a cause of illness.

RACE AND SOCIOECONOMIC STATUS

Earlier we noted that race and socioeconomic status (SES) are important factors in understanding social stress. Here we touch on some observed connections between stress and health related to these two factors.

---

[4]For a review of confounding variables, see Rabkin and Struening (1976b).

First, lower SES typically translates to more hassles in living, and more time spent just trying to arrange for basic living necessities. Housing is often substandard and includes numerous harmful conditions, such as fire hazards (poor wiring and refuse, for example) and a high density of rodents and insects. Housing and communities tend to go together. That is, poor housing typically exists in poorer communities. These communities carry additional risks because of higher crime rates, threat of attack, and the presence of more physical hazards such as toxins and pesticides. Further, there is generally more crowding in the community in general and in housing in particular, and a correlated rise in noise. Crowding usually translates to a variety of uncomfortable if not unwanted contacts with people whose behavior may range from the only mildly eccentric to the outright threatening. In general, there is a clear and simple relationship between social class and health outcomes: lower SES is associated with more negative health (Taylor, 1997).

Several minority groups are found disproportionately in lower SES. Nearly 33% of African-Americans are found in lower SES, but only about 11% of the white population occupies lower SES. Minority groups are more frequently refused important services, including access to financial institutions and resources to acquire more adequate housing. Minority groups also are more frequently either not insured or underinsured for medical needs. They often find it difficult, then, to avail themselves of direct care for pressing medical emergencies and are even less likely to be able to obtain preventive medical services. In spite of efforts in the United States to reduce disparity of treatment in social programs for culturally diverse groups, there are still many signs that equality is a goal yet to be reached. On virtually every major index of health status, African-Americans show lower standing than the white population. Worse yet, differences in morbidity and mortality appear to be widening, not narrowing (Taylor, 1997).

Lesley Slavin's group proposed a multicultural model of stress (shown in Figure 8-1) that examines many variables related to stress in minority groups (Slavin, Rainer, McCreary, & Gowda, 1991). Their model is based on the cognitive-transactional model developed by Richard Lazarus' research team (Lazarus & Launier, 1978). Slavin's group defines **culture** as "the thoughts, beliefs, practices, and behaviors of a group of people" as they relate to the group's history and social, religious, economic, and political organization (p. 156). Four points highlight the unique circumstances that expose minority members to stress. First, the smaller the minority group, the more likely an individual will be exposed to stressors related to acts of discrimination and racism. Second, oppressed groups will experience acts of discrimination with great regularity. Third, related to SES, the poor and politically weak will experience stronger stressors. Fourth, some stressors will occur that are directly related to the unique cultural customs of the group.

COPING WITH SOCIAL CHANGE

The complexity of social change precludes giving specific recommendations, as we might with more specific stresses. Social change is global, pervasive, insidious, and constant. As several writers have suggested, change may be the most constant part of our environment. Accepting the fact of change may be an important first step in coping with it. Preparation and self-education are also vital. The well-read, socially alert, and culturally aware person may have the greatest likelihood of managing innovation, technology, and lifestyle choices with the least amount of stress. Ostrich-like responses to unwanted change do nothing.

FIGURE 8-1

A multicultural model of stress incorporating transactional–relational themes from Lazarus (shown in the upper area). Culturally relevant aspects of stressor events and the appraisal process are shown in the lower shadowed area.

SOURCE: Slavin et al., 1991.

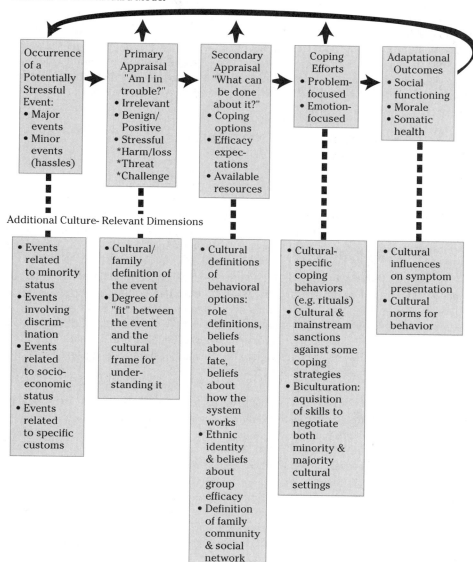

Elements of the Standard Model

| Occurrence of a Potentially Stressful Event:
• Major events
• Minor events (hassles) | Primary Appraisal "Am I in trouble?"
• Irrelevant
• Benign/ Positive
• Stressful
*Harm/loss
*Threat
*Challenge | Secondary Appraisal "What can be done about it?"
• Coping options
• Efficacy expectations
• Available resources | Coping Efforts
• Problem-focused
• Emotion-focused | Adaptational Outcomes
• Social functioning
• Morale
• Somatic health |

Additional Culture- Relevant Dimensions

| • Events related to minority status
• Events involving discrimination
• Events related to socio-economic status
• Events related to specific customs | • Cultural/ family definition of the event
• Degree of "fit" between the event and the cultural frame for understanding it | • Cultural definitions of behavioral options: role definitions, beliefs about fate, beliefs about how the system works
• Ethnic identity & beliefs about group efficacy
• Definition of family community & social network | • Cultural-specific coping behaviors (e.g. rituals)
• Cultural & mainstream sanctions against some coping strategies
• Biculturation: aquisition of skills to negotiate both minority & majority cultural settings | • Cultural influences on symptom presentation
• Cultural norms for behavior |

Stress-inoculation methods may also help (Meichenbaum & Jaremko, 1983). This approach focuses on imagining worst-case scenarios that might induce a high degree of stress. The assumption is that once you have anticipated your worst fears and thought about strategies for managing them, you will manage the situation better when it happens. In addition, change will be easier to tolerate because you have already worked out the emotional side of it.

An early report, *Healthy People,* presented several ways for people to cope with social stress (Institute of Medicine, 1979). These included belonging to a group, having acceptable substitute activities available, having ready access to advice, having someone to talk to about personal troubles, and having an education. Belonging to a group is important for social support (Cohen & Wills, 1985). Social support is helpful when one makes stressful decisions such as quitting smoking and going on a diet. Conversely, lack of social support may contribute to psychological disorders (Leavy, 1983).

RELIGION AND BELIEFS: INFLUENCE ON COPING AND HEALTH

For some period of time, discussing matters of religion in the context of health was almost taboo. The past few years have seen a resurgence of interest in the buffering effect of religion in coping with stress and maintaining health. A survey reported by Levin & Puchalski (1997) showed that nearly 80% of Americans believe in the power of God or prayer to improve the course of illness. Just a few years ago, only 3 medical schools offered classes on religious issues, but now nearly 30 schools do.

Religion probably works through cognitive belief systems to influence (1) the perception or appraisal of certain events, (2) the method of coping with stressors, and (3) use of certain health-promoting or -maintaining behaviors (Dull & Skokan, 1995). At the personal level, religion provides an assumptive world view that helps individuals construct logical accounts for events happening to them. These accounts do not have to be logical in any objective sense, only logical in a personal, subjective sense. Quite often these logical accounts include assumptions about the degree of control one may have over an event or even the need to control ("It's God's will for my life") an event. People often also construct a just world view using tenets from their belief system, which helps them maintain optimism in the face of some of the most traumatic events.

Religious beliefs are widely used to cope with stressful situations such as grief after loss of a loved one. To the extent that the practice of religion can be a form of coping strategy, it would be expected to have a positive effect on stress physiology and immune competence. Religious beliefs also are known to influence certain health practices (Dull, 1995). In some cases, the outcome is to promote positive acts. In other cases, it may be restrictive, reducing the likelihood of engaging in high-risk behaviors (promiscuous sex, addictive drugs, or smoking, for example) by "keeping pure the temple of God" (paraphrased). Finally, religious beliefs seem to provide a strong, durable sense of personal identity that is not shaken by traumatic events. Although scientific data is sparse on exact links between stress, health, and religious beliefs, there is a strong sense that a holistic view of the person must incorporate religious beliefs and practices as an important ingredient in the person's appraisal processes and coping strategies.

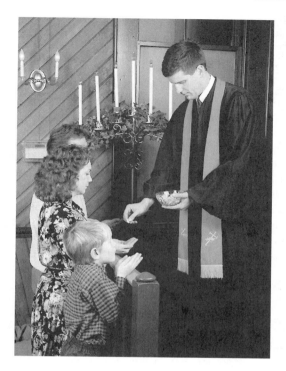

The social support, stable tradition, and belief structures provided by organized religions seem to provide many people with added means for coping with stress.

COPING WITH VICTIMIZATION

America—the land of the free, land of opportunity, play, and the biggest shopping malls in the world. America beckons many tourists to experience its pleasures. Yet, some European countries are rewriting America's slogans. "America—Deathtrap Under the Palms": so blared one headline in a German paper after a spate of separate victimizing crimes against tourists claimed three of its citizens.

April 1993: Special-education teacher Barbara Meller Jensen, along with her children, just wanted to experience some American culture on their holiday. They strayed off I-95 near Miami in their rented car. Within minutes Jensen was dead, murdered in front of her children in a so-called "bump-and-run" robbery.

After the Jensen murder, investigators discovered that local thugs were using the unique license plates of rental cars to locate targets. The tags were like neon signs inviting a hit. Visitors, whether American or foreign, typically carry a lot of money and are particularly vulnerable as strangers in the area. Steps were taken to correct the license plate spotlight, but it was in no sense a complete or permanent solution.

January 1996: A German vacationer is beaten to death near Key West.

February 1996: A Dutch tourist is shot to death in a Miami gas station.

As in many cases like this, the effects of crime reach out to others and endure (Hepburn & Monti, 1979). Barbara Jensen's family and friends, also victims, must suffer the consequences of this senseless crime for years.

Current crime statistics reveal both good and bad news. The good news first: Violent crime dropped more than 12% during 1995, the biggest drop since the Bureau of Justice began its surveys (1997). Now for the bad news: Crime creates more than 38 million victims each year, a figure that includes 9.6 million (25%) violent crimes and 28 million (74%) property crimes.[5] Nearly 2.6 million aggravated assaults and 21,937 murders occurred in 1994. Still in 1994, 432,000 women were forcibly raped or sexually assaulted. Nearly 33,000 men also were raped or sexually assaulted. Material loss from all types of robbery is more than $10 billion annually. Corporate and white-collar crime bilks untold billions through coercion, extortion, and fraud. Terrorism, something that used to happen only in other countries, has also become part of America's wounded psyche.

Great as the immediate physical and material losses may be, the aftermath of crime produces even more pervasive and debilitating effects. Call it "mind-rapes"—the unwanted, continual forced entry into one's consciousness of the memories, feelings, pain, and terror of the event. For many, this continual intrusion into the inner sanctum of the mind is the greater crime and the source of recurrent stress (Janoff-Bulman, 1988).

POSTTRAUMATIC STRESS DISORDER: A FIRST LOOK

Traumatic events may include natural disasters, murder, rape, combat, accidents, or terrorism. Still, there are common traits that typify victims' reactions, called *posttraumatic stress disorder* or PTSD for short (American Psychiatric Association, 1994). Four signs lead to the diagnosis of posttraumatic stress disorder (PTSD). First, evidence must exist of a recent stressor in which the person experienced or witnessed events that involved actual or threatened death or serious injury. Second, the victim relives the event through dreams, intrusive thoughts, or feelings that the traumatic event is happening again. Third, the victim avoids stimuli associated with the event and experiences numbing of responsiveness, which may appear as decreased interest in activities, detachment from others, or flattening of emotional affect. Finally, the person may show two or more symptoms of heightened arousal, including startle responses, sleep disturbance, survival guilt, or cognitive impairment, among others. The symptoms of rape-trauma syndrome are the same as those of PTSD (Burgess, 1983).

FEAR—THE VICTIM'S JAILER

The most pervasive psychological effect of trauma is fear. An assault or robbery does not even have to take place for fear to weave its web. Berg and Johnson (1979) speak of the **"fear-of-crime" syndrome** (p. 58) and of "self-defined prisoners," (p. 59) who no longer have safe havens when crime follows them into their homes. Fear becomes their jailer and gatekeeper, shutting off free access to an outside world that still beckons but is too frightening to explore. Personal freedom seems limited, because victims generally feel compelled to alter patterns of social, market, and work behavior (Brooks, 1981). They feel constant vigilance is necessary to ensure that personal injury or loss does not occur

---

[5]These figures are for people 12 years and older only, so they do not include crimes committed against younger children.

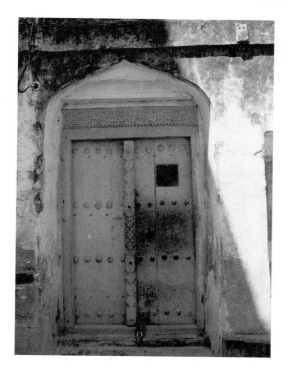

For many people, homes are as much prisons as retreats; they may only feel safe when tightly locked and barred inside.

again. Disillusionment about society in general and justice in particular become enduring attitudes. Victims expend mental energy in conflict that could be used for creative pursuits. In effect, fear changes the victim's reality.

VICTIMOLOGY: INVESTIGATING CRIMINAL-VICTIM RELATIONSHIPS

Criminologists are specialists who investigate the relationships between social systems and criminal behavior. Another group of specialists, **victimologists,** try to discover the factors that contribute to people becoming victims (Schafer, 1977).[6] Among many questions raised by these investigators, three are central. One issue is **risk:** What factors predispose some individuals to be targets of crime? A second question has to do with **prevention:** What can be done to educate people to reduce their risk? Another is *coping:* What can be done to help victims put their work, social, family, and personal lives back together?

The Question of Risk: Who Are the Victims?

Victims of crime exist in every segment of society, though some groups are more vulnerable than others. The term **vulnerable** refers to groups with shared demographic or personal characteristics who are susceptible to becoming victims through no fault of their

[6]Victimology is the science that explores the role of the victim in crime.

own (Galaway & Hudson, 1981). Several demographic traits are associated with higher risk for violent crime. The most important traits include age, race, and gender, but SES and marital status also provide clues to vulnerability.

AGE Younger persons have a higher likelihood of becoming victims, probably because of mobility and social behavior. However, the elderly experience more anticipatory fear and are more likely to feel the effects of victimization because of their relative lack of power (Berg & Johnson, 1979).

ETHNIC GROUP Blacks are more likely to be victims of robbery and assault compared with whites. Recent data on murder revealed that 48% of the victims were black and 48% were white (Bureau of Justice, 1997). Based on absolute number, then, there is no difference. However, based on population percentages, blacks appear to be relatively more vulnerable to murder.

MARITAL STATUS Unmarried people have a greater risk of becoming victims than married people, generally because of socializing activities. On the other hand, married people generally spend more time at home or work than on the move.[7]

SOCIOECONOMIC STATUS People of lower SES and unemployed people have a higher risk of becoming victims than those of higher SES and employed people.

SEX Men are at higher risk than women. This finding mirrors the patterns previously described: the most vulnerable people are young, unmarried, unemployed males, especially black males, who may be in the wrong place at the wrong time. Young males may be at higher risk, but females report more fear of victimization.

Prevention: How to Avoid Becoming a Victim

To be sure, modern living entails risks. Still, the likelihood of serious loss or injury from personal crime is less than that from driving a car. Further, a few simple steps can be taken to reduce the risks of becoming a victim. In other words, *reducing risk does not require monumental changes in lifestyle, only subtle shifts in habits.* This notion, that reducing risk does not require major lifestyle changes, is *the single most important idea* in this entire discussion.

Lifestyle Assessment

Lifestyles are significant factors in personal crime because lifestyles relate to being in places and situations with high *opportunities* for criminal actions. *Lifestyle* refers to routine work or leisure activities (Hindelang et al., 1978). A lifestyle assessment may be helpful, then, to understand how personal behavior alters environmental risks.

The first step is to identify personal habits of shopping, socializing, and movement in your locale. Habits by definition are automatic and require little or no conscious attention. Keeping a diary for one or two weeks may bring unattended trouble spots into focus. By cross-checking habits against the risk information that follows, you may see that certain adjustments are desirable.

---

[7]Schafer (1977) presents information that disputes this general pattern. He suggests that both the number of criminals and the number of violent crimes is largest among married persons. The argument, though, uses frequency rather than proportional statistics; this casts doubt on the argument. Schafer qualified the argument as pertaining to violent crime and not to all instances of victimization.

ADJUSTING TIME Overall, violent crimes are more likely to take place during the day than at night, but rapes and sexual assaults are more likely to take place between midnight and 6 A.M.

ALCOHOL USE Alcohol plays a significant role in criminal acts. Most importantly, *the contribution of alcohol to the risk of criminal assault comes as much from the victim as from the offender.* Alcohol affects decision-making processes and lowers important protective social inhibitions. Steele and Josephs (1990) call this an "alcohol-induced myopia." It appears to contribute to provoking criminal attacks or increasing the likelihood of injury or both.

AVOIDING HIGH-RISK PLACES Two places are notably high-risk: home and the street. About 25% of violent incidents occur at or near home. However, crimes occurring in these two arenas are dramatically different. Assaults in the home are most often crimes of passion, committed by a spouse, lover, or friend after a serious domestic conflict. These crimes have a high injury rate because the partner tends to react with physical aggression.

Criminal assaults on the street are often crimes of profit or power (territorial imperatives) precipitated by strangers experiencing personal frustrations (Schafer, 1977). Street assaults can be avoided largely through adjusting time schedules, using modes of transportation that avoid prolonged contact on the street, and traveling in groups.

TAKING SELF-PROTECTIVE MEASURES After a crime has occurred, victims frequently replay the episode and second-guess their reactions to the event. They wonder what they could have done differently. The basic principles of self-protection can be summarized briefly. Where profit seems to be the motive, it is less risky to let the thief carry on without resisting. When engaging in self-protection, physical counterattack more than doubles the risk. The most successful means of warding off attacks include verbal resistance through threats of detection, persuasion, or talking the offender out of committing the crime (20% injury rate, 80% injury free); evasive action (16% injury rate, 84% injury free); and simply yelling or screaming (36% injury rate, 64% injury free) (Hindelang et al., 1978).

ADJUSTING DAILY ACTIVITIES As noted earlier, only minor behavior adjustments are necessary to reduce risk. For example, you should vary routine market behaviors (shopping for food, clothing) instead of maintaining a rigid schedule. Also, shop during the day or early evening hours. Adjust job-related behaviors so hours of transit and mode of transit are optimal. Leave the office early to take a crowded metro, not late when you will be traveling alone. Attend social activities (such as movies and dining out) in small groups. On university campuses, late-night escort services are common to enable people to move about with safety. If one exists, consider making use of it when appropriate.

BARRIERS TO EFFECTIVE PREVENTION

Three psychological processes seem to influence both the risks we take and the stress reactions we experience from victimization. These are cognitive appraisals, beliefs, and emotional reactions. Cognitive appraisals include evaluating the risk of becoming a victim and making causal attributions about crime. Beliefs refer to our readiness to act based on the perceptions that our behavior will be beneficial in some respect. Fear is the emotional reaction of primary concern, as noted earlier.

Misattributions About Crime

Three faulty attributions play a crucial role in leading people to think that their risk for harm is not as great as it actually is. These attributions involve *local versus distant distribution* of crime, *local versus outside involvement,* and **self-blame** for cause of the crime.

MISATTRIBUTION 1: CRIME IS WORSE ELSEWHERE On average, people think crime is a big problem elsewhere, but not in their community. This is true even where crime rates are high, such as in urban inner-city districts (Hindelang et al., 1978). People are more likely to evaluate threat in their community as less than that in other communities even within their city. This misattribution may enable people to diffuse threat so it will not be a constant burden. It may also contribute to reduced vigilance, which increases the risk for subsequent victimization.

MISATTRIBUTION 2: OUTSIDERS ARE DOING IT People tend to attribute crime in their area to outsiders. Using data from a Florida sample, Schafer (1977) showed that the majority of offenders (61.5 %) lived only a few miles and a few minutes from their victims. Worse yet, 45% of murder victims and 68% of rape and sexual assault victims were related to or knew their assailant.

MISATTRIBUTION 3: I AM TO BLAME The process of self-blame has been the subject of much research over the past two decades. At least two motives affect the way people cope with serious accidents, injuries, or illness. The first, described in the work of Lerner, suggests that people need to maintain their belief in a just world (Lerner & Matthews, 1967; Lerner & Simmons, 1966). This motive subscribes to the belief that people get what they deserve and deserve what they get. Misfortune cannot be just random. Therefore, if something bad happens, the victim must have done something to deserve it.

TABLE 8-1
Relationship between sexual assault or rape victims and offenders

VICTIM-OFFENDER RELATIONSHIP	PERCENT OF RAPES/SEXUAL ASSAULTS
Intimates	24.0
Spouse	7.3
Ex-spouse	<0.1
Boy-/girlfriend	14.3
Other relatives	<0.1
Acquaintance/friend	40.0
Stranger	32.0

The second motive, described in the work of Elaine Walster, concerns the perception of control over the environment. Walster (1966) suggests that most people attribute blame to a victim to reassure themselves that they will not be likely to suffer the same misfortune. The basis of the reasoning is, again, that if the event is unpredictable or uncontrollable, it could happen to anyone, including themselves, at any time. Therefore, the victim must have had something to do with the accident.

Whether an individual *personally accepts blame* for a misfortune depends on the person's perception of control. If the victim perceives that he or she had control over circumstances leading up to an incident, the victim is more likely to engage in *behavioral self-blame* (Janoff-Bulman, 1988). This usually allows the victim to retain belief in the utility of preventive behaviors. *Characterological self-blame* occurs when the victim believes some enduring trait contributed to the incident. This usually involves self-esteem deficits and consequent depression. Bulman and Wortman (1977) also observed cognitive reappraisal. Some people evaluate the outcome as desirable. They may believe that "God is testing me," or "It really is a blessing in disguise," or "I know I will grow a lot because of this."

Attributing personal blame adds a significant load to the coping process and may interfere with recovery from life-threatening assaults and illness. Denial of blame may be a necessary short-term defense after a traumatic event. Continued denial, on the other hand, may interfere with assessment and implementation of adaptive changes in the lifestyle that contributed to the risk in the first place. Denial may also impair the healthy sense of caution needed to live safely and securely.

Beliefs About Personal Vulnerability

Beliefs about crime are also important. Beliefs are predispositions to act in certain ways based on positive and negative evaluations of people, places, and things. Our belief about vulnerability in particular is paramount. Beliefs about vulnerability may change behavior in one of two ways. First, belief in continuous vulnerability may heighten fear, and thus become disabling. Taken to the extreme, it approaches a paranoid-like state, a "bunker mentality," that may produce undesirable side effects, such as depression and disorientation, while placing unnecessary limits on personal freedom. On the other hand, people who believe that they are invincible tend to take unnecessary risks. Such people are likely to scorn suggestions to assess their lifestyle and to ignore most of the preventive actions suggested earlier. Beliefs can increase or decrease the likelihood of engaging in preventive behaviors, and they can help or hurt coping efforts in the aftermath of crime.

COPING WITH THE AFTERMATH OF CRIMINAL ASSAULT

As noted earlier, the effects of a criminal attack can be revealed in PTSD. Even in the absence of clinical PTSD, sleep disorders, anxiety attacks, and changes in appetite may occur. Compulsive lock checking, becoming housebound, and experiencing feelings of extreme terror may go on for weeks or months.[8]

---

[8]Studies of victims reveal that the mental maelstrom following a personal assault or loss may last up to three years. Severity of the crime and personal characteristics of the victim influence duration.

Reconstructing Assumptive Worlds

Another significant change occurs in the aftermath of traumatic events. Schemata constructed through experience are damaged, if not destroyed (Janoff-Bulman, 1988). Victims lose their sense of control and invulnerability. They feel their world is no longer safe and benevolent. The most important assault, the most hurtful injury, is to their schema of self-worth and self-acceptance. One important part of recovering from a traumatic episode is to reconstruct one's assumptions about the world in as coherent and positive a way possible.

Managing Fear from Victimization

The most powerful emotion victims feel is fear. Fear is a complex response that includes thoughts, feelings, and bodily reactions. It generalizes to encompass people who look similar to the offender and places that remind the victim of the original situation. Eliminating fear thus requires methods that will deal with these three channels of involvement and that can help the victim deal with generalized fears.

The most successful method for treating specific fears over the past few years has been systematic desensitization, which will be discussed in detail in Chapter 12. Another technique that may help combat fear is rational-emotive therapy. Rational-emotive therapy assumes that irrational thoughts bolster the fear and underlie self-limiting behavior. As practiced by Ellis (1962), the therapist attempts to point out the link between the person's emotions and thought processes. The goal is to replace irrational constructs, which stand in the way of healthy behavior, with rational assessments.

Another technique is stress inoculation, a multimodal method that combines several specific techniques. Stress inoculation attempts to get the individual to deal with small fears one at a time. A program can be structured so that success in dealing with little fears is almost a sure thing. As successes build, the person gathers resistance so that larger fears do not seem as overwhelming as before. As the process continues, larger fears become more manageable, until the person can deal successfully with the normal range of activities and people. This technique will be discussed in more detail in Chapter 12.

One behavioral manifestation of fear is avoidance of people, places, and things that remind the victim of the original event. This is anticipatory fear. Any behavior that leads to fear reduction is more likely to be repeated. Thus, avoidance behaviors are likely to increase after the assault. This is generally unnecessary, but it constitutes a restriction on personal freedom that should be considered. Positive assertion to gradually increase the frequency and range of encounters with people and social situations is one approach that can be used.

Active Mastery: Keys to Coping with Victimization

In the preceding sections, we reviewed positive steps to reduce stress and develop active coping skills. These steps were lifestyle assessment based on knowledge of personal and environmental risks; inspection of cognitive misattributions; evaluation of potentially misleading beliefs; and coping with fear. In addition, we may consider environmental design (or lack thereof, such as poor street lighting) that contributes to increased risk. Another strategy is to seek restitution through a state victim assistance program. Finally, many local organizations provide educational and counseling programs that speed recovery and help reduce future risks. It appears that people who ignore or avoid such assistance may continue to be at risk compared with those who use these services. For example, one group of victims decided not to participate in a prevention education-counseling program. Three years later, this same group had burglary rates almost three times greater than normal (Schneider & Schneider, 1981).

SUMMARY

In this chapter, we have traced briefly the concern for social stress and social stability in early research and theory. This work identified several primary conditions (such as poverty, overcrowding, racism, and unemployment) thought to be the origins of frustration and stress in modern society. The following is a summary of the major points made in the course of the discussion.

- Road rage or aggressive driving is probably symptomatic of the frustration that people feel in a complex society. It may also be a crude expression of personal freedom that goes with the power of the car and the freedom of the highway.
- One recent theory suggests that lifestyle incongruity plays a role in social stress and ultimately lower health. Lifestyle incongruity is the disparity between the desire for market goods and the ability to acquire them.
- Social causation theory suggests that low-status groups have higher rates of disorder because they encounter harsher conditions associated with their status.
- Among the major sources of social stress are dislocations and frequent relocation, dehumanizing institutions, lack of efficient human service delivery, and rapid spread of technology.
- Rapid social and technological changes appear to be very powerful stressors for many people.
- Psychosocial research on social stress has focused on life-change stressors. The notion is that whenever we must make some change in life circumstance, it requires adaptive energy.
- The Social Readjustment Rating Scale is a widely used measure of life-change stressors. Social readjustment is the intensity and length of time required to adapt to a life-change event.
- If people experience several life-change events in a short period of time, there is an increased likelihood of overall poorer health in the time that follows the life-change events.
- Although early retrospective research pointed in the direction of a link between life-change stress and poorer health status, later prospective research showed that the link was much weaker than earlier thought.
- Research on SES shows a very simple and direct connection; that is, lower SES is associated with higher levels of stress and more negative health outcomes.
- Recent evidence points to the fact that active involvement in religion and acceptance of a religious belief system may serve to buffer the person against the effects of stress. However, the relations are complex and simple answers do not seem to be readily available.
- Coping with rapid social change often confronts us with a range of value conflicts that present difficulty, especially for the unprepared. Preparation for change through self-education, stress inoculation, and value clarification are among the various methods used to deal with social change.

- Another significant source of stress in urban areas is victimization. Many people live with the fear of assault, and home may become a type of self-imprisonment.
- Information on risk factors shows that young, unmarried, unemployed black males have the highest risk, although the impact of victimization is probably most keenly felt by women and the aged.
- Prevention involves lifestyle assessment to identify habitual behaviors that may place the person at risk. Changing lifestyle to reduce risk often takes only very minor changes.
- Both misattributions and faulty beliefs tend to prevent effective coping behaviors. Critically examining problematic causal attributions and beliefs can help to reduce risk.
- Additional coping strategies may be appropriate for dealing with fear. Fear can be reduced through desensitization and rational-emotive therapy.
- Stress inoculation may be used to reduce the potential for overwhelming stress.
- Positive assertion and social action are also helpful in removing the restrictive effects of fear. The key is to obtain active mastery of one's environment through personal and social actions designed to reduce risk.

CRITICAL THINKING AND STUDY QUESTIONS

1. Compare and contrast the different theories that try to explain how social conditions contribute to stress. What appear to be the key assumptions of these theories?
2. How do social drift, social causation, and social selection models differ in explaining the higher concentration of disorders in low-SES groups?
3. What was the rationale and overall method behind the development of the Social Readjustment Rating Scale?
4. What are the strengths and weaknesses of the arguments that life-change stress is linked to negative health outcomes? Try to answer this question both in terms of logic and in terms of empirical data.

KEY TERMS

anomie
criminologist
culture
demoralization
Dodge-Martin theory
"fear-of-crime" syndrome
life-change and illness
Life-Change Unit
    (LCU)

lifestyle
lifestyle incongruity
posttraumatic stress
    disorder
prevention of
    victimization
risk of victimization
self-blame
social causation

social drift
social readjustment
Social Readjustment
    Rating Scale (SRRS)
social selection
stress inoculation
victimologists
vulnerability

WEBSITES social sources of stress

URL ADDRESS	SITE NAME & DESCRIPTION
http://cpmcnet.columbia.edu/dept/ rosenthal/Guide5.html	☆Women's Health Resources on the World Wide Web. Extensive link site for women's health issues
http://www.nih.gov/od/odp/whi/	Women's Health Initiative. Information on the current 15-year research program
http://www-hsl.mcmaster.ca/tomflem/ menshealth.html	Men's Health Links
http://www.who.ch/	World Health Organization. Access to information on global distribution of diseases such as HIV
http://hanksville.phast.umass.edu/misc/ NAresources.html	Index of Native American Resources on the Internet
http://www-hsl.mcmaster.ca/tomflem/ firstnations.html	First Nations Health Links. Access to websites with information on Native American Indian health issues

CHAPTER 9

Environmental Stress:

Disasters, Pollution, and Overcrowding

Man's attitude toward nature is today critically important simply because we have now acquired a fateful power to alter and destroy nature.

RACHEL CARSON

QUESTIONS

- How may environmental change relate to stress?
- What are some plausible explanations for environmental stress?
- What are the identified different types of environmental stress?
- How do natural disasters typically affect human mood, thought, and behavior?
- Is there an identifiable reaction sequence to natural disasters?
- How do technological disasters differ psychologically from natural disasters?
- What have we learned about stress reactions from Buffalo Creek and Three Mile Island?
- What are the various coping strategies used to deal with disasters?
- What are the psychological effects of noise pollution?
- What are the psychological and physical health consequences of air pollution?
- How does overcrowding function as a stressor and what are the consequences for health?

Probably no disaster of the past century has touched America's conscience like the Oklahoma City bombing. Pictures of billowing smoke and the incredible ruin to a once-stately building are still vivid in our memories. For most, though, the indelible memories are those of the walking wounded trying to get away from the awful destruction; rescue personnel rushing victims to medical treatment; the especially powerful picture of firefighter Chris Fields carrying the body of 1-year-old Baylee Almon; and pictures of suspects flashed on TV news bulletins as the massive search for those responsible swung into high gear. Only later did we find out just how devastating the blast had been: 168 dead, including 19 children, and more than 675 injured (Gleick, 1996). In a matter of seconds, the $2\frac{1}{2}$-pound bomb brought down not just the federal building; it brought down America's pride and shattered attitudes of invulnerability. For many, Oklahoma City was emblematic of the heartland, main street America. Worse yet, the masterminds apparently walked the same main streets; they were us.

Natural catastrophes and technological and terrorist disasters produce intense suffering for living victims, survivors who must rebuild shattered lives and reconstruct dreams around a new reality. Less intense, though no less real, is the stress endured by the worried well—those who wait and wonder when they might also be caught up in the maelstrom of a major disaster. Schemata that once were organized around the notion of a safe, supportive habitat may be reorganized around imminent danger and the awesome power of natural or technological forces. The more ruinous outcome, then, may be the effects such disasters have on long-standing perceptions.

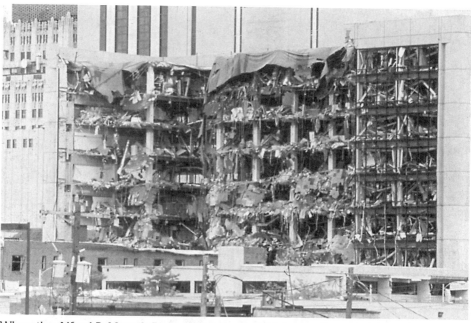

When the Alfred P. Murrah Federal Building in Oklahoma City was destroyed by a terrorist bomb, the repercussion in America's psyche was even more profound perhaps than the blast itself.

In recent years, we have identified several stressors that occur because humans have altered, exploited, or dumped on their environment. Following a major disaster, it is small consolation that the environmental alterations were intended to shelter and protect humankind. We also combat air and noise pollution in crowded urban areas. Chemical wastes dumped into streams and on once-virgin soil endanger the earth's species. Toxins created to control pests infiltrate the food chain.

The study of environmental stress deals with natural, technological, and social disasters. The results of this study should provide answers to pressing questions. What differences in individual perceptions and thoughts turn disaster into defeat for one but challenge for another? What environment-behavior interactions are most likely to increase physical illness, emotional distress, and mental disturbance? What promising applications emerge from the study of environmental stress? Can we learn how to design self-control procedures so people will be less wasteful of natural resources? Can we discover ways to intervene in the environment without disrupting habitats and destroying nature's balance? Answers to these questions could reduce both strain on the environment and the psychological impact of environmental stressors.

The purpose of this chapter is to provide a perspective on stress generated by the most commonly encountered environmental stressors. One important part of this discussion will focus on posttraumatic stress disorder, a severe psychological syndrome that can endure years after the trauma. We will consider stages in personal reaction to trauma, as well as the recovery process. To begin, a few definitions are in order.

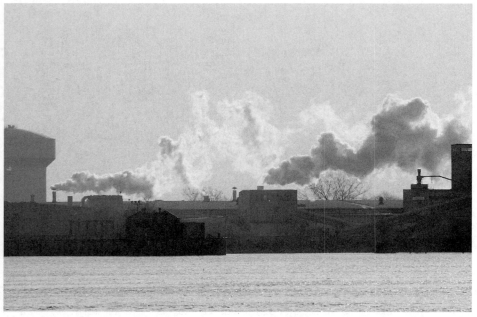

Although serious work has been done to clean up the environment, we still pollute our roads, rivers, and meadows with the byproducts of an industrial society.

ENVIRONMENT AND ECOLOGY

Some terms commonly encountered in environmental stress literature are **environment, habitat,** and **ecology.** Environment refers to surroundings, the physical space that we perceive and in which we behave. Habitat is where a particular animal resides. The natural habitat for a trout is the lake; for deer, the forest. Humans are gregarious creatures. We are fond of living together, sharing companionship and trading services. The village, small or big, is our natural habitat. Still, humans are endlessly adaptable. We can survive over a much wider range of climates and conditions than any other animal (Moran, 1981).

The term ecology refers to a distinct branch of biology that studies relationships between living organisms and their environment. The relationship between an organism and the environment is reciprocal, an exchange that goes on over several cycles. To illustrate, some years ago hunters in the Southwest received bounties for killing pests. As a result, coyotes and wildcats became rare in and around the Kaibab forest of Arizona. This produced a rapid increase in the deer population. Deer overgrazed the land, which destroyed ground cover and increased erosion. Tragically, thousands of deer died for lack of food.

Mounting concern for ecology may be due in part to our harmful environmental manipulations. We are not content to build shelters to protect us from the elements; we believe we can and should harness and control the elements as well. To exercise control, we seed clouds, drill wells, drain swamps, build dams, design earthquake-proof

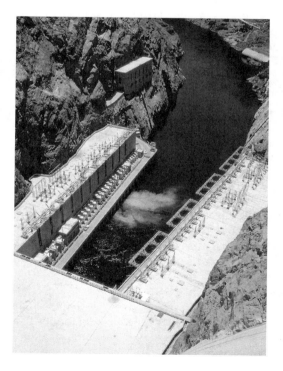

Hydroelectric plants, such as the Hoover Dam or the new China project, may supply many benefits for citizens, but the environmental and wildlife consequences can often be both unpredictable and tragic.

buildings, burn off forests, and harness nuclear energy. As we change the environment, though, we change relationships between animals, humans, and their environmental niches. Some of these changes are beneficial, but some are not. Examples of injurious influences on the ecology of an area are abundant. The Aswan Dam, built to control floods along the Nile and provide hydroelectric power, had devastating effects on fish and fishing all along the river's course. Acid rain, mass destruction of the Amazon forest, and extinction of many species caused by civilization's encroachments on natural habitats furnish other examples. Viewed in this light, disturbing the ecological balance can produce powerful sources of stress for many organisms.

THEORIES OF ENVIRONMENTAL STRESS

Numerous theories seek to explain environmental stress. These include **arousal theories,** learning theory, **behavior constraint theory, ecological theory,** and **environmental stress theory.** Environmental stress theory integrates Hans Selye's general adaptation syndrome with Richard Lazarus's cognitive-transactional theory. In Table 9-1, I have summarized the core notions from a select group of these theories.

Arousal and Stimulation Theories of Stress

One way to view the relationship between the environment and human behavior is in terms of the amount of stimulation the environment provides. These so-called arousal theories are relatively simplistic. Still, some support exists for the notion that stress varies with level of arousal. For example, Albert Mehrabian and James Russell (1974) tried to identify the dimensions that best describe any environment. They found this could be done with just three dimensions: pleasure, dominance, and arousal.

The major idea common to arousal theories is that different degrees of stimulation produce varying degrees of arousal. Very intense stimulation, such as a rock band rehearsing in the upstairs apartment, probably will lead to too much arousal and feelings of distress. On the other hand, very low levels of stimulation, such as stimulus deprivation, can result in too little arousal and feelings of boredom.

Wohlwill's (1974) **adaptation level theory** suggests that each person has a preferred and optimal level of stimulation. This optimal level varies among people; some people prefer more stimulation than others. Optimal levels also vary within people over time; we prefer more stimulation at some times than at others. Finally, the current level of preferred stimulation is a result of adaptation; we adjust the value we place on stimulation because of continued exposure. Whether something is understimulating or overstimulating depends on the current level of adaptation. For example, after spending an intense day at an amusement park, you might consider a comedy movie boring. Conversely, after being confined in a hospital for an extended time, you might think that same movie very entertaining.

Conditioning and Environmental Stress

Learning models have been widely used to explain adaptive behaviors, including adaptation to stress. Byrne and Clore (1970) proposed a **classical conditioning theory** that includes a role for conditioning attitudes, something not included in the original theory. Attitudes are predispositions to act in certain ways. Specifically, Byrne and Clore proposed that attitudes are conditioned to distinctive environmental stimuli and, as a result,

TABLE 9-1

Comparison of key features of environmental stress models

STRESS MODEL	DEFINITION OF STRESS	SOURCE(S) OF STRESS	MODEL'S STRENGTHS	MODEL'S WEAKNESSES
Arousal theories	No specific definitions provided but suggests stress is negative reaction to variations in stimulation	Overarousal Underarousal Mismatch between preferred arousal and current level of stimulation	Main constructs are easy to grasp Seems easy to operationalize and test empirically	Extremely simplistic view of stress Places major emphasis on stimulation Ignores biological factors Largely ignores cognitive-appraisal factors Little extensive or intensive testing to verify theories
Conditioning theory	Faulty conditioning arousing negative attitudes and/or conditional emotional responses	Presence of any conditional stimuli that evoke negative attitudes or emotions	Empirically based Clear operational definitions for basic terms and procedures Extends classical model to arena of cognitions	Mostly indirect rather than direct testing Limited in scope Does not provide integrated view of biological or social variables
Behavior constraint model	No specific definition provided	Real or perceived limits on behavior	Incorporates three well-defined and tested constructs in coherent theory Empirically based	Indirect evidence rather than direct tests Limited in scope Seldom used
Ecological theory	No specific definition provided	Behavior settings or factors, such as undermanning	Incorporates social/normative notions of relations between settings and behavior Has led to variety of applications for environmental design	Limited in scope Little or no consideration of biological factors. Little interest in individual or cognitive variables Difficult to test
Environmental stress theory	Combination of the biological and cognitive models of Selye and Lazarus	Real or perceived psychosocial pressures	Encompasses a broad range of variables, from biological to psychological and social	An eclectic theory, taking the best of current theories Not directly tested but logically synthesized

become tinged with positive or negative values. If an attitude is associated with an event, recurrence of the event may evoke a stress reaction through the associated attitude.

For example, a child goes to a doctor's office and receives a painful injection. The office and other related stimuli (doctors, nurses, uniforms, odors) become signals for pain. Later, when the child expects to return to the office, a strong negative emotional response occurs. Based on this emotional response, a negative attitude forms: "I don't like that place."

In the Byrne and Clore model, pain from the injection is an unconditional stimulus, while fear and avoidance are part of the unconditional response. The office is the conditional stimulus, which was neutral before the injection. Afterward, it takes on the power of the unconditional stimulus and produces fear and avoidance, the conditional or learned response. Fear and avoidance may occur even when the doctor's office is only symbolically represented in conversation.

The Behavior Constraint Theory

On occasion, the environment can produce effects over which we have little or no control. Severe storms, hurricanes, and blizzards are forces that usually require a "ride-it-out" response. Under such conditions, behavior is constrained, or limited. However, according to the behavior constraint model, the limits imposed on behavior need not be real limits; they can be imaginary as well. If we merely *believe* the situation is out of control, our behavior will be as limited as if we really do lack control.

According to Judith Rodin and Andrew Baum (1978), three steps lead to behavior constraint: perceived loss of control, psychological reactance, and a feeling of learned helplessness. The notion of **reactance** is that people do not like feeling out of control, so they take steps to regain control. When people try to regain control but repeatedly fail to do so, they may develop learned helplessness (Seligman, 1975). Learned helplessness is a condition in which a person could exert control but does not because of previous failures. In emergency situations, such as natural and technological disasters, people may give up because they feel there is nothing they can do. Although the behavior constraint model contains some interesting elements, it is seldom used in environmental psychology.

Behavior Settings and Ecological Psychology

Roger Barker (1968) advocated an ecological view of environmental stress. The key concept in his theory was **behavior settings.** A behavior setting is a culturally determined physical milieu that calls for certain fixed patterns of behavior. These include group behaviors as well as individual behaviors. For example, a church is a behavior setting that has several predictable behavior patterns. Classrooms and restaurants are other examples, as are business and faculty meetings. Knowing the setting enables one to predict with some certainty what behavior should occur. Change the setting, and the behavior also changes.

Related ideas in Barker's theory include undermanning and overmanning. For example, amusement parks can be "overmanned" when large crowds exceed the park's capacity. In such circumstances, people may feel frustrated and stressed. In large universities and large classes, students may feel left out, uninvolved, and anonymous. On the other hand, in smaller universities and smaller classrooms, students may feel involved and worthwhile. Barker's model has proven useful in studying stress in business, mental institutions, schools, and churches. It has also been helpful in suggesting ways to engineer the environment to eliminate or reduce stressors.

Environmental Stress Theory

Environmental stress theory combines the best of both Hans Selye's general adaptation syndrome and Richard Lazarus's cognitive-transactional theory. Andrew Baum's research group analyzed environmental stressors, such as the Three Mile Island incident, in terms of these two theories (Baum, 1990; Baum, Singer, & Baum, 1981). They concluded that the cognitive processes suggested by Lazarus and the physiological arousal proposed by Selye occur consistently in several environmental stress situations, including catastrophic events, noise, and crowding. This suggests that a specialized theory of environmental stress does not add much explanatory power, if any, to that provided by these two well-known and well-researched models. Figure 9-1 shows the two theories in integrated form (Fisher, Bell, & Baum, 1984).

CATEGORIES OF ENVIRONMENTAL STRESS

Work on environmental stress has focused on several major stressors. There is, first, the short-term catastrophic disaster, which affects few people. Its effect on the environment and people is usually severe, but such events tend to happen infrequently. Natural, technological, and social disasters[1] fit this category.

A second category, ongoing, chronic stressors, affect many more people daily but in less severe ways. Further, their effects may not appear for years. Fisher and his colleagues labeled these **background stressors** (Fisher et al., 1984), whereas Holahan (1986) labeled them **ambient stressors. Noise pollution, air pollution, chemical pollution, crowding,** and **commuting** are examples of this type of environmental stress. The remainder of this chapter focuses on the most important environmental stressors.

NATURAL DISASTERS

When Hurricane Andrew approached the heavily populated east Florida coast, everyone knew it had the potential to be a killer storm. Peak wind velocities were clocked at 164 miles per hour. Early warnings and precautions by area residents served to prevent heavy loss of life. Still, no one was fully prepared for the magnitude of the loss that came from this display of earth's fury. Even as the storm left to continue its devastation in Louisiana and another hurricane, Iniki, ravaged Hawaii, survivors could do little more than look on with a mixture of shock, grief, and awe at what had taken place in so short a time: 63,000 homes destroyed; 250,000 people homeless; 38 dead. We may never have a completely accurate account of all losses, but estimates suggest that it will take years and cost more than $20 billion to help homeowners, businesses, and government rebuild.

---

[1]The term *social disaster* is my own. It refers to those events that do not readily fit the natural and technological categories, but nonetheless share the elements of unpredictability and lack of control and produce a powerful impact on people's lives. The Jonestown suicides and the Oklahoma City bombing belong in this category.

FIGURE 9-1

The environmental stress model proposed by Fisher, Bell, and Baum.

SOURCE: Fisher, Bell, and Baum (1984).

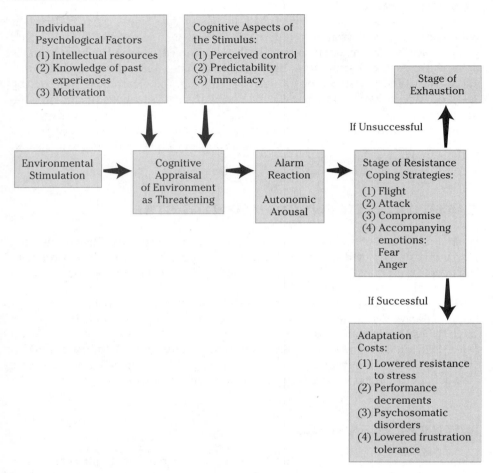

Following a disaster of this magnitude, survivors find their usual comfortable existence replaced by discomfort, severe deprivation, and physical fatigue. Lengthy periods of cleanup, recovering personal effects from the devastation where possible; enforced relocations that sometimes become permanent; rebuilding; caring for sick or injured family members; and arranging for the burial of deceased family members are some of the activities that consume enormous amounts of physical and psychological energy. Media coverage from Mexico City and Armenia following devastating earthquakes vividly illustrate some of these conditions and reactions.

Beyond mere physical loss and privation, though, disasters like Hurricane Andrew have both obvious and hidden psychological effects. In Chapter 1, I noted that stress most often results from events that are uncontrollable and unpredictable. Natural disas-

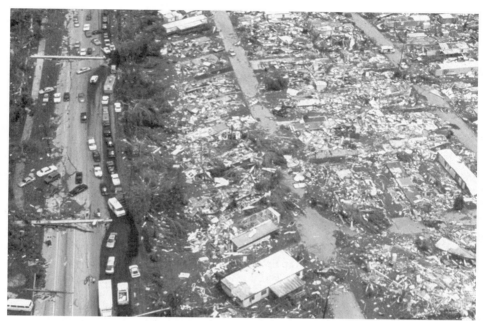

The devastation produced by natural forces such as Hurricane Andrew can bring on very strong emotional reactions.

ters fit this pattern very readily. Consider, for example, nature's lottery, the tornado. No matter how sophisticated modern weather reporting may be, warning that a tornado is approaching is all that can be done. Where and when that tornado will touch down is anyone's guess. Since natural disasters are also largely uncontrollable, people may feel they are at the mercy of forces beyond their wildest imagination.

Many studies carried out worldwide over the past 25 years provide insights about what can be expected from such catastrophes. In brief, the experience of shock and grief is nearly universal, and survival guilt also occurs. Fear of a recurrence of the dread event may erode decision-making ability and interfere with appropriate problem-solving behavior. Sleep disturbances are common, as is loss of appetite. To deal with anxiety and depression, disaster victims often increase their use of alcohol, cigarettes, sleeping pills, antidepressants, and tranquilizers (Joseph, Yule, Williams, & Hodgkinson, 1993). More detail will be provided later about psychological and physical symptoms, but here we will describe the global stages and patterns of reaction to disasters.

Stages of Reaction to Disasters

Disaster studies reveal a typical sequence that victims go through as they come to grips with what has happened. In general, three distinct stages appear—the *impact* period, lasting only as long as the disaster event itself; the *recoil* period, lasting in some cases for several days; and the *post-trauma* period, lasting up to a lifetime (Leach, 1995). In the impact period, victims are often overwhelmed by sensations never before encountered. This may include the awful feeling of a once-sturdy house being ripped to shreds, acrid smoke and searing heat from a firestorm, or a bridge's sudden heaving and shifting. The impact period is typically short, especially in catastrophes like tornados or earthquakes.

Often overlooked, though, is a second group of casualties, the rescue squads. Rescue workers are not just heroes or stoic troopers doing their jobs. Their shock may be different, and it typically does not hit until they move into the disaster area and begin their work. Still, the psychological impact for emergency personnel is no less real. One of the worst traumas for rescue workers is when they rush to the scene of a disaster only to find that one of their own family members has been killed or seriously injured.

The recoil period occurs after the primary threat is over, but the survivors now face a second wave of threats. Only after the intense mental and physical struggle to survive is past may they realize just how hungry, exhausted, and frayed they are. At this time, survivors try to take stock of what has happened, all the while not fully recognizing the magnitude of their loss or understanding how hard the road to recovery will be. For the moment, they may appear stunned, dazed, and confused. Their confusion is due in part to the fact that a future that once seemed secure is now hopelessly muddled. A common defense pattern during this time is denial. Some feel that what they just lived through is only a dream, not something that really happened. They fully expect to awake and find that the disaster really never happened, at least not to them—but of course it did.

To add insult to injury, it is just about this time that forced evacuation brutally destroys their protective illusions and forces them to accept a harsh reality. This often means the beginning of a long-term disruption in family organization, routines, and intimacy. Relocation usually means smaller living quarters, more crowding, greater isolation

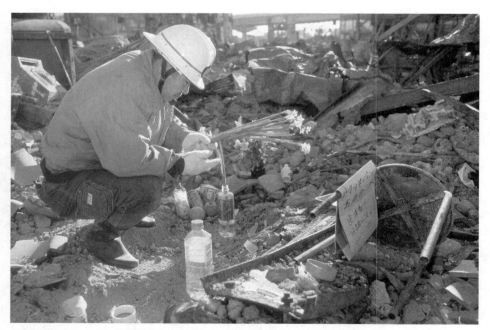

Amidst the personal tragedies that occur in natural and man-made catastrophes, the stress experienced by rescue workers is often overlooked.

from friends and other social support groups, and food and water shortages (Riad & Norris, 1996). When families have been embedded in closely networked communities, disruption typically extends to the social life of the community as well.

Some survivors will recover their ability to reason, plan, and problem solve more quickly than others. Those who can get involved more quickly in meaningful activities tend to suffer lower degrees of stress. This may explain one observation in traditional families, namely that men who quickly go back to work often display fewer symptoms of stress and recover more quickly than their wives, who remain in or near the disaster area in shelters or emergency housing. Finding more time on their hands, those left behind spend the time brooding on the negative events that have just occurred.

Many will also begin to show the first signs of emotional venting. For some, it will be the first time they let down and cry. Other common emotions include residual fear, anxiety, and anger. One behavior noted in this period is the compulsion to talk. Some survivors seem to need to tell everyone, to talk incessantly about what they have just endured (Leach, 1995).

In the post-trauma period, people have survived the disaster and the basic threats. Still, survivors often experience both physical and psychological disorders following their confrontations with disaster. Symptoms of PTSD may last for years, as shown by one study of survivors of a terrorist attack (Desivilya, Gal, & Ayalon, 1996). In this case from 1974, Palestinian terrorists attacked an Israeli town on the border with Lebanon. They seized 120 high-school children and held them for 16 hours. During that time, 22 children were killed, and many more were wounded. After 17 years had passed, the research team tracked down 76 survivors of the attack and obtained data on frequency of PTSD symptoms. Thirty-nine percent of the survivors still experienced up to four symptoms; 52% reported between 5 and 8 symptoms; and 9% still suffered most of the classic PTSD symptoms. Studies of Vietnam combat veterans show that 15% continue to suffer chronic PTSD even though the war has been over for more than 20 years (Bremner, Southwick, & Charney, 1995).

Patterns of Reaction During Disasters

Leach (1995) believes that disaster victims can be grouped according to specific patterns of responding to the initial impact. The first group remains relatively calm, lucid in their thinking, and calculating in their actions. As Leach noted, these people are often called the "supercool." From 10 to 20% will fall into this group.

The second group will appear very dazed and confused. Their thinking processes will typically be faulty or impaired, and they will not be able to plan in a coherent way. Their behaviors may seem robot-like, and they will show clear physical symptoms of high anxiety. About 75% of victims fall into this group.

The third group will actually show a variety of inappropriate behaviors that increase their risks. Some seem frozen in time and space: Even though they should move out of harm's way, they remain immobile, perhaps simply waiting for the inevitable. Others may engage in very dangerous behaviors, as some did after the Oakland/Berkeley Firestorm (Koopman, Classen, & Spiegel, 1996). People tried to get close to the fires, even if it meant crossing police barricades to get into a blocked-off area. These dangerous behaviors were often part of the victims' dissociative responses (described next) to the catastrophe. About 10 to 15% fall in this group.

Effects of Natural Disasters

Many psychological and physical symptoms appear after a natural calamity. Psychological symptoms include initial panic, anxiety, phobic fear, vulnerability, guilt, isolation, withdrawal, depression (including some suicide attempts), anger, and frustration, as well as interpersonal and marital problems (McLeod, 1984). Sleep disturbances, disorientation, and loss of a sense of security may occur for a time. Some people report that they continually relive the agony in their dreams, as though they cannot escape from the horror. The severity and duration of these effects seem to depend on the magnitude of the loss.

Following the Oakland/Berkeley Firestorm, investigators examined a reaction that commonly occurs in response to disasters, the **dissociative response** (Koopman et al., 1996). The *dissociative response* includes numbing of responsiveness, and detachment usually expressed as **depersonalization** and **derealization.** *Depersonalization* occurs when victims experience themselves as strangers, detach from their bodies, or feel that this must be happening to someone else. About 25% of earthquake survivors, 31% of accident survivors, and 54% of airline-crash survivors experience depersonalization (Koopman, Classen, Cardeña, & Spiegel, 1995). *Derealization* is the feeling that what happened took much longer than it did or did not really happen, or the event is distorted in hallucinations and delusions. A dissociative reaction is more likely to occur when the victim is a woman who has been exposed to a severe calamity and who has a prior history of stressful events.

The symptoms described in the two preceding paragraphs fit the pattern of posttraumatic stress disorder (PTSD), a syndrome discussed in Chapter 8. Following Hurricane Andrew, a survey of mental disorder among a small sample of adults found that 36% met the criteria for PTSD, 30% suffered a major depression, and 20% experienced anxiety disorders (David et al., 1996).

One important question is why some people experience severe symptoms of PTSD while others do not. This has led to a search for the etiological (causal) factors in PTSD. Based on an extensive review of this issue, Bremner's group concluded that various early stressors increase vulnerability to later PTSD (Bremner et al., 1995). Early stressors that have been linked to PTSD include childhood abuse and neglect, family alcoholism and mental illness, poverty, and poor academic performance, among others. This link suggests that early exposure does not lead to resilience, as some have argued, but to increased sensitivity to stressors.

Children are just as prone to stress reactions as adults, as one team has found (LaGreca, Silverman, Vernberg, & Prinstein, 1996). Their study among 3rd- to 5th-grade children showed that 30% had severe symptoms of PTSD. The researchers also tried to develop a model that would predict children's reactions to disasters. They found that five variables could predict about 40% of the variance in children's long-term (7-months post-trauma) reactions. The five variables, shown in Figure 9-2, are (1) exposure to traumatic events during and after the disaster; (2) demographic traits; (3) occurrence of major life stressors; (4) availability of social support; and (5) type of coping strategy used. In more specific terms, more severe symptoms of PTSD were associated with (1) greater threat of death during the disaster or loss and continued disruption following the disaster; (2) minority (Hispanic or African-American) status; (3) higher rate of major life events (such as death, hospitalization); (4) less social support from parents and friends; and (5) use of blame/anger and withdrawal as a coping defense.

FIGURE 9-2

Conceptual model for predicting children's reactions to natural disasters. PTSD = posttraumatic stress disorder.

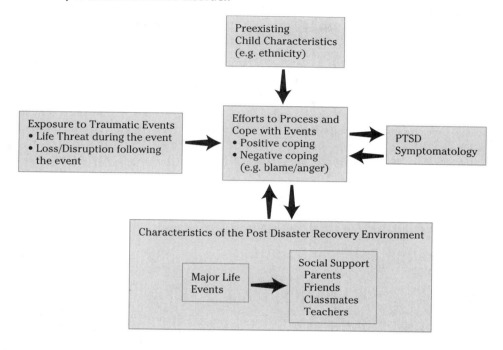

While most clinicians accept PTSD as a reliable description, McFarlane (1988) warns against its uncritical acceptance. He pointed to the lack of research supporting the contention that different types of traumatic events produce the same outcome. McFarlane studied a group of Australian fire fighters who fought a disastrous bush fire. Core signs of PTSD—intrusive thoughts and recurrent intense images—appeared in one group not diagnosed with PTSD. In spite of the cognitive disruption, they showed no significant long-term disability. Instead of finding survival guilt and detachment, McFarlane observed the opposite: namely, many fire fighters became more socially involved following the disaster. Finally, a comparison of fire fighters diagnosed with PTSD with fire fighters without PTSD showed little difference in morbidity. McFarlane questioned whether these core symptoms are sufficiently specific to be helpful diagnostic criteria.

Physical symptoms following a natural disaster include increased fatigue, headaches, colds and other illnesses, and weight loss from both sleep and eating disturbances. The amount of physical illness, though, is much less than what might be expected. One possible explanation for this is that the short-term, acute nature of disaster stress triggers the body's natural self-defense mechanisms. Because the stress is over quickly, lowered resistance and exhaustion do not occur (Baum, 1990). This is also consistent with the observation that the severity and duration of both psychological and physical effects depend on the significance of the loss produced by the disaster.

The symptoms reported here also appear to be nearly universal. The Sri Lanka cyclone of 1978, for example, provides one well-documented, confirming case study (Patrick & Patrick, 1981).

THE AFTERMATH OF MOUNT SAINT HELENS

One of the most widely publicized natural disasters was the eruption of Mount Saint Helens on May 18, 1980. The 9600-foot mountain, located in the southwestern part of the state of Washington, exploded with a force that lifted a cubic mile of debris from its peak.[2] The force of the eruption hurled ash as high as 50,000 feet into the atmosphere and covered several thousand square miles with volcanic ash. Nearly 300 people were working, camping, or sightseeing near the volcano. More than 200 escaped or were rescued, although 2 of these died later. Another 60 persons died or disappeared and are presumed dead (Murphy, 1984).

Shortly after the eruption, a team of investigators collected data from cities and towns in the impact area (Pennebaker & Newtson, 1983). What they found confirmed

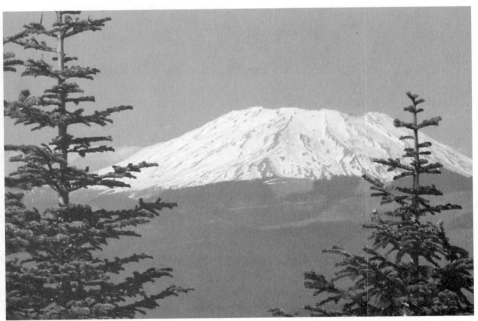

When Mount Saint Helens erupted, it laid waste to many square miles of forest lands and turned many people's lives upside down.

[2]To appreciate the volume of a cubic mile of earth, consider this. A cubic mile of earth is equal to 5.5 billion cubic yards. Most standard gravel trucks carry approximately 14 cubic yards of dirt. If you could line up enough trucks to haul away all the debris from Mount Saint Helens, it would take a string of 390,741,623 trucks. If you could fill one truck every ten minutes, working 24 hours a day, it would take 7434 years to do what Mount Saint Helens did in a matter of minutes!

earlier findings. The data showed a pattern of initial short-term panic with little or no long-term effect. Within the first 24 hours, outgoing telephone calls ran a full 100% above normal levels, jamming phone lines in the process. This level of activity subsided quickly, however.

Both physical symptoms and negative emotional moods occurred at a higher rate than in a normal population, but the frequency of symptoms varied with both proximity and temporal factors. People living in a dangerous area while trying to deal with the day-to-day necessities of living reported fewer physical and emotional symptoms. Once again, involvement in planful activities seemed to be protective. These people were also less willing to provide information to interviewers, which suggests that their anxiety levels were still high. The investigators concluded that these people had not allowed themselves time to work through their feelings about the disaster. As time went on, people in the dangerous areas became more willing to talk. Most residents showed few effects of the eruption in a follow-up survey about a year later.

Shirley Murphy (1984) studied victims of the Mount Saint Helens eruption to assess how quickly and completely people recover from the effects of a natural catastrophe. Murphy classified victims into four categories. One group consisted of victims who had suffered the *presumed* loss of a relative or close friend. The second group had suffered the *confirmed* loss of a relative or close friend. The third and fourth groups had lost, respectively, permanent or vacation homes. A fifth group, which served as a control group, suffered no loss at all.

Murphy found that bereaved victims reported higher levels of emotional stress and poorer mental health status compared with other victims. But they did not seem to suffer any poorer physical health than the group that had experienced no loss. Those who had relatives or friends *presumed* dead appeared to show the most distress when interviewed. They talked about how "waiting was agony," how they went on "hoping, yet knowing they were dead," and that "it's hard to come to terms with no body" (Murphy, 1984, p. 212). People who lost permanent homes reported levels of stress similar to those of the bereaved group, but they reported no greater physical or emotional difficulties than the control group. These people also experienced greater amounts of anger, blame, and dissatisfaction with financial aid for rebuilding than any other group. Those who lost vacation homes did not show differences from the control group on any of the measures. Most victims reported that they felt only partially recovered even 11 months after the disaster.

TECHNOLOGICAL DISASTERS

Tuesday night, September 27, 1994: The ferry *Estonia* loaded its 1051 passengers and hundreds of cars in Talinn, Estonia, on the Baltic Sea. At the outset, it looked like any other early fall evening and another routine run to Stockholm, Sweden, one of three runs made every week. The ship was a high-tech, well-designed marvel with all the safety features known to the industry. Maintenance standards were high and the ship had been inspected twice in that same month. This night, however, would prove to be a very different, and deadly, night.

The weather was bad, with 62 mile-per-hour winds and 32-foot seas, but it was still nothing unusual for this time of year (Jackson, 1994). Most of the passengers had turned in around 8:30 p.m. because of the bumpy seas. Shortly after midnight, the ship began taking on water through the seals around the bow door. Miscalculating that the water was only rainwater, the crew activated bilge pumps but did not carry out any site inspection. This proved to be a fatal error in judgment. Within minutes, the ship was taking on large amounts of water, and beginning to roll heavily onto its left side. Some survivors estimated that it took less than 15 minutes from beginning to end. The marvel of engineering now rested on the bottom of the ocean in 260 feet of cold water.

Of the 1051 passengers who boarded, only 139 survived, most of them young men who had the strength to survive the frigid waters of the north seas for 3 to 4 hours before rescue ships and helicopters began arriving. They also described the scene as the ship was sinking: "It was the law of the jungle," one said, with no time for gallantry (Jackson, 1994). Perhaps the most horrible, haunting memories came from the screams of women and especially the wailing of children crying for help and unable to save themselves. A few of the survivors displayed dissociative reactions, denial, and inappropriate affect. Others showed signs of anxiety and depression. One interesting reaction among several of the survivors was just wanting to hold someone, anyone's hand, or hug and be hugged as though they could not get enough physical contact (Taiminen & Tuominen, 1996).

The Nature of Technological Disasters

Technological disasters share several characteristics with natural disasters. They tend to be unpredictable and uncontrollable and can produce intense physical suffering, psychological stress, and social disruption. In fact, one must look to the very worst of the natural disasters to find destruction on a par with the disasters of Hiroshima and Nagasaki, the Vietnam War, or the Bhopal (India) tragedy.[3] Most technological disasters subject people to acute stress because they last only a short time. Still, certain types of technological disasters can produce stress effects over long time-frames. The incident at Three Mile Island probably has passed into memory for those living outside the region. For those living in the immediate vicinity, however, it continues to be a source of fear.

In other ways, technological disasters are very different from natural disasters. Technological disasters usually result from human miscalculation, carelessness, and greed. Sometimes they result from flagrant disregard for the value of human life as compared with the corporate balance sheet. They are, in a word, preventable. From the vantage point of hindsight, at least, it seems that someone could have done something to prevent these disasters from happening. It is difficult to accuse a Supreme Being of malice when a tornado strikes, but sins of human error are not so easily forgiven. To the victim, human error demands that someone must pay. It is hardly surprising, then, that more anger and resentment follow technological disasters than natural disasters (Lystad, 1985). Our sense of control is also threatened. We think that what we create, we also control. After a technological disaster, it is indisputable that what we created, we could not and did not control.

---

[3]The Bhopal tragedy of 1984 resulted from the release of deadly methyl isocyanate fumes from the Union Carbide plant. It left 250,000 scarred, blinded, or disfigured, and more than 2500 dead.

BUFFALO CREEK AND THREE MILE ISLAND

Few technological disasters have been more extensively studied than the Buffalo Creek flood of 1976 and the nuclear accident at Three Mile Island of 1979. These studies reveal patterns of physical and psychological symptoms similar to those found following natural disasters. They also suggest that the effects of technological disasters are more long-term than those of natural disasters.

The Buffalo Creek Flood

The Buffalo Mining Company built a dam of coal slag to control flooding in towns along the Buffalo Creek Valley in West Virginia. In February 1976, after rains had swollen the creek behind the dam, the dam collapsed. In 15 minutes of unbridled fury, the wall of water destroyed the town of Saunders and several other valley settlements. Over 5000 people were left homeless, while 125 would never come home again. The physical and psychological effects, still evident two to four years later, included (1) anxiety, grief, and despair; (2) apathy and withdrawal; (3) depression; (4) stomach problems; (5) anger and rage; (6) regression in children; (7) nightmares and sleep disturbances; and (8) survival guilt. Some combination of these symptoms occurred in roughly 80% of the adults and 90% of the children.

The Three Mile Island Nuclear Accident

Among the most frightening of disasters is a nuclear plant explosion or meltdown. Many movies have exploited the theme and graphically depicted visions of wholesale destruction that might transpire. In spite of assurances of safety from various sources, many people remain unconvinced. Until the meltdown at the Chernobyl nuclear power plant in 1986, the world had witnessed only limited danger from nuclear accidents. The immediate reaction to the Chernobyl meltdown was largely restricted to medical and technical aid. It did not include studies of the psychosocial impact, as has occurred in other nuclear accidents. As a result, Chernobyl can only stand as a grim reminder of the horrendous forces and frightful damage that could engulf the world with a full-scale meltdown. Unlike Chernobyl, Three Mile Island was extensively studied from a psychosocial view.

The incident began when the reactor dubbed Unit 2 malfunctioned and radioactive gases escaped into the atmosphere. The crisis lasted several days, with evacuations and disruption of life in the immediate region. Plant personnel quickly brought the reactor under control and reduced the potential for serious danger. Still, the threat of radioactive leaks continued for some time. It was more than a year before workers could clear contaminated water and gases from the building and erase the threat entirely.

Several studies in the years following the accident reported that psychological distress increased. There were more physical complaints and increased physiological arousal as indicated by levels of adrenaline in urine samples. Residents who had little or no social support showed more evidence of stress than those who had strong support (Baum, 1990; Fleming, Baum, Gisriel, & Gatchel, 1982). This finding again confirms Cobb's notion that social support operates to buffer the effects of stress (1976).

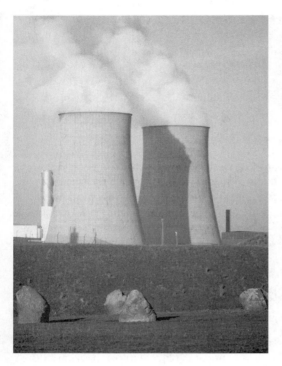

Nuclear power plants, such as Three Mile Island in the U.S. and Chernobyl in the Ukraine, have experienced technological failures exposing residents to harmful radiation. Such disasters are often more difficult to deal with because human error is usually involved.

Love Canal: The Silent Killer

In contrast to dramatic disasters, Love Canal was a silent killer. Its onset was slow and insidious, and most people were unaware that anything was wrong. Love Canal was a 16-acre chemical dump site for the Hooker Chemical Company of Niagara Falls, New York. The company used the abandoned canal to dispose of nearly 20,000 tons of chemical wastes over a period of roughly ten years, ending in 1953. Hooker Chemical then covered the canal and sold it to the local school district for $1. Families built homes on the site over the next 20 years. But no one told them the open field in their midst contained the seeds of deadly destruction; it was to be a park for the children (Gibbs, 1983).

Officials did not begin to investigate the problem seriously until 1976, and they did not take any substantive action until 1978, when they developed a relocation plan that allowed 237 families at the center of Love Canal to seek homes elsewhere. Unfortunately, 700 families on nearby streets were not included in the relocation plans. They were left alone to worry about their safety and their fate.

Residents were frightened, frustrated with the lack of action by government offices, and angry at the coverup that had occurred in years past. The most extreme frustration and anger arose when residents felt they had no control and when no progress was evident. Many residents reported feeling helpless and trapped.

Perhaps the most difficult problems were due to uncertainty and lack of information. Residents feared for their own safety and that of their young children. They also feared that pregnant women would bear deformed children. Pregnant women and children under the age of two were the only residents "officially" declared at risk in the area. Officials knew that chromosome damage and ovum damage could result. Yet no one had any concrete answers to the residents' questions.

As Lois Gibbs reports, many people threatened to take their lives because of inability to deal with the constant stress. Several people tried and succeeded. Gibbs (1983) also said that "it [was not] uncommon to watch my neighbors, who before Love Canal were calm, easygoing people, throw books at officials, use profanity in public, or threaten officials with physical harm at heated public meetings" (pp. 123–124).

COPING WITH THE EFFECTS OF DISASTER

While it is one thing to identify the problems resulting from natural and technological disasters, it is another to provide information about how to cope with disasters. At least one team of investigators attempted to address this issue. Another team found that survivors of a natural disaster may come out of the experience with much better coping skills than they had before the disaster (Quarantelli & Dynes, 1977). The following information is based on a composite of findings from studies reported earlier.

Psychological Triage: Managing the Aftermath of Disasters

Leach (1995) provides insights into the kinds of activities that help victims in the first hours after a disaster. They include identifying those who appear the most dazed and impaired and attending to them quickly. It also helps to identify skills and knowledge that can be useful to the group of survivors. When survivors can themselves become involved in useful activities that aid recovery, it tends to have a therapeutic effect on them and speeds the process of recovery. In cases where emergency personnel are delayed in getting help to the disaster area, it may also be beneficial to use a roll call to identify people's presence and the extent of injury. Leach points out that the roll call can help people re-establish their personal identity and gives them a connection to others. Roll-call information can also be extremely valuable to emergency workers when they do arrive.

Coping with Nuclear Disaster: Lessons from Three Mile Island

Following the Three Mile Island incident, an investigative team headed by Andrew Baum studied the coping strategies used by residents in the vicinity (Baum, Fleming, & Singer, 1983). Baum's team asked a small sample of people to describe the coping strategies they used over the months following the accident. The research team used a scale that measured the extent to which each person used an emotion-control coping style as opposed to a problem-control coping style (Folkman & Lazarus, 1980). They defined **emotionally focused coping** as a strategy in which a person tries to control and release negative feelings (such as anger, frustration, and fear) provoked by the incident. **Problem-focused coping** was defined as a strategy in which a person tries to develop concrete plans of action and exerts as much direct control as possible.

Based on this initial assessment, Baum's group classified each person as high or low for emotionally focused coping and high or low for problem-focused coping. Then the group counted the number of symptoms reported for each coping style. People who were *low* on emotionally focused coping reported nearly three times the number of symptoms compared with those who were high on this trait. People who were *high* on problem focused coping reported nearly three times the number of symptoms compared with those who were low on this dimension.

This suggests that, in disaster situations, the most effective strategy is to focus first on ridding oneself of any negative emotions. Victims should seek ways of bringing emotions out in the open and avoid locking them up inside. In addition, victims probably should not be concerned about trying to control through direct problem confrontation. This advice does not apply to all stress situations, though, for a specific reason.

The investigative team reasoned that a disaster such as Three Mile Island confronts people with a situation that is inherently uncontrollable for anyone without technical training. Attempts to assert direct control, then, seem to add stress by increasing personal feelings of frustration at not being able to do anything about the disaster. In other stressful situations, such as interpersonal conflict, a problem-solving approach may be the most effective means of managing the stress.

Information seeking is also a highly visible coping strategy in disaster situations. Uncertainty is a major cause of stress; obtaining relevant and concrete information can help reduce uncertainty. The problem is that information provided during and after disasters may be inaccurate, unclear, and confusing. This was the case with much of the information supplied during the Love Canal controversy. People often received mixed messages on health problems, relocation efforts, economic support, and so forth. In this situation, people who sat back and waited were often better off than those who actively pressed for information. Thus, officials charged with the responsibility of providing information should be careful to provide only information that is accurate and clear.

The Crash of Flight 232

A clinical intervention study following the July 19, 1989, crash of United Airlines Flight 232 at Sioux City, Iowa, confirmed several of these issues (Jacobs, Quevillon, & Stricherz, 1990). News coverage of this crash was extensive, due in part to the time that elapsed between the first warnings that the plane had lost hydraulic power and the actual crash. The pilot displayed courage and calmness through the ordeal, and his heroic efforts enabled 184 passengers to survive.

Jacobs, Quevillon, and Stricherz (1990) were part of the mental health disaster team whose responsibility was to provide crisis counseling for the families and friends of passengers on Flight 232. Their article provides insights into the difficulties of critical-incident stress debriefing and makes suggestions for mental health disaster planning in the future. Medical response to the disaster was superbly handled, but provision of emotional support to the families was hindered by diffusion of responsibility and official misinformation.

During the chaotic morning following the crash, the team received four different reports on the imminent arrival of family members. First, it was reported that 100 family members would arrive, and the team called in the 80 mental health counselors needed to deal with that number. Then the airline reported that only 7 family members were arriving; as a result, half the counselors were sent home. Shortly afterward, 100 family members were expected again, and the counselors were called back. Less than 10 minutes later, the 7 family members arrived.

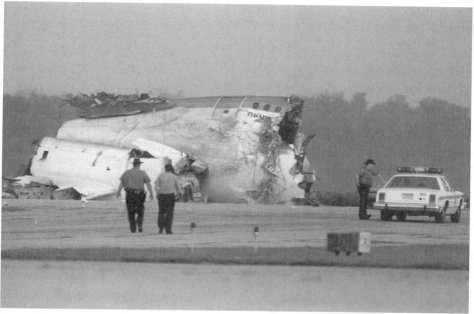

Sioux City police stand guard over the fuselage of United Airlines Flight 232. The pilot's courage in crisis is credited with saving 184 of the 300 passengers.

The press, however unwittingly, also contributed by publishing inaccurate information. Incorrect lists of passengers led to confusion, with alternating hope and grief. One man noted that his loved one's name did not appear on the list, and his hope for her safety was reborn. Only 30 minutes later, he had to be told of her death.

NOISE POLLUTION

Urban residents often seek the silence of forest and field as a vacation from the din of traffic, the clatter of jack hammers, and the roar of airplanes. The fact that people try to escape noise, reduce noise, or engage in political battles to control noise suggests that the properties of noise are unpleasant. In extreme cases, people even kill because of noise. Such was the case one warm summer night.

A normally quiet and responsible young man, Mike came home from his night-shift job tired and looking for a peaceful night's sleep. He awakened to the sounds of loud music, laughter, and talking at a nearby party, a party to celebrate Kelly's 21st birthday. Mike asked the party crowd to quiet down, and heated words passed between Mike and Kelly. After some shoving, a chase, and another shouting match, Mike ran to his apartment, retrieved a gun and shot Kelly to death. Noise does not usually produce such extreme outcomes, but it is a source of stress for millions of people each day.

As the case of Mike and Kelly illustrates, noise is a relative matter. One person's noise is another person's music. There may be individual differences in sensitivity to noise that also influence response (Topf, 1989). We usually define noise in terms of the effect it has on people. More formally, *noise* is unwanted sound. We perceive noise as an unwarranted, offensive, and mostly uncontrollable intrusion on our peace.

The three dimensions of sound most closely related to whether we perceive it as noise are intensity, predictability, and controllability. The measure of intensity is the decibel (dB), a standard that provides a physical reference for measuring and comparing sounds. Normal conversation is about 60 dB. Street noise is about 80 dB. Rock bands often play at from 120 dB to 140 dB. Auditory pain begins to occur around 100 dB. Permanent damage can occur with sustained exposure to sounds above 100 dB, such as those encountered in foundries. The U.S. Occupational Safety and Health Administration (OSHA) has set a 90-dB ceiling for business and industry, but more than half the production workers in America are exposed to sound levels that can produce hearing loss. Table 9-2 lists decibel levels for sounds people commonly hear at home and at work.

Generally, predictable noise is less disturbing than unpredictable noise. People can adapt readily to the effects of consistent, predictable noise. For example, most people who have grown up in Chicago around the elevated trains can sleep through the night without great difficulty because they have adapted to the noise. A person moving to Chicago from a rural area might have great difficulty sleeping at first.

An isolated event dramatically illustrated the importance of predictability and adaptation. One night, police stations along one train route in Chicago were inundated with

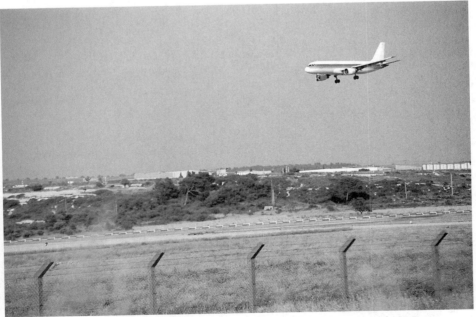

Large jets making their approaches and takeoffs over heavily populated areas produce a high level of noise pollution in spite of noise abatement procedures.

TABLE 9-2
Decibel levels for common sounds at home and work

SOURCE	DECIBEL LEVEL	EFFECT
Rocket engine	180	
	160	
Aircraft carrier deck	140	Intense pain
Emergency sirens at 100 feet		
Rock concert/discotheque	120	Moderate auditory pain
Automobile horn at 3 feet	110	
Off-road motorcycle		
Garbage truck	100	Beginning of pain
Subway station	90	Maximum OSHA level
Lawn mower/outboard motor		Hearing damage begins
Noisy restaurant	80	
Freeway at 50 feet	70	Interference with use of phone
Washing machine		
Normal conversation	60	
Residential street noise	50	Quiet
Living room with TV on		
Refrigerator	40	
Library		
Whisper at 15 feet	30	Very quiet
	20	
Broadcasting studio	10	Barely audible
	0	Threshold of hearing

calls from curious residents. "What happened?" "I know something is wrong, but I don't know what it is. Can you help?" The explanation turned out to be very simple: A power outage had shut down the trains! People awoke because of the silence. The more unpredictable and inconsistent the noise is, the more stressful it is. When it is predictable, we can adapt to it, anticipate it, and thus minimize its impact.

Finally, when we can control noise, it is less aversive than when we cannot control it. Consider this example: Your radio is playing loudly when someone suggests looking for a different station. If someone else dials in a new station, you probably will react more negatively to the white noise between stations than if you do it yourself. Muting switches are built into some stereo receivers to avoid this very problem, an example of engineering to control the aversive properties of noise.

Research shows that noise impairs performance in schoolchildren (Bronzaft & McCarthy, 1975). It reduces the production efficiency of factory and clerical workers.

Noise also increases certain types of illnesses, although the evidence for this is often weak. Nonetheless, gastrointestinal disturbances such as ulcers, vasoconstriction, higher blood pressure, and increased secretions of catecholamines (adrenaline and noradrenaline) occur consistently in association with high levels of noise (Cohen, Evans, Krantz, & Stokols, 1980). After a review of literature on noise exposure and subjective reactions, Job (1988) concluded that the findings are similar across different nationalities using different measuring techniques.

Even if noise is not strongly linked to health problems, it may have severe disruptive effects on social behavior. Noise apparently causes distortions in our perceptions of other people. It may affect our liking or disliking another person (Siegel & Steele, 1980). In addition, research confirms that noise tends to increase the likelihood of aggression, but this may only occur when a person is already angry. Thus, noise may facilitate, but not instigate, aggression (Konecni, Libuser, Morton, & Ebbesen, 1975). When Mike shot Kelly, something that happened earlier that day might have annoyed Mike; the noise of the party may only have provided the excuse for ventilating anger. By the way, a jury later found Mike innocent.

COPING WITH NOISE POLLUTION

Numerous techniques are available to deal with noise. In ecological terms, we call these *noise abatement procedures*. Noise control techniques can be divided into two broad categories. One approach is to control noise at the source. This would involve stricter laws and enforcement for mufflers on trucks, automobiles, and motorcycles. Quiet airplanes would have to be designed, and quiet office equipment, typewriters, and printers would have to be built. Even then, we could not effectively eliminate all unpleasant sounds that are part of modern industrial society.

The second general approach is to engage in better environmental design for work and living space that minimizes the potential for intrusion of unwanted sounds. Increased thickness of walls, with attention to economically feasible soundproofing, may go a long way to reducing the side effects of noise. Thicker carpets, acoustic dampening on ceilings, sound-absorbing wall surfaces, curtains, and plants may reduce the spread or influx of sound.

Masking, which uses a desirable sound to drown out an undesirable sound, is sometimes effective. Some masking may occur without design, such as the masking that occurs from heating and ventilating fans. Masking also may be by design. Offices use music to reduce background noise, and you might use the stereo to mask street sounds at home. It is possible that people use personal portable stereos (cassettes and CDs) to help block out unwanted sound. These sound sources give people control over the type and volume of music they hear. This in turn makes the sound environment predictable.

AIR POLLUTION

The Taj Mahal is one of the world's great architectural achievements. Design of the building took 7 years, and construction took nearly 22 years. More than 20,000 workers labored year-round to complete the project. It was finished in exquisite detail with precious and semiprecious stones inlaid in marble. Now, a massive effort is under way to restore, preserve, and save the Taj Mahal from destruction. It is slowly being eaten away by corrosive air pollutants from a nearby power plant.

Although air pollution does not seem to cause the psychological distress that disasters, crowding, or noise do, it is nonetheless important. At least three harmful effects are related to air pollution. First, it directly threatens human and animal health. Second, air pollution can have sweeping effects on the environment through a variety of atmospheric and climatic changes, including ozone depletion, smog, and acid rain. Third, air pollution has the potential to harm and destroy buildings through corrosive effects, as illustrated by the Taj Mahal.

One problem with air pollution is that it is not always detectable to the senses. The most apparent sign of air pollution is smog, the haze we can see on the horizon. We can smell air pollutants, such as gases from automobiles, smoke from processing plants, and odors from smoking tobacco. Other pollutants, such as carbon monoxide and radon gas, are undetectable to either the eye or the nose. Airtight homes and super efficient office buildings illustrate this problem. Such buildings can be more polluted inside than outside, yet the owners are not aware of it (Cullen, Cherniack, & Rosenstock, 1990a, 1990b).

The Air Pollution Syndrome

The health hazards of air pollution are well known. At the extreme end of the spectrum, from 50 to 90% of cancer cases may result from air pollution. In the United States alone, health officials estimate that 140,000 deaths result from air pollution each year. In Mexico City, with a population of 18 million people and dense industrialization, 100,000 people die each year from air pollution, 30,000 of whom are children. Fisher's group reported that one breath of air in an average city contains 70,000 dust and dirt particles; just living in New York City is equivalent to smoking 38 cigarettes a day (Fisher et al., 1984).

Doctors have identified an **air pollution syndrome (APS)** (Hart, 1970). The syndrome includes headaches, fatigue, insomnia, depression, irritability, eye irritation, and stomach problems. Fisher's team also provided a short but detailed summary of additional health hazards from air pollution (Fisher et al., 1984). Long-term exposure to carbon monoxide, for example, can result in headaches, epilepsy, memory disturbances, visual and auditory impairments, Parkinsonism, and physical fatigue. In addition, carbon monoxide deprives body tissue of oxygen, a condition known as hypoxia. Particulates, such as those emitted from smokestacks, exhausts, and other sources, include lead, mercury, and asbestos. These pollutants can cause cancer, anemia, and respiratory and neural problems. Psychiatric problems are also aggravated by air pollution, as indicated by increased hospital admissions.

Air pollution has other effects as well. Human performance suffers as pollutants increase. Reaction time, attention, and perceptual motor deficits occur. It is possible that such effects contribute to the frequency of automobile accidents in heavily congested cities. Air pollution also may change social behaviors, including increasing aggression.

Involuntary (Passive) Smoking

Among the most divisive issues in recent years involves the rights of nonsmokers and smokers and the issue of **passive smoking.** Several studies have shown that inhaling the smoke from someone else's cigarette can have detrimental health effects. Breathing rate, heart rate, and blood pressure increase. The Surgeon General and the National Academy

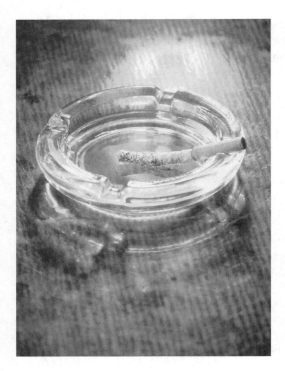

The smoke given off by a burning cigarette carries even more toxic byproducts than the smoke inhaled by the smoker.

of Science both published reports in 1986 stating for the first time that passive smoke inhalation causes disease (Fielding & Phenow, 1988). They singled out the increase in risk for lung cancer as the most notable.

In their review of this issue, Fielding and Phenow (1988) compared mainstream smoke, inhaled by smokers, with sidestream smoke, the aerosol given off by the end of smoldering tobacco. They noted that sidestream smoke "has a higher pH, smaller particles, and higher concentrations of carbon monoxide, as well as many toxic and carcinogenic compounds" (p. 1452). Among the strongest evidence suggesting a direct association between passive smoke inhalation and disease is the dose-response relationship. Risk increases (response) with increased exposure (dose) on a continuum that includes low-dose smokers (one or few cigarettes per day). One widely used short-term urinary marker, cotinine, correlates positively with increased exposure to tobacco smoke. In addition, evidence exists of respiratory disorder as measured by reduced expiratory volume and flow and of upper-respiratory problems in both adult and child nonsmokers living with smokers.

Combining the results of several studies, the best estimate of the relative risk for lung cancer is 1.34.[4] Compared to unexposed persons, then, exposed individuals are at increased risk for lung cancer. This estimate may seem small, but the cost in human lives is not, as Fielding and Phenow point out. Of the 12,200 annual deaths from lung cancer, 2500 to 8400 deaths may be attributable to involuntary smoke inhalation.

---

[4]Recall that relative risk as defined in Chapter 2 is the ratio of disease in the exposed group to disease in the nonexposed group. Thus, a relative risk of 1.34 means that if 500 nonexposed people showed clinical signs of lung cancer, 670 exposed people would show signs of lung cancer.

STRESS AND OVERCROWDING

The management, or mismanagement, of space frequently contributes to stress. Perhaps the most important issue in this context is that of overcrowding. Researchers use two terms, **density** and *crowding* when discussing overcrowding (Baron & Needel, 1980). Density is the physical condition of overpopulation. Crowding, on the other hand, is "a psychological state characterized by stress and having motivational properties (e.g., it elicits attempts to reduce discomfort)" (Fisher et al., 1984, p. 216).

To illustrate density, consider that in a city the size of San Francisco one can encounter 300,000 people in a 15-minute walk. Calcutta, India, has inner districts that are among the most densely populated in the world, with nearly 35,000 people per square kilometer. That is equivalent to 35,000 people in the space of five square blocks! That is density. However, even where the population is very dense, some people may not feel crowded. Without doubt, a complex web of psychosocial factors produces the subjective feeling.

The effects of overcrowding on human behavior can be summarized as follows:

1. High density frequently produces negative moods. This is true only for men, as women appear to have negative moods more frequently in low-density conditions. This suggests a *socialization* process that differs for males and females (Freedman, 1975).
2. Physiological arousal—as measured by higher blood pressure, skin conductance, sweating, and increased cortisol and epinephrine output—

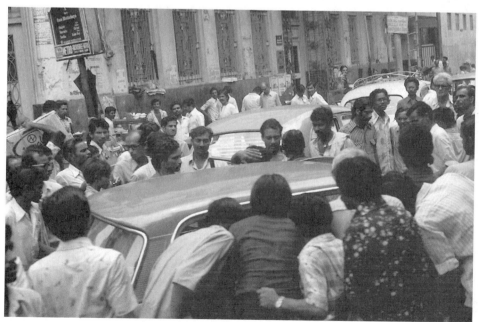

Calcutta, India: Crowding may influence social behavior, but people can adapt to crowding.

occurs in a variety of laboratory and natural settings under conditions of crowding. One study of commuters noted that the intensity of arousal, however, depended on the degree of control that commuters had in choosing their space on the train (Lundberg, 1976). This suggests that the effect of crowding is dependent on how the person appraises the *controllability* of the situation.

3. Illness increases as density increases, as studies of prison inmates, college students, and naval crews show. The types of illnesses reported are not serious, but the frequency increases.

4. Overcrowding also may increase withdrawal and aggression. Withdrawal responses include lower levels of eye contact and maintenance of greater interpersonal distance (Baum & Koman, 1976). If aggression increases at all, it does so only in males. The findings are somewhat weak and inconsistent on the latter issue.

Most negative outcomes of overcrowding are consistent with the cognitive-transactional model and the idea of loss of control. As Baum and Valins (1979) noted, overcrowding generally leads to an increase in unwanted interactions, which itself is a basic loss in controlling the range and quality of interactions. Fisher and his colleagues also saw stimulus overload and behavior constraint as potentially contributing factors, but these are still consistent with the cognitive model (Fisher et al., 1984). Loss of control could mediate physiological arousal, leading to increased sympathetic arousal and illness.

Coping with Crowding

At least two different means of coping with overcrowding have been suggested. The first focuses on environmental design aimed at reducing the feeling of crowding. Bright colors, wall decorations, higher ceilings, and rectangular rooms can increase the perception of space and reduce the feeling of crowding. Design of space to stir symbolic and affective qualities can also be helpful, especially in major metropolitan areas (Stokols, 1980).

The second approach focuses on the feelings of anxiety or apprehension felt by people in situations of crowding. One study used three different techniques to reduce anxiety in commuters (Karlin, Katz, Epstein, & Woolfolk, 1979). The three techniques included relaxation training (discussed in Chapter 11), cognitive reappraisal, and imagery (both discussed in Chapter 12). The results suggest that each technique provided some help, but cognitive reappraisal produced the most positive results.

Commuting in Urban Environments

Commuting may be one of the more stressful experiences for urban workers living in the suburbs. Above and beyond the time and expense of commuting, commuters face the daily hassle of traffic jams; accidents; rude, if not hostile, aggressive drivers; and competition for right-of-way, position at stop lights, access to freeway ramps, and parking. Research shows that commuting stress increases with the volume of traffic, changes in the weather, and two-lane or curving roads (Stokols & Novaco, 1981). Several factors affect commuting stress, including personality and the degree of control the person can exert in crowded conditions.

SUMMARY

This chapter has reviewed the status of research on stress and health related to environmental factors such as disasters, pollution, and crowding. While disasters typically produce more intense but acute (short-term) stress, pollution and crowding generally produce less intense but chronic (long-term) stress. The major points made in this chapter are summarized below.

- Although we tend to think of human operations on the environment as done to improve the quality of life, some alterations of the environment actually can disturb sensitive balances with disastrous effects for wildlife, humans, or both.
- One group of theories on environmental stress focused primarily on the need for a personal optimum level of arousal. Too much or too little stimulation could prove stressful for certain individuals based on their own adaptation level.
- Environmental stressors are grouped as natural disasters, technological disasters, and background stressors such as noise and air pollution.
- Negative health effects of natural disasters generally include short-term disturbances in eating, sleeping, and physical fatigue, with some increase in the frequency of normal illnesses.
- Psychological effects may include recurrent fear, survival guilt, depression, and increased dependence on drugs.
- The overall reaction pattern to a disaster has been described as a three-stage process beginning with impact, recoil, and post-trauma. Still, there are individual differences in reaction to disaster stress.
- One effective coping strategy during a disaster is to become involved in small tasks that serve to restore order, especially those tasks that help friends and neighbors.
- Technological disasters differ from natural disasters in that there is a human element involved in the origin of the disaster. This typically provokes more intense anger and blame reactions than is seen with natural disasters.
- Coping with disasters may be categorized as emotion-focused versus problem-focused. Emotion-focused coping works to control and release negative feelings while problem-focused coping tries to develop a concrete plan of action to exert more direct control.
- Emotion-focused coping tends to work better when we can exercise little direct control as with the overwhelming force of nature. Problem-focused coping may work best with interpersonal stressors where rational decision making can be implemented with some degree of direct control.
- Noise pollution may lead to mild impairments in cognitive function, and it tends to elevate blood pressure and increase circulating hormones such as adrenaline and noradrenaline.
- Air pollution does not seem to have the psychological effects that other environmental stressors do, but it is associated with a variety of respiratory ailments as well as cancer.
- Passive smoking is inhaling side-stream (second-hand) smoke. Sidestream smoke is actually even more toxic than the smoke inhaled by the smoker. Passive smoking is associated with increased risk for respiratory ailments and cancer in a dose-response fashion.

CRITICAL THINKING AND STUDY QUESTIONS

1. Compare and contrast the features of the environmental stress models. What do you see as the relative strengths and weaknesses of the respective models? Is there any model that stands out as a stronger model? If so, which one, and why?

2. Disaster rescue workers probably suffer significant stress in the course of doing their duty. How might their stress be different from that of a victim's family? Would you expect the rescue worker's stress to be more or less problematic to deal with, and how might you go about providing psychological aid to rescue workers?

3. Why would technological disasters lead to different types of reactions than natural disasters? Does this difference suggest that there might have to be differences in agency responses to help disaster survivors?

4. What evidence is there linking background stressors (noise and air pollution, for example) to negative health outcomes? What is your assessment of the strength of this evidence?

KEY TERMS

adaptation level
    theory
air pollution
air pollution syndrome
    (APS)
ambient stressors
arousal theory
background stressors
behavior constraint
    theory
behavior setting

chemical pollution
classical conditioning
    theory
commuting
crowding
density
depersonalization
derealization
dissociative response
ecological theory
ecology

emotionally focused
    coping
environment
environmental stress
    theory
habitat
noise pollution
passive smoking
problem-focused
    coping
reactance

WEBSITES environmental stress

URL ADDRESS	SITE NAME & DESCRIPTION
http://www.trauma-pages.com	☆David Baldwin's Trauma Info Site. Perhaps the most comprehensive site available for disaster links, support, and materials
http://www.cmhc.com/guide/anxiety.htm	Mental Health Net: Posttraumatic Stress Disorder (PTSD)
http://www.dartmouth.edu/dms/ptsd/	National Center for PTSD
http://gema.library.ucsf.edu:8081/	Global Emergency Medicine Archives
http://www.fema.gov/	Federal Emergency Management Agency. Information on how to get or give help in emergencies/disasters
http://www.disaster.net	The Internet Disaster Information Network

PART FOUR

Coping, Relaxation, and Imagery

CHAPTERS

CHAPTER 10

Coping Strategies:
Controlling Stress

The bow always drawn soon breaks.
GREEK PROVERB

QUESTIONS

- How should we define coping?
- What is the difference between problem-focused and emotion-focused coping?
- What personal resources are important to successful coping?
- How does social support influence coping efforts?
- What is the difference between combative and preventive coping?
- What coping techniques are most important?
- How do people differ in their unique coping styles?

The Tour de France is undeniably one of the world's premier sports events. Each year, about 200 cyclists put their bodies to the ultimate test of endurance, covering about 2500 miles in three weeks. On top of the physical wear and tear of time trials and the exhausting climbs out of grade mountain passes, these elite cyclists are exposed each day to many social pressures as well. Thousands of fans press for autographs, and an aggressive press corps wants the latest word on race strategy or insights into the mental state of the contenders.

In the midst of this, Miguel Indurain captured the attention of the world not just for his five straight victories, but for the way he handled all the pressures. Whether mounting the podium to accept another yellow jersey or meeting the demands of fans and reporters, he always appeared perfectly calm and composed. At times, one had to wonder if the Tour Indurain was any different from the private Indurain stretched out in a lounge or on family holiday.

COPING CAMEOS: STRUGGLES AND STRATEGIES

Not everyone deals with daily pressure with the same grace that marked the career of Indurain. Consider these additional coping cameos, starting with a pair of highly visible athletes who became linked in a lurid competitive intrigue. Tonya Harding made headlines around the world after members of her entourage conspired to assault and cripple her rival Nancy Kerrigan. In the weeks that followed, there were numerous stories of

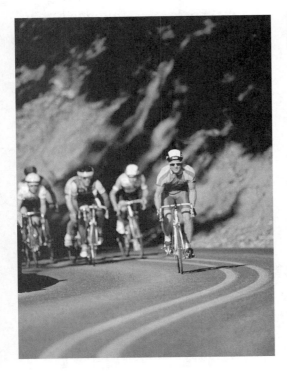

Professional cyclists have daily pressure both on and off the race course.

clashes between Harding and the press. Often, Harding appeared to lose her temper and lash out at members of the press. Later, when a broken shoelace threatened to prevent her from competing at the Olympics, Harding became visibly distraught and tearfully pleaded with the judges for time to make repairs. Meanwhile, after weathering the initial shock from the assault, Kerrigan seemed to deal with her uncertain situation and the demands of fans and press in a composed way.

For Todd and Ann Marie, life had been every couple's dream. Their parents managed successful businesses. School had been a breeze, and both had been popular members of their class. They expected marriage to be the beginning of a life distinguished by adult career successes, punctuated by fun and romantic interludes. The birth of their first child burst the bubble, leaving them shocked and dismayed for a time. Their child, far from being perfect, was mentally handicapped and would require substantial care throughout life. Todd and Ann Marie drew strength from their religion and support from their family and friends in the church. Before long, they came to accept their child as a precious gift from God, one that only needed to be nourished and cherished.

A modestly successful farmer, frustrated with government agricultural and taxation policies, became involved in a tax protest group. The federal government charged him with issuing illegal sight drafts[1] and income tax evasion. He lost his farm, and, after a short flight to avoid prosecution, his freedom. When it came time to appear in court, he refused to walk, talk, or cooperate with authorities. Officers rolled him into court on a

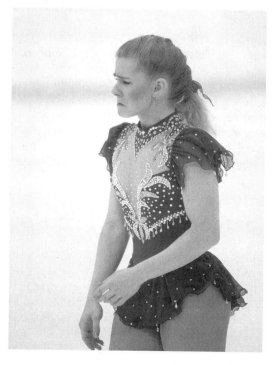

Tonya Harding, who was under great pressure at the Olympics, seemed to lose her composure when faced with setbacks.

[1]Sight drafts were a form of currency (checks) that protest groups used to challenge the authority of the federal government to issue currency, but the government regarded sight drafts as counterfeit.

handcart. Still, he refused to open his eyes or talk to the judge. He seemed to think that he could avoid reality by simply shutting it out.

Jan Kemp blew the whistle on preferential treatment of athletes at the University of Georgia. At the outset, it was a case of a teacher's conscience asking for academic honesty and integrity. Kemp could not have anticipated the shock waves that would reverberate through the academic and athletic communities. Along the way, she decided to take on the Cyclops of big-time college athletics through legal means. It cost Jan her job, placed her career in jeopardy, nearly destroyed her family, and led to two suicide attempts. During the trial against the university, Jan described herself as shy but courageous. A journalist called her another "Iron Magnolia," a nickname previously used in reference to Rosalyn Carter. *Sports Illustrated* described Jan as tough and resilient (Nack, 1986). In the end, Jan Kemp won a moral and legal victory with reinstatement to her job and a major damage award. Her methods of coping with this threat were not always positive. Still, she met the challenge and won the battle.

These coping cameos were real dilemmas faced by real people. Each was trying in some fashion to offset stress that accompanied a unique situation. These people used an assortment of coping strategies, both positive and negative, to manage pressures. We may not agree with the way they met their personal threats, but each was successful to some degree.

Several issues are important as we begin this discussion of coping. What accounts for individual differences in coping styles? What factors enable some people to cope so admirably while others struggle so much to win out over adversity? How may our study of stress help us better understand the ways people find to confront the slings and arrows of everyday existence?

These cameos also highlight several problems in the literature on coping skills. What does it mean to say that we "cope" with stress? Should we evaluate coping solely in terms of outcome? In other words, should we make no distinction between positive and negative strategies and judge only whether the strategy led to success? Do certain coping strategies work best in specific situations, or are there general coping methods?

In the pages that follow, we will discuss several issues in coping, including how to define the term and how to classify **coping strategies.** One typology in particular will provide the organizing structure for much of the chapter. We will also examine **coping resources, coping behaviors,** and **coping styles** that help or hurt coping efforts. We turn our attention now to these issues.

COPING TERMINOLOGY: ORIGINS AND DEFINITIONS

The phrase "to cope with" is a British colloquial expression. It means literally to confront an adversary or obstacle head-on, or to contend with some foe successfully, on equal terms. "To cope with" also means to be a match for someone or something that is a threat (*Webster's,* 1979). The term seems admirably suited to a discussion of stress, since stress is usually viewed as an adversary or something that threatens our psychic safety.

We all contend with stress in one form or another and more or less on a daily basis. Yet it seems clear that we do not always cope with stress on equal terms; we are not always successful with our coping efforts. This may be because we do not know what the source of stress is, because we do not have the weapons to combat stress, or because we have not learned how to use the coping weapons that are available.

In one early attempt to define **coping,** Folkman and Lazarus (1980) suggested that coping is all the cognitive and behavioral efforts to master, reduce, or tolerate demands. It makes no difference whether the demands are imposed from the outside (by family, job, or friends, for example) or from inside (while wrestling with an emotional conflict or by setting impossibly high standards, for example). Coping seeks in some way to soften the impact of demands.

Kenneth Matheny and his coworkers reviewed a large body of coping research and arrived at a similar definition (Matheny, Aycock, Pugh, Curlette, & Silva-Cannella, 1986). They defined coping as "any effort, healthy or unhealthy, conscious or unconscious,[2] to prevent, eliminate, or weaken stressors, or to tolerate their effects in the least hurtful manner" (p. 509). One aspect of this definition deserves comment—that is, coping efforts are not always healthy and constructive. People sometimes adopt coping strategies that actually get them into more difficulty. One example is the person who embezzles money to solve personal financial problems. Coping efforts may have a positive goal, but the outcome of faulty coping may be anything but positive.

This points to a sticky problem in terminology: When we speak about coping, we must be careful to note whether we are talking about the process of coping or the outcome of coping. Prior research has not always kept these two facets separate. Rudolph, Dennig, and Weisz (1995) try to introduce some order into the picture by talking about *coping episodes,* which include three components, a *coping response,* a *coping goal,* and a *coping outcome.* In this view, a **coping response** is any deliberate action, mental or physical, that occurs in response to a perceived stressor and is directed to changing the external event or internal state (p. 329). A **coping goal** is defined as the objective to be achieved by engaging in the coping response. Typically, the goal is to eliminate, reduce the level of a stressor, or transform the stressor. Finally, a **coping outcome** is the direct consequence, be it good or bad, of the coping response.

COPING CATEGORIES: PROBLEM-FOCUSED VERSUS EMOTION-FOCUSED COPING

In the years since Selye's (1956) stress research began, researchers have tried to classify different types of stress. Their aim was to snatch order from the midst of chaos and allow research to proceed in a more systematic fashion. The same is true for coping research. Several groups have provided classifying schemes to bring some order to coping research. To begin, we will revisit a simple two-category scheme encountered in earlier chapters, as provided by Folkman and Lazarus.

In Folkman and Lazarus' view (1980), one way that we may cope is by trying to change the self-environment relationship. This type of coping is **instrumental** or *problem-focused* coping. One of Jan Kemp's strategies to restore academic integrity was to use the legal system as a problem-solving strategy. Consider as another example a family member trying to care for a chronically ill loved one. The care-giver may seek advice

---

[2]Their use of the term *unconscious* is seen by some as muddying the water, though, since coping seems to suggest more planful activities. In clinical terms, unconscious activities may be regarded as the classic defense mechanisms. This is an issue that is still not satisfactorily resolved.

from medical people, read various instructive materials, and attend group sessions to learn how others provide care. These efforts may enable the care-giver to reduce, if not master, the pressure of taking care of the sick person.

A problem-focused approach seems most rational, but stress often sparks strong emotional reactions and conflicts. Coping must then work to lessen emotional pain and distress. Folkman and Lazarus called this **palliative** or *emotion-focused* coping. Imagine that a spouse has just learned that his or her mate intends to file for divorce. The spouse typically feels a great sense of loss, perhaps pangs of guilt for the marriage's failure, and some uncertainty and confusion about the future. In the first few weeks after learning of the divorce, more often than not the spouse will try just to cope with the overwhelming sense of hurt and wounded pride.

These examples make it plain, though, that the two strategies are not independent of each other. The care-giver often has to deal with intense emotions even as additional problem solving goes on. Imagine that the care-giver watches a degenerative disease (Alzheimer's or terminal cancer) gradually rob the loved one of ability to live a normal life. No matter how rational the care-giver is, there will be many times when direct and immediate action must be taken to relieve the emotional pain. Similarly, after dealing with the emotional wound, a forsaken spouse may use several highly rational problem-solving strategies, such as retaining legal counsel, to dissolve the marriage in an orderly way.

The weaknesses inherent in simple dichotomies have lead other researchers to consider more extended classifying schemes. Here, we will briefly consider the two most integrative efforts, one from Menaghan (1983) and one by Matheny's group (Matheny et al., 1986). Elizabeth Menaghan suggested that coping can be considered in terms of three higher-order issues: coping resources, coping strategies, and coping styles. *Coping resources* are the supply line for coping strategies. They are the physical, personal, and social assets that a person brings to the situation. *Coping strategies* are direct plans and actions used to reduce or eliminate stress. To the extent that plans imply an objective, this is comparable to coping goals, while actions are comparable to coping responses. The Matheny group concentrated primarily on coping strategies. Their scheme, described below, may be viewed then as an elaborated subset of Menaghan's scheme. *Coping styles* are stereotypic or habitual ways to confront a crisis.

COPING RESOURCES: ASSETS AND SUPPORT

Effective coping depends on having certain resources ready to supply the effort. These resources may be personal traits, social networks, or physical assets. Among the most important personal traits are self-efficacy, optimism, perception of control, and self-esteem. Jan Kemp embraced the virtues of honesty and integrity both for herself and for her students. She had a quiet courage that saw her through the toughest time of her life. Social resources include family, friends, job, and extended local agency networks. Todd and Ann Marie used an important social resource, their church support group, to help them cope with the demands of their handicapped child. Physical resources include good health, adequate physical energy, functional housing, and minimum financial stability.

Personal Traits: Self-Efficacy and Optimism

What we think of ourselves—self-concept—is shaped by past experiences, but it also powerfully influences how we deal with current stressors. Self-concept also shapes our expectations for success in the future. The business world uses a slogan to the effect that success breeds success. The flip side suggests that failure is a slippery slide to nowhere. This business insight has its parallel in coping efforts. Past coping success feeds a positive self-concept. This makes dealing with current stressors easier and usually sets an expectation for success in the future. Past failure tends to feed a negative self-concept. Failure makes current coping efforts more difficult, and may set an expectation of failure in the future. Coping research uses several constructs to explain this process, but we will discuss just two ideas encountered earlier, self-efficacy and dispositional optimism.[3]

As noted in Chapter 3, Bandura (1977) talked about a self-referent belief called self-efficacy, or the belief that one can control events or cope with stressful demands. In Bandura's view, our mastery expectations affect whether we will or will not initiate a coping strategy as well as how persistent our coping efforts will be.

Self-efficacy is part of the secondary appraisal we make in response to a perceived stressor. A secondary appraisal answers the question about whether we have the skills needed to cope with current demands. Strong belief in coping efficacy usually leads to lower stress levels, while a weak belief in coping efficacy usually leads to higher stress. Bandura and his coworkers confirmed this principle, and they observed several other negative outcomes as well. In addition to experiencing higher levels of subjective distress, people with a weak belief in coping efficacy have increased autonomic arousal and elevated plasma catecholamine secretions (Bandura, Reese, & Adams, 1982).

People can also make faulty appraisals, which tend to produce undesirable outcomes, such as anxiety and behavioral dysfunction. Matheny and his colleagues use the common magnifying glass as an analogy (Matheny et al., 1986). When you look through one end of a magnifying glass, everything seems much larger. If you look through the other end, however, everything appears much smaller. People with strong coping-efficacy appraisal may see demands as small because they see their skills as more than adequate for anything. On the other hand, people with weak efficacy may see demands through a magnifying lens even when the demands are objectively small. Further, they may see their coping skills through the dwarfing lens even when an outsider would see the person's skills as good.

A strong sense of self-efficacy may foster positive health outcomes, including enhanced immune system function (Wiedenfeld et al., 1990). The success of several intervention strategies appears to depend on changes in perceived self-efficacy (O'Leary, 1985).[4] These include smoking-cessation and pain-management programs. Diet and exercise regimens following heart attacks may also depend on changes in self-efficacy. As O'Leary points out, though, actual competence is not as important as the perception of efficacy. Self-efficacy is not a fixed trait; it can change with new experiences.

Self-esteem is also an important personal resource, but it is not synonymous with self-efficacy. *Self-esteem* means to accept and have high regard for oneself. Presumably, self-esteem should increase with boosts in perceived self-efficacy. Indirect support for

---

[3]These concepts were discussed in Chapter 3 as cognitive processes that influence appraisals. Here, we focus primarily on their contribution to coping.

[4]This suggests that self-efficacy is not a fixed trait but can be changed as a result of experience.

this notion comes from research that shows good copers have a higher sense of self-worth than poor copers (Witmer, Rich, Barcikowski, & Mague, 1983).

Dispositional optimism is the expectation that good things will happen. Optimism is a perceptual filter that colors many situations in their best light, while pessimism colors situations darkly. Scheier and Carver (1987) believe optimism is a personality trait that can have a powerful influence on coping. Their research suggests that optimists are more likely than pessimists to rely on coping methods that produce better outcomes and that lead to more favorable outcome expectancies. Optimists, as well, are more likely than pessimists to persist in their coping efforts (Scheier, Weintraub, & Carver, 1986). A study of female executives in Canada revealed that high optimism predicted a reliance on more practical social support, acceptance, and expressiveness when coping with job pressures (Fry, 1995). Overall, the optimistic women were less likely to suffer blows to self-esteem when confronting work pressures and they were less likely to show signs of burnout. This work on optimism and the earlier work on self-efficacy suggest that efforts to improve both traits can have a positive effect on coping.

Social Support: Structures and Functions

Social support has emerged as a major resource for effective coping. The evidence suggests that social support makes only a small contribution to coping efforts by itself, but it is very important when combined with other coping techniques. Social support may help people cope with stress through indirect or direct action (Cohen & Wills, 1985). The indirect effect is called the buffering model. Here, social support does not do anything directly to reduce or eliminate stress. It only shields the person from the negative effects of stress.

On the other hand, social support may be valuable and beneficial in its own right, providing people with a sense of direct control over stress or ensuring multiple ways to act against stress. As one example, consider a person who wants to challenge a large corporation that is polluting the environment. Trying to take on the task alone might be futile, but with the help of some social agency, the effort may result in major changes in the corporation's activities. This may reduce or eliminate a major source of stress not just for that person but for many other people in the vicinity as well.

Whether social support works as a stress buffer or stress terminator, people engage in an ongoing dialog, implicitly or explicitly, with the units of social support (family, friends, job, and church, for example). This dialog involves an exchange of both positive and negative information between the person and the social unit. The information exchange may inspire positive coping or it may have a disregulatory effect on coping (Leavy, 1983).

Sheldon Cohen (1988) believes that social support must be defined by structure and function combined (Cohen & Syme, 1985; Cohen & Wills, 1985). In Cohen's view, there are informal and formal social structures. Family, friends, and co-workers are examples of informal structures. Most social agencies and the church are examples of formal structures. Religious groups provide very strong social support systems. Social networks function to provide emotional support, give information and advice, or help devise a problem-solving strategy.

There is evidence that quantity of support is not as important as quality of support (Schultz & Saklofske, 1983). This is based on evidence that people with extensive, but low-quality, support report feeling lonely more often than people with less, but high-quality, support.

Additional evidence suggests there are significant gender differences in quality of social support. Compared with women, men typically have a more extensive support network, but the support tends to be more superficial. Conversely, women typically have a more limited network, but it is also more intimate and intensive (Shumaker & Hill, 1991). For most males, their intimate and intensive support most frequently comes from their spouses, while women generally have several friends outside the marital unit that serve this function. Finally, women typically use their support systems more effectively during crises, while men are less likely to use theirs.

Certain stressful situations may benefit more from social support than others. This is especially true when the stressor comes from having to care for young or old family members with a chronic illness or some other limiting condition (Shapiro, 1983). Families with handicapped children, for example, often benefit from social support groups that can exchange information on care-giving techniques as well as help the emotional turmoil that goes with being a care-giver (Kirkham, Schilling, Norelius, & Schinke, 1986; Yablin, 1986).

AIDS and ARC patients also experience more distress when they believe that less support is available (Zich & Temoshok, 1987). In the San Francisco Men's Health Study, Robert Hays and his colleagues were concerned about levels of depression in gay males (Hays, Turner, & Coates, 1992). They observed that the men in their sample were slightly more depressed than normal, but their depression was not clinically severe. Two factors were highly important to this group in buffering against stress and depression. These factors were the quality of social support received and the informational support provided.

Unfortunately, building good social support networks is more difficult than learning how to use relaxation or how to control weight. Intervention strategies may have to adopt a long-term approach and focus on various social skills, including openness and commitment in personal relations. Information on social agencies may be important as well, but this information usually needs to be specific to the problem that the person is dealing with at the time. Finally, intervention strategies may have to be gender appropriate, since it appears that men are less likely to have effective social support systems compared with women.

COPING STRATEGIES: COMBATIVE AND PREVENTIVE COPING

The second coping resource involves coping strategies that we have learned to use through experience, by observing others using a novel coping strategy, or by reading instructive material on coping techniques. There are far too many coping strategies to discuss in one chapter. To simplify, I will use the framework provided by Matheny's group (Matheny et al., 1986). Matheny's team based their classifying scheme on a meta-analysis of coping studies. (A meta-analysis, discussed in Chapter 2, is a quantitative method to summarize the results of many studies and to examine patterns of outcomes from these studies.) Matheny's framework appears in Table 10-1.

First, coping strategies may be grouped into two broad categories called combative coping and preventive coping (Matheny et al., 1986). **Combative coping** is a provoked reaction to some stressor. The intent is to suppress or terminate the stressor. In the terminology of classical learning theory, combative coping is intended to effect an escape

TABLE 10-1
Preventive and combative coping methods

PREVENTIVE STRATEGIES	COMBATIVE STRATEGIES
1. Avoiding stressors through life adjustments	1. Monitoring stressors and symptoms
2. Adjusting demand levels	2. Marshaling resources

3. Altering stress-inducing behavior patterns	3. Attacking stressors
	   a. problem solving
	   b. assertiveness
	   c. desensitization

4. Developing coping resources
   a. physiological assets
   b. psychological assets
      confidence
      sense of control
      self-esteem
   c. cognitive assets
      functional beliefs
      time-management skills
      academic competence
   d. social assets
      social support
      friendship skills
   e. financial assets
	4. Tolerating stressors
	   a. cognitive restructuring
	   b. denial
	   c. sensation focusing
	
	5. Lowering arousal
	   a. relaxation
	   b. disclosure
	   c. catharsis
	   d. self-medication

SOURCE: Adapted from Matheny et al. (1986).

from an aversive event. This makes combative coping sound like an inferior form of coping. But in some cases, we have no choice.

For example, we may get caught by a natural catastrophe, a flood or an earthquake. All that we can do, then, is seek to minimize the effect of this stressor. Consider another example. A young woman meets a young man and after a short courtship marries him. He has all the attributes she has hoped for and they settle into what seems like a happy marriage. Shortly, however, he displays a pattern of physical abuse that slowly escalates to frightening levels. Given the absence of any prior signs of this violent streak in her husband, she has no choice now but to use a coping strategy that is primarily reactive.

On the other hand, **preventive coping** is proactive. It tries actively to prevent stressors from ever appearing. In classical learning terms, preventive coping is avoidance learning. We learn to anticipate the onset of an aversive event and respond in advance to prevent its appearance. To illustrate with an actual case, a young woman, Leah, was involved in a relationship with a young man, Rick. The relationship grew increasingly serious. As Leah got to know Rick's family better, though, she saw signs of danger. The father often engaged in verbal and psychological abuse of his wife and daughter. On several occasions, Leah saw Rick repeating the father's pattern, verbally abusing his own mother and sister. Leah took decisive steps to leave the relationship to prevent any repetition of this pattern with her.

Matheny's group found evidence for five general types of combative coping strategies: monitoring stress, marshaling resources, tolerating stressors, attacking stressors, and lowering tension. **Stress monitoring** involves being aware of tension when it occurs and recognizing the source. This is a necessary first step to being able to use other coping strategies. It includes being sensitive to physical changes and signs of tension in muscles and viscera. The second combative strategy is *marshaling resources,* which includes organizing one's personal and social resources. We may also simply *tolerate stressors,* somewhat like enduring slivers in the hand. Instead of digging them out, we let them work their way out. For mild or some moderate stressors, this approach may work adequately and it reduces the effort required for coping. Still, this approach is viewed as a bunker mentality that simply hopes to ride out the barrage. It is not likely to help with most moderate and severe stressors.

When we try to completely eliminate a stressor, we are using the strategy of *attacking stressors.* This is often done by using problem-solving skills, seeking relevant pieces of information, using social skills prudently, or being assertive as necessary. One subtle method of attacking stressors is **cognitive restructuring.** To do this, we must examine thought patterns that are negative, self-defeating, and self-limiting. Often this method requires some outside help, because we have difficulty seeing the flaws in our own thought patterns. Among the cognitive restructuring strategies used for this purpose are self-instruction training and rational-emotive therapy (RET).

The fifth combative strategy is to *lower arousal* by using relaxation techniques (described in Chapter 12) or by reducing stimulation. It is important to note once again that not all coping strategies yield positive outcomes. Consider the following example of a coping strategy that is used by some people to lower arousal and anxiety, but that can increase risks in a very serious way.

Although this example is taken from research conducted among gay and bisexual men in San Francisco, it has implications for heterosexual activity as well (Folkman, Chesney, Pollack, & Phillips, 1992). Folkman's research group looked at risky sexual behavior in the context of a stress-coping model. Prior research suggested that sexual contact may be used by some people as a tension-relief strategy. Unfortunately, this strategy may also lead to an increase in the number of sexual partners, which greatly increases the risk for AIDS.

Folkman's group did not find a link between amount of stress and a person's tendency to engage in unprotected sex. However, the person's habitual method of stress coping did have an effect. Subjects who reported that they used sex as a stress-coping strategy were much more likely to engage in unprotected sex during periods of stress. This suggests that intervention programs to prevent AIDS should account for the unique coping strategies of the clients. In addition, the program should teach alternative coping strategies that will reinforce self-protective health behaviors.

In the analysis provided by Matheny's group, four preventive coping strategies emerged. These are identified as making life adjustments to avoid stressors, adjusting demand, changing stress-inducing behaviors, and developing more personal coping resources. One life adjustment to avoid stress is to leave an unrewarding job, or change careers altogether. We may adjust demands by knowing when to say no, and not feeling guilty about saying no. Buying expensive gifts for the family beyond one's financial means may lead to combative coping, as when the bill collector shows up at the door. Adjusting the demands to meet resources prevents that from happening.

We may change stress-inducing behaviors by getting rid of Type A tendencies, or reducing impulsiveness that gets us into trouble in interpersonal relations. An anxiety-prone person may look for ways to temper hyperreactivity. We may work on building personal coping resources by improving self-efficacy, by learning time-management skills, or by cultivating extended but high-quality social networks. Although time management may not seem as crucial as other coping skills, King, Winett, and Lovett (1986) showed that time management can serve as an effective coping strategy leading to reduced stress. McLaughlin, Cormier, and Cormier (1988) also showed that dual-career women frequently use time management and that it is positively related to better marital adjustment and lower levels of stress.

COPING EFFORTS: WHAT CAN YOU DO TO COPE WITH STRESS?

Coping behaviors may be external (actions) or internal (cognitive), positive or negative, approach (active) or avoidant, direct or indirect (Rudolph et al., 1995; Suls & Fletcher, 1985). They may include seeking help, seeking information, or diverting attention. Whatever their nature, coping efforts have one primary function: to prevent, eliminate, or reduce stress. The extensive literature on coping reveals no less than a dozen behaviors that may be used for this purpose. The discussion in this section follows the summary of Matheny's group, with examples, supporting evidence, and types of training procedures added (Matheny et al., 1986). The first four coping efforts—tension reduction, cognitive restructuring, problem solving, and use of social skills—showed the strongest effect on coping outcome.

Tension Reduction: The Aspirin Therapy for Distress
The most commonly used coping skill is **tension reduction.** Tension is a physical warning that something is wrong. It usually means that an event in the environment or an unresolved internal conflict has increased physiological arousal to uncomfortable, if not harmful, levels. Tension can perpetuate stress even after removal of the stressor, so reducing tension can have positive outcomes. We may attain tension reduction through such methods as progressive relaxation, meditation, or autogenics.[5] Matheny's group found that relaxation was the most widely used single treatment procedure and had the greatest positive effect on coping outcome. Many clinicians recommend relaxation for a wide range of stress-related conditions, including migraine headaches (Sorbi & Tellegen, 1988).

Cognitive Restructuring: Changing Perceptions
Cognitive restructuring changes the meaning of an event or changes perceptions of personal adequacy to handle a situation. Coping efforts typically involve an anticipatory process that begins before actually meeting a threat or stressor. Consider people thinking about impending surgery. They may dwell mentally on the upcoming procedure day after day until their anticipation becomes anticipatory anxiety. This is especially true when people have heard stories—no matter that the stories may be more myth than fact—about the likely discomfort, pain, or nausea associated with a medical procedure. This is why ruminations[6] can become the Achilles' heel of coping efforts.

---

[5]These techniques are described in more detail in Chapters 11 through 13. Instructions for relaxation practice are given in the appendix.
[6]Ruminations are repetitive thoughts, going over the same event again and again.

Anticipatory anxiety occurs more often in younger patients and in those who have higher trait anxiety (Jacobsen, Bovbjerg, & Redd, 1993). Children waiting for dental work, for example, report many "catastrophizing" thoughts that increase their anxiety and make the dentist's work more difficult. Still, some children use positive coping strategies spontaneously (Branson & Craig, 1988). Their cognitive efforts include positive self-talk ("I tried to think good thoughts"), thought stopping (eliminating bad thoughts), and emotional control cognitions ("Try not to worry"). They also seek information and support from the dentist, engage in attention diversion, and practice relaxation or deep breathing to reduce tension.

Fernandez and Turk (1989) showed that cognitive coping strategies are effective in alleviating pain.[7] Klingman (1985) provided training in cognitive-behavioral coping to girls preparing for inoculation against rubella. The girls showed lower levels of anxiety and were more cooperative compared with girls in a control group who received only technical information.

Shelley Taylor's (1983) theory of cognitive adaptation integrates many important components of coping with threatening events. Taylor argued that readjustment to threat involves three general themes. First, we look for meaning in the experience. We may even change the meaning of an event after reflection or after obtaining a different perspective from a friend or confidante. Next, threat often makes us feel insecure about our control or efficacy. So we try to regain mastery over the event and over life in general. Finally, because threat often attacks self-esteem, we may try to enhance self-esteem through positive self-evaluations.

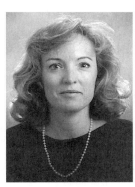

Shelley Taylor, author of the cognitive adaptation theory, has contributed a great deal to our knowledge of stress, coping, and health outcomes.

Clinical interventions commonly use rational-emotive therapy and stress inoculation to bring about cognitive restructuring. In Matheny's meta-analysis, cognitive restructuring was second only to relaxation training in frequency of use. It also had the highest positive effect on coping outcome, matching the strength of relaxation training as an intervention procedure.

Humor may be a means of restructuring perceptions of stressful events. The prominent personality theorist Gordon Allport (1937) discussed the role of **humor** in personality. He considered humor a prime correlate of insight. People can reformulate ordinary problems and misfortunes through humor. They gain a new perspective, a novel frame of reference. Consistent with Allport's view, individual differences exist in preference for humor, as do gender differences in the type of humor used to cope with stress (Schill & O'Laughlin, 1984). Rod Martin and Herbert Lefcourt (1983) discovered that humor moderates the relation between negative life events and mood disturbance. Fry (1995) also found that female executives with a strong sense of humor weathered daily hassles in their business and personal lives better than did those with a low sense of humor.

[7]This study was discussed in Chapter 2.

Problem Solving: Rational Steps to Stress Reduction

Many events are stressful because they involve elements of problem solving that we are ill-prepared to handle. When we can solve a problem readily, we either experience just a little stress or we experience only a challenging stress. When the solution to the problem eludes us or involves competencies that we do not possess, considerable stress is likely to occur. Jan Kemp (see page 288), employed extensive problem solving by retaining a lawyer and following a legal process to reach a solution. Bandura (1989) suggested that people who believe in their problem-solving ability remain more effective analytic thinkers in difficult situations. Success in problem solving, then, may feed back to increase self-efficacy.

One might learn problem solving as a general strategy. On the other hand, one might learn specific problem-solving strategies for specific issues or situations. Maura Kirkham and her colleagues adapted a general problem-solving model called SODAS to help mothers of handicapped children (Kirkham, Schilling, Norelius, & Schinke, 1986). **SODAS** is an acronym for **S**top, **O**ptions, **D**ecide, **A**ct, and **S**elf-praise. In the process, first Stop and identify the problem. Then, list all the solution Options. Next, Decide which option is probably best. Outline a step-by-step plan to implement the decision and then Act. Finally, reinforce yourself for solving the problem with Self-praise. Most often, problem-solving classes focus on specific issues, such as study skills, weight control, escaping cycles of abuse, single parenting, effective parenting, and so forth.

Social Skills: Communication and Assertion

Problems with interpersonal relationships create many stressors. We may read signals of friendliness as overtures for intimacy and then get hurt. We may talk too much, listen too little, and hear even less. We may seek positive evaluations to bolster our self-esteem, then fail to respond positively to the efforts of someone trying desperately to please us. Each of these situations involves social skills, the ability to navigate the troubled waters of interpersonal exchange in a mutually satisfying way (Marsh, 1988; Richmond, McCroskey, & Payne, 1987). Practicing social skills should enable us to achieve needs and goals in a way that does not harm others in the process. Social skills training includes interpersonal communication (Hargie, 1986; Mader & Mader, 1990), intimacy and self-disclosure, and **assertiveness,** among others (Cotler & Guerra, 1980; Zuker, 1983). As a group, social skills may positively influence coping outcomes, but they do not contribute greatly to coping success when learned as simple separate interventions (Matheny et al., 1986).

Positive Diversions: Filling Time Constructively

Positive diversions, also called **attention diversion,** use constructive activities to divert attention from painful or distressing thoughts. For example, a widow who takes on volunteer service may find that the new involvement reduces the frequency of memories of the spouse who died recently. Hobbies such as music, reading, acting, and exercise can also serve this purpose. Diversions may be useful in situations of uncertainty. For example, waiting for a call that means getting a special job can be difficult, especially if one conjures up cognitive scripts that anticipate a negative outcome. A similar situation exists when waiting for results from medical tests or when dealing with a family member with long-term illness.

Open and Closed Systems: Letting Out or Holding In

Another coping effort involves **self-disclosure** and **catharsis.** *Self-disclosure refers* to being open as a person, being able to share thoughts and feelings with others. *Catharsis* means release of or purification of emotions. In clinical practice, it means bringing un-expressed, repressed emotions into the open so they can be dealt with directly. Closed-in people often suffer because they distance themselves from social support by their behavior. Also, they are like a dam stopping up a huge reservoir of emotionality. When emotion finally breaks out, it does so in a torrent instead of a controlled release. However, Irving Janis (1983) cautions that high disclosure can be harmful if it leads to demoralization.

The ideal is to maintain a balance between control and expression of emotions. Extreme or inappropriate emotions need to be controlled to some extent, whereas less extreme and appropriate emotions can be expressed more openly. The process of **ventilating emotions** can have a therapeutic effect and reduce stress. Similarly, self-disclosure can be beneficial if it is not too rapidly paced or done under duress.

Seeking Information: Ignorance Is Not Bliss

Information seeking is a very important cognitive skill when dealing with uncertainty. People using this skill aim to obtain information that will reduce uncertainty and the stress that goes with it. Patients considering a doctor's advice for elaborate tests may ask friends for information about the doctor, about the tests, or even about where to get more information (Horn, Feldman, & Ploof, 1995). They may go to the library to read about symptoms, treatments, and prognosis before undergoing the lab tests. This can be beneficial and reduce stress in certain situations. In other situations, it may increase stress.

Stress Monitoring: Keeping an Eye on Distress

One train of logic suggests that being oblivious to stress is desirable. Another suggests that being aware of stress is of importance to survival. The argument for stress monitoring depends on the notion that awareness of stress is necessary to identify sources of stress in events and people. This view is consistent with a control theory of stress management (Suls & Fletcher, 1985). If we can identify stress-inducing events and people, then presumably we can engage in problem-solving behavior that will reduce, if not eliminate, stress from these sources. If we cannot, then disregulation may occur, leading to even more stress.

Stress monitoring includes awareness of increasing tension in muscles. This signal should enable us to take steps to halt or reduce the tension (Suls & Fletcher, 1985). The exercises used in progressive relaxation focus attention on tension and develop awareness of the contrast to relaxation. Stress monitoring also involves awareness of one's optimal range of stimulation.

Matheny's group found that stress monitoring could sensitize people to the existence of stress. In this case, the effect on coping efforts was negative. Suls and Fletcher (1985) studied coping with painful medical procedures, and their analysis provided some insights into this phenomenon. They showed that when monitoring focuses on threat, it increases distress. On the other hand, when monitoring focuses on sensory information, it does not. Further, if stress monitoring includes constructive efforts, such as identifying problem spots and engaging in problem solving, then the process can have a positive effect on coping outcome.

Assertive Behavior: Standing Firm, Not Angry

Many people encounter stress in normal transactions because they lack assertion skills. When someone cuts in line at the theater ahead of a nonassertive person, instead of gently but firmly asserting the social norm of turn taking, the nonassertive person may say nothing. The event, though, may fester inside the person, welling up as a seething anger directed toward others. This cycle may also lead to lowered self-esteem. Learning appropriate assertion can help remove this source of distress (Cotler & Guerra, 1980; Zuker, 1983).

Negative Coping: Avoidance and Withdrawal

Avoidance or withdrawal is another coping strategy commonly used to protect against unwanted emotions. A person using avoidance usually seeks to eliminate stress by physically or mentally leaving the scene. People may avoid seeing a doctor for fear of hearing bad news. They may avoid the banker for fear of being pressured about a loan or an overdrawn account. Students may skip class for fear of bad news on a test. Avoidance is not reality oriented and, when used to the extreme, it can interfere with effective stress management. Further, excessive avoidance may feed back negatively to lower self-esteem and self-efficacy.

Suls and Fletcher (1985) provided evidence from a meta-analysis of coping literature that avoidant strategies show their strength compared with other coping strategies only in the short run. For instance, immediately after the appearance of a stressor, avoidance is superior to attention strategies. Yet, within from two to six weeks, the pattern reverses when attention strategies become superior. The researchers suggest that this may be due to a time lag required to marshal resources to begin a more direct attack on the stressor.

Denial and Suppression: Intrapsychic Defenses

A person may escape mentally through **denial** or suppression. These control procedures usually seek to eliminate unpleasant emotions. In Freud's popular theory of personality, denial and suppression had a special name—*defense mechanisms.* Denial ignores a stressor, and suppression pushes the event deeper into the morass of the unconscious. These two defenses constitute a refusal to accept objective reality for what it is. At the same time, these cognitive escape routes can be helpful when life-threatening illnesses first appear (Druss & Douglas, 1988). It is also a major, possibly necessary, stage in grieving.

Mardi Horowitz (1979) wrote extensively about the psychological responses to serious life events. He outlined the signs and symptoms of denial that occur in stress reactions; these appear in Table 10-2. Despite its helpfulness in some situations, denial may be self-defeating. Extreme denial may prevent healthy coping and slow down progression to other stages of adjustment to and recovery from emergency situations. The more denial or suppression distort reality, the more likely the outcome will be negative.

Another intrapsychic defense is **intellectualization,** a process that translates feelings into thoughts. The thought process blocks out feelings we do not want to deal with immediately. Clinical theory treats denial as a primitive defense and intellectualization as a more mature means of defending against unwanted emotions (Vaillant, 1977). A major problem exists when people intellectualize to such an extent that they filter all feelings through the rational net and thus can never express their emotions.

TABLE 10-2
Signs and symptoms of denial phase of stress response syndromes

SIGNS	SYMPTOMS
Perception and attention	Daze Selective inattention Inability to appreciate significance of stimuli
Consciousness	Amnesia (complete or partial) Nonexperience
Ideational processing	Disavowal of meanings of stimuli Loss of reality appropriacy Constriction of associational width Inflexibility of organization of thought Fantasies to counteract reality
Emotional	Numbness
Somatic	Tension-inhibition–type symptoms
Actions	Frantic overactivity to withdrawal

SOURCE: Horowitz (1979).

Negative Coping: Escape Through Self-Medicating

Finally, some people cope through **addictions** or *self-medication* behaviors. Using tranquilizers, alcohol, and other drugs to reduce arousal or blunt the effect of stress falls in this category. Excessive use of medications for pain relief is also negative coping, although it is a fairly common solution. Even children dealing with dental or arthritic pain reported taking medicine as a likely means of coping with pain (Branson & Craig, 1988).

Although self-medication may be viewed as successful coping from a personal point of view, it is really a negative coping effort. The long-term effects are generally self-defeating, and the behaviors themselves entail more risks and health hazards. Sorbi and Tellegen (1988) showed that migraine patients reduced their use of medications following either cognitive stress-coping training or relaxation training. They also increased assertive and problem-solving behaviors and reduced depressive reactions.

Structuring: Putting It All Together

Structuring refers to ways in which we assemble or organize coping resources, then use these resources in anticipation of a stressful event. Stress inoculation is a technique that serves this purpose.

COPING STYLES: REACTIVE AND PROACTIVE COPING

People are creatures of habit much more so than they like to think. This is true with coping efforts as well. A stereotypic or habitual reaction to stress is called a coping style. An early view of coping styles suggested that people are either *proactive* or *reactive* (Adams,

Hayes, & Hopson, 1976). A **proactive** person is one who acts early to prevent stress from developing. A **reactive** person cares little for preventive efforts and just reacts instinctively when stress occurs. Some people become counter-aggressive in the face of threat while others become submissive.

In a study of women coping with the stress of abortion, Cohen and Roth (1984) saw a parallel pattern. Some women were approachers: They seemed to feel that doing something was better than doing nothing. Some were avoiders: They seemed to think that they could wait out the problem before they could directly beat the problem.

The previous differences focus primarily on coping behavior. It is possible to identify coping styles by cognitive habits as well as by behavior. One distinction is between the reflective and the impulsive type person. The reflective person typically seeks information, problem solves, and plans carefully how to deal with a stressor. The impulsive person, on the other hand, is more likely to react quickly and emotively—a "shoot from the lip" style—without thinking much about the likely outcome.

Another cognitive style that is receiving much attention is a person's attributional style. Some people make an external attribution when anything goes wrong. That is, they blame something or someone other than themselves. This tends to blunt the impact of any stress that might come from the blunder. Others make an internal attribution— that is, they blame themselves. This only tends to add to their stress. As noted in Chapter 3, Martin Seligman's group believes that one cognitive style in particular, the pessimistic explanatory style (PES), is linked with several poor outcomes. The PES combines an internal attribution for negative outcomes that is stable over the long-term, as well as global. A PES says, "I am the cause of the problem [internal] because I am always [stable] incapable of managing any [global] of my affairs." In contrast, someone else might think that the problem occurred only because of a temporary lapse in judgment (a transient, not a stable, cause) having to do with a small area of skill (a specific, not a global, flaw).

BUILDING COPING SKILLS

Stevens and Pfost (1984) identified eight components of typical stress management programs: stress information, assessment, relaxation training, cognitive restructuring, problem solving, time management, nutritional counseling, and exercise planning.

The preceding chapters provided essential principles and theories about stress and health. This information should enable you to identify sources of stress in family, school, social, and work environments. You should recognize the attitudes, beliefs, behavioral patterns, and high-risk behaviors that can add to stress. You should also understand how these sources of stress alter internal functions and thus can damage the body. These ideas form the foundation of any informed, focused stress-management program. They also provide a sound base for implementing a personal health program.

Although space does not permit thorough discussion of stress assessments, your instructor may include stress assessments as class activities. In this chapter, we identified coping resources and behaviors to manage stress and reduce risks. Subsequent chapters will show how specific techniques work, including the rationale, theory, and supporting research. The first set of techniques presented will be *stress-management skills*. The second set deals with *personal health-programming skills*.

One widely used and generally applicable stress management technique, progressive muscle relaxation, is presented in Chapter 11. Relaxation is a tension-reduction skill. Several methods build on relaxation training, including cue-controlled relaxation, differential relaxation, and desensitization. In Chapter 12, we will discuss imagery procedures, including autogenics, desensitization, cognitive restructuring, and stress inoculation. We will review meditation and biofeedback in Chapter 13. Chapter 14 describes student survival skills and time-management techniques, and Chapter 15 discusses nutrition, diet, and exercise.

SUMMARY

In this overview of coping, we have looked at terminology, categories, and methods of coping. The major points are summarized below.

- Coping is any effort to prevent, eliminate, or reduce stressors, or to tolerate the effect of stress with minimum harm.
- Coping responses are deliberate actions that occur in response to a perceived stressor.
- Problem-focused coping attempts to change the self-environment relationship. In other words, this form of coping works to resolve any conflict or problem that may exist between the self and others (interpersonal stress) or between the self and agencies.
- Emotion-focused coping seeks to lessen emotional pain or discomfort due to the presence of a stressor.
- Effective coping depends on having resources and strategies. In addition, coping styles often determine immediate reactions to stress. Coping resources are physical, personal, and social assets used to confront stress.
- Among the personal resources are self-efficacy and optimism. Self-efficacy is a self-referent belief that we can act with some degree of mastery or control on our environment. People higher in self-efficacy tend to experience less stress while people low in self-efficacy tend to experience more stress.
- Dispositional optimism is the expectation that good things will happen. Optimists tend to perceive situations differently than pessimists. Optimists also tend to use better coping techniques and they persist longer with their coping efforts.
- Social support is important to effective coping, but it is the quality of the support—not mere quantity—that is most important. Building good social networks is one method of improving coping efforts.
- Coping strategies are the plans and actions we use to manage stress.
- Coping styles are the habitual ways we confront stress. Combative coping is a provoked reaction to a stressor, while preventive coping is proactive. That is, proactive coping seeks to prevent stressors from appearing in the first place.
- Learning new coping skills adds to our personal resources. Problem-solving ability is an important cognitive skill that usually requires high-quality information, and seeking information in general appears to be an effective coping strategy.
- One cognitive coping strategy involves restructuring. With this method, we change the meaning of stressors so they become less threatening, or possibly even challenges.

- Social skills may be important as a group, but individual social skills (such as assertiveness) do not seem to enhance coping significantly. The practical implication is that one should work on a range of social skills instead of depending on just a few.
- Negative coping strategies, such as withdrawal or denial, may be helpful in short-term coping, but long-term coping depends on more mature coping strategies.

CRITICAL THINKING AND STUDY QUESTIONS

1. How should we define coping? Is it satisfactory to define coping solely in terms of outcome? That is, if the coping effort gets rid of the stressor, does it really matter if the coping method was negative itself?
2. If you were coping with an environmental threat, such as a hurricane or a possible nuclear accident, how would you probably best cope with the situation? How would this differ from coping with news of a serious personal illness or some interpersonal conflict?
3. Why is self-efficacy considered an important personal resource? How does it influence the coping process?
4. What is the difference between combative and preventive coping? Are there times when combative is better than preventive coping? Why? Are there times when preventive coping is preferred to combative? If so, why?
5. Consider a recent stress episode that you went through, and try to imagine how you might use one or more of the techniques (cognitive restructuring or problem solving, for example) to deal with the stress episode. How would these methods differ from what you actually did at the time of the episode?

KEY TERMS

addiction	coping resources	palliative coping
assertiveness skills	coping response	positive (attention)
avoidance	coping strategies	diversion
catharsis	coping styles	preventive coping
cognitive restructuring	denial	self-disclosure
combative coping	humor as coping	self-esteem
coping behaviors	behavior	social support
coping (defined)	information seeking	stress monitoring
coping goal	instrumental coping	tension reduction
coping outcome	intellectualization	ventilating emotions

WEBSITES coping strategies

URL ADDRESS	SITE NAME & DESCRIPTION
http://www.uib.no/STAR/	☆STAR (Stress and Anxiety Research Society). Stress and coping newsletter and journal
http://imt.net/~randolfi/StressLinks.html	One of the most impressive link sites to many other Stress Management sites
http://www.hypnosis.com/	Hypnosis website with information and links
http://www.nlpinfo.com/	The NLP Information Center (NIC). Central site for Neuro-Linguistic Programming
http://www.mindtools.com/	Mind Tools. A site devoted to various coping skills, such as problem solving, stress, and time management

CHAPTER 11

Progressive Muscle Relaxation:

Premises and Process

The real task is to succeed in setting man free by making him master of himself.

ANTOINE DE SAINT-EXUPÉRY

QUESTIONS

- What is the rationale behind Progressive Muscle Relaxation?
- How is the autonomic nervous system linked to the relaxation response?
- Does relaxation only reduce arousal or does it also change cognitive processes?
- What are the optimal conditions for learning how to relax?
- What is the process for learning relaxation?
- How can you get relaxed faster?
- When is it appropriate to use relaxation on a real problem?
- Is it possible to get relaxed on cue?
- Can relaxation be used for just a select muscle group?

While teaching off-campus courses in stress management and personal health, I have encountered several interesting and unusual cases for which relaxation offered relief. One involved a person I'll call Elaine. She suffered from chostochondritis, or Tietze's syndrome,[1] an affliction that leaves the front walls of the chest inflamed and irritated. The effects of the inflammation can be very powerful and frightening. People afflicted with chostochondritis may think they have a heart problem or a serious stomach disease. Women are more frequently afflicted than men, and the condition may intensify with tension and overwork.

When I first met her, Elaine had been suffering from this condition for nearly a year. During that time, she had obtained medical diagnosis and treatment. X ray examination of the chest, stress tests, electrocardiograms, and other examinations revealed no physical cause. The attending physician diagnosed the condition as chostochondritis and recommended that Elaine use a heating pad whenever possible and take three aspirins four times daily. After complying with this medical regimen for a time, Elaine reported that "the chest pains continued. It was as if I were having a heart attack many times a day, although I was relieved to know this wasn't my problem."[2] Further tests for stomach and colon disease were negative, and the doctor prescribed a stronger drug. Unfortunately, nothing seemed to work.

At the beginning of the stress management class, I assigned each student the task of researching a stress situation or personal health problem. Then each student was to design a program to reduce stress or improve health or both. Meanwhile, we began training the relaxation response.

During class discussions, we pieced together some vital bits of information about times and places when Elaine's chest pain seemed most likely to strike. She worked as a real estate appraiser and reported that both mental and physical stressors occurred frequently. Almost always, the most severe inflammation occurred during these periods of severe work stress. Because of this, the condition seemed to occur much more regularly than not. The recognition that stress was somehow related either to the onset or the intensification of the condition suggested that it might respond to a stress management technique such as progressive relaxation.

Therefore, we used a structured approach to introduce relaxation exercises in relation to the physical condition. First, Elaine practiced relaxation, using techniques described later in this chapter, until she could induce relaxation very rapidly. Simultaneously, she monitored the frequency, intensity, and duration of the attacks. Finally, Elaine was instructed to begin the relaxation response whenever she recognized the presence of stress during the day. Over a five-week period, she reported that the frequency of attacks decreased to near zero. Even when an occasional attack occurred, it was much less intense and was over much quicker than those she had suffered prior to the training. This outcome is nearly as important as the decrease in frequency of attacks. Elaine's case showed how effective the relaxation technique can be. In approximately seven weeks, it had eliminated a painful affliction that had lasted nearly a year.

[1]Technically, the term *Tietze's syndrome* designates the condition when local swelling occurs, something that does not occur in chostochondritis.

[2]Personal statement supplied by the student with permission to publish.

The purpose of this chapter is to provide an overview of the rationale for and practice of **progressive muscle relaxation (PMR)** as a tension reduction technique. Several methods of stress management build on this skill, including **cue-controlled relaxation, differential relaxation,** and desensitization.

PROGRESSIVE MUSCLE RELAXATION: THE PROMISE

Few techniques have proven as powerful and generally applicable as the relaxation technique. It has withstood the test of time, as well as stiff competition from the new kid on the block— *biofeedback*. The advantages of relaxation are many. Relaxation can be used in the privacy of one's home or exported to the office. It can enter the boardroom or the courtroom. You can take it on the road during rush-hour traffic or settle jittery nerves at 30,000 feet. Without fanfare and public recognition, it debuted at Wimbledon, restoring smoothness to tense muscles and accuracy to a champion's service.[3] It also got a novice skier down a terrifying ski slope in Utah.

Relaxation procedures can be used to treat both migraine and tension headaches (see Carlson & Hoyle, 1993, for a review), hypertension (McCubbin et al., 1996), pain, insomnia (JAMA, 1996), tension headaches, test anxiety, performance anxiety, flight phobias, and Raynaud's disease (Pinkerton, Hughes, & Wenrich, 1982). Reviews of clinical applications reveal that relaxation is also useful for children suffering from stress-related symptoms (Smith & Womack, 1987). It is being used to help people deal with claustrophobia while undergoing magnetic resonance imagery (MRI) scans (Lukins, Davan, & Drummond, 1997). Bruning and Frew (1987) suggest that relaxation is a stress management technique in its own right, with the power to lower arousal indicators of stress. Thomas Burish and his research group used relaxation training to reduce the side effects of chemotherapy in cancer patients (Burish et al., 1988). This is only a partial list of applications.

There are numerous relaxation techniques. These include PMR or abbreviated PMR, autogenic training, the relaxation response, Transcendental Meditation, and hypnosis. Autogenic training, an imagery-based procedure, came from Johannes Schultz's work during the early 1950s (Schultz & Luthe, 1959). The relaxation response (not to be confused with PMR) derives from Herbert Benson's interest in Transcendental Meditation (1975). We will discuss autogenics in Chapter 12 and the relaxation response in Chapter 13. Hypnosis can be regarded as a relaxation technique only with a very broad definition of relaxation. Still, some clinicians use hypnosis in this way. I note these variations on the relaxation theme to make an important point: *The particular form of relaxation you develop is probably unimportant.* I say "probably" because we cannot state with confidence that all relaxation procedures are equivalent or interchangeable (Smith, 1988). Nonetheless, most research shows that they have similar results in practice. The most important issue is that you develop at least one tension-reduction skill to a level of practical proficiency.

The technique described here, progressive muscle relaxation, has other names, including progressive relaxation and deep muscular relaxation. It has grown steadily in

---

[3]The procedure referred to here is differential and graduated relaxation, which will be discussed later in this chapter.

popularity since its founder, Edmund Jacobson, first wrote about it in 1938. Jacobson took great care in developing progressive relaxation, although his procedure as first developed is generally considered cumbersome to use. As time passed, many clinicians added to and refined the practice while providing a massive body of supporting data. Because of this, it is now possible to provide clear, detailed instructions on how to practice and apply PMR. The gold standard for relaxation training is Bernstein and Borkovec (1978), which reduced the sessions and muscle groups involved, leading to the term abbreviated PMR or APMR. Still, the technique generally is just referred to as PMR. As a result of such developments, learning relaxation does not require one-on-one, high-cost therapy. With careful attention to a few guidelines and some diligent practice, most people can begin to practice PMR in a short time.

It is important to note that relaxation training involves more than just learning how to relax. It includes learning to spot signs of stress in mind and body and to connect these signs to the conditions present in your environment. Ultimately, it also includes learning to apply the skill selectively to a variety of situations and individual muscle groups.

FROM PROMISE TO PREMISE

Relaxation training relies on a simple assumption: You cannot be relaxed and tense simultaneously. In spite of the apparent simplicity of this statement, there is much more to it than that. Tension and relaxation are body states that correspond to two parts of the nervous system, the sympathetic and the parasympathetic. Since we discussed how these two autonomic components operate in Chapter 5, we will only review here the elements relevant to the relaxation technique.

Recall that when we are in an aroused state, as when threatened, afraid, angry, or excited, the sympathetic nervous system is in control. This is the emergency system, or the *fight-or-flight* system. Blood rushes from the digestive tract to provide energy to important muscle groups, such as the arms and legs. Heart rate increases, and blood pressure usually rises as well. During aroused states, the body burns energy at a tremendous rate. Breathing rate increases, and sweating may occur. Sympathetic arousal, then, is a tearing-down process.

During sympathetic arousal, *muscle tension increases dramatically*. This tension is not an all-or-nothing affair, though. Depending on the type of stress, only certain muscle groups may tense. Which group tenses usually depends on factors unique to your body and your way of dealing with stress. Some people feel tension in the back, some in the forehead, some in the neck, and so on. Also, muscle tension varies on a continuum from slight to extreme, depending on the severity of the stressor.

Conversely, when we are in a quiet, relaxed state, such as in sleep, the parasympathetic system is in control. Heart rate slows, blood pressure normally drops, and breathing becomes slow and easy. Blood returns to the center of the body for digestion and energy storage. Muscle tension decreases, and people generally report a feeling of muscular heaviness or relaxation. This is a building-up or restoring process.

Parasympathetic processes are the opposite of sympathetic processes. In technical terms, these two systems are reciprocally inhibitory; that is, they tend to inhibit each other alternately. In less technical terms, when one system is loud, the other system tends to be quiet. When one is dominant, the other tends to be subordinate. Both systems typically are not highly active at the same time.[4] Again, in behavioral terms, you cannot be tense and relaxed simultaneously.

This relationship seems intuitively obvious, even simple. Jacobson recognized this but took it a step further. He claimed that we could directly control the balance in the autonomic nervous system through behavior. In making this claim, though, he challenged established scientific theory. The prevailing scientific view held that the autonomic nervous system, which controls nearly all life-support functions, is an *involuntary* system. Scientists assumed it was involuntary because the processes continue whether we are asleep or awake. On the surface, this logic seemed acceptable.

Still, a long history of observations and research began to expose the label's fallacy. One line of evidence came from joint American and Indian research teams who studied the remarkable Yogis of India. These investigations revealed that Yogis could produce extraordinary changes in body processes. They survived burial for two or three days through heart slowing (not heart stopping) and respiratory control. They regulated body heat to withstand freezing temperatures with scant clothing. They altered brain waves through self-induced trances. Investigators agreed that the Yogis showed clear control capability, even though the mechanisms were not immediately obvious (Anand, Chhina, & Singh, 1961a; Bagchi & Wenger, 1957).

The dilemma was clear: What should be done with the theory of the involuntary nervous system? True to the scientific spirit, numerous investigators conducted more controlled studies and confirmed that these responses could be controlled voluntarily (Kamiya, 1969; Miller, 1969). It was Jacobson who put two and two together in the relaxation training program. Very simply stated, *relaxation is a voluntary behavioral method of controlling the reciprocal relationship between the excited and calm sides of your autonomic nervous system.* You can put the parasympathetic system back in control through practiced relaxation. When the sympathetic system is loud—your stomach is tied in knots, your muscles are tense, or a headache makes your head feel like a drum—you can quiet it down behaviorally.

A COGNITIVE-BEHAVIORAL VIEW OF RELAXATION

Before moving on to relaxation procedures, we must discuss a theoretical controversy about what occurs during relaxation practice. Smith (1988) challenged the popular notion that relaxation primarily reduces arousal. Smith believes that this arousal model of relaxation is more incomplete than incorrect. He also questioned the interchangeability assumption proposed by Benson (1975). This is the notion that various relaxation techniques are interchangeable and will lead to identical outcomes. Smith's **cognitive-behavioral theory of relaxation** attempts to round out the incomplete arousal model of relaxation.

Smith proposed that three cognitive processes are involved in relaxation: focusing, passivity, and receptivity. Focusing is the ability to maintain attention to a single stimulus for an extended period. Passivity is the ability to stop customary goal-directed activity or analytic pursuits and become inactive for a time. Receptivity is the ability to tolerate and

---

[4]There are certain times when both systems are highly aroused simultaneously, but these departures from the rule do not alter the basic notions presented here (Berntson, Cacioppo, & Quigley, 1991).

be open to uncertain or paradoxical experiences. According to Smith, learning relaxation involves altering cognitive schemata in many ways.

These cognitive schemata include the notion that being a productive, valued member of family and society requires constant activity, wage-earning, and social involvement. Inactivity is nonproductive, if not a sign of laziness. In this view, we exaggerate the value of those behaviors that directly lead to goal attainment. We devalue, if not ignore, indirect behaviors, such as restoring energy and creativity through diversions. As relaxation progresses, convergent cognitive structures emerge that support the value of focusing, passivity, and openness. In addition, divergent cognitive structures that interfere with relaxation slowly dissipate.

Positive relaxation experiences provide support for convergent structures. As practice continues, the ability to control arousal provides more positive feedback. In addition, the person becomes aware of differences between relaxation and tension both sensorily and cognitively. Cognitive structures emerge, allowing one to label and articulate changes that accompany relaxation. Simultaneously, the person abandons irrational or incorrect cognitive structures that interfere with relaxation. The result is a changed set of beliefs about self and the value of activity versus passivity. In Smith's model, arousal is controllable, but it is only one component in a complex process of cognitive change.

Although Smith believes a family resemblance exists between the relaxation techniques, he also thinks the techniques differ greatly in demands on the cognitive system. Progressive muscle relaxation is concrete and undemanding, whereas meditative techniques are more demanding. He suggests that the more demanding techniques are also more threatening and take longer to learn. Still, people who begin with a concrete method probably will progress to more complex cognitive structures. Until recently, though, clinical research showed little concern for theoretical niceties such as those contained in Smith's view.

FROM PREMISE TO PREPARATION

Clinicians believe four conditions are important prerequisites for successful relaxation practice:[5] setting, mood, preparation, and medical precautions.

Arranging the Setting

Where you practice relaxation can affect success and consistency. First, *select a comfortable room where you can isolate yourself from family or friends for a while.* The room should be properly ventilated in the summer and adequately warm in the winter. Use a comfortable chair that provides support for the entire body. A recliner is ideal, but avoid the fully reclined position; the temptation to sleep may interfere with learning. Some clinicians insist on a hard, straight-backed chair for initial training. The reason is that *you should practice relaxation for the first few weeks with an optimal level of self-awareness and observation.* Extended use of the technique requires that you can recognize the difference between muscle tension and relaxation. That awareness cannot come if you are nearly asleep.

---

[5]A detailed set of instructions appears in the Appendix. Other methods for presenting instructions (audiotapes, for example) are also discussed there.

The room in which you practice should be quiet and free from distractions. Disconnect the telephone if possible; otherwise ask a family member to answer the phone immediately. Try not to worry about missed phone calls. Recognize that you have a right to privacy and a right to time for yourself. You can choose not to have that privacy invaded.

With family members, it is probably best to appeal to their understanding by explaining what you are doing and why it is important. Enlisting family support can help reduce the likelihood of chance interruptions. This may work well with older children but not as well with younger children. Here, a simple matter of timing may suffice. Try to practice during their naps or after they have gone to bed in the evening.

An important condition for early success is consistency. *Practice relaxation exercises twice daily at roughly the same time each day for the first three to four weeks.* This will increase the likelihood of success and speed development of the skill. Be flexible in applying this rule. Some books recommend even more daily practice, up to four times per day. Experience suggests that such a recommendation is hard to follow because of its sheer impracticality. Further, no evidence suggests that you will progress faster with more sessions.

Finally, *use background music during practice if you wish.* The right type of music can foster a sense of tranquility and aid relaxation. Quiet classical or easy-listening music is probably preferable. Clinics often use "nature" music, such as sounds of wind and seashore and calls of whales and porpoises. Whatever you choose, play it at a low volume so you will not be attending to the music more than to the relaxation exercise.

Cultivating a Positive Mood

Approaching daily practice in the right frame of mind is important both to objective success and to the subjective sense of satisfaction. The following are the most important rules for setting the mood.

CULTIVATE A SENSE OF PASSIVE ATTENTION Learning to be adept at relaxation requires a balance between attention and quiescence. The key to using relaxation anywhere is that you can read muscle tension whether it is loud or soft. The sequence of instructions is designed to attain this outcome, especially in the early stages of practice. Muscle tension is the body's red-light warning system that indicates when you are under stress. Passive attention is necessary for learning to discern when tension is present. Strained attention relegates everything else to secondary importance and adds more tension to the system. Passive attention can be likened to listening with an inner or third ear; it goes on with no conscious thought.

DO NOT TRY TO MAKE RELAXATION HAPPEN This is not a task like jogging. You do not have to sweat and strain to master relaxation. It is not a technique to beat into submission. It is, instead, a technique that comes quietly and gently.

DO NOT HURRY Relaxation is not like lunch hour, to be rushed through to get back to more important things. It is more like prayer and meditation. It is like lying on a beach soaking up rays or lounging in a boat listening to the lapping of gentle waves. At these moments, time is the least important condition of existence. As you become more skilled, you may come to regret that tranquility must be abandoned for the clamor of the real world. Getting through the exercises is not important, but experiencing the moment is.

DO NOT USE DRUGS Although certain drugs may help you relax, drugs will interfere with the primary goal of relaxation training: learning to recognize muscular tension that signals stress. Tranquilizing drugs, for example, depress normal brain function. Thus, it may be more difficult to recognize *real signals* of body tension as opposed to *noise* generated by the drugs. Developing sensitivity to body signals will be harder, not easier. If you are on medication by doctor's order, wait until you are off to begin relaxation.

TRAIN FIRST; APPLY LATER A major mistake in developing a technique like relaxation is trying to use it on big jobs right away. Then, when it doesn't work, for whatever reason, one tends to blame the technique and quit. This can lead to frustration—and possibly feelings of helplessness and hopelessness. Master the technique and its extensions before moving on.

DO NOT BE AFRAID OF DIFFERENT FEELINGS The practice of relaxation can produce anxiety and other novel sensations. Among those who learn relaxation, about 40% experience some anxiety. To explain, the experience of very deep relaxation can produce a feeling of loss of control and strong feelings of fear. It appears that the thought of losing control frightens some people. We do not know how to explain *why* they feel this way, only *that* they do. The feeling generally passes quickly as they experience the benefits of relaxation. Relaxation may not be the method of choice when there is a personal history of extreme anxiety reactions (Heide & Borkovec, 1983).

Clients also report feeling they will not be able to come back. The sensation of deep relaxation seems to them like a hypnotic trance with no one around to guide them back. In reality, coming out of relaxation is no more difficult and no more aversive than waking up from a nap. In many ways, the heavy feeling and tranquil state of mind are similar to feelings enjoyed in a nap state. Although you may experience the sensations as different, you may come to welcome and enjoy these sensations before long.

Taking Proper Medical Precautions

Persons with physical conditions such as severe back injuries, recent muscle strains, or broken bones should exercise caution. *Ask your physician if it is safe to engage in an exercise that will place a moderate strain on bones and muscles.* With strains or broken bones, you may have to wait for complete healing before beginning your practice. For severe back injuries, procedures such as autogenics (see Chapter 12) or Benson's relaxation response (see Chapter 13) may be suitable. Benson's technique is meditative, passive, and intuitive and thus eliminates any muscle tension exercise.

Also, persons with a history of heart difficulty should seek advice from their physician before beginning. Problems may occur when there is a history of heart difficulty combined with a current severe cold, especially a cold with chest congestion. Deep-breathing exercises could be painful, leading to anxiety, which in turn could aggravate a heart condition.

RELAXATION: THE PROCESS

Relaxation exercises follow a sequence of alternating tension and relaxation in 16 muscle groups. Self-Study Exercise 11-1 shows a typical sequence beginning with the hands and arms. This sequence can be altered to suit personal preference. Some people feel more comfortable working from head to feet, while others may work a reverse sequence from feet to head. There is no evidence that one sequence is better than another. Also, the number of muscle groups may vary depending on grouping. Some clinicians suggest that the tongue and jaw muscles should be treated as separate groups. Again, there is no evidence that this is crucial to success.

Tension-relaxation cycles should be about 30 seconds each, with slightly more time given to relaxation than to tension. Early sessions may require from approximately 45 to 75 minutes to finish. Later, much less time is needed for relaxation. Adept practitioners

---

SELF-STUDY EXERCISE 11-1

Learning Relaxation Skills
Sequence for relaxation practice
1. Preferred arm
2. Alternate arm
3. Preferred hand
4. Alternate hand
5. Shoulder muscles
    a.   Preferred-hand side
    b.   Alternate side
6. Neck muscles
7. Forehead, eyes, scalp
8a. Jaws and mouth
8b. (Tongue, optionally, as extra step)
9. Breathing—chest and trunk
10. Stomach
11. Lower back
12. Buttocks
13. Preferred thigh
14. Alternate thigh
15. Preferred foot and calf
16. Alternate foot and calf

Additional reminders:
2 sessions per day, same time, same place
3 repetitions for each muscle set
10–15 seconds for tension sets
15–20 seconds for relaxation sets
45–75 minutes for the first few sessions
Sessions will be greatly reduced in length after the first few sessions.

---

can reach complete body relaxation in from 5 to 15 minutes. Reducing time also requires shortcut techniques that will be described later.

As a first step to making relaxation a useful stress management technique, it is important to spend the alloted time studying the difference between tension and relaxation. *These differences in muscle sensations exaggerate the signals that occur during stress.* Studying these contrasts develops sensitivity to signs of tension and adds to the utility of relaxation.

Frequently, people report feeling pressured, but they do not know why they feel that way. They also do not seem to know the source of the pressure. This may be because they do not hear the warning signals from their body. Even when they do hear, some do not understand the connection to what is going on around them. When you can detect subtle changes in muscular tension, you can also look for the event that triggered it. When the alarm sounds, the natural response should be: Who is present? What is the situation? What is the theme of the conversation? Money? Sex? Control? How am I responding? Defensively, aggressively, angrily? Has this cycle happened before? In this way, the red-light warning system can help us detect the sources of stress.

A TENSION-SCANNING EXERCISE

To aid this learning, carry out a simple exercise for a full week. Make a mental note each day that you have one personal project to do: namely, *tune in* to signs of muscular tension. During this week, observe body tension reactions all day, not just during relaxation. Carry a small notebook or diary with you. Whenever you spot signs of muscular tension, record the time, place, and people involved. If you cannot do so immediately, then record it as quickly as possible without disrupting your normal routine.

The event may be loud and long or quiet and short. It may involve many muscle groups or only an isolated muscle. Yet it will result in noticeable change. Look for signs of tension: neck muscles cramping, shoulder muscles knotting up, lower back muscles tightening, knotting or butterflies in the stomach, forehead muscles tensing, jaws clenching, teeth grinding, fists doubling, breathing increasing, and heart pounding. The objective is to learn how to identify tension signals in the real world before you become distressed or physically sick.

MOVING ON: WHEN CAN I DO SOMETHING WITH IT?

One practical problem is how to know when it is suitable to move on. First, allow at least two weeks for basic practice before proceeding. Second, gauge the depth of relaxation and your satisfaction with it. In clinical research, formal procedures exist to do this, but this is unnecessary in practice. You should experience both deep relaxation and personal pleasure with relaxation before applying the skill. Third, monitor the amount of time it takes to become relaxed. You should become relaxed in less than 30 minutes before trying advanced procedures.

GETTING RELAXED THE FAST WAY

If you had to spend 30 minutes to become relaxed every time and needed a recliner and quietness, you might question how useful the technique could be. As you will see, you can reduce tension quickly and quietly through a combination of techniques that make a total package of relaxation training.

First I will describe a method of relaxing entire groups of muscles together. Then we will discuss a method called **cue-controlled relaxation.** With this method, a single word that you associate with relaxing can be your password to reduced tension. Later, I will describe how to relax one muscle group by itself through the technique of differential and graduated relaxation.

RELAXING A GROUP OF MUSCLES

The 16-step sequence described earlier relaxed each muscle as though separate from other muscles. It is possible, however, to relax groups of muscles together. Typically, we use 5 stages to reduce the time to relaxation. Two stages reduce the number of muscle groups, and 3 stages reduce the amount of voluntary muscle tension.

From Sixteen to Eight Steps

For the first few days, relax (1) both arms together, (2) both hands together, (3) both shoulders and neck muscles, (4) the forehead with scalp, jaws, and mouth together, (5) both chest and stomach muscles, (6) lower back and buttocks together, (7) both thighs, and (8) both calves and both feet together. The 16-step procedure is now 8 steps. This phase usually requires about five days. Self-Study Exercise 11-2 shows the steps to take.

At first you may encounter difficulty with tension-relaxation contrasts. The arms, hands, and legs are probably the easiest. Continue to study the contrasts in tension and relaxation. Some people have difficulty with the head muscles because several very different muscles are in this group. If you encounter this, continue to relax the muscles in this group as separate muscles. Practice with the other combined muscle groups until you are successful, then return to the head muscles. Once again, there is no evidence that a rigidly prescribed sequence is the one and only one right way to do this.

Now Softer on the Tension

The next step is to reduce the intensity of tension in the tension-relaxation cycle. Instead of tensing the biceps very tightly, tense them only a moderate amount. For all muscle groups, lower the amount of tension without reducing the amount of time in the tension cycle itself. Also, do not change the relaxation cycle in any way.

To help with this step, imagine muscle tension on a 100-point scale. The high end of the scale corresponds to the highest tension, such as when you are arm wrestling with a friendly competitor. The low end corresponds to the deepest relaxation, such as when you are stretched out in an easy chair. For the first step in tension reduction, imagine what your muscles would feel like at the 75-point mark on the scale and try to tense to about that 75% level. The scale is very subjective and personal with no absolutes. This

SELF-STUDY EXERCISE 11-2

Guide for Reduction Steps in Relaxation Practice

First reduction set
1. Both arms
2. Both hands
3. Shoulder and neck
4. All head muscles
5. Chest and stomach
6. Lower back and buttocks
7. Both thighs
8. Both feet and calves

Second reduction set
1. Both arms and hands
2. Shoulders, neck, and head
3. Chest, stomach, lower back, and buttocks
4. Thighs, feet, and calves

Additional reminders:
2 sessions per day, same time, same place
3 repetitions for each muscle group
10–15 seconds for tension sets
15–20 seconds for relaxation sets
25–35 minutes for the first few sessions
Sessions will be reduced in length after the first few sessions.
Reduce tension about 25% after reaching criterion before going on to the second set.
Reduce tension about 25% more at the end of the second reduction set.
Reduce tension about another 25% and practice to criterion. Go on to cue-controlled relaxation.

step may seem paradoxical, but the rationale is simple: ultimately, you should be able to sense tension whenever and wherever it occurs.

To do this, you need to sense subtle tension just as easily as nagging tension. When you can spot the whispers of stress as readily as the shouts, you will begin to realize the benefits of relaxation. Reducing tension voluntarily in these exercises will teach you to discriminate between degrees of tension.

There is another important reason for reducing tension. The portability of relaxation depends on your ability to become relaxed quickly. When you have finished reducing the muscle groups to four, you should have phased out the intense tightening routine. From that point on, you will return to the tension cycles only when you need a booster.

From Eight Muscle Groups to Four

Self-Study Exercise 11–2 also guides you through the second reduction set. The procedure is the same as before. Try to relax all the muscles in a group together. Again, if you have any difficulty with a group of muscles, go back to the previous mastery step for that muscle group. The idea is to be flexible; the rules are not absolute. There is nothing wrong with using nine muscle groups in the first reduction phase or five muscle groups in the second phase. Allow yourself freedom to read your body, and adjust the groupings so they feel right. This phase should take another five to seven days.

Even Softer on the Tension
At the end of the first reduction phase, you reduced voluntary tension to about 75% of maximum. The goal now is to reduce it even further. Try to imagine how your muscles would feel when tensed to about 50% on the scale. For another week, use this 50% standard for the tension phase.

Now Ever So Softly
The last step is to reduce the level of induced muscle tension to about 25% of the original level. Try to imagine the 25% level on the scale, and tense to that level. This may take another three to five days. You should still reach deep relaxation, and you should become relaxed as quickly as before. You may find that you can achieve deep relaxation in from 5 to 15 minutes. If so, congratulate yourself and feel well rewarded for your efforts.

To review, progressively reduce the number of steps to reach relaxation by grouping muscles together. Also reduce the amount of voluntary muscle tension as follows:
1. Reduce from 16 muscle sets to 8 muscle groups over five to seven days. When you can relax as quickly and almost as deeply as before, go to step 2.
2. Reduce the amount of artificially induced muscle tension to about 75% of the original level. Practice until you can relax as quickly and deeply as before, then go to step 3.
3. Reduce from 8 muscle groups to 4 muscle groups over five to seven days. Practice until you can relax quickly and deeply, then go to step 4.
4. Reduce the amount of artificially induced muscle tension to about 50% of the original level. Practice until you can relax as quickly and deeply as before, then go to step 5.
5. Reduce the amount of voluntarily induced muscle tension to roughly 25%.

TERRIFYING SLOPES: RELAXATION TO THE RESCUE

Life can have its terrifying moments, even when you are having fun. Such was the case when I combined a business trip with some skiing pleasure on the slopes at Park City, Utah. Although I had been on skis just once before, the morning went wonderfully. After lunch I somehow ended up on a slope that completely disappeared from view. It had beautiful moguls—many, many moguls, tightly packed and small. For me, it was too much too soon. The end was a humbling slide on my posterior, skis in hand, while supportive souls in the lift above found their afternoon lightened by this comic sight. Yet the real terror was still ahead.

A quick search of the trail map revealed a green-marked trail, the beginner's route down the mountain. I settled back, relieved that I would have a pleasant cruise to the bottom, where I could count my ego losses, reconstruct my self-image, and prepare for a frontal assault on the mountains another day. At first the trail looked like a gentle, slowly winding descent down the mountain. Of course it wasn't really the easy trail. It was only the easiest from that part of the mountain.

My partner and I skied past a rope tied with red flags and signs warning of danger. Beyond was a sheer, ice-packed slope that looked as though it went straight down. It had just one purpose: to convey any object in a straight line as fast as possible to the bottom. Only later did I learn that it was the downhill race course. For now, that sheer cliff was beyond the rope, and here where I was skiing, that beautiful trail still stretched out gently in front of me. It vanished around a cluster of trees ahead. That could only mean one thing—the *real* trail must continue somewhere beyond and to the side of this ice sled of a downhill course. But, disappearing around the trees wasn't half of it. The trail wound around those trees and disappeared—right onto the top of the downhill course. Now there was no way back, around, or down . . . except!

My terror was complete. I had never seen anything like this. My partner gave a brief reassuring smile and a "See you at the bottom" salute. He pointed his skis down the slope and gracefully rounded a ridge at the bottom before I could even consider what to do. If only I could be off this mountain that fast.

My problem was with my body and my mind. Both had to be calmed before I could get down that hill. My mind was a jumble of thoughts. My body felt like muscular pretzels. Every inch was in knots except my knees, which wouldn't stand still for anything.

I went through two processes to get down that mountain: thought stopping and muscular relaxation. The mental process combined rational problem solving and an emotional control process to drive the frightening, self-defeating thoughts out of my head. The relaxation process was to get my body under control. If you watch professional skiers, you realize how fluid and loose they look. Whether it is Michael Jordan doing a spectacular slam dunk, or Pete Sampras making a reflex shot at the net, muscular tension is the athlete's enemy.

Because I had practiced the technique before, it took just a moment to achieve relaxation, even on this mountain slope. I concentrated on the major tense spots—my stomach, shoulders, and legs. Finally, I planned a path down the mountain that included several traverses. This helped mentally as well, because I recognized that I could control my speed with this technique. It seemed like an eternity, but I still must have spent several minutes transfixed in the middle of that course thinking and relaxing. Then I began the trip down. The first traverse and turn were tense, but I felt the ski edges bite and carve the way they should. My confidence went up, and the next turn was crisp and clean. It now seemed more like fun, and before I knew it, there was the bottom of that once terrifying slope. I must have felt some degree of arrogance, then, because I turned and gave a defiant salute to the mountain. I also praised myself for a victory over both the physical elements and the fear that only moments before had been my oppressor.

These are obviously not the conditions in which you should practice relaxation the first time. Once you have developed the skill, though, you may be surprised where you can take relaxation. This incident illustrates two different procedures: cue-controlled relaxation and differential relaxation. In the next few pages, we will examine these techniques to see how they might operate in stress management.

RELAXING WITH A WORD

Most instructions for relaxation suggest that you use a cue word with breathing—for example, "Breathe out, and as you do, say 'Relax.'" This instruction forms the core of cue-controlled relaxation. The secret of the technique is simple: the repeated connection between a cue and a response makes it possible for the cue to produce the response automatically. A familiar example may help to illustrate this point.

When you were born, many cues, such as words, did not have any real power to control or change your behavior in and of themselves. Through a long process of learning, words become connected to important events in such a way that they now alter your behavior as directly as the events themselves did.

"Stop!" and "No!" mean nothing to an infant. Along the way, many connections will be made between such commands and something dangerous the child is doing. When children first touch a hot stove, they encounter a powerful incentive to withdraw the hand—burning pain. Pain usually leads to quick and durable learning. If the parent is nearby, the child may hear a loud "No, no!" just before touching the stove. If so, a quick yet permanent connection may be built between the command and the dangerous event. Over time, many repeated connections between a cue (such as parents' warning words) and some dangerous event (such as running into a heavily traveled street) will occur. Children's ability to control their behavior will increase as they internalize additional examples of cue-response connections. It may not happen on the very first try, but it will come with time.

You may have seen another step in the development of personal control after an incident of this type. The child approaches the stove again and reaches toward the stove. Then the child stops, looks at the parent, and says "No" aloud. The word is now an internalized controlling cue. The child does not need to be burned, punished, or even warned repeatedly to avoid hot stoves and onrushing cars.

The process of using a word to control relaxation is much the same. Relaxation is the response we want to control. The cue word is the signal that triggers the response of relaxation. At first, the cue word may have only a general meaning. After you repeatedly link the cue to relaxation, you can use it to induce relaxation directly. Instead of several tension-relaxation cycles, you simply say the word and relax.

What's the Word?

The particular word you use is not important, although you should avoid words that occur in routine conversation. Some people use words like *peace, quiet, easy,* or *warm.* Some select a word that is similar to a **mantra,** a sacred, privileged, and secret word. Whatever word you choose, make sure that when you breathe out, you use that word only.

Beginning Cue-Controlled Relaxation

Learning cue-controlled relaxation is usually easier than the steps you have taken to learn relaxation. There is nothing special to do except practice breathing out and using the chosen cue word. You will find brief instructions in the Appendix after Chapter 15.

Repeat the cue-controlled sequence for approximately one week. Start each relaxation period with breathing-cue word cycles. Complete each period by using the tension-relaxation cycles to achieve relaxation if necessary. When you can reach from about 50 to 75% of the relaxation you normally reach with the tension-relaxation method, you can move to the next step. You should not expect to achieve the depth of relaxation that you achieve from tension-relaxation cycles. The use of cue-controlled relaxation does not demand complete relaxation because complete relaxation would be detrimental to its everyday use.

Using Cue-Controlled Relaxation

In addition to knowing how to produce cue-controlled relaxation, you need to know where and when to use it. Earlier in this chapter, I suggested that you keep a diary noting times, places, and people involved when you felt tension. If you did this, you should have some useful information by now to tell you where and when to practice cue-controlled relaxation. First, categorize the diary incidents of stress on two dimensions (home and work or home and school, as appropriate). Then go through the events and evaluate the corresponding levels of tension (high or low). The correct classification of home, school, or work should be automatic. The correct classification for level of tension is entirely a subjective judgment.

To classify tension, start with the event that produced the most intense muscle tension. Then find the event that produced the lowest muscle tension. Use these extremes to scale and categorize the remaining events. After you do this, you are ready to apply cue-controlled relaxation to a real situation.

Select a situation from the low-tension/home category. It is best to pick one that happens regularly so you can practice more often and soon. The next time the event occurs, prompt yourself to use cue-controlled relaxation. Take a deep breath, hold for a moment, and release it completely while you say to yourself your personal cue word. Nobody needs to know that you are cuing relaxation. In fact, it is probably best to avoid telling other people what you are doing. In the middle of an intense exchange, it might irritate others more than relieve them. You should notice a decrease in the intensity of your arousal. Most people report a *rush* of relaxation and a reduction in anxiety.

The positive effects should be even more pronounced in interpersonal relationships and problem-solving situations. Amid interpersonal conflict and crises, extreme arousal and tension reduce our ability to think clearly and to respond sensitively (Bandura, 1989). Arousal may also interfere with our ability to read verbal and nonverbal nuances in messages from others involved in the conflict. We may become defensive, responding

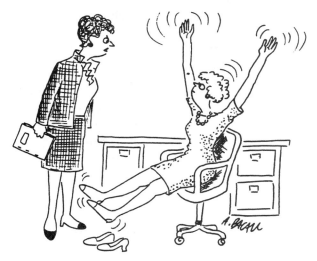

"Would you mind not going through your stress-reduction exercises while I'm reprimanding you?"

to protect our ego and personal needs instead of listening to the needs revealed by others. Then the outcome is predictable. We miss possible solutions to the problem or overlook important clues to what the other person is really saying. Thus, we may bring tension back into the situation. Decreasing tension by cue-controlled relaxation should help prevent this defensive posturing and garbled communication.

It should now be obvious why complete relaxation is not the goal of cue-controlled relaxation. Complete relaxation would not be constructive in the middle of an interpersonal conflict or a crisis. It helps your spouse or supervisor little for you to say, "Excuse me for a few minutes while I relax." During a major exam, you want to control extreme tension, but you still want some arousal. The goal is to bring tension back to an optimal, moderate level. After gaining success with a home stressor, go on to other situations for practice.

CUE-CONTROLLED RELAXATION AT SCHOOL OR WORK

After success at home, go back to the diary and identify stressful situations that occur regularly at school or work. The principle is the same as before: Find a situation that will allow you to practice cue-controlled relaxation with a high degree of frequency, but one that does not have high tension. One such situation for students is the midterm exam.

When you recognize that tension is developing, use cue-controlled relaxation. Go through the same procedure as before: Take a deep breath, hold it momentarily, let the breath go, say your personal cue word to yourself, and relax. If necessary, repeat the cycle.

Make a mental note of the effect. If you succeeded in relaxing, work with this situation until you feel you can control your tension as needed. Then do the same with other events in that category. If you did not feel a sense of moderate relaxation and some relief, reexamine the incident. Perhaps the situation was more stressful than you originally judged. Perhaps this particular episode was more stressful than it usually is. If the former, reassign the situation to the *high-tension* category and pick another event. Return to this one later. If the episode became more stressful than usual, continue with it, especially if you attained at least some degree of relaxation.

After you succeed with both home and school (or work) low-tension stress situations, move on to the high-tension stressors. It may be helpful to reexamine the situations you originally placed in the high-tension categories. First, judge whether you can make finer distinctions among the events. If so, separate the moderate stressors and work with them in the same way as before. Finally, pick a tough stressor from the school or work list. After you succeed with one of your toughest stressors, you should be close to having a useful stress management technique.

A final word of caution is in order. Cue-controlled relaxation is not a panacea. It will not make up for lack of training in areas of technical or professional expertise on the job. It will not solve problems of insensitivity, lack of impulse control, or incompetence in other people. No matter how reasonable, calm, and in control you are, this will not necessarily make other people more reasonable, calm, and controlled. However, cue-controlled relaxation may help you assess when circumstances are out of your control. Then, instead of dumping pressure on yourself, you may recognize that long-term and group goals need to be negotiated. Further, you may see when you need to go to some-one else for help. It is important to recognize that admitting you need outside help does not mean admitting defeat; this is more properly recognizing the limits of human ability, an important part of realistic self-appraisal. The popular "Serenity Prayer" expresses the message well: "God grant me the serenity to accept the things I cannot change, the courage to change the things I can, and the wisdom to know the difference."

DIFFERENTIAL AND GRADUATED RELAXATION

We now turn to differential and graduated relaxation, a technique that can be used in private or in public to reduce stress-induced tension and physical fatigue. This tech-nique is widely used by professional athletes such as tennis players to reduce muscle tension and restore fluidity to serves and volleys. The technique depends on two es-sential skills: the ability to scan muscles to judge which muscle group is tense, and the ability to relax that muscle group to the level that is desirable and suited for the situ-ation. While this may seem like a tall order, you will see that you have done much of the work already.

Mental Scanning for Tension

Scanning your body for tension should be almost second nature by now. Mental scan-ning for tension should be like a CB scanner, quietly but automatically exploring body channels until it finds a signal. Reducing tension on a graduated scale should be possi-ble as well, because you have practiced reducing tension to 75%, then 50%, and finally 25% of maximum tension.

Relaxing One Muscle Group

An example may help show how differential relaxation can be used. When driving in heavy traffic to meet a deadline, I sometimes find my right shoulder muscle growing very tight. I might just ignore it at first, but I soon realize that tension will make me more tired and may interfere with concentration. It also takes the pleasure out of driving.

In a situation like this, we do not want to reduce general arousal, as should occur with cue-controlled relaxation; we just want to reduce the tension in that one muscle group. Most importantly, we want to control the depth of the relaxation. Too much relax-ation while driving could be dangerous. Similarly, when playing tennis or basketball, we want to maintain some muscle tension, but we want fluid tension. This is why the proce-dure is called *differential and graduated relaxation*.

To develop this skill, look again through your diary and judge whether one muscle group becomes tense more frequently than others. Then practice relaxing that muscle group only. Tense one muscle by itself, then relax. Make sure you are working only on that muscle and do not worry about the rest of your body. When you can achieve deep relaxation, work on graduated levels of relaxation. Try to scale tension relaxation as you did before and reduce tension first to 75%, then to 50%.

It is not necessary to produce deep relaxation with this procedure. Most clinical studies suggest that you will not be able to do that anyway. If you achieve relaxation even in the 50% range, you are probably doing very well. A 50% reduction in muscle tension will usually suffice for practical applications of the technique.

Two other techniques can be combined with relaxation for better control. One is to attach a novel cue word to the muscle group. If you are typically only concerned with one muscle group, this can be quite effective; just be sure to select a unique cue word. Combine deep breathing and the cue word with practiced relaxation of that muscle group. With enough practice, you can reduce tension in one muscle the same way you reduce general tension—with a word. You can regulate the depth of relaxation by repetitions of breathing and cue control.

A second technique is to use visual imagery. Form a mental picture of something unique—for example, see yourself with that shoulder muscle in a whirlpool bath, with warm jets of water pulsing the muscle. See yourself receiving a massage. This is similar to the autogenic procedure, which makes extensive use of visual imagery.

When you tense the muscle during practice, the image should not be present. Just as you relax, call up the image and make it as strong as possible while you continue to relax. Another technique is to prepare slides or cut pictures from a magazine to pin on the wall. Close your eyes during the tension phase. Open your eyes and look at the picture during the relaxation phase. Try to lock the picture in your mind so it can be called up quickly and vividly. If you know you are good at imagery, this technique may be right for you. If you have difficulty forming mental images, it might be better to stick with the cue-word technique.

After some practice at home, the next step is to apply it on the go. Use your diary again. Do you still have events to deal with that are suitable targets? Maybe you play bridge regularly and find your neck muscles tense during keen competition (or because your partner does not always play well). This social situation might be a good candidate for differential relaxation.

Differential relaxation can be used in many situations. As noted earlier, this technique has found widespread acceptance among professional athletes, who need to maintain fluid muscle control even in the midst of intense competition. You can use it while driving, flying, or skydiving. Mountain climbers even use it while climbing. You might find it more useful on the tennis court or in a staff meeting.

To conclude, be sure the relaxation procedure you use is situationally appropriate. You would not want to go into a deep state of relaxation while driving. After a long, pressure-packed day at the office, deep relaxation may be very pleasurable. Differential relaxation may not be desirable in a staff meeting if general anxiety is the problem; cue-controlled relaxation would be better. Intense cramping in the neck during an exam calls for differential relaxation. The next chapter discusses extensions of the imagery technique and how to desensitize specific fears.

SUMMARY

In this chapter, we have introduced the rationale and method to learn your first coping skill, progressive muscle relaxation. Although this technique is a general tension reduction skill, it can be applied in a wide variety of situations that include anxiety and/or fear as well as for some basic problems like difficulty failing asleep. The following were among the major points made in the course of this chapter.

1. Progressive muscle relaxation (PMR) training is a technique first developed by Edmund Jacobson in 1938. It is one of a school of techniques that uses relaxation as a way to reduce tension that can come about from a variety of stressor situations.

2. Learning PMR should lead to better awareness of the signs of stress the body sends us. In this sense, learning PMR helps us to identify the events that lead to stress.

3. PMR is based on a basic notion derived from the reciprocity between the sympathetic and parasympathetic nervous systems. Simply stated, you cannot be tense and relaxed at the same time. If you learn how to relax, you can behaviorally switch off the tension associated with sympathetic arousal.

4. Learning PMR may involve fundamental changes in the cognitive system, including focusing, passivity, and receptivity.

5. Four conditions are important for successful practice of relaxation. These are setting, mood, preparation, and medical precautions.

6. The setting should be conducive to quietness and be absent of distractions or interruptions.

7. The mood should be passive instead of aggressive. You cannot make relaxation happen by energetic willing or forceful attention.

8. Do not rush to use PMR before you have learned it well. In other words, train first, apply later.

9. Make sure that there are not medical conditions that preclude use of relaxation training.

10. PMR works through 16 muscle groups with alternating tension and relaxation cycles. Early sessions may take from 45 minutes to more than an hour. Later sessions can be substantially reduced so that relaxation can be induced in as few as 5 to 15 minutes.

11. Reducing the time required to get relaxed involves grouping muscles and relaxing them at the same time. The 16 muscle groups can be reduced first to 8 and then to 4 groups.

12. Relaxation can be induced by a cue, a unique and private word associated with relaxation itself. In this way, mild forms of relaxation can be induced almost instantly, even in very public places, through covert repetition of the cue word.

13. A final refinement of the relaxation technique is to learn to relax a specific muscle and to do so to a desired level. For example, this technique is used by professional athletes who may get "tight" in the midst of competition.

CRITICAL THINKING AND STUDY QUESTIONS

1. What is the rationale of relaxation for control of tension as it relates to the operation of the nervous system?

2. What are some of the stress-related disorders for which PMR has proven effective?

3. How useful is PMR in the real world of business and sports? Stated in other terms, how is it possible to make PMR a portable but private technique?

4. Are there specific tensions, stressor events, or other problems for which you think PMR might be useful? How would you outline a program for yourself to make use of PMR? Remember the cardinal rule: learn first, apply later.

KEY TERMS

cognitive-behavioral
    theory of relaxation
cue-controlled
    relaxation

differential (and
    graduated)
    relaxation
mantra

progressive muscle
    relaxation (PMR)

WEBSITES progressive muscle relaxation

URL ADDRESS	SITE NAME & DESCRIPTION
http://www.cybertowers.com/selfhelp/index.html	Self-Help & Psychology Magazine. A site with a guided meditation section
http://www.fitnesslink.com/mind/meditate.htm	Online directions for learning relaxation and deep breathing

CHAPTER 12

Cognitive and Imagery Techniques:

Autogenics, Desensitization, and Stress Inoculation

All our interior world is reality—and that perhaps more so than our apparent world.

MARC CHAGALL

QUESTIONS

- What role does mental imagery play in relaxation techniques?
- What is autogenic relaxation?
- How does the autogenic technique compare to PMR?
- What are the basic exercises of autogenic relaxation?
- What stress-related disorders may be treated with autogenics?
- What is desensitization?
- How can desensitization be used to manage fears?
- What are the three keys to desensitization?
- What is Eye Movement Desensitization and Reprocessing?
- How does cognitive restructuring work to reduce stress?
- What is stress inoculation?

T om was a 28-year-old who had suffered several years with severe colitis.[1] For nearly seven years, he had gone from doctor to doctor seeking a physical remedy. He had even checked into the nation's most prominent medical facility for a lengthy series of tests. Still, the answer seemed to elude him, while the abdominal pain and diarrhea frequently disabled him. The first time he called me, it was for help with the colitis. Soon it became obvious that Tom's colitis was just one branch in a maze of symptoms, a complex set of anxieties and fears that prevented him from enjoying life to the fullest.

In addition to colitis, Tom had a phobic fear of meeting customers in the store where he worked. His most debilitating fear, though, was the obsession that he would be stricken by a heart attack while out with friends. This fear stemmed from a previous social engagement when he became highly aroused in the presence of a young woman. Tom found the intensity of the arousal very frightening, but that was not the worst of it. He felt guilty because of his passion and feared the woman would reject him. The result was a terrifying panic attack with hyperventilation, which can feel like a heart attack. Unfortunately, Tom gave the worst possible interpretation to the symptoms—that he had a serious heart problem. From this he reasoned that he could not ask anyone to marry him, and, at 28, became a recluse with little or no social life.

This was not the end of the symptoms, however. Tom could seldom relax and had extreme difficulty sleeping. He also had a pervasive pattern of obsessional thinking that influenced all his actions. While at work, he was obsessed with the thought that he had left the windows open or the gas range turned on at his apartment. He thought the landlord would find out and evict him. At night, he worried that he had left a labeling machine on at the store. In his mind, he saw this machine kicking out pricing labels all night, engulfing the store in a billow of paper. The only logical consequence, it seemed to him, was that he would be fired as soon as he showed up for work. At times these thoughts overwhelmed him, and he would leave home in the middle of the night and walk nearly one mile to the store to reassure himself that the machine was off.

Dealing with pervasive anxiety, deep-seated fears, and panic requires more than just relaxation. It requires some way of restructuring irrational thoughts and attitudes that prompt self-defeating, self-restricting behaviors. In this chapter, we will describe several techniques for dealing with fears and anxieties. First, we will discuss **autogenics,** a variation of the relaxation technique.[2] Then we will discuss **desensitization,** one of the most useful techniques ever developed for dealing with specific fears and obsessional thought patterns. Later, we will discuss a new, controversial technique called **eye movement desensitization and reprocessing (EMDR)** that is being advocated as a major new treatment for PTSD. Finally, we will examine **stress inoculation training (SIT),** a technique that prepares a person to deal with stress in advance.

IMAGERY: THE CORE OF RELAXATION

In many clinical studies of relaxation and meditation, investigators have tried to discover what clients are doing internally, what they are thinking or saying to themselves to bring on deep, quieting, satisfying states of relaxation. A common thread that ran through

---

[1]"Tom" is a pseudonym. While Tom was my client, he related numerous specific fears that sometimes incapacitated him. Colitis is also called "irritable bowel syndrome."

[2]Some people prefer to think of autogenics as a self-hypnosis technique.

client reports was the clients' use of mental pictures or images. For example, one person might picture a peaceful, sunlit beach and hear soft waves lapping and cries of sea gulls. Another might imagine being on a mountain peak looking out over a vast, beautiful, unspoiled wilderness and hearing the wind murmur through the pines.

A similar thread has been discovered in studies of Eastern mystics. Indian Yogis, for example, use a variety of imagery techniques to gain control over mind and body. During religious ecstasies, they produce a brain wave called **alpha,** a slow (12 to 14 Hz) wave form that occurs between the alert waking state and the first stages of sleep. Joe Kamiya (1969), a pioneer biofeedback researcher, showed that people could learn to control alpha rhythms with **biofeedback.** During his research program, Kamiya noted that many subjects used some form of visualization to keep alpha high. It is possible that concentrating on these mental pictures allowed subjects to control alpha moreso than did the specific biofeedback procedure.

AUTOGENICS: IMAGERY-BASED RELAXATION

Autogenic therapy (*autogenic* means self-produced) is a relaxation technique that emphasizes imagery and self-suggestion. The German psychiatrist Johannes Schultz introduced autogenics in 1932, and since that time, it has been the relaxation method of choice in Europe. According to Schultz and his protégé, Wolfgang Luthe (1969), autogenics is a means of maintaining the internal psychophysiological balance of the body. Schultz and Luthe also maintain that autogenics allows a person to plumb the depths of the unconscious.

The major appeal of autogenics is that it is simple for beginners wanting to learn a basic tension-reducing method. Because of this, it is often used as a home-based exercise in combination with other clinically guided techniques for treatment of anxiety disorders (Stoyva & Carlson, 1993). At the same time, autogenics is complex enough to permit skilled users to employ the more arcane aspects, presumably to tap the hidden recesses of their psyches. A cautionary note is important here: Advanced autogenics usually requires professional guidance to use it safely and effectively! If you relish the thought of exploring autogenics in more depth after this basic introduction, you are encouraged to seek out a professional autogenic therapist rather than trying to proceed on your own.

The training procedure for autogenics bears some resemblance to procedures for deep muscular relaxation, but differences do exist both in practice and in application. Relaxation training is a very active muscle exercise procedure that teaches the person to recognize differences between tension and relief. In autogenics, the goal is to develop an association between a verbal (thought) cue and the desired body state of calm; there are no active physical exercises as such. Although autogenics focuses on body posture, imagery, and self-instructions, the body still remains passive.

Preparing for Autogenic Training

Just as one takes certain steps to prepare for relaxation, Schultz and Luthe suggest several preconditions for successful autogenic training:

1. A high degree of motivation and willingness to follow the instructions exactly.
2. An adequate degree of self-direction and self-control.
3. Use and maintenance of correct body posture.

4. Reduction of external stimuli and mental focusing on internal physical and mental states.
5. Use of monotonous, repetitive input to the various senses.
6. Concentration on somatic processes to produce an inward-focused consciousness as opposed to an outward-focused consciousness.

According to Schultz, if the person meets these six conditions, he or she will soon attain a feeling of passivity, an almost vegetative state of mental activity that melts into altered consciousness.

The last two conditions are really outcomes of autogenic training, not steps in preparation. They are signs of success when the person adheres to the instructions.

7. The emergence of an overpowering, reflexive psychic reorganization.
8. The occurrence of disassociative and autonomous mental processes, leading to change in ego functioning and dissolution of ego boundaries (Pelletier, 1977).

Students of autogenic training must be prepared to accept the altered state of awareness, look for it, and perhaps even long for it. Otherwise, its appearance may be regarded as something to be feared and rejected instead of welcomed. This could interfere with continued progress in autogenic training, if it does not result in the pupil's discarding the technique altogether.

Luthe (1969) discusses a type of reflex motor tremor that occurs during early training called the **autogenic discharge.** Crying spells may also occur during training. These are instances of emotional catharsis for pent-up mental tension. The reflex motor tremor closely resembles the strange sensations that some people report in progressive muscle relaxation.

Maintaining passive concentration during practice is important to continued progress in training. Therefore, when these strange sensations occur, try not to fight them. Let them pass as part of the process, and judge them as signs of progress, not failure.

The preparation rules discussed for relaxation also pertain here. That is, choose a time and place for comfort and isolation. Reduce external distractions by disconnecting the phone or having calls intercepted. Remove tight-fitting clothes or jewelry, and prepare your mood for passive attention to the exercises.

Autogenic Body Postures

For relaxation training, you typically use a recliner in a partial reclining position. In autogenics, you may use one of three body positions, none of which matches the PMR posture. These are (1) lying down, (2) seated with back support, and (3) seated without back support.

In the first position, lie on your back on the floor with pillows or blankets to cushion your head and knees. If you use a pillow, make it a shallow pillow so that your head will be cushioned without misalignment with your body. Arms should be at your sides, with hands near your thighs and palms turned up. Your legs may be slightly apart, with toes pointed away from the body. Avoid using a bed so you do not fall asleep during training.

The second position requires a chair with a high, straight back. A chair with arms is fine but not necessary. Position yourself back in the chair so both your back and your head are supported. Keep your head aligned straight over your neck and back; avoid letting it fall to either side, because correct alignment with the body axis is important to success. Arms can be supported either on the arms of the chair or in your lap if you do not use an armchair.

The third position uses a stool or low-backed chair. With either type of seat, sit forward on the stool or chair. Support your arms on your thighs, your hands dangling loosely over your knees. Your head may come forward over your chest but should not touch. Keep your feet about shoulder-width apart and just slightly forward of the knees.

The image of the doll suggested by Schultz and Luthe may help you visualize this position. Imagine you are a big rag-doll puppet with a string attached to the top of your head. The string pulls you upright in the chair. Because you are a rag doll, you will be completely limp, legs and arms dangling with no tension. Then, imagine that the string breaks. What would happen to the doll? The head, neck, and shoulders would collapse forward. This is the posture you want. Again, take care that your head does not roll so far forward that you restrict breathing.

In the seated positions, you will not attain the degree of muscular relaxation that occurs while reclining, because the muscles must continue to support the body. Still, you can obtain adequate relaxation if you concentrate on proper body position. If you sense that you are tensing to support yourself in a seated posture, check to be sure that your alignment is correct. Whichever position you choose, stick with that position in the early stages of training until you see results. The only exception to this is that some exercises specify a particular position. Later, you can switch from one position to another.

Learning autogenics is broken down into two phases; phase 1 has six elementary exercises, and phase 2 has six advanced exercises. Specifically, the basic exercises emphasize body sensations to establish balance and rhythm in the autonomic system. In the second phase, imagery exercises emphasize mental capacity to form, hold, and manipulate mental images of external objects. Do not rush through the exercises, and do not move to the second set until you have reached the criterion described at the end of the instructions for the first set.

The Six Primary Exercises of Autogenics

Autogenic training begins with 6 staged exercises that concentrate attention on different parts of the body or on different sensations. Here are the basic exercises and instructions that support the practice of autogenic relaxation.

STAGE 1: ARM AND LEG HEAVINESS Concentrate first on the arm that is your active arm. (If right-handed, start with the right arm; if left-handed, start with the left.) Repeat silently to yourself as you concentrate on the arm:

- "My right (left) arm is heavy."

Do this from 3 to 6 times in a 30- to 60-second period. Close your eyes if you wish. When finished, shake yourself out of any lethargy and open your eyes. In autogenic terms, this is called *cancellation*. Then switch to the other arm. Repeat the instruction, using the rule of 3 to 6 repetitions in each 30- to 60-second interval. Then repeat the process for each leg using the instruction:

- "My right (left) leg is heavy."

Finally, do the limbs together using the sequence indicated in these instructions:

- "Both my arms are heavy."
- "Both my legs are heavy."
- "My arms and legs are heavy."

Remember to use *cancellation* after each sequence before moving to the next stage.

STAGE 2: ARM AND LEG WARMTH In the second stage of the exercise, concentrate on the sensation of warmth. It is not uncommon for people to experience feelings of warmth during the previous heaviness exercises. Now, the specific focus is on warming the body, which feels like a spreading sensation of warmth throughout the body. Repeat the general procedure used in stage 1, but with modified instructions. If it helps, use a mental image such as the warm sun on a beach, or imagine soaking in a hot bath. The instructions follow this form:

- "My right (left) arm is warm."
- "My right (left) leg is warm."
- "Both my arms are warm."
- "Both my legs are warm."
- "My arms and legs are warm."

With each exercise, be patient until you experience the comfortable, pleasant sensations of warmth and heaviness. You may need anywhere from 4 to 8 weeks to learn to produce warmth in the limbs (Pelletier, 1977). It may be several months before you can produce the entire range of experiences with ease and speed.

The speed with which you develop the skill depends on how consistently you practice. In autogenic training, regular practice is from 1 to 6 sessions per *day*, with each session lasting from 10 to 45 minutes. Expect early sessions to take from 40 to 45 minutes. The norm is 2 or 3 daily sessions, but you may use more if you have time. Still, you will make rapid progress by practicing twice daily. Later, you may experience the full benefits in as few as 10 or 15 minutes.

STAGE 3: HEAVINESS AND WARMTH IN THE HEART In the third stage, extend the heaviness and warmth exercises to heart processes. The instruction is:

- "My heartbeat is regular and calm."

Do this for 2 or 3 minutes, repeating the instruction at regular intervals. You may want to hold your hand over your heart so you can feel changes occurring. Also, for this exercise, you may use the reclining position. Remember, always use cancellation between each instruction and stage.

STAGE 4: PACED RESPIRATION After focusing on heaviness and warmth in the heart region, the exercises concentrate on measured or paced respiration. Paced breathing can have a very calming effect on the mind. With intense attention, it takes on a rhythmic, trancelike quality. Many groups have used breathing as a means to enhance muscular relaxation and mental tranquility. You can alternate between the two self-instructions listed here:

- "It breathes me."
- "My breathing is calm and relaxed."

Repeat these instructions 4 or 5 times in about a 90- to 150-second period. Mental visualization of an image may also help. For example, you might visualize waves rolling in on the beach and pace your breathing to each wave that breaks. With this exercise, you may notice significant gains in anywhere from 1 to 5 weeks.

STAGE 5: ABDOMINAL (SOLAR PLEXUS) WARMTH In the fifth exercise, you try to induce warmth in the abdominal region. The focus of attention is the solar plexus, the upper abdomen just above the stomach but below the heart. The instruction used for the heart can be used with only minor modification:

· "My solar plexus is warm."

It is important to note that you are not trying to warm the surface of the skin. The intent is to produce warmth deep inside the upper abdominal cavity. Warming the solar plexus has a soothing effect on the activity of the central nervous system. It will also enhance muscular relaxation, and it may cause drowsiness. These effects may be related to parasympathetic nervous system activity. For example, imagining warmth in the abdomen may induce increased blood flow to the center of the body and reduce muscle tension. Thus, the verbal cues of autogenics may behaviorally switch the autonomic system from sympathetic arousal to parasympathetic calmness.

STAGE 6: A COOL FOREHEAD The last basic exercise is to practice cooling the forehead. The instruction is:

· "My forehead is cool."

The other exercises have focused on warmth or heaviness, but this one tries to induce a feeling of coolness on the forehead. This exercise may require the prone posture. If you work at this exercise too quickly, you might experience light dizziness or even fainting. Start slowly, then, with no more than 2 or 3 repetitions over about 20 to 30 seconds. Later, you can build up to 4 or 5 repetitions lasting from 2 to 4 minutes.

Sometime during the first year, most people reach a point where they can complete all 6 exercises in less than 5 minutes. As noted earlier, you should not expect this to occur in less than about 2 months. Some exercises may not feel right until much later, while others, such as breathing, may feel right much sooner. When you reach this level of proficiency, though, you should stay in the state of autogenic meditation from 30 minutes to an hour.

Beginning Autogenic Visualization

Although basic exercises use very little imagery, visualization is an integral part of advanced autogenics. According to Schultz and Luthe, the purpose of visualization exercises is to capture and hold images long enough to assess their effects on consciousness. Some clinicians feel the assistance of an autogenic therapist is necessary at the beginning of this sequence. Therefore, the following discussion will be descriptive only. It is not intended as a guide to the practice of advanced autogenics.

LOOKING AT YOUR FOREHEAD The first exercise rolls the eyeballs upward as though looking at the back of the forehead. Many meditators use this eye position. It usually increases brain alpha and enhances a trancelike state.

IMMERSING THE MIND IN COLOR In the second exercise, the pupil picks a favorite color and tries to "see" that color. Imagine a room without form or dimension. Then imagine that room bathed in a favorite color. The color fills the entire visual field and saturates the mind. If pupils master this exercise, they are ready for more complex images.

Autogenic therapists suggest that different colors have different effects. For example, purples, reds, yellows, and oranges may induce warmth. Blue and green, on the other hand, more frequently induce coolness. Still, the colors most likely to induce a mood may depend on personal factors.

From this point on, the pupil can begin to visualize more complex shapes and colors. For example, pupils might visualize bright white clouds against a blue sky. Then they could visualize moving clouds. Next comes simple geometric forms such as squares, triangles, and circles. After this, pupils can try many different manipulations. They can fill the forms with color and change them. They can zoom in so the forms fill the entire mental frame, then draw back to view them from a distance. The intent is to become familiar with the ability of the mind to manipulate images of form and color.

FOCUSING ON OBJECTS   In this exercise, the autogenic student chooses an object to visualize against a dark void. They might pick a vase, the mandala,[3] the Oriental symbol of unity, Greek theater masks, or silhouettes. The choice of object is personal but should be kept simple. This stage of training can take much more time than previous stages.

TRANSFORMING ABSTRACTIONS   This exercise concentrates on some abstract idea, such as truth, love, justice, or freedom. The intent is to obtain a mental image of an idea and transform it into a concrete symbol. You may hear a word, such as love, and see a symbol that represents unity better than any dictionary could. This is the meaning of transforming abstractions. This stage takes from two to six weeks.

TRANSCENDING FEELINGS   Previous exercises involved some form of visual or auditory imagery. This exercise requires the pupil to concentrate on a feeling, an arousing emotion, just as though something external started it. Imagery still plays a role, but imagery is only a tool in this exercise. It is the feeling that is important. Seeing oneself on top of a mountain peak overlooking a vast wilderness may be associated with joy, contentment, or ecstasy. Vivid erotic fantasies may occur as though one is a part of the scene.

The intent of this exercise is to explore the role that personal involvement plays in emotionally loaded transactions. It provides practice in detecting switches from reality to fantasy. If successful, we could begin to plumb psychic depths and gain insight into conflicts and tensions that we create. Then we should be able to manage stressful events more effectively. Finally, we should be able to maintain better physiological balance conducive to good health.

VISUALIZING OTHERS   In the last stage of imagery practice, the task is to visualize other people. At first, pupils should focus on innocuous people who are at some personal distance. Then they may visualize more important people, such as peers, colleagues, and family members. With progress, these significant others include people involved in previous conflicts. As pupils visualize these troubled transactions, they should work to achieve a vivid image of the person and the setting. The intent is to revive the former emotions. This training provides valuable insights into feelings toward others. It may also help change one's attitudes toward others and, thus, one's perceptions of them.

---

[3]The mandala, or circle, is a universal religious symbol.

In sum, autogenic exercises intend to provide a means of self-regulation and self-study. Through the power of imagery, a person can attain a balance between the arousing influence of the sympathetic and the calming effect of the parasympathetic. One line of speculation suggests that this is because the right side of the brain, which controls the autonomic nervous system, is also the creative, holistic, imagery-processing side of the brain. Thus, we may have a way to tell the autonomic system how fast we want the body to run. The exercises may also provide a way to bring intense feelings closer to the surface so we can neutralize, if not eliminate, the seeds of conflict that keep the body aroused.

Autogenics for Coping and Wellness

A word of caution is needed before we discuss autogenic successes and failures. A recurrent script in clinical practice reads something like this. A new therapeutic technique seems to bring hope for helping people resolve personal dilemmas. A rush of research on physical and mental ailments takes place, and we hear glowing reports of great success. Soon someone "markets" the technique with great fanfare, and people jump on the bandwagon. After more careful and dispassionate observation, others find the practice is far less of a panacea than formerly claimed, but it has a special clinical niche that it fills with some success. Unfortunately, great expectations followed by a negative press and eroding confidence can destroy the credibility of the practice even for that special niche.

At first, numerous studies showed that autogenic practice could have a positive effect on health problems. Luthe (1969) provided an example in the treatment outcomes for 78 patients. These patients received 8 weekly sessions of group training. The clients presented several complaints, including anxiety and phobic and hysterical disorders. Of the 78 patients, 10 (12%) showed very good improvement, and 20 (26%) showed little or no change. The remaining 48 clients showed good improvement. Luthe and Blumberger (1977) summarize many successful applications of autogenic therapy.

In reviewing research on autogenics, we may be astonished by the success it has enjoyed over the years. Yet we may be disconcerted by the elixir-like quality of the claims for autogenics. Investigators claim success for autogenics in rehabilitation of neurologically impaired patients or in curing cancer (Simonton & Simonton, 1975). They suggest that autogenics is a viable treatment for epilepsy or alcoholism, for reducing smoking, for curing sexual dysfunction, and for tension headaches (Anderson, Lawrence, & Olson, 1981) or blood pressure (Watanabe et al., 1996). Foerster (1984) reported success with a group of leukemia patients restrained in a germ-free environment. In contrast to the Simontons' claims of a cure for cancer, Foerster just wanted to help patients accept their treatment and adjust to treatment restraints with minimal distress.

Charlesworth, Murphy, and Beutler (1981) also used autogenic training to help nursing students manage anxiety associated with their medical training, including reducing test anxiety. They reported modest success in achieving these goals. Their treatment was a multimodal package combining autogenics with several other components (such as relaxation, imagery, and desensitization). In this context, it is impossible to separate the contributions of the different components.

Clinicians now are more skeptical of the exuberant claims for autogenics. Still, this should not lead to its casual dismissal, because, despite its failures with certain disorders, autogenics still may have a niche to fill as a valuable coping technique. It appears to enjoy some success for treating panic disorders (Sakai & Takeichi, 1996), and it may be useful for chronic headaches (ter Kulle, Spinhoven, Linssen, & van Houwelingen, 1996).

MANAGING SPECIFIC FEARS

While relaxation and autogenics may be used for many stress and health problems, another group of stress problems requires different approaches. This is especially true for extreme anxiety and specific fears, as illustrated with Tom's situation. For these people, it is more than just being anxious or fearful. It is the knowledge that anxiety and fear always exist that keeps them captive in a world with invisible bars. It is knowing that no matter how silly or irrational, their thoughts cannot be driven from consciousness. It is wrestling with the mental distress, behavioral restrictions, and social confinement that fear brings.

Fear of any kind produces behavioral changes, physical reactions, and thought processes. Behavior motivated by fear is usually some type of escape or avoidance seeking to get away from the feared object or event. Physical reactions range from cold sweat and light-headedness to chest pains, nausea, and fainting. Thought processes include recurring images of a feared scene, feelings of unworthiness and being out of control, and fear of going crazy. There are different types of fears. First, *simple fear* is alarm or fright at some real or imaginary danger. The most severe fear is a **phobia,** the irrational but persistent fear of some specific object or situation. **Anxiety** is the feeling of impending doom without knowing when, where, and how the doom will occur. When it is severe, anxiety can render a person incapable of speech, movement, or coherent thought (Scrignar, 1983). **Panic attacks** are the most severe anxiety reactions. During a panic attack, the person experiences a sudden onset of terror or apprehension of doom (American Psychiatric Association, 1994). In addition, physical changes occur, including sweating, faintness or dizziness, shaking, nausea, rapid pulse, shallow breathing, and hyperventilation.

The most common phobia is **agoraphobia.** The word is from the Greek, *agora,* for marketplace. It is fear of the marketplace, of open, public places. Agoraphobia often makes an individual housebound. **Social phobias** involve an irrational fear of situations that expose the person to public observation and possible embarrassment. A very common social phobia is fear of speaking or performing in public. Another common social phobia afflicts men who are afraid to use public urinals. **Specific phobias** include fear of animals, such as dogs or snakes; fear of closed spaces, such as elevators and tunnels; and fear of heights, such as tall buildings and flying. As Scrignar (1983) pointed out, such fears can interfere with travel, personal relationships, vocations, and even recreation.

Anxiety seems to be the core of obsessive-compulsive disorders. An obsessive-compulsive disorder has two components. First, recurrent and persistent thought patterns (obsessions) emerge that cannot be voluntarily stopped. Second, repetitive behavior patterns (compulsions) seem to occur almost automatically.

Tom's obsessive thought was that he had not shut off the gas stove. Several times he walked to work only to have fear compel him to walk home, check the stove, and return to work late. His solution was simple, if ineffective: get up an hour earlier to check the stove more often—sometimes 15 to 20 checks—and still get to work on time.

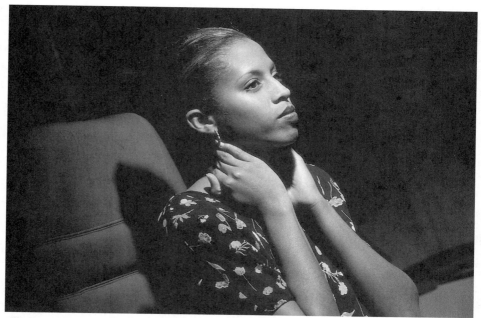

For some people, flying—or even the thought of flying—is enough to bring on high levels of fear, sometimes enough to result in nausea and fainting.

MANAGING SPECIFIC FEARS WITH DESENSITIZATION

In recent years, desensitization has proven very effective in dealing with recurrent fears. One clinical group even automated it to improve efficiency in treatment delivery (Thomas, Rapp, & Gentles, 1979). Joseph Wolpe (1958), a South African psychiatrist, developed the procedure in the 1950s. Wolpe worked for several years with phobic and obsessive-compulsive clients using traditional psychoanalytic therapy. He became concerned about his low rate of success in curing his patients. Wolpe was not alone, though, since other clinicians noted their own lack of success as well.

After reading a wide range of experimental literature, Wolpe became convinced that phobic and obsessive-compulsive disorders could be treated using recently developed behavioral theories. The behavioral model argues that phobic and compulsive disorders are learned disorders that can be unlearned. Wolpe (1958) detailed the desensitization procedure in his now classic book *Psychotherapy by Reciprocal Inhibition*. Reciprocal inhibition means that the two branches of the autonomic nervous system stop each other in turn. When the sympathetic system is aroused, the parasympathetic is quiet, and vice versa.

Wolpe accepted the idea that relaxation is a behavioral switch that turns off sympathetic arousal, but he went far beyond this. He reasoned that the power of an event to incite fear can be controlled by manipulating the intensity of the feared event. This, he proposed, can be done through mental imagery. If the person relaxes while imagining a mildly feared object, the object will become associated with relaxation instead of fear.

Gradually, more intense images of the feared object can be presented until the person can stay relaxed while imagining the object they fear most. The term *desensitization,* then, means removal of the sensitizing power of a feared object. In this way, we can counter-condition or unlearn fear.

THE THREE KEYS TO DESENSITIZATION

Desensitization requires three elements: training in deep muscular relaxation, construction of a hierarchy of feared objects or events, and imagining the feared objects while in a state of relaxation. In the previous chapter, we discussed the rationale and procedure of relaxation training. The next few pages will explain the remaining two keys to the method.

Constructing a Ladder of Fear

The second step in desensitization is to build a stimulus hierarchy. Think of this as a ladder of feared objects. The low rungs hold less feared objects, and the highest rungs hold the most feared objects. The rationale for building this hierarchy can be explained as follows.

Fear of objects can be controlled by maintaining physical distance. If you are afraid of heights, the solution is to stay off tall buildings. If you are afraid of snakes, you stay away from the areas where they live. You restrict the amount of time spent in elevators if you are afraid of closed spaces.

Psychologically, fear decreases as objects or events become less and less similar to the original. For example, assume someone is deathly afraid of rats or mice. The person might maintain physical distance from rodents by having frequent visits from the local exterminator. The person could also stay away from pet shops or laboratories, where rats and mice might be on display. Now assume that this person goes to a theater to see a movie. Much to the viewer's dismay, the action takes the characters into a dark basement where rats run across their feet. A movie with rats may be too realistic and result in tension. Now suppose I showed this person an abstract representation of a rat (Figure 12-1). In all likelihood, the person would experience very little anxiety because the artwork is so different from the real thing.

In more formal terms, this is the principle of **stimulus generalization.** Simply put, stimulus generalization occurs when someone responds in the same way to similar objects. The more similar the objects, the more likely the same response will occur. Rats, mice, and possibly gerbils could all produce the same fear response. Rabbits and guinea pigs probably would not because of major differences in appearance and meaning. The abstract rat would be even more unlike the real thing than a rabbit or a guinea pig.

Thus, the likelihood that similar objects will produce the same response is not all or nothing. It is a generalization gradient that describes objects in terms of degree of similarity. Figure 12-2 shows one fear gradient of generalization. Objects at one end of the scale, rats and mice, are very similar. At the other extreme are less similar objects. The vertical scale shows the probability of a fear response. As objects become less and less like rats and mice, the fear response is less and less likely to occur.

Building a ladder of fear, called a stimulus hierarchy in technical terms, is building a generalization gradient. We place objects on all rungs of the ladder in order of increasing fear response, with the real thing at the top of the ladder.

FIGURE 12-1

An abstract representation of a rat.

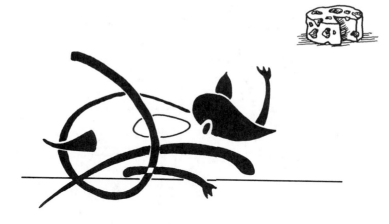

FIGURE 12-2

A stimulus generalization gradient for the feared stimulus of rats.

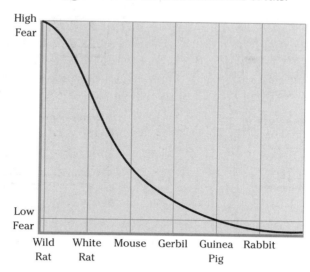

FIGURE 12-3

Fear ladders for the common fears of flying and public speaking.

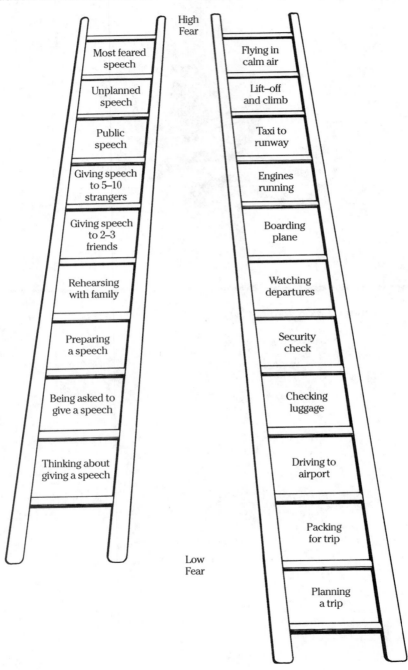

Figure 12-3 shows examples of fear ladders for flying and for public speaking. By starting at the lowest level, you can control fear and keep it at a distance psychologically, so that calm prevails instead of tension.

Generally, we cannot use the real objects or events, but that is where visualization comes in. As we well know, the mind can replay images of feared objects. These images are the mental videotapes of anticipated encounters. They contain threat and arouse fear as though the object is there. As noted earlier in Chapter 3, research shows that the brain does not distinguish between a real and an imagined event (John, 1967). This is why the process of imagining a feared event can produce the positive effects observed in this procedure. Desensitization uses a controlled, voluntary replay of images to maintain psychological distance from the object and thus keep fear at manageable levels.

When we imagine the object on the lowest rung of the fear ladder while staying relaxed, stimulus generalization also works in our favor. The association between calmness and the first object spreads to the second rung on the ladder. Then the second object arouses less fear than it did before, even though we have not yet paired it with relaxation. As we climb the ladder, we can handle more feared items because we have already desensitized them somewhat by the spread of relaxation from lower rungs. Finally, we can handle the most feared event. At this point, we have desensitized the object, and fear should no longer occur when the object is present.

Here are some rules of thumb for building a hierarchy or fear ladder. First, keep the length of the ladder at about 15 rungs. You could brainstorm until you have between 20 and 25 items at first. This is important because you may have to drop some items later. Second, place the most feared object or event at the top of the ladder. Third, try to think of an object far enough from the top so that it will produce very little tension. Put this event on the bottom rung of the fear ladder. It is important, though, that the object has some similarity to the highly feared object. You cannot just select any object to fill this bottom rung. Finally, select objects to fill the middle rungs.

SELF-STUDY EXERCISE 12-1

Constructing a Fear Hierarchy

For this exercise, think about things you would like to do but feel you cannot do because of overwhelming fear. Perhaps you would like to audition for a role in a dramatic production but feel terribly frightened by performing in public. Numerous examples of the kinds of things people often fear have also been cited in the text. After identifying one fear that you would most like to conquer now, follow the guidelines provided over the next few pages and set up your own fear ladder. If at first you cannot think of a fear that seems terribly important, you may want to look back at items you designated as major stressors in Chapter 1 on the chance that one or more of these items has a significant core of fear involved.

After you finish the fear ladder, go through the objects—from bottom to top—as you have placed them on the ladder. Try to visualize each object or event as vividly as possible. Note the amount of tension you feel, and decide whether you placed all the items in the right order. If you find a pair in which the lower object produces more tension than the next higher one, reverse the order or think about using a new object to fill that rung.

If you want to be really precise, assign the lowest rung on the ladder a scale value of 1 and the top rung a value of 100. Then assign values to the other objects to reflect the relative increase in fear you feel when going from low to high. Clinicians call this the **subjective unit of distress (SUD).** For example, the distance from the first object to the second may deserve a scale value of 5 units because it requires only a small jump in fear. The next object might deserve a scale value of 15 because moving up requires a larger jump in tension. You can play with the objects in your hierarchy until you have rated all the rungs on the scale, and all rungs are spaced about the same distance apart.

Some pairs of items may be too close to each other on this scale. If so, go back to the pool of objects you chose at the beginning. The objective is to have about 15 items, with equal distances between each object in terms of the amount of fear produced. Just as climbing a ladder should allow the same amount of movement (equal distances) from rung to rung, subjective distress should change by the same amount as you move up the ladder.

You might express fear of dogs on a continuum that progresses from seeing a dog at a distance to petting a dog. Fear of leaving home to be in large open areas (agoraphobia) might be expressed in blocks or miles from home and in the number of family members present versus being alone. For the person with agoraphobia, being alone in the marketplace is more fear-provoking than being there with a number of supportive family members. Claustrophobia (fear of closed-in spaces) can be scaled in terms of the size of the space and the amount of time spent there. You might scale fear of flying in terms of making flight arrangements, going to the airport, watching planes take off, boarding a plane but not flying, taxiing to the runway but not taking off, and finally taking off in a plane. These are examples of common fear ladders.

Before you take the final step, a few comments are necessary on how to present the items to yourself. As noted before, you do not typically work with real objects. There *are* methods that do so, and even Wolpe's technique can be modified to do so. When we conduct desensitization with the real object, it is called **contact desensitization** or **in vivo desensitization.** The latter means desensitization performed in the natural environment.

The two methods commonly used to present the fear stimuli are emotive imagery and pictorial representation. Which method is better for you depends most on how visual or how concrete you are. If you have good powers of visual imagery, you should start with emotive imagery. If you need more concrete stimuli and do not consider yourself a good visualizer, the pictorial method may be best.[4] Either way, the method should not change the outcome.

EMOTIVE IMAGERY   In desensitization practice, the **emotive imagery** technique is the standard, and it works something like this. Imagine a scene from the fear ladder as though you are drawing a mental picture of it or playing a mental videotape. Make a conscious effort to picture the scene as vividly as possible. The scene usually has emotion associated with it, but be passive in this regard. In other words, you should not try to force a feeling into the scene, nor should you try to block feelings that well up.

In the clinical setting, it is the clinician's job to prompt images with verbal phrases that help make the mental image more vivid. This luxury is not available in your home. Some people find that a verbal cue for each rung of the ladder written on a sheet of paper is all that is necessary. Others record prompts on a tape recorder to have an elec-

---

[4]You can also use autogenic exercises to increase your ability to visualize.

tronic stand-in for the clinician. Whatever the method, know what objects or scenes you want to use before you begin a relaxation session. It is easy to do this because you need to visualize no more than three to four objects from the fear ladder in any given session.

PICTORIAL REPRESENTATION The method of **pictorial representation** uses drawings, pictures, or slides to present feared scenes. It is possible to mix drawings and pictures. Drawings make it easy to obtain some remote symbols of feared objects. Some years ago, a student of mine was distraught about a rodent phobia that had been her nemesis since she was about six years old. With my direction, she carried out a self-conducted desensitization program beginning with only line drawings and pictures. For the lower rungs of the fear ladder, she used line drawings like the abstract rat in Figure 12-1 and cartoons of rats and mice. Blurred and dark pictures of rats were just below the middle of her fear ladder. She placed more vivid color pictures just above the middle. Pictures of people holding rats were near the top. Scenes of this nature can be presented by either slides, drawings, or photos. Mixing hard copy drawings and photos is not a problem, but I do not recommend mixing slides with hard copy. It is best to keep the presentation method and medium as uniform as possible.

EYE MOVEMENT DESENSITIZATION AND REPROCESSING

Very few techniques for treating anxiety disorders have arrived with as much fanfare or generated more excitement than the method devised by Francine Shapiro (1995, 1996) called eye movement desensitization and reprocessing (EMDR). Shapiro apparently conceived the method when she noticed her own anxiety subside as she moved her eyes back and forth in a scanning motion. The technique has been touted as an important therapy for PTSD and other anxiety disorders with promises of virtually immediate and permanent cures. Since its inception, more than 20,000 therapists have become licensed to practice EMDR. Now advocates suggest that EMDR may be useful for generalized anxiety disorders, eating disorders, substance abuse, excessive rage, learning disabilities, or even paranoid schizophrenia. We will look at the actual method first, and then look at recent critical evaluations of its claims.

The method is complex, but the key ingredients involve visualizing traumatic episodes, verbalizing and rating negative emotional reactions, verbalizing desired positive emotional reactions, and practicing eye movement while visualizing a traumatic event. Rating the negative emotions is done using the SUDS method described earlier in the chapter. Eye movement is carried out by following the therapist's finger as it sweeps rhythmically right to left at about 2 strokes each second. The scene is visualized during about 12 to 24 sweeps or for about 6 to 12 seconds. Then, the client is asked to blank out the scene and report their SUDS rating again. This procedure is repeated until the SUDS rating falls to a level indicating low anxiety. As Shapiro (1996) points out, the technique includes components of exposure, desensitization, cognitive restructuring, and rehearsal. It is difficult, therefore, to make conclusions about what the effective ingredient is in the treatment program.

The method has drawn criticisms from the beginning, including concerns that the method lacks a coherent rationale and what is presented is more mystifying than clear

SELF-STUDY EXERCISE 12-2

Practicing Desensitization

At this point you are ready to take the final step to practice relaxation while imagining the objects on the fear ladder. To proceed, first prepare your quiet retreat as though you were going to engage in a regular relaxation session, but omit background music for desensitization sessions. Then choose the three or four images you will use for the session. Next, induce a deep level of relaxation and maintain it for a short time.

When you feel comfortably relaxed, stir yourself enough to imagine the first item on the fear ladder. Concentrate on the image so it becomes as vivid as possible. While you try passively to remain relaxed, scan your body for signs of tension. Hold the image for approximately one minute. After this time, if you feel no disturbance in relaxation, stop the image and continue to relax for a few seconds. Repeat the imagery of the first rung one or two more times, then go on to the second rung of the fear ladder. Repeat the process through the set of objects selected for the session.

If you experience disruption in relaxation (tension increases) at any time while imagining an object, *stop the imagery immediately!* Reinstate deep relaxation and enjoy it for about one or two minutes. Next, go back down the ladder one rung to the previous object. Imagine the scene again while relaxing. If you have already progressed to about the third or fourth image, stop on that positive note and wait another day to resume. If the disruption occurs early in the session, you may try the image again or return to an image from the previous day's session that you successfully imagined. Sometimes you have to back down the ladder two steps, but usually you can manage setbacks by going back just one step.

Do not worry about these slight regressions; they are typical of the process. They only suggest that you moved up the ladder too quickly or that you tried to take a bigger emotive step than you thought. After two or three tries, if you cannot get past this event, you may need to insert one or two more rungs from your first pool of items.

In each session, you should work with no more than three or four scenes and present each image two or three times. Typically it takes about three weeks to desensitize all the objects on the hierarchy. This depends, though, on the nature and intensity of the fear. Some hierarchies might be completed in as little as one week, whereas others might take six weeks or more.

When you have finished the procedure, test yourself in the real world. It is advisable, though, to *proceed slowly.* For example, a common tactic for people afraid of heights is to go to the second floor of a mall where they can look over an open court to the first level. Many malls have multiple levels that permit the person to move up one floor at a time. To the extent possible, try lower items of the hierarchy in the real world first. After testing yourself at this level, test yourself with more items from the upper range before trying the item highest on the ladder. Using the fear of heights example again, the person may go out on the top of a building that has an observatory, and gradually select higher buildings, such as the observatory on top of the Empire State Building. This is equivalent to in vivo desensitization. Although in vivo desensitization may be necessary with severe phobias, desensitization through emotive imagery is typically enough to eliminate fear of the real event.

(Lilienfeld, 1996). Several efforts have been made to provide a theoretical model in terms of conditioning, distraction, or orienting responses (Armstrong & Vaughan, 1996). In the meantime, numerous summary analyses have appeared that try to evaluate the overall effectiveness of the technique. Shapiro (1996) asserts that the method is more difficult to teach than first thought, and that problems in outcome are more likely due to lack of quality in clinical standards or lack of methodological rigor or both.

In one extensive review of EMDR, the authors arrived at several conclusions, none of which is entirely positive to EMDR (Lohr, Kleinknecht, Tolin, & Barrett, 1995). They concluded that verbal reports of anxiety are typically reduced, but behavioral and physiological indices of anxiety show little effects from treatment. Further, they concur with Dunn's direct test that eye movement itself is not an essential component in the treatment, leaving one to wonder what the effective ingredient may be (Dunn, Schwartz, Hatfield, & Wiegele, 1996). David Wilson's group found evidence that some relaxation components (slowed respiration and heart rate, lower blood pressure and galvanic skin response) are associated with eye movement, indicating that the mechanism of EMDR may be virtually identical to that of desensitization (Wilson, Silver, Covi, & Foster, 1996). Given ingredients that are comparable to more common forms of graded exposure (including desensitization), it appears that EMDR is unique in title only and its effectiveness no greater, if even equal, to that of the earlier techniques.

COGNITIVE RESTRUCTURING

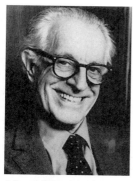

Albert Ellis developed rational-emotive therapy, which has been applied to cognitive coping skills.

Cognitive restructuring is most closely associated with the work of Albert Ellis (1962). Ellis assumed that irrational, self-defeating thoughts and beliefs, combined with catastrophizing behavior, lead to increased personal distress. To eliminate this distress, Ellis believed that the cognitive system must be restructured with positive, self-supporting, and reasonable patterns of thinking. Decker, Williams, and Hall (1982) compared one group who had undergone a 12-week training program of cognitive restructuring with a no-treatment control group. They showed that the treatment effectively reduced stress and irrational beliefs. Unfortunately, their study used intact groups instead of random assignment. Also, using a no-treatment control group does not eliminate the explanation of suggestion and expectation: Because subjects in the cognitive restructuring group expected to receive a treatment that had potential for success, this expectation could account for the improvement.

Heimberg (1989) reviewed several methods, including cognitive restructuring, used to remove social phobias. Most studies showed substantial improvement after treatment. However, the designs used were rarely strong enough to conclude that cognitive restructuring produced the change. The outcomes might also be explained by reduced fear of self-evaluation, lowered self-awareness (or manageable self-consciousness), and habituation of somatic arousal. These outcomes also result from desensitization and relaxation components, which are often unsystematically mingled with cognitive restructuring. Taylor's (1996) meta-analysis shows that cognitive restructuring combined with exposure provides the greatest overall success for treatment of social phobias.

One major component of cognitive restructuring is self-talk or **self-statement modification (SSM).** Self-statement modification assumes that anxious people carry on private monologues that include "I can't" or "I'm bad" statements. David Dush and his associates conducted a meta-analysis of 69 studies that focused on self-statement modification as the primary method of treatment (Dush, Hirt, & Schroeder, 1983). Most of the studies reviewed dealt with test anxiety, speech anxiety, and unassertiveness.

The analysis suggested that SSM produces substantial gains compared with no-treatment controls, but only modest gains compared with placebo controls. When clients received personal treatment, the gains were almost double that achieved when clients were treated in groups. The authors noted another interesting outcome. Gains were extremely large in all studies conducted by Meichenbaum compared with studies by other investigators using Meichenbaum's variation of SSM. This may reflect expertise, investment, or interest. The authors also noted that the effects of SSM have declined over the years, which may add strength to the interest explanation for differences in treatment outcomes.

Another result confirms earlier clinical analyses: Self-referred clients showed much larger gains than volunteers or referred clients. The finding that personal motivation is important to success in therapy is an extremely robust one, having been replicated over many years and many studies. It was also found that short-term interventions proved effective, casting doubt on the cost-effectiveness of long-term treatments. Desensitization was effective, but not as effective as SSM. Finally, relaxation training did not prove successful compared with SSM for this group of problems.

STRESS INOCULATION: PREPARING FOR STRESS

When confronted with diseases of epidemic proportions, medicine developed inoculation procedures. A doctor injected a vaccine into the body in a controlled amount. The body, through the immune system, reacted to the presence of the germ cells by developing antigens to fight the disease. In other words, the body acquired immunity to the disease so that any future exposure would not be as likely to make the person sick.

Stress inoculation, the brainchild of Donald Meichenbaum (1977), adopts the same notion, but the "germ" is psychosocial stress and the vaccine is exposure to low doses of stress in controlled conditions.[5] Meichenbaum believed that if people receive low doses of psychosocial threat combined with skills to deal with that threat, they develop resistance to the effects of stress. Later, when exposed to stress, they seem to have an immunity, and psychosocial stress does not seem to disturb them.

There are now many success stories in preventing stress among adult patients facing surgery or childbirth or preparing for painful medical tests. People with phobias, test anxiety, social shyness, speech anxiety, depression, anger, and chronic pain also respond positively to stress inoculation training (Janis, 1982). It appears to help those who are in conflict after making difficult career decisions and those who have decided to file for divorce. Further, it may be helpful in dealing with problems of recidivism in dieting and nutrition improvement, smoking, and alcohol consumption (Janis, 1982).

Stress inoculation training (SIT) involves three distinct phases: education, rehearsal of coping skills, and graded exposure to stressors combined with practice of coping

---

[5]Seymour Epstein was among the first to emphasize self-pacing and exposure to small doses of threat. He helped develop coping skills in men who routinely engaged in dangerous activities such as parachuting and combat flying.

skills (Meichenbaum, 1977). The goal of the educational phase is to provide understanding of the nature of the stress response and normal stress reactions. This information must be specific to the major current or anticipated stressor.

For example, people facing surgery or the death of a loved one can obtain information on what to expect. They can prepare for the emotional and physical reactions that are likely to occur. Surgical patients seem to endure better any disruptive emotional and physical effects, whether anticipated or real, when they have such information (Janis, 1982). With reassurances provided in SIT, they can shed feelings of self-efficacy. Because of this, stress inoculation may change the extent to which a person feels in control of a threatening situation.

In the second phase, SIT teaches specific techniques to deal with particular situations. The techniques may include, among others, relaxation, cognitive rehearsal, thought stopping, and self-instructions. Georgiana Tryon (1979) reviewed thought-stopping research covering a wide range of designs. Much of the research occurred in clinical settings with less than adequate controls and small samples or samples of size one. The target of the treatment usually was obsessive thoughts. While the technique has shown some success, it remains unproven that thought stopping is the most effective means to deal with intrusive thoughts.

Meichenbaum listed a variety of self-instructions that can be used in various situations. For example, in preparing for some type of provocation, a person might mentally rehearse these statements:
- "This is going to upset me, but I know how to deal with it."
- "Try not to take this too seriously."

When the situation is a confrontation, an appropriate self-instruction might be:
- "If I get mad, I'll just be banging my head against the wall. So I might as well just relax." (Meichenbaum, 1977)

Cognitive rehearsals effectively change perceptions and attitudes that initiate and perpetuate stress interpretations.

The third phase involves applying the new coping skills to a graded series of imaginary and real stress situations. For example, assume a manager has had difficulty providing candid periodic evaluations of employees. The manager might prepare for an upcoming meeting by imagining an evaluation session in process. Aspects of the situation that produce fear might be desensitized, and tense interactions might be met with cue-controlled relaxation. The manager might mentally rehearse self-instructions for interactions that often undermine the integrity of the process. In this way, when the real sessions take place, the manager is more likely to conduct them in a calm, professional fashion.

Does Stress Inoculation Work?

Novaco, Don Meichenbaum's associate, provided some of the best examples of stress inoculation. Novaco (1977) suggested that we fan the flames of anger with self-statements made in tense situations. For example, police dealing with rioters or involved in crowd control are under immense pressure. Anger may kindle very quickly. One impulsive move prompted by frustration can lead to counterattack and disastrous consequences. The riots during the 1968 Democratic Convention in Chicago amply illustrate this point.

In Novaco's educational scheme, he conceptualized anger in terms of a sequence of events that involve cognitive appraisal and physical arousal. When physical arousal occurs, the brain probably will interpret the arousal as due to real danger or threat. When this happens, one tends to label the opponent in a negative, perhaps even demeaning, way. Then the antagonists may play out anger-attack scripts in the mind. This drives the physical system to even higher levels of arousal. The higher the arousal, the more likely that some word or action will trigger the anger-attack schema.

In the second phase, Novaco taught relaxation training and self-instructional rehearsal. The person learns how to self-prompt with statements about the sequence of events that will occur. He or she also learns thought-stopping statements to interrupt the labeling process and the arousal spiral. Finally, in the third phase, the person imagines various anger-arousing situations. Then, he or she cognitively rehearses coping with such provocations through relaxation, deep breathing, and self-statements (Meichenbaum, 1977).

Much of the information provided earlier in this book is equivalent to the first inoculation phase. Its primary purpose is to inform you of the internal processes and situations that lead to stress interpretations and reactions. Information on methods makes up the second part of this book. This is the foundation of coping skills necessary to manage stress. The third phase, graded exposure, is something you must do yourself.

How Does Stress Inoculation Work?

Researchers are still evaluating SIT. One research group compared SIT with a standard psychotherapy procedure combined with medical interventions (Foley et al., 1987). The group's clients, 40 multiple sclerosis patients, received a five-week training program. The SIT group showed significantly lower depression, state anxiety, and subjective stress. Members of the SIT group also improved their problem-focused coping efforts. They maintained the first three improvements at six months, but their problem-focused coping had declined. The psychotherapy group did not show any change on these measures.

It is possible that type of training may interact with client characteristics. This principle is well understood in college life, where the method of delivering instruction may interact with traits of the student. One theory of anxiety suggested that people experience anxiety differently. That is, some people may experience anxiety largely as cognitive distress, whereas others may experience anxiety primarily as somatic disturbance and arousal (Heimberg, 1989). If so, cognitive interventions may be better for those who experience anxiety primarily in the cognitive mode. Relaxation or arousal-reducing therapies may be better for those who experience anxiety in the somatic modality.

This notion received some support from the work of Elizabeth Altmaier and her colleagues (Altmaier, Ross, Leary, & Thornbrough, 1982). They assigned subjects to either a cognitive restructuring treatment, a coping-relaxation treatment, a typical stress inoculation program, or a no-treatment control. They also assessed differences in cognitive-somatic anxiety, but they assigned subjects to treatments without regard to type of anxiety. Their results partially confirmed the hypothesis. Cognitive anxiety subjects responded favorably to stress inoculation and cognitive restructuring, whereas relaxation was least effective for them. Somatic anxiety subjects, though, responded about equally well to all treatments.

Much of the early research treated SIT in total and took reported successes at face value. A research team led by Daniel West carried out a detailed analysis of the components of stress inoculation training (West, Horan, & Games, 1984).

They reasoned that because SIT is a complex program combining multiple treatments, any single treatment or combination of treatments could account for positive outcomes. West's team randomly assigned 60 acute care nurses to five groups, one of which was a control group. They designed the four experimental groups to isolate the relative contribution of the different SIT components. One group received education only. The second group received education plus coping skills training. The third group received education plus exposure, and the fourth group received the customary three-step procedure. The dependent variables included state-trait anxiety, assertiveness, job tension, burnout, life satisfaction, and blood pressure measures.

The results of this study were very instructive. First, compared to the control group, all the treatment groups improved on the dependent measures. Second, *the component most consistently associated with positive outcomes was the coping skills training step.* Coping skills subjects improved significantly compared with subjects who received no coping skills training. Further, all dependent measures improved in coping skills groups. Yet, when coping skills were excluded, only two measures changed. These changes were still visible at follow-up. For subjects not receiving coping skills training, however, the improvements obtained on only two measures had disappeared at follow-up. The authors concluded that coping skills training is the major active ingredient of stress inoculation training.

SUMMARY

In this chapter, we discussed four techniques that use imagery and cognitive representations of stress situations. The rationale and strengths of these various approaches is summarized below.

1. Autogenics, a variation of deep muscular relaxation, is relatively passive and incorporates explicit imagery exercises. It uses a mental focusing approach as compared to the active muscular tensing and relaxing used in PMR.
2. Developing imagery skills helps in applying autogenics to anxiety and stress problems. Further, autogenics can enhance the practice of other stress management skills, such as desensitization and stress inoculation, that also include significant imagery components.
3. Although many claims are made that autogenics is successful for a variety of stress and health problems, the data is not as strong as it is for PMR.
4. Desensitization may be used to treat anxiety, specific fears, and panic disturbances. It can be tailored to individual situations and fears, and it does not need a professional therapist to be used successfully.
5. Desensitization can be carried out in the privacy of one's home and requires no equipment other than the capacity to use mental visualization. It is a natural extension of relaxation training for dealing with specific fears.
6. The three components of desensitization include learning PMR (Chapter 11), building a ladder (low to high fear) of images related to a specific fear, and associating items on the hierarchy with relaxation.
7. A variant of desensitization, EMDR, appears to work through mechanisms similar to those of desensitization. Still, there is an ongoing controversy about how sound the procedure is and differing opinions about the strength of the data used to support EMDR.

8. Cognitive restructuring is a method intended to alter irrational, self-defeating thoughts.
9. Self-statement modification is a cognitive restructuring procedure that tries to replace negative talk with positive, self-enhancing talk.
10. Stress inoculation is the preventive, immunizing branch of stress management. It teaches people first how to anticipate stress transactions, then how to defuse the potential for stress by rehearsing statements and behaviors that can be carried out in real-world situations.
11. By building up doses of mentally rehearsed stress conditions through stress inoculation exercises, the individual can deal more effectively with a variety of stressful situations.

CRITICAL THINKING AND STUDY QUESTIONS

1. What is the general rationale and procedure of autogenics? What are some of the pros and cons that should be considered in a critical evaluation of autogenics?
2. What is a phobic fear? Have you noted any fears in the book's exercises that you really want to get under control? If so, use the guidelines presented in the chapter to begin managing fear.
3. What is the rationale of desensitization? From a learning point of view, what is presumably happening as you combine an imagined item with relaxation?
4. What is the rationale of the fear ladder? In other terms, how does the fear ladder take advantage of generalization to eliminate fear?
5. What is the rationale of cognitive restructuring? How is it represented in self-statement modification and stress inoculation?

KEY TERMS

agoraphobia
alpha
anxiety
autogenic discharge
autogenics
autogenic therapy
biofeedback
cognitive restructuring
contact desensitization
desensitization

emotive imagery
eye movement
   desensitization and
   reprocessing (EMDR)
in vivo desensitization
panic attack
phobia
pictorial representation
self-statement
   modification (SSM)

social phobia
specific phobia
stimulus generalization
stress inoculation
   training (SIT)
subjective unit of distress
   (SUD)

WEBSITES cognitive and imagery techniques

URL ADDRESS	SITE NAME & DESCRIPTION
http://www.nacbt.org	☆National Association of Cognitive-Behavioral Therapists
http://www.emdr.com/frmain01.htm	The EMDR home site and link to the international association
http://www.cmhc.com	☆Mental Health Net. Many resources for a variety of anxiety disorders

CHAPTER 13

The Concentration Techniques:

Meditation and Biofeedback

One night ... being kept awake by pain, I availed myself of the stoical means of concentration upon some different object of thought.... In this way I found it possible to divert my attention, so that pain was soon dulled....

IMMANUEL KANT

The systematic approaches to relaxing and treating anxiety, described in the previous two chapters, are mostly products of modern technological culture. They mesh well with the Western penchant for scientific study and treatment of mental and physical health problems. Still, a long tradition of altering and controlling internal body states reaches back to the dawn of recorded history. The most prominent of these, the Yogi tradition of deep **meditation,** has its roots in ancient Hindu society. We cannot discuss at length the sequence of events that led from the Western "discovery" of Eastern yoga to practical coping methods. But even the most cursory historical sleuthing reveals a fascinating story with intriguing vignettes and startling insights.

THE MYSTERIOUS GOD-MEN OF INDIA

From the time the British first landed in India to the modern day, reports have filtered out of India about Yogis who could control their bodies to a degree never before believed attainable. For nearly half a century, Western scientists observed these mysterious "god-men" of India (Brent, 1972). What they explored and observed with scientific methods led to changes in our notions of how the mind and body interact.

For example, there were sensational reports of gurus who could reduce heart rate to the point of total cessation. In a type of suspended animation, they could be buried alive for days (Hoenig, 1968). The mystery of how they could control heart function is now partially solved, but having explained it does not detract from the sheer wonder that they could do it at all (Anand, Chhina, & Singh, 1961b). Other reports told of Yogis who could control blood flow to their bodies so they could withstand severe cold.

What is the secret behind these Yogic practices? And what can we learn, if anything, that is useful for modern living? To answer the first question, we must look at Yogic meditative practice. In the process, we will study **Transcendental Meditation (TM),** a meditative procedure widely recognized in Western cultures. In addition, I will describe Herbert Benson's **secular meditation** (1975).

To answer the second question, we must look at how the West has placed meditation under the scientific microscope. One outcome of this laboratory close-up is **biofeedback,** once touted as a high-tech alternative to years of religious discipline. In the last section of this chapter, we will discuss the more common biofeedback procedures. Finally, we will consider empirical evidence on the merits of biofeedback and how it may complement the other coping techniques described.

THE HIGHROAD OF MEDITATION

In ancient Hindu society, meditation was the highroad to spiritual enlightenment. Religious literature shows that meditation often occupied a position on a par with sacrifice and prayer. It was a means to an end, a concentrative method for withdrawing from the world of illusion, escaping the cycle of rebirths, and obtaining union with the oversoul.

The Yoga System of Meditation
One prominent system that featured various meditative practices was Yoga, which literally means "union." The first systematic record of the Yoga way of life is the *Yoga-Sutras,*

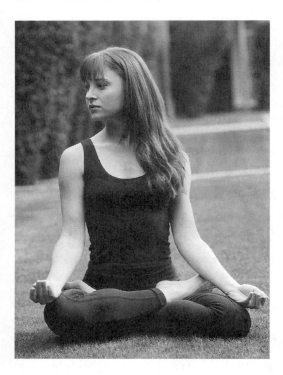

Yoga meditation usually involves sitting in the lotus position and focusing concentration on a sacred word or some object to bring the mind under control.

a manual written by Patanjali about 200 B.C.E.[1] The *Yoga-Sutras* reveal a philosophy with strict ethical and moral codes of conduct. It prescribes an ascetic lifestyle and teaches a set of rigorous physical and mental exercises.

The practice of Yoga is an eightfold pathway, beginning with ethical teachings to (1) restrain antisocial and selfish behavior and (2) ensure positive conduct.[2] Then the student of Yoga learns (3) postures, (4) control of breathing, and (5) withdrawal of the senses.[3] The physical path of postures and strenuous exercises has become associated with Hatha Yoga. Breathing exercises consist of learning how to inhale, hold the breath, and exhale with control (Behanan, 1964). Through these exercises, a person can gain control of the body and then also control the mind. Still, control of the mind is the province of (6) meditation, (7) contemplation, and (8) isolation.[4] The intent of Yoga in this life is to recondition the mind to release creative energy and free the person from chains of unconscious impulses and bondage to the senses.

[1]A controversy exists among scholars of the East as to the exact time frame of Patanjali's life and the date of the *Yoga-Sutras.* The dates range from the third century B.C. to the fourth century C.E. The date above comes from the thoughtful analysis of Dasgupta in *A History of Indian Philosophy.*

[2]The negative ethical code was *yamas* and the positive ethical code was *niyamas.* These were the first two steps in Yogi practice.

[3]The postures are *asanas,* breathing rituals are *pranayamas,* and withdrawal is *pratyahara.*

[4]Meditation is *dbarana,* and contemplation is *dbyana.* Isolation is the final release, called *samadhi.*

Science Tunes In to Meditation

While philosophers wrote about the Yoga system for years, the Western scientific community discounted, if not ignored, most of the claims for altering heart rate, changing body temperature, fire walking, needle penetration without bleeding, and altering consciousness. Scientific interest dawned in the 1950s, when investigative teams set out to verify the claims. Before this, however, a French cardiologist, Thérèse Brosse, traveled to India in 1935, anticipating later efforts to understand Yoga methods. Brosse carried a portable electrocardiograph to measure Yogis as they tried to control their heart activity. One of the published EKG records showed heart potentials approaching zero. Her work gave credibility to the scientific study of Yoga practice and had a major impact on the next team that made a similar trip, over 20 years later.

The team of Wenger and Bagchi (1961) traveled in India for five months in early 1957. The purpose of their trip was to test "various claims of voluntary control of autonomic functions and [record] physiological changes during Yogic meditation" (p. 312) . In observations of 45 Yogis, they observed temperature control, voluntary regurgitation, heart control, increased systolic blood pressure, and lower skin resistance. They concluded that the Yogis were controlling heart processes through muscular control and breathing but not through any direct control. Later studies of a Yogi at the Menninger Clinic in Topeka, Kansas, supported this conclusion (Green, Green, & Walters, 1972).

Wenger and Bagchi also attempted to measure arousal in the sympathetic nervous system in beginning and advanced students of Yoga. The Yoga school claimed for centuries that the practice of meditation benefits both the mental and physical life of the practitioner. If this claim is true, Wenger and Bagchi reasoned, there ought to be some correlate in lowered activity of the sympathetic system. Wenger and Bagchi compared the physiological recordings of the Yoga group to an American control group. The results were somewhat surprising. On 7 of the 11 measures, the Yoga group showed *higher* sympathetic activity during yoga meditation than the American control group. If meditation was aiding in coping with stress, it was not apparent in these observations. Still, Wenger and Bagchi recognized the limitations of their method and urged others to carry on research to understand the changes associated with meditation.

Western society has been most fascinated with **alpha,** a brain wave consistently produced by Yogis during periods of meditation. Zen monks practice a form of meditation derived from the Indian Buddhist tradition. They also show increased alpha during meditation (Kasamatsu & Hirai, 1963). More will be said about the alpha rhythm later in this chapter.

TRANSCENDENTAL MEDITATION: A WESTERN MANTRA YOGA?

During the 1960s, political, social, and religious activism were at a fever pitch. It was the decade of Students for a Democratic Society (SDS), hippies, communes, resistance to the war effort in Vietnam, and Transcendental Meditation (TM). TM is an adaptation of Mantra Yoga tailored to Western sensibilities. The Maharishi Mahesh Yogi, TM's founder, cut out nonessential elements of traditional Yoga practices. He also stripped TM of theological significance so it could be marketed as a secular practice. He and his organization took steps to ensure that no one connected TM with hypnosis, autosuggestion, or any of the then-popular encounter groups.[5] At one time, TM may have had between 500,000 and 1 million followers. They established and continue to operate a university with its own curriculum, and now maintain a website to provide ready access to information on TM programs and research.

The practice of TM is remarkably simple, although the formal initiation cere-monies make it seem mysterious and complex. The normal format of instruction in-cludes three sessions. After an opening information session, students attend a more de-tailed instructional session at which a commitment to practice TM is made. The final session is an initiation ceremony where the guide aids students in choosing their **mantra,** a secret word that should not be divulged to anyone else. From this point on, the person practices TM alone.

The guidelines for practicing TM are sparse. A person practices from 20 to 30 minutes per day twice a day. The preferred time for practice is just before breakfast and just before the evening meal. During meditation, the person takes a seated position on a bed or on a floor cushion. TM prefers the lotus position, the posture of "physical centeredness." Re-search shows that this position is the most relaxed of any seated position (Shapiro & Zif-ferblatt, 1976). Practice usually occurs in a setting free of distractions. During meditation, the person typically closes his or her eyes and repeats the mantra continuously. The pur-pose of this mental focusing is to prevent thoughts of object attachment or concern with mundane matters. Thus, the use of the mantra is similar to the practice of visual focusing used in other circles. Zen monks concentrate on a **koan,** an unsolvable riddle, to help fo-cus the mind and ultimately to drive the mind beyond itself (Kapleau, 1966).

TM Under the Microscope

Shortly after TM appeared in America, the team of Robert Wallace and Herbert Benson (1972) put TM under the scientific microscope. They used instruments that permitted continuous recording of blood pressure, heart rate, temperature, skin resistance, and EEG. They also measured oxygen consumption and carbon dioxide elimination. An-other measure, blood-lactate, was of special interest because of its presumed connec-tion to anxiety.

Wallace and Benson observed 36 subjects whose experience in the practice of TM ranged from one month to nine years. After a brief period to adapt to the laboratory sit-uation, each person provided data over three 20- to 30-minute periods before, during, and after meditation. The results showed reduced oxygen use, a marked decrease in blood-lactate, increased skin resistance, and intensification of the alpha wave. These re-sults closely paralleled those obtained in the earlier field studies of Yoga and Zen monks.

Based on their observations, Wallace and Benson suggested that TM is a fourth state of consciousness, which they called a "wakeful, hypometabolic" state. It is different from any of the three primary states of consciousness—waking, sleeping, or dreaming—although it shares some similarities with each. Wallace and Benson called it "hypometa-bolic" because energy expenditure goes down. Because several physiological indicators related to stress and anxiety decreased during meditation, Wallace and Benson argued that TM could be used to ensure better mental and physical health.

---

[5]I once attended meetings given by a TM instructor to introduce and initiate a group of people into the prac-tice. The statements on the origins of TM represent the position of TM as presented in these meetings.

Dillbeck and Orme-Johnson (1987) conducted a meta-analysis of 31 studies that used TM. They also found consistent evidence for lowered somatic arousal combined with increased alertness, as compared with eyes-closed resting. The paradoxical states of lower energy expenditure and higher alertness (associated with increased cerebral blood flow) are consistent findings across the years (Jevning, Wallace, & Beidebach, 1992). A more recent meta-analysis of several hundred studies adds support to the contention that TM (1) reduces physiological arousal during practice, (2) decreases trait anxiety, (3) increases indicators of mental health, and (4) reduces drug use and abuse (Alexander, Robinson, Orme-Johnson, Schneider, & Walton, 1994).

Numerous reports during the 1970s extolled TM's virtues. It was the mental supercure for drug dependency and smoking. It could increase IQ, control depression, reduce anxiety (including death anxiety), aid self-actualization, and manage job stress (Boerstler, 1986; Delmonte, 1984; Dillbeck, Aron, & Dillbeck, 1979). Vietnam veterans could manage posttraumatic stress syndrome using meditation (Brooks & Scarano, 1985). Another study, using a variant called *mindfulness meditation,* showed success in self-regulation of pain (Kabat-Zinn, Lipworth, & Burney, 1985). A best-selling book praised TM and suggested that a fulfilled society would result if everyone practiced TM (Bloomfield, Cain, Jaffe, & Kory, 1975).

Subsequent research led to skepticism about the claims for TM, including the notion that meditation produces a unique state of consciousness. One study showed that meditators spend significant time in sleep stages and in alpha, which do not necessarily qualify as unique states of consciousness (Pagano, Rose, Stivers, & Warrenburg, 1976). Another study failed to find any reduction in physiological indicators of anxiety during a stress test (Lintel, 1980). It should be noted that TM claims for reduced physiological arousal are usually based on observations made during meditation and not while under stress itself. Holmes and colleagues found that meditators had lower somatic arousal, but they also showed that TM did not reduce arousal any more than simply resting did (Holmes, Solomon, Cappo, & Greenberg, 1983).

Puente and Beiman (1980) tested TM head-to-head against self-relaxation, PMR combined with cognitive coping skills, and a waiting-list control. TM clients had higher cardiovascular stress responses following treatment than before and their cardiovascular stress responses were worse than the waiting-list group. Both relaxation groups showed significant decreases in their cardiovascular stress responses (Puente & Beiman, 1980). Thus, if TM has any positive effects, they apparently cannot be attributed to a unique ingredient. TM's benefits are more likely the result of a nonspecific component similar to that found in other relaxation procedures.

Many TM studies suffered from methodological flaws, which only added to the skepticism. They often lacked control groups, or failed to control for expectation effects by using an untreated control but not a placebo control. Finally, the studies frequently mixed meditation with other forms of relaxation training, which makes it difficult to assess the contributions of TM itself.

Still, some people point to the fact that TM is easy to learn and practice. Further, the results may be as good as from any general relaxation procedure (Throll, 1982). Data reviewed by Alexander's group suggests that TM may reduce hypertension and mortality in the elderly, leading to fewer clinic visits and lower medical care costs (Alexander et al., 1994). Therefore, there is no good reason not to use it. As with other methods, however,

TM is not a panacea: It cannot be all things to all people for all situations. In addition, TM does not have the clinical track record of PMR, especially when PMR is combined with cue-controlled, differential relaxation and desensitization.

THE RELAXATION RESPONSE: SECULAR MEDITATION

After studying TM for some time, Herbert Benson became convinced that the active agent in TM is general relaxation. From this, he reasoned that we do not need either the physical exercises of PMR or the initiation rites of TM to relax. Benson (1975) then developed the secular meditation procedure described in *The Relaxation Response*.

In brief, Benson (1975) felt that four basic ingredients are necessary to cultivate the relaxation response. In his view, these elements contain no cultural, religious, or philosophical prejudices, thus the name *secular meditation*. The four elements are as follows:
- a quiet environment
- an object on which to focus mentally
- a passive attitude
- a comfortable position (pp. 78, 79)

A quick inspection shows secular meditation's similarities to both progressive muscle relaxation and autogenics. A quiet setting is vital for any of the relaxation-concentration exercises described earlier. A comfortable position is also important, although the actual position probably is not. In PMR, it was a semi-reclined, seated position. In autogenics, it could be any one of three positions. Benson recommends a sitting position, but other positions may be used, including the lotus position. However, any position that is conducive to sleep should be avoided.

In TM, mental focusing results from silently repeating the mantra, the sacred word. Many other methods also result in focused attention. Autogenics used color and form. In PMR, it was alternating states of tension and relaxation. Symbols, such as the mandala, may be especially good choices for mental focusing. The Eastern symbol of unity might serve just as well. Another ancient practice is to focus on the navel, the forehead, or the inside of the eyelids. You can choose nearly any word, sound, symbol, or object and obtain the same relaxing result. Benson recommended a rhythmic breathing cadence with the word "one" repeated each time you breathe out.

Benson also recommended use of a thought-stopping technique to control intrusive thoughts during early practice sessions. For a short time, repeat the word "No" each time an intrusive thought occurs. This should enable you to eliminate unwanted thoughts and return to focused concentration. If the cue word is strong, you could eliminate the intrusive thought with breathing cycles: Each time you breathe out, repeat the cue word.

All relaxation procedures emphasize a passive attitude. In fact, attitude seems to be the most important thing in producing alpha during meditation (Shapiro & Zifferblatt, 1976). Attempts to make relaxation happen will only destroy the effort. Simply allow it to happen. Even if you do not attain deep relaxation at first, do not struggle to do so. Continue in quiet contemplation until the end of the session. Deeper states of relaxation will come eventually.

Benson's secular method may produce the same positive benefits that occur with PMR, autogenics, and TM. Benson (1975) says that the relaxation response "can act as a built-in method of counteracting the stresses of everyday living which bring forth the fight-or-flight response" (p. 111).

Although clinical research has not tested secular meditation as extensively as PMR, it may be possible to extend the procedure somewhat. For example, Benson's procedure recommended using a cue word in connection with breathing. This was the backbone of cue-controlled relaxation, the ability to relax anywhere. Intuitively, secular meditation could follow the same procedure and thus cover the same range of stressful situations. Still, we must emphasize that we do not know precisely the effective ingredient of cue-controlled or differential relaxation. Further, little research exists to suggest whether secular meditation can be used effectively in this way. Thus, the generality of secular meditation is mostly a matter of guesswork, and any extensions must be attempted on a strictly experimental basis.

BIOFEEDBACK: ELECTRONIC EUPHORIA OR PRACTICAL TOOL?

Even as field and laboratory investigations exposed meditation to critical analysis, other researchers were looking at new ways of producing altered states of consciousness. There seemed to be two different lines of reasoning that supported this effort. One view was largely rooted in theory building. It assumed that science ought to do its best to explore and explain the conditions that lead to physiological and brain-wave changes in meditation. A second practical, if not mystical, view suggested that there ought to be some way to produce the changes more directly without going through 20 years of asceticism. Yet it was not clear how this could be done. Then several investigators thought they had found the answer in biofeedback. Through 1985, over 2400 journal articles and 100 books provided the best laboratory and clinical evidence available (Hatch & Riley, 1986).

Putting Information Back into the System

Biofeedback has historical roots in *cybernetics,* or communication and control science. The mathematician Norbert Weiner (1954) defined *feedback* as regulating a system by putting back into the system information about its past performance. Biofeedback uses a special type of information—information about the performance of the biological system. Whenever we obtain information about how our body is working by making internal signals externally visible, we are using biofeedback. George Fuller (1977) defined biofeedback in a more formal sense as "the use of instrumentation to mirror psychophysiological processes of which the individual is not normally aware and which may be brought under voluntary control" (p. 3).

An Overview of Biofeedback Procedures

In practice, biofeedback has very few components. First, we must decide on the physiological system to be changed. Then we must identify a body signal produced by that system. Finally, we must use a detection device that can read, amplify, and display the body signal. (See Figure 13-1.) We may adjust the output of the detection display from time to

FIGURE 13-1
A biofeedback system usually includes (1) a sensing device that reads body signals,
such as electrodes; (2) a filter/amplifier system to select the right signals and
convert the body signal into an electrical signal; and (3) a display device to make
the signal visible to the person.

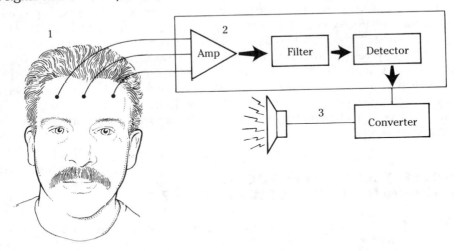

time so we force larger and larger changes in the body response. When the learner
reaches the desired state (for example, reliable production of alpha or elimination of
headaches), we typically fade out the feedback system. Then we try to transfer control
of the body response to cognitive or behavioral cues or both.

Body signals can be displayed with lights or meters, with sounds or strip charts. Any
method is acceptable as long as it tells a person when the desired internal state is present. Some clinicians devised novel displays of body messages. In one case, a model train
provided feedback. The train ran slowly as alpha first appeared and picked up speed as
alpha grew stronger. Conversely, when alpha disappeared, the train stopped. Another
team, working with children who were polio victims, used muscle signals to light up a
clown's face (Stern & Ray, 1977). No matter how we choose to display body signals, the
purpose is the same: to enable the person to connect the internal change to a behavior,
a thought, or an image. By engaging in the same activity later, it may be possible to re-
produce the internal state voluntarily.

LISTENING TO YOUR BODY

There are now numerous biofeedback techniques that make many internal responses
visible. The procedures most often used are electromyography **(EMG),** electroencephalography **(EEG),** skin **temperature,** galvanic skin response **(GSR), blood pressure,** and heart rate **(cardiovascular)** feedback.

FIGURE 13-2

Location of measuring electrodes for EMG biofeedback in muscle tension at (1) the frontalis muscle, (2) forearm, and (3) the trapezius. The labels on the electrodes indicate the active (A) and ground (G) electrodes.

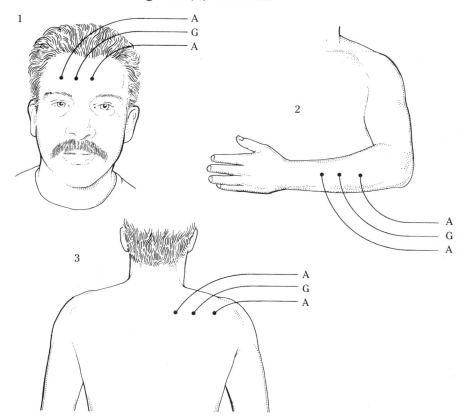

Listening to Muscle Tension

As muscles contract, they give off an electrical signal that can be detected through small electrodes. Electromyographic feedback amplifies this signal and provides information on the amount of muscle tension. Visual feedback is most often a dial somewhat like an ammeter that shows when a battery is charging (high tension) or discharging (low tension). We typically provide auditory feedback in one of two ways. In the first method, a single tone goes on when muscle tension is too high and off when muscle tension drops to an acceptable level. In the second method, a tone is on when muscle tension exceeds a certain level and increases in loudness as muscle tension increases. As muscle tension drops, so does the loudness of the tone, until it turns off when muscle tension is under the desired level again. This method is very effective when used to aid relaxation training.

Electrode placement depends on the physiological response to be changed. (See Figure 13-2.) If the intent is to aid general relaxation, either the trapezium muscles of the shoulder or the forearm site is appropriate. If the intent is to reduce tension headaches, then clinicians prefer the frontalis muscle location on the forehead. EMG biofeedback has proven very useful in the treatment of different types of headaches, but it is most often used with **tension headaches.** It is also used for neuromuscular rehabilitation of stroke victims. It may be useful in the treatment of lower back pain, but the efficacy of biofeedback for chronic low back pain is still in doubt (Nouwen & Bush, 1984).

EEG Feedback: The Alpha Wave Revisited

The brain emits tiny electrical discharges just as muscles do. In 1928, Hans Berger showed that these minute currents could be amplified and displayed in graphic form on a machine that he invented, the electroencephalograph (EEG). The process is still somewhat troublesome, however, because of the care that must be taken to get accurate recordings.

In most clinical settings, EEG recordings come from electrodes placed on the surface of the skull. This means that the electrodes pick up the combined activity of thousands, if not millions, of cells located just below the electrode. Uniquely different

FIGURE 13-3
The different stages of sleep and dreaming are marked by differences in brain waves as shown in these EEG records. Deep sleep is marked by slow, large amplitude waves. Dream sleep has the added feature of rapid eye movement (REM) shown here in the bottom line.
SOURCE: Courtesy of T. E. LeVere.

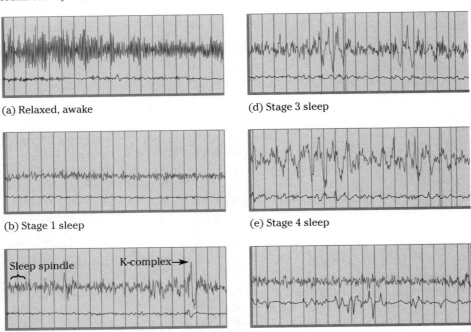

(a) Relaxed, awake

(b) Stage 1 sleep

(c) Stage 2 sleep

(d) Stage 3 sleep

(e) Stage 4 sleep

(f) REM, or "paradoxical" sleep

brain waves—alpha, beta, theta, and delta—reflect different states of consciousness. Alpha reflects a relaxed, meditative state; beta is present during alert waking stages. Theta reflects states such as daydreaming or a hypnogogic state, and delta waves reflect deep sleep. (See Figure 13-3.)

Sensing devices can be "tuned" to see a certain brain wave. Assume, for example, that clinicians want to feed back information on the alpha wave. They set the detection device so that it filters out any brain wave below 8 Hz and above 12 Hz. When the filter detects a brain wave within this window, that brain wave can be amplified and used to turn on a tone or a light. For EEG feedback, an auditory signal is most frequently used.

EEG recording is difficult to carry out at home. Care must be taken in placement of electrodes, and they must be coated with a special electrolytic gel to get good readings. Although new techniques now make the process easier and more reliable in the clinic, these techniques are not likely to filter down to the home market for some time.

Most importantly, EEG biofeedback has few clinical uses. It may be useful in the treatment of insomnia and epilepsy. Some studies showed improvements in concentration, attention, and shifting awareness. Yet the potential for self-management seems even more limited than for clinical applications. Even the hoped-for electronic euphoria, equivalent to the Eastern mystical trance, did not appear.

Temperature Biofeedback: Keeping Cool

The body regulates temperature by changing the amount of blood flowing in the extremities. Surface blood vessels expand or contract in response to environmental conditions and internal demands. When the vessels relax, they permit more blood to flow, thus raising body temperature. When the vessels contract, they restrict the volume of blood, thus lowering body temperature.

The Yogis of India apparently had very fine control of blood flow. In one report, a Yogi could raise the temperature in his right earlobe several degrees and simultaneously drop the temperature of the left earlobe by an equal amount. Clinical applications usually target finger temperature. This method may be used to treat **migraine headaches** and a rare disorder called **Raynaud's disease** (Blanchard & Haynes, 1975; Rose & Carlson, 1987). Further, it may be useful to treat irritable bowel syndrome, a disorder associated with distress (Blanchard, Schwarz, & Radnitz, 1987).

In temperature biofeedback, the detection device is a small electrode, called a thermistor, that measures finger temperature. Feedback may be visual or auditory or a combination of the two. Multicolor displays that change to yellow and red as the temperature goes up are very effective. Care must be taken to move the electrodes from finger to finger and from hand to hand as learning takes place. This is to ensure that the person learns a global response that warms the whole hand. Huge temperature changes may be possible in a single finger. But unless the person can warm the entire hand, the change will not be enough to alter the main symptom that needs to be controlled, such as migraine.

Visual imagery, such as that used in autogenics, aids in the process of changing skin temperature. The Menninger Clinic reported using autogenics in combination with biofeedback. Researchers suggested that the cognitive aspects of autogenics can be guided by biofeedback, while biofeedback aids in producing the desired physical change more rapidly (Green et al., 1973).

The Telltale Skin

When a person has an emotional reaction, a subtle but telltale change occurs in the skin. The skin's resistance goes down so that it conducts an electric current more readily. This is the principle behind the lie detector test. The galvanic skin response (GSR) may measure several different underlying processes; it may be related to increased moisture, sympathetic activity, or other processes. Generally, increased emotionality is associated with heightened sympathetic activity. One common outcome of autonomic arousal is perspiration. Moist skin helps conduct more current relative to dry skin.[6]

Few biofeedback procedures depend on the GSR. Clinicians typically use it to help people who are insensitive to internal changes. Finally, it may be helpful for sorting items in a desensitization hierarchy.

Changing Cardiovascular Activity

Obtaining a reliable measure of cardiovascular activity is in some ways even more difficult than obtaining reliable brain-wave measures. People have learned how to control blood pressure and heart rate. Unfortunately, the gains are often statistically significant but clinically meaningless. These methods seemed at first to have great utility for people with hypertension, cardiac arrhythmias, and other heart problems, but the instrumentation was complicated and expensive. Also, most gains obtained with biofeedback, such as reduction in blood pressure, could be obtained through relaxation or EMG biofeedback or both (Lustman & Sowa, 1983). It seems, then, that a practical, useful cardiovascular biofeedback system is still somewhere in the future; and even should it become available, it might not produce clinically meaningful changes.

BUT IS IT GOOD FOR ANYTHING?

Among the many questions raised about the promise of biofeedback, three are crucial. The first is whether people can learn to alter specific internal functions with biofeedback. The answer is an unqualified yes. The second question is whether biofeedback is useful for treating a variety of stress and health problems. The best answer is a qualified maybe. The third question is whether biofeedback's success comes from unique properties not present in other procedures. The answer is, mostly, no. The more scientists examined biofeedback, the more it appeared to share common elements with relaxation and cognitive restructuring procedures. The following is a brief summary of biofeedback's major successes and failures.

Biofeedback for High Blood Pressure

At first there was great hope for biofeedback as a treatment method for high blood pressure. Typically, subjects can reduce both systolic and diastolic blood pressure to a degree that is not due to chance factors. Still, the results are often not clinically meaningful because the amount of change is so small and/or the training does not have a long-term effect. Where large changes do occur, it is usually because blood pressure was extremely high at the outset. In addition, the new blood pressure levels generally are still above safe levels.

---

[6]A crude, but effective, analogy is to think of getting a jolt of electricity standing on a dry floor. Then imagine getting the same current standing in water. Water conducts the current more readily.

Biofeedback may help subjects reduce blood pressure more than relaxation does, but both procedures lead to lower levels (Engel, Glasgow, & Gaarder, 1983). One study showed that biofeedback and relaxation are equally effective and that both maintain lowered blood pressure up to a year after treatment (Walsh, Dale, & Anderson, 1977). Blanchard's research group conducted studies of hypertensive patients on medications (Blanchard et al., 1986; Blanchard et al., 1989). The group obtained a highly significant result showing that thermal biofeedback was successful in 65% of the cases, compared with 35% of those on relaxation training. Interestingly, their thermal biofeedback training combined autogenic phrases for warming hands. Still, professionals disagree on the issues of permanence and superiority.

Excedrin Headache #27 or EMG Headache #1?

The use of biofeedback for treating headaches has been very popular. Most frequently, the targets are either tension headaches or migraine headaches. Tension headaches may occur because of prolonged muscle contractions that result from some type of stress. Migraine headaches are most often attributed to vasoconstriction (Cohen et al., 1983). Typically, clinicians used EMG biofeedback for tension headaches and skin temperature biofeedback for migraine headaches (Budzynski, Stoyva, & Adler, 1970).

One extensive study compared relaxation and biofeedback in treatment of three headache groups: migraine, tension, and a third group whose members suffered both migraine and tension headaches at different times. Relaxation alone led to significant improvement in all three groups, but biofeedback led to significant additional gains. In the tension-headache group, 73% improved greatly, and 52% in the migraine group improved greatly (Blanchard et al., 1982). Further studies by Blanchard's group showed that successful treatment with long-term maintenance can be attained with very little contact (Blanchard et al., 1988). Blanchard's group has also shown that children with migraine can be more effectively treated with thermal biofeedback plus PMR than with any other type of treatment, including pharmacological means (Herman, Kim, & Blanchard, 1995). One interesting finding is that younger children appear to have greater reductions in migraine than older children (Herman, Blanchard, & Flor, 1997), which contradicts the notion that biofeedback requires a more mature level of cognitive development to be successful.

Evidence reviewed by Stanley Chapman (1986) called into question the prevailing notion that migraine calls for thermal biofeedback and tension headache calls for EMG biofeedback. He noted that migraine patients improve as much with EMG biofeedback as they do with thermal biofeedback. Also, the bulk of evidence does not support the contention that biofeedback is superior to relaxation in the treatment of headaches. Most negative outcomes with biofeedback occurred in studies with better controls, clearer diagnostic criteria, and longer adaptation periods and baselines. Finally, Chapman suggested that investigators provide little evidence that their subjects have really learned biofeedback when they maintain that biofeedback has been the effective agent.

In spite of the successes, there is still reason to doubt that biofeedback is necessary. For example, a study by Theodor Knapp (1982) showed that both biofeedback and cognitive coping skills can reduce frequency, duration, and intensity of migraines. In addition, the patients reduced medications after either treatment. The Colorado group headed by Thomas Budzynski concluded one report by noting that "EMG training [for tension headaches] alone is not effective in all cases" (Budzynski, Stoyva, Adler, & Mullaney, 1973). Robert Stern and William Ray (1977) suggested that the real benefit of biofeedback in the treatment of tension headaches may be that it teaches people to recognize signs of tension in body muscles so that they can begin relaxing immediately. Thus, biofeedback is probably not essential for control of headaches, but it may be an important element in education. Silver and Blanchard summed up the situation even more bluntly: In clinical tests comparing biofeedback with other procedures, there is no consistent advantage for any treatment (Silver & Blanchard, 1978).

A Cure for Cold Hands and Feet?

Raynaud's disease involves greatly restricted peripheral blood volume that causes the person to feel uncomfortably, if not painfully, cold. Usually this coldness occurs in the hands or feet or both, although the face and tongue also may feel cold at times. Both cold outside temperatures and emotional stress can trigger attacks (Pinkerton, Hughes, & Wenrich, 1982). As the attack progresses, the affected area may change color from whitish to cyanotic blue to bright red.

Clinicians often use temperature biofeedback to treat Raynaud's syndrome. One research group compared finger temperature biofeedback with frontalis EMG biofeedback or autogenic training (Freedman, Ianni, & Wenig, 1983). The patients treated with finger temperature biofeedback showed a significant reduction (92.5%) in symptoms compared with the other two groups (32.6% and 17%, respectively). This difference was still significant one year later at follow-up. On the negative side, David Holmes (1981) conducted a thorough review of the literature on biofeedback, including the treatment of Raynaud's disease. He concluded that scientific support for the effectiveness of biofeedback in the treatment of Raynaud's disease, migraine, or hypertension is inconsistent.

There are many other uses for biofeedback to treat other ailments and medical conditions, but reviewing all these uses is beyond the scope of this book. Stern and Ray's book, *Biofeedback: Potential and Limits* (1977), is an easy-to-read yet comprehensive early review of biofeedback research.

BIOFEEDBACK: THE FINAL SCORE

In spite of the attention and great expectations, biofeedback has not lived up to its promise as a treatment technique or as a coping procedure. Independent reviews of biofeedback have provided comparable sobering conclusions. Turk's research group concluded that biofeedback has no demonstrated superiority over procedures such as relaxing or cognitive coping skills training. In addition, these procedures can be carried out with much less cost and effort than biofeedback (Turk, Meichenbaum, & Berman, 1979). Turk's group also noted that many biofeedback clients use cognitive controls and instructional sets to obtain successful outcomes.

Carol Schneider (1987) tried to provide evidence for the cost-effectiveness of biofeedback. Unfortunately, her review clouded issues by using relaxation training as the primary intervention, assisted by biofeedback as a learning strategy. The review also mixed studies that have clear cognitive stress management components; this makes it difficult to evaluate the contribution of each discrete treatment component. Cost-benefits assessment in this quagmire cannot be applied meaningfully to a single component.

Thomas Burish (1981) looked at EMG biofeedback specifically for stress-related disorders. He concluded that biofeedback has not proven effective in reducing either internal or behavioral reactions to stress. As he stated:

> It may be naive to think not only that a biofeedback procedure aimed at changing the EMG level of a specific muscle group will produce a general (i.e., multi-system) relaxation effect, but also that any type of relaxation strategy will *by itself* produce and maintain a permanent change in stress-related symptoms if the nature and intensity of the stressor is not modified. (p. 418)

Lawrence Simkins (1982) asked the rhetorical question "Is biofeedback clinically valid or oversold?" He pointed out that many studies have internal flaws that fail to eliminate alternate explanations, especially the placebo effect. In addition, many studies use small samples and lack adequate controls. Simkins concluded that we probably expect too much from biofeedback. Effective stress management and personal health maintenance must incorporate cognitive, attitudinal, and lifestyle changes as well.

It is important to note that biofeedback can play an important part in teaching people how to read the signals of their bodies, including signals of tension. On this issue, no disagreement exists. When used as an educational and counseling ally, biofeedback can be very helpful (Schneider, 1987; Winfield, 1983). There is also no dispute that biofeedback can produce some positive outcomes. The point is that *it is not absolutely necessary to use biofeedback to produce these positive results.* If we could shift focus from biofeedback as a primary treatment or coping strategy and focus instead on the information gained from biofeedback that can be used in other ways, then this procedure should find an honored and rightful place with the other techniques described here.

SHOULD I TRY BIOFEEDBACK?

Whether you should try biofeedback depends on several factors, such as (1) the intended use; (2) the nature and severity of the symptom to be treated; (3) prior treatment history, if any; and (4) the demonstrated usefulness for treating the target symptom. There are various uses for biofeedback. For example, you can obtain more objective ratings of anxiety using EMG biofeedback to help build a fear ladder for desensitization. You can improve your ability to tune in to body signals. You should be cautious, though, if you intend to use biofeedback to alter a symptom that has medical implications. The more serious the symptom, the more cautious you should be. Also, if you have never received treatment for the symptom, you should have a medical examination first.

Anyone proposing use of biofeedback should first seek evidence that biofeedback is successful for the target symptom. In the absence of this evidence, biofeedback should not be used. If you do decide to use biofeedback, set realistic goals. Do not expect to make global changes in health problems. Also, do not expect biofeedback to cure everything. As suggested before, typically you need to combine biofeedback with lifestyle change and cognitive coping strategies to obtain satisfactory long-term results.

SUMMARY

In this chapter, I reviewed the status of several popular methods for coping with stress and improving health. These methods included variations of meditation and the western technology called biofeedback. Several major issues were raised as summarized below.

1. The Yogis of India have practiced different forms of meditation for centuries. They were the first to demonstrate to the western world that many of the so-called involuntary systems of the body could be influenced by concentrative methods of meditation.

2. The method of Mantra Yoga, repetition of a personal sacred word, became very popular in the U.S. in the procedure called Transcendental Meditation. It has been touted for a number of problems including tension reduction and control over addictions.

3. Herbert Benson modified TM to a practice he calls secular meditation. This method requires very little external trappings, just the motivation to practice the technique on a regular basis until mastered.

4. Evaluated in historical and personal perspective, the many claims for positive outcomes from meditation seem sound. Meditation may produce certain desirable, even sought after, altered mental and physical states.

5. From a scientific point of view, the changes associated with meditation are not unique to it. Other procedures, such as deep muscle relaxation and autogenics, can produce the same positive results.

6. There is a fair amount of research supporting meditation methods, such as TM, but the applications are more difficult to evaluate. Thus, meditation seems more limited in comparison to previously mentioned procedures.

7. Benson's secular meditation is easy to learn, and the guidelines are simple.

8. The high-tech solution to meditation, biofeedback, has expanded far beyond its original boundaries. The most common types of biofeedback include EMG, EEG, GSR, temperature, and forms of cardiovascular feedback.

9. Stress symptoms most frequently treated with biofeedback include migraine and tension headaches, hypertension, and chronic pain.

10. While biofeedback may yield positive results for some people in certain situations, most practitioners are no longer as enthusiastic about biofeedback as they once were.

11. The more sobering findings suggest that biofeedback does not always result in clinically meaningful change; the results do not always last; cheaper and easier techniques are as successful; and other techniques often must be added to obtain satisfactory results.

12. In spite of these qualifiers, biofeedback may be valuable for education and symptomatic relief if the person takes certain precautions.

CRITICAL THINKING AND STUDY QUESTIONS

1. How did science first become involved in the study of Yoga meditation? What were some of the paradoxical findings that required us to rethink our view of mind-body links?
2. If you were approaching meditation from a detached scientific perspective, how would you evaluate the strengths and weaknesses of meditation for stress management in general?
3. What if any personal situations might be appropriate for the use of one or more of the methods discussed in this chapter? How might you go about applying the method to your situation?
4. What is the scientific status of biofeedback now? What do you see as the strengths and weaknesses of biofeedback for altering body processes?

KEY TERMS

alpha	EMG biofeedback	secular meditation
biofeedback	GSR biofeedback	(Herbert Benson)
blood pressure	koan	tension headaches
biofeedback	mantra	temperature biofeedback
cardiovascular	meditation	Transcendental
biofeedback	migraine headaches	Meditation (TM)
EEG biofeedback	Raynaud's disease	

WEBSITES the concentration techniques: meditation and biofeedback

URL ADDRESS	SITE NAME & DESCRIPTION
http://www.cmhc.com/guide/pro10.htm	☆Mental Health Net. Site devoted to biofeedback and neurofeedback
http://www.achenet.org/	American Council for Headache Education. Information on origins, prevention, and treatment of headache pain
http://freud.tau.ac.il/~biosee/	Clinical Psychophysiology and Biofeedback Homepage
http://www.aapb.org/index.htm	Association for Applied Psychophysiology and Biofeedback
http://www.spiritweb.org/spirit/yoga/overview.htm	An extensive collection of materials and links for various Yoga practices
http://www.kevala.co.uk/yoga	International Yoga School. Information on Yoga methods and holistic therapies

Student Stressors, Nutrition, and Exercise

CHAPTER 14

Student Survival Skills:

Transitions and the Paper Chase

Human history becomes more and more a race between education and catastrophe.

H. G. WELLS

QUESTIONS

- What are the common stressors encountered by college students?
- How does the transition to college contribute to stress?
- What are the more important stressors for minority students and international students?
- What are some ways to deal with test anxiety?
- Why is time management an important stress management skill?
- What are the more common ways that we waste time?
- How can we find out where our time goes?
- What are the guidelines for good time management?

The university environment confronts students with many new pressures, some expected, some unexpected. College is a time of many transitions. It marks a rite of passage from the ambiguity of adolescence to the clear and certain expectation of responsibility as an adult. It is a time when many profound choices that shape a person's career goals and professional identity must be finalized. Also, the difficult arena of interpersonal and intimate relationships must be navigated more or less on one's own, far from the watchful eyes and usually sympathetic guidance of parents. Some women attending university will find that the hallowed halls of ivory are far less sanctuaries than hunting grounds where they may fall prey to sexual violence. College also is the crucible in which lifelong habits of work, duty, and integrity are tempered for use in the student's chosen career.

A GALLERY OF STUDENTS AND STRESSORS

During my 30-some years in education, I have observed many students under more or less severe stress. Typically, I have been more interested in the nature of their response to stress than the nature of the stressor itself. These biographical vignettes give only small portions of the flavor—some bitter, some sweet—of students coping with stress. The names are fictitious, but the incidents are very real.

There is probably nothing so alarming as having to confront a major illness and surgery at a 20-something age. Alan was, in most respects, a typical student working more hours than he probably should to pay for college, while trying to balance class demands with the lure of social life. As part of his full-time load, he was in my pressure packed statistics-methodology class, a course that involved learning skills in research design, statistical problem solving, and computer data analysis. The workload included exams as well as several major data sets to be analyzed. Because of the amount of material to be covered, there were constant deadlines that added to the pressure.

Somewhere in the middle of this, Alan discovered that he had to be hospitalized for about two weeks to undergo major surgery and recuperation. For some, this would be enough to end the academic term right there. But not for Alan. He mapped out a plan that included getting advance assignments from his instructors and turning in work that was already assigned before entering the hospital. He used his recovery period to keep reading and doing assignments that he could work on at home. When he returned, he immediately made up the one missed exam in my class, and turned in all his data assignments. For all intents and purposes, he had never missed a beat.

Compare Alan's response to Donna's. Donna was also working at a part-time job while going to school. Late in the term, she came down with a nasty bout of flu that took her out of classes for just two days. Still, this setback seemed almost catastrophic, and from her point of view, she could never recover. Although she had missed only one test and had just one data set overdue, she was ready to abandon the entire term, a decision that could also cost her all the tuition for the term with nothing to show for it.

Another young woman, Sarah, responded more like Alan. She was near the end of her college career, needing only a few more classes to graduate. Sarah hoped that by taking two of those classes during summer, she could finish in the fall term and not have to return for the spring. At this point in early June, she was nearing the end of her first pregnancy, and she was obviously excited about the prospect of her child's birth. If the doctors were right, the baby should come no more than two weeks after the end of class. The class in Abnormal Psychology met five days a week at 7:30 A.M. Yet Sarah was there everyday, on time, for the duration of the class—more or less. On several occasions, she left looking pale, and I knew from earlier discussions that she was battling another bout of morning sickness. When it came time for the class to take a break, I would find her lying down on one of the hard hall benches. Somehow, she felt that she should apologize for leaving the class in the middle, but then she would come back after the break to continue. Throughout the session, she took her tests on time, even giving her oral report when scheduled. For her, the challenges that lay ahead seemed to energize and propel her.

A TYPOLOGY OF STUDENT STRESSORS

In the early chapters of this book, we identified what most people consider as major stressors. Similar work has been carried out in the university setting to identify what students feel are their most important stressors (Gray & Rottman, 1988; Tyrrell, 1992). There are similarities in both environments, but there is enough that is unique in the university setting to reveal different stressors as well. In the next few sections, then, we will describe some of the more common college stressors, and we will try to provide some guidelines on how to cope with them. For the sake of convenience, I will discuss stressors in three broad groups. First, we will look at common stressors from the personal and social arena, such as **loneliness** and intimacy. Second, we will look at issues of adjustment and acculturation stress among different ethnic groups. Finally, we will examine several common academic stressors such as test anxiety.

Personal and Social Stressors:
Transitions, Loneliness, and Relationships

Among the most important personal and social stressors are transition issues, the most obvious leaving home, siblings, and long-time friends. There are also many stressors having to do with transitions into the new environment, including making new friends, periods of loneliness, and managing romantic relationships.

In a study of female students, the top 20 stressors included 5 relationship issues—being rejected, breaking up, unfaithfulness of an intimate partner, broken engagement, and unwanted pregnancy (Frazier & Schauben, 1994). The two most frequent stressors were test pressure and financial problems. Although these two events were the most frequent, the most powerful stressors were death of a parent or partner and an unwanted pregnancy. Frazier and Schauben found that the more stress and the more powerful the stressors (for example, rape, bereavement, or relationship breakup), the more the students were likely as well to report serious psychological symptoms (for example, depression, hostility, paranoia). At the severe end, rape survivors reported highest symptom levels.

LONELINESS Many students find the transition to university life complicated by periods of loneliness. Loneliness is described as an "unpleasant experience that occurs when a person's network of social relationships is significantly deficient in either quality or quantity" (Blai, 1989, p. 163). It is not necessary to be alone to be lonely; as an old adage suggests, we can be lonely in a crowd. Students, seeing others around them who are happy and enjoying the companionship of various friends, while they themselves have few if any friends, may be among the loneliest.

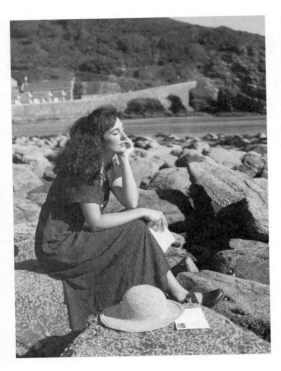

One stressor cited by students is loneliness as they leave old friendships behind and try to find new friends in the hustle and bustle of college life.

Loneliness can influence both psychological well-being and physical health. People who report being lonely also report more depression, dependence on drugs as escape, and higher blood pressure. There is evidence that loneliness is associated with higher risks for heart disease, lower immunocompetence, and lessened longevity, and increased risk for recurrent illness (Hafen, Karren, Frandsen, & Smith, 1996).

The extent of loneliness is dependent on a number of personal as well as external factors. Personal factors refer to personality traits, interpersonal style, and social skills that make it more or less easy to form new and lasting relationships. People who are shy, unassertive, and lacking in self-esteem typically have more difficulty making friends than those who are outgoing and self-confident. External factors include the size of the university and the types of activities and services provided. In general, large universities tend to produce more feelings of isolation and anomie, which translates more often to feelings of loneliness.

There are several ways to attack the problem of loneliness. These include both changes in attitude and changes in behavior. First, university communities typically have a large number of resources to help students explore personal growth issues. If shyness or lack of assertion seems to be playing a role in loneliness, then investigate courses or workshops that may help change either of these patterns. If interpersonal skills seem to be part of the problem, look for help in that area. Also, although you may have moved to a new community for your university career, stay in touch with friends from high school days. These relationships can provide continuity in the midst of change, a touchstone of the familiar that will take the edge off the strange new world of college.

Second, becoming involved in familiar activities can help. For example, if your lifestyle prior to college included church attendance, then investigate local churches to find one compatible with your beliefs. Many churches located in college communities have college and/or young career groups where new friendships can be formed in a more supportive environment. Getting involved in volunteer activity, either through the church or through local social agencies, is also a way of overcoming loneliness. The gift of giving of yourself often leads to very satisfying relationships.

Third, learn to appreciate solitude as a time of personal creativity and increased self-understanding. You do not have to always be attached or in a relationship to be fulfilled. Being alone can provide many rewards if you use that time to develop skills, avocations, and hobbies. A friend of mine had a very productive career, but his avocation was playing guitar. In order to keep his skills at a high level, he spent many hours alone, as many do in the performing arts community.

Finally, many students find great comfort in keeping and caring for a pet. This may not be possible in a dorm room, but it can be in an apartment. Pets are the best natural Rogerians: that is, they give unconditional love and regard in the simplest possible terms. It is always so refreshing to see the exuberance in my dog when I get home at the end of the day. Every day, his greetings are unbounded expressions of joy that seem to occur no matter how positive or negative my own mood is at the time. There is evidence that pets are therapeutic in a variety of ways, and thus can provide benefits to their owners with or without loneliness at stake.

FINANCIAL PRESSURES Financial pressures are consistently mentioned by students as one of their ongoing major stressors. In many cases, the pressure is not just paying college expenses, but managing finances to cover both essentials and wants. Rising costs of tuition and books (essentials) is enough pressure in most respects. Analysis of cultural changes, however, suggests that students now expect they should also be able to have the latest in fashion, good (if not new) cars, electronic equipment, and party money while they go to school. This attitude adds even more pressure, which usually translates to working more hours to generate income, even though study time and focus on school may suffer.

Spending habits can combine with certain risk factors to create more difficulties for the college student. Some people are impulsive shoppers, who forget any budget restraints when the notion strikes them to hit the mall. Others shop on occasion-setters. A family birthday becomes an occasion to shop, not always just for the family member but for themselves as well. Spring, fall return to school—any number of events may become occasions for shopping. Still other people shop when they get depressed. Sometimes, the buying spree may be viewed as therapy, but more often than not it is an automated (subconscious) reaction to the negative emotion rather than a deliberate coping response.

Several changes in attitude and behavior may be needed to stay on a sound footing while in school. First, it is generally wise to set a budget and stick to it. Some people find this distasteful, but the financial consequences of not doing so can be disastrous. On the other hand, getting into the budget habit can provide very important benefits in the long run.

Scott Burns, a financial-page columnist, talked about his own failure to budget early in life, and what one habit in particular would have meant to later financial security. He smoked two to three packs of cigarettes per day through his 20-something years, and did not quit until he was about 34. He reckoned that if he had put the roughly $6 per day spent on cigarettes into a savings account, he would have accumulated over $30,000 by the time he quit. If he then had rolled the savings into higher-yield stock funds, he calculated that he would have accumulated nearly $650,000 in a retirement account by his early- to mid-60s. The same thinking could apply to that CD you just have to have, or the parties three times per week that can drain from $15 to $20 each time.

University counseling centers may offer courses on managing finances, as well as more personal interventions for impulsive spenders. More people are finding the plastic jungle distasteful and are cutting up their credit cards. In general, more credit cards do not equal better credit, so resist the temptation to take every credit card offer that comes along. Multiple credit cards can become a slippery slope to overwhelming debt. Too many people have gotten caught when they run each of their cards out to the limit, and then find that the minimum payment that once seemed so easy to make is now eating huge hunks of their resources. If you would like to know what your spending personality and risks may be, you can follow the instructions at the website listed in Self-Study Exercise 14-1.

SELF-STUDY EXERCISE 14-1

Healthy Money Management
http://www.healthycash.com/center

Stress Among African American, Mexican American, and International Students

Studies among Mexican American students show that their major stressors revolve around acculturating to a new environment, feelings of not belonging, and perceptions of discrimination (Vázquez & García-Vázquez, 1995). Acculturation refers to changes in behavior and values that result from coming into extended contact with members of another culture. For the most part, American university culture is dominated by Anglo-European values and codes of conduct. Still, there are no major differences in acculturation stress between different generations of Mexican American students, and most report that they can adopt a bicultural style with little or no difficulty. Further, the students in the Vázquez and García-Vázquez study reported that they used direct planning and accessing of their social network (talking with friends or relatives about a problem) to cope with stress in the university setting.

Stress among African American students appears to be higher than among their White or Mexican American counterparts. Removal from family and locale is reported to represent a significant problem, and financial problems are also severe. Inner-city working class students seem to suffer the most acculturation stress at the university level (Young, Ekeler, Sawyer, & Prichard, 1994).

Acculturation stress probably is at its peak with international students. Not only do they experience more severe disruption in family ties, but they often confront a strange environment with language barriers that make the transition even more difficult. The disruption in family ties is described as a profound sense of loss (Sandhu, 1995). Compounding the problem is that return to the homeland typically is not possible on a routine basis because of the high costs of transportation. Many must delay return until they complete their studies several years after arrival. One study among Chinese students found that they resort to many different means to cope with the extreme acculturation stress felt at American universities (Situ, Austin, & Liu, 1995). They may use rituals, isolation, rebellion, and even innovation to circumvent immigration laws to be able to stay with their studies.

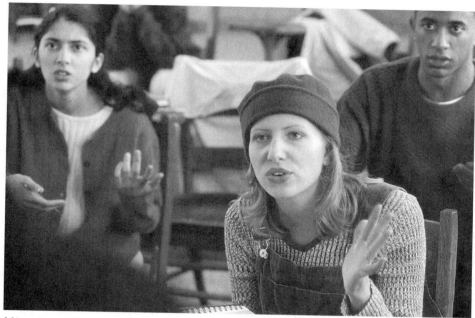

Minority and international students may find a very different culture from what they expected, making their adjustment more strained than that of others.

Academic Stressors: Test Anxiety, Workload, and Time

Students report a common core of specific academic stressors. These include pressure over grades, academic standing, cheating, major term papers, red tape involved in registering and getting financial aid, course and career decisions, finding a job after graduation, the volume of work in courses, fear of falling behind in course work, and time pressures (Frazier & Schauben, 1994; Gray & Rottmann, 1988). Space does not permit talking about all the specific stressors, but two in particular seem noteworthy: **test anxiety** and time management. The remainder of the chapter will be devoted to these two topics. Although the space allocated to time management in a college setting is considerable, the utility of good time-management skills cuts across many areas of life from family and homelife to your chosen career.

EVALUATION STRESS: TEST ANXIETY One of the most pervasive fears among students concerns the near crippling anxiety over taking tests and the subsequent performance feedback. Some anxiety (arousal) can be helpful in test taking, but too much anxiety can be very detrimental. Very often, students with test anxiety fear that they will do poorly—even when there may be evidence to the contrary—and that their career plans will be thrown into a tailspin. They complain of more than just the usual nervousness, and may feel sick to the stomach, break out in a cold sweat, or even feel that they might faint. Test anxiety is typically thought to be a type of state anxiety. In other words, it is limited to a given few situations. It is typically not trait anxiety, which is a stable characteristic of the person that is common to many different situations.[1]

[1]Chapter 4 detailed the differences between state and trait anxiety.

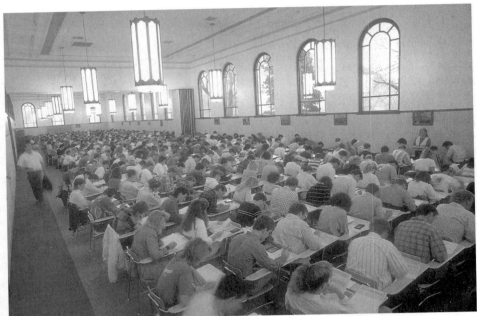

Many students experience uncomfortable levels of anxiety over tests. To deal with this, most universities offer a variety of college skills classes to help students overcome test anxiety.

Dealing with test anxiety typically involves repelling an attack on several fronts. First and foremost, there is nothing like preparation to help lower the stress of test taking. This typically means working at the course on a consistent basis rather than cramming the night before a test. Learning theory suggests that distributed practice (spacing out study sessions over time) will be more efficient than massed practice. Well-timed brief reviews of material are also much better than a single intensive review the night before the exam. The rule of thumb is to spend about 15 minutes reviewing material from the class you attended about 6 hours earlier. For example, if you had a psychology class at 2:00 in the afternoon, and you have study time scheduled around 8:00 in the evening, taking 15 minutes to review what was covered that day will give more benefit than even an hour spent later on the same material the night before the exam. Of course, if you can do both—review briefly along the way and do a thorough review prior to the exam—that is best. What you need to avoid is trying to get all the learning done in one long session just before the exam.

Second, develop an attitude of healthy, realistic self-appraisal. Do not put pressure on yourself by trying to achieve unrealistic goals. It is perfectly appropriate to keep trying to do better; it is unhealthy to work yourself into a state of high anxiety because you want an A in biochemistry and you have generally never gotten more than a C in science lab classes. My academic Achilles' heel is language. I have a tin ear and a lead tongue. I know that, so even though I continue to try to become more fluid in several languages, I do not dump pressure on myself because the effort does not go smoothly all the time.

Third, find out what academic survival-skill classes are taught at your university. In many university settings, the counseling center offers workshops that explore the topic of text anxiety. Several techniques that we have talked about already are often at the core of a text-anxiety program. Cognitive restructuring may help you identify any irrational beliefs you may have about your test performance. It may also allow you to engage in covert self-instruction sequences that promote calming thought patterns for test taking.

Another skill is deep breathing and cue-controlled relaxation. If you go into a test with some apprehension, just before the test is handed out, do a deep breathing or cue-controlled sequence. Nobody around you has to know it is even happening. You may also use an imagery method to promote calming. This can also be done in the middle of the test if anxiety reappears. Remember, you do not want to get rid of all anxiety, only the high levels of anxiety.

If fear of a test is extremely difficult to handle, bringing nausea and dizziness, you may want to use the desensitization method. Construct a hierarchy of least- to most-feared test situations. Then pair the items on the hierarchy with relaxation—in your room, of course—until you can emotively image the most fearful test scenario without disturbing the relaxation. Some combination of these techniques will typically help you win the battle against test anxiety.

Finally, learn test-taking strategies. Talk with other students and instructors so that you can cultivate some sense of test-taking savvy. Here are just a few tips that I pass on to my students to help with objective tests. First, pace yourself by dividing the time about equally for each question. A 50-minute class with a 50-item test is easy: 1 minute per question. If you struggle with 1 question, instead of getting frustrated with that question, leave it and move on. Answers to other questions may come quickly. When you have gone through the test once, then go back and use the remaining time to deal with the difficult questions. Sometimes you will find that later questions actually jog memories that will help you go back and recognize the answer to the question that troubled you earlier.

Second, if you see an answer that reads "All of the above" or "None of the above," then treat each of the other answers as simple true-false statements. It may help to put a "T" or an "F" beside each statement as you read it. When you are done, if all of the statements have a "T" beside them, you know the "All of the above" answer is correct. This also works well for options like "Both A and C are correct."

TIME MANAGEMENT FOR STUDENTS

Remember those childhood days when time passed without a care? Remember how all those childhood activities—playing house or going fishing—were seldom calculated in terms of time? True, our parents were constantly reminding us of time: "Be home for supper." "Be in by 10:00." "You have to have your homework done by 6:00 or you can't watch TV." No matter. When we were engrossed in pursuits of the imagination, time did not seem to matter.

If anything, time hung heavy. School days could wear on and on. Waiting to become an adult seemed like a trip down the long road of eternity itself. And being an adult meant being on your own and being able do with your time what you wanted.

How times change! Now time passes too quickly. Now there is never enough time. If only we could have a 36-hour day! But time is a fixed commodity. Therefore, it is not how much time we have but how we use it that makes the difference. And, perhaps most crucial, it is not so much the absolute standard of time that pushes us, but how we think about time that pressures us.

WHY STUDY TIME MANAGEMENT?

According to Jack Ferner (1980), **time management** is "efficient use of our resources, including time, in such a way that we are effective in achieving important personal goals" (p. 12). Some people have already acquired good time-management skills, but others need to spend time developing them. Time management is an important stress management skill because it allows us more discretionary time, as will be explained later.

Time management also can produce positive outcomes for students in an academic setting, reducing the likelihood of their dropping out and raising grade point average by small amounts (Bost, 1984). One study used a critical-incident technique to study this issue. Students ranked setting goals as the second most important factor related to success in college. Time management was ranked the fourth most important factor. Conversely, the students ranked failure to engage in good time management as the second most important factor in academic failure (Schmelzer, Schmelzer, Figler, & Brozo, 1987). What was the most important? It should be no surprise: failure to study.

There are several reasons why time management is also central to the relationship between stress and health. First, using some rather simple time-management techniques can improve personal productivity. The net effect is to provide more discretionary time for social pursuits, family, exercise, recreation, and hobbies. Lack of time for personal pursuits tends to be one of the most frequently cited stressors.

Second, it has become almost a truism that modern society is time driven, if not time obsessed. We studied the Type A personality in Chapter 4. Another group, those high in need for achievement, may even feel annoyed when their watches stop running (Webber, 1972). Society's preoccupation with time may also be a sign of much that is wrong with the way value is calculated. All too often, value is calculated in terms of money, power, and position, all of which generally require hard work and long hours. A study of time management may help us rethink long-standing attitudes towards time.

For example, we hear the cliche that *Time is money,* but this often translates to more impersonal and driven behaviors with negative consequences. An alternative, more positive attitude, is to think that *Time is a resource.* This notion is reminiscent of the famous Will Rogers saying about land: "Buy it. It is one thing they're not making any more." Like land, time cannot be manufactured. We each come into the world with exactly the same amount of time: 24 hours per day, 8736 hours per year. If time is conceived as a resource, the proper way to get the most out of it is through wise management. The applicable slogan is " Work smart, not hard."

Still, time management should never become a goal in itself. Time management is a tool to be used for a short while to reset priorities and recast inefficient work habits. When the job is done, it should be put on the back shelf until needed again. If time management ever starts managing you, throw it out!

SEVEN DEADLY SINS OF TIME MISMANAGEMENT

Before discussing how to manage time, it is necessary to know how you may be mismanaging time. This involves taking a personal inventory of your time expenditures. In this way, you gain a sense of what needs to be changed and what should stay the same. More details on how to do this will be given later. For now, consider these sins of omission and

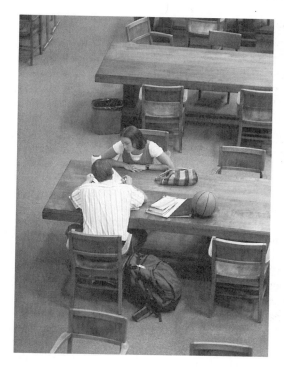

Although socializing is an important part of the college experience, when serious study needs to be done, it is usually preferable to eliminate as many distractions as possible.

commission that drain off time. The most common time-management sins are confusion, indecision, diffusion, procrastination, avoidance, interruptions, and perfectionism.

Confusion: Where Am I Going?

When people complain that they are wasting too much time but are not sure where their time is actually going, you can be fairly sure they do not know where *they* are going. In Lewis Carroll's *Alice's Adventures in Wonderland* (1865/1966), Alice and the Cheshire Cat have a dialogue that aptly captures this dilemma. Alice has come to a fork in the road where she is confused about what to do next. Spying the Cheshire Cat in the tree, she asks:

> "Would you tell me, please, which way I ought to go from here?"
> "That depends a good deal on where you want to get to," said the Cat.
> "I don't much care where," said Alice.
> "Then it doesn't matter which way you go," said the Cat. (p. 89)

Time management depends on knowing where you want to go. Failing to know where you want to be in the next few months and years may be the single biggest error in time management.

Indecision: What Should I Do?

The second major error in time management is **indecision,** or failing to make a decision that needs to be made. It has been noted that there is no such thing as indecision; there is only the decision not to decide. In any case, indecision is the hidden foe of effective time management.

Indecision often translates to handling tasks several times instead of once. It also tends to increase confusion and tension, because the decision is easily put off but not so easily put away. It is still there, waiting to be made, playing on the back roads of the mind even while other tasks are pressing. Indecision robs us of the freedom to focus, to relax, to create. Also, the inability to make decisions may be behind other problems in time management, such as procrastination, creating and allowing interruptions, and avoidance of duties.

Indecision may stem from many psychological factors. Stress may intrude from some other area of life and erode decision-making capabilities. Indecision may be due to lack of interest in the task, a failure of motivation. Indecision may also result from a deep-seated fear of making the wrong decision. Finally, it may result from lacking the information necessary to make a good decision; in this case, however, indecision may be acceptable and wise.

Diffusion: Mental and Physical Overload

Diffusion is the attempt to do far more than is necessary, perhaps even more than is possible. It is having too many irons in the fire. Mental diffusion produces ineffective problem solving, lack of concentration, and poor motivation for even the simplest tasks. Trying to keep up with all one's duties then takes its toll on the body in physical fatigue, and on the mind on what Charles Kozoll (1982) called the **battered mind syndrome.** This syndrome is marked by (1) many thoughts at once, (2) pervasive worry about what remains to be done, and (3) loss of focus on what can and should be done as pressures mount.

Diffusion typically results from not knowing your own limits. It also results from not knowing when and how to say no to requests from your friends and colleagues. In some cases, the two may be related—that is, the inability to say no may be due to your not knowing your own limits.

Procrastination: That Will Keep for Another Day

Procrastination is the thief of time, the cardinal sin of time mismanagement. Procrastination has been defined as putting off until tomorrow what you should do today. Robert Rutherford (1978) discusses two excuses that seem to keep a person from going to work: "I wish" and "I just can't get started" (p. 28). The "I wish" excuse usually entails wishing not to have to do the work or wishing for some type of miracle that gets the job done. In essence, it removes the responsibility of making something happen. The second wish is a type of self-fulfilling prophecy. It turns self-deceit into reality, which in the end is a self-defeat.

Laura Solomon and Esther Rothblum (1984) were concerned about the observed relationship between procrastination and poor college performance. The results of their study suggested that procrastination is more than just weak study habits and poor time management. One significant component that appeared in a large group of students was task aversiveness. In another, smaller group of students, the factors contributing to procrastination included such cognitive and affective components as irrational ideas, low self-esteem, depression, anxiety, fear of failure, and lack of assertion. Solomon and Rothblum suggested that this group of students would probably need to consider more than just time management in order to get past the procrastination problem.

Eliminating habitual procrastination requires some remedial action. For a while you should note which tasks you keep putting off. Then look for a common pattern in these tasks. One simple rule is to do the things you do not like first, so that the aversive task is no longer hanging over your head. Another effective strategy is to break big jobs down into smaller units that are easier to finish. Some people make a self-contract that allows them an indulgence or reward for finishing tasks, especially the unpleasant tasks.

Avoidance: Escape to Fantasy Land

People find many ways of avoiding work. They stretch coffee breaks or wander the halls looking for someone to talk to, presumably on business. They daydream, or read material—books or magazines—they really do not need to read. They dwell on trivial aspects of organizing their work, constantly cleaning their desk or files. They write and rewrite letters or memos in the name of perfection. In fact, they are probably avoiding some other task they do not want to do. If you catch yourself frequently saying that you are a perfectionist, consider whether you are also avoiding by overdoing.

Interruptions: Getting Started Is the Hard Part

One of the most frustrating time-killers is the unscheduled interruption. Phone calls, a friend dropping in for a chat in the middle of a study session, and so-called emergencies all represent disruptions to the normal flow of work. Charles Hummel (cited in Posner, 1982) said that tension exists between the urgent and the important. Important tasks—like the term paper—virtually never have to be done right away, today, or even this week. On the other hand, urgent tasks and crisis require instant action. We may be prone to treat the slightest upset in an intimate relationship or an overheard piece of gossip about us as a crisis that demands immediate attention. The problem is that the crisis diverts attention from the work plan and disrupts the schedule. But the crisis also becomes an excuse. Important work is not done. It's all right, though: There was an emergency!

Interruptions are perhaps most damaging to complex projects, where larger blocks of time are important to the flow of thought and sequential thinking. Creative writing and computer programming are two examples of such projects. These jobs involve a warm-up period to establish a rhythm. Interruptions require additional time to reorient and warm up again.

Perfectionism: I Was Raised a Perfectionist

You have probably heard it many times: "I'm a perfectionist." LeBoeuf (1979) points out that a perfect golf score is 18, whereas an excellent golf score is 72. No one seriously expects to attain perfection in golf, but people set equally unrealistic standards for other aspects of their lives. **Perfectionism** may have a place, but perfectionism for the sake of perfection is about as useful as rewaxing the whole car because you missed a tiny spot the first time. This type of perfectionism is really little more than compulsive overdoing.

The challenge is to draw the line between the necessary and the excessive, between quality that will return dividends and meticulousness that will never be noticed. Remember the law of diminished returns: Up to a point, the extra effort will be worthwhile. After that point, no amount of extra effort will produce any gain. (See Self-Study 14-2.)

POSITIVE TIME MANAGEMENT

Having identified your most common errors of time management and studied your personal use of time, it is now time to think about how errors can be reduced or eliminated.

Priorities: The Solution to Confusion

"You have to have your priorities straight!" This saying is overworked, but nonetheless true. The best solution for confusion is to set goals and reevaluate those goals periodically. There are a few basic guidelines for setting goals. First, establish clear, achievable goals. Second, assign a priority to each goal. Third, identify small tasks, related to your

SELF-STUDY EXERCISE 14-2

Finding Time-Management Weaknesses

We often think of time as a constant. In purely objective terms, this may be more or less true, but our subjective perception of time is often distorted depending on what we are doing. Subjectively, we stretch out tedious or boring periods and foreshorten periods filled with excitement (McConalogue, 1984). As a result, we can be very far off the mark if we depend on our subjective time estimates to tell us where our time is going. If you find yourself at the end of the day asking yourself where the time went, you may benefit from a time study. A time study seeks answers to three basic questions: What do you do? When do you do it? How much time does it take?

A simple way to obtain this information is to keep a daily log in which time periods are listed down the left side of the page and days across the top. Use periods as short as 15 minutes or as long as 1 hour, depending on the type of work you are doing. A 30-minute period will probably work for most purposes.[2]

Divide each day into two columns, one for the type of activity, the other for the people present. Jot down a short reminder of the activity you carried out during each period and note the people present. If the activity continues for more than one period, either fill successive periods with ditto marks or leave them blank until the activity changes.

After you have collected at least one week's information, begin searching for patterns. First, set out all non-work blocks of time, including commuting to and from classes or your job. Second, label all the nondiscretionary time—time determined by class schedule, work schedule, job requirements, or family-related functions. Be careful here: Do not label time as nondiscretionary just to be rid of the responsibility of managing it more effectively. Third, identify discretionary time—that is, time under your own control. Fourth, look at discretionary time to see where wastes are occurring and improvements need to be made.

If you see blocks of discretionary time broken up by interruptions, identify the people (yourself included) or events responsible for those interruptions. You may see a simple plan of action to correct the situation. If you find that a great deal of time is spent in nonproductive commuting, you may be able to transform it into productive time by listening to tapes of class notes, language review, or audio books.

goals, which can be carried out in short work periods. Fourth, set target dates for completion of the smaller tasks. Finally, reevaluate your goals periodically. Even if you have a personal five-year plan, you may need to reevaluate it each year.

Goals should be clear and achievable. While dreams may be the stuff of progress, unrealistic dreams generally produce only disillusionment and lowered resolve. Set your goals for three distinct time frames: long-term, medium-range, and short-term. Long-term goals should answer the basic questions: "Where do I want to be in five years and what do I have to do to get there?" Medium-range goals should address the issue of "Where do I want to be next year at this same time?" If you are under 25, you may want to use shorter periods, say three years for long-term goals and six months for short-term goals.

Regardless of your age, you usually have to break short-term goals down into more tangible tasks. First, for each week set attainable, concrete objectives that provide for some progress toward the major goal. Second, make a daily "to do" list to organize both personal and school time. These lists do not have to be written formally, but the most efficient corporate executives report doing so. They write their "to do" list before leaving the office, later in the evening before retiring, or in the first few minutes after reaching the office.

[2]Typically, each page will contain the record for one week. However, some people feel that weekends, or at least one of the weekend days, should be unstructured and will use only the five weekdays, or six days at most.

The Pareto Principle

The **Pareto principle** is named after an Italian economist and sociologist, Vilfredo Pareto. His idea is captured in the phrase *the vital few and the trivial many.* The **vital few** means that 20% of your goals (the few) contain 80% of the value—they are vital. The **trivial many** refers to the fact that 80% of your goals (the many) account for only 20% of the value—they are trivial. To manage time effectively, invest time in proportion to value—in other words, invest in the few goals with much meaning.

The way to solve this problem is to list what you want to accomplish in long-term, intermediate, and short-term periods. Then arrange the list from most important to least important. Finally, distribute most of your time among the few items at the top of your list. Let the things at the bottom of the list go if time does not permit and they are not required by an instructor or job supervisor.

Goals set at one time do not stay valid for all time. Re-evaluation is essential to avoid working toward the wrong things. Buzz Aldrin, one of the first astronauts to set foot on the moon, learned this the hard way. He suffered a nervous breakdown shortly after his return to earth. In his autobiographical account, he revealed that he forgot there was life beyond the moon! He had focused his attention so exclusively on going to the moon that he forgot to think about what he would do afterward. Whether you are graduating from college, completing a major project, or retiring, it is important to re-evaluate and have a plan, formal or informal, for what comes next.

Pruning and Weeding

The solution to diffusion is to prune the unnecessary and weed out the unattainable. This may require you to focus on which specific tasks are necessary to reach the goal you have set. For example, some people become pack rats when it comes to paper, reading and filing reams of material. Then they go through a time-consuming panic of cleaning files when things pile up. Learn to handle the material once and decide if it is important or not. Extract what is necessary from the important material, and keep only what is essential. Agendas for meetings past are not essential. Keeping copies of outgoing correspondence for potential information is usually a waste of time but the practice may be essential if it concerns a legal matter.

Most importantly, learn to say no to requests for involvement in other activities. As pleasant as it might be to be all things to all people, it is better to be the best for yourself and your family, even if that means being best in a more limited arena of activity.

If you find you are having difficulty saying no, examine the reasons. Is it fear of being left out or being less liked? If so, put these hidden assumptions to a test. Recall the times you did say no and examine the outcomes. You will probably find that the results were not as disastrous as you had imagined. Maybe the failure to say no is due to lack of assertiveness: You want to say no but cannot. Consider taking an assertion training class or reading a book on assertion.

Getting Started: Breaking the Procrastination Habit

One common cause of procrastination is that the procrastinator views the job as too big to fit available time. The logic then seems to be, why start? The solution is to break the task down into smaller parts. Writing a term paper, for example, can be segmented into doing background work, reading, organizing, drafting, and rewriting. Even the background work can be broken down into smaller components. A 15-minute period here and there can be used to check references, obtain books, and copy journal articles for later reading. Once procrastinators view a job this way, they will see many more shorter periods of time as useful, and getting started becomes easier.

Structure your work situation to provide cues that help get you started rather than add to inertia and lethargy. Your office should be an office, not a lounge or recreation room. Work cues should facilitate paying attention without strain while minimizing distractions. It may be nice to have a cozy office, but too many nonwork cues, such as popular magazines and pictures of the family vacation, will only sidetrack you. These cues become conversation pieces when other people come in, extending the interruption even longer. If a computer game constantly lures you, remove it from your computer. You do not have to destroy it completely: Download it to a floppy disk and send it to your parents. You can reload it later when time permits the diversion.

Finally, do not mix functions in your work area. If you read to fall asleep, do so only in bed, never in your study chair and only with non-technical material. If you find yourself getting sleepy every time you try to read, you probably have your cues mixed. Your mind is telling you that reading is a signal for going to sleep, when you actually need to stay alert. The general idea is to strengthen the cues most conducive to efficient work habits.

Concentrating: Zeroing in on Essentials

Getting started is only one part of the battle in effective time management. Two other issues must also be confronted. One is concentrating on the job long enough to complete some whole unit or stage of the task. The other is sticking with the task until it is done.

The ideas discussed earlier (controlling the cues in your work area and reducing distractions) will help you with concentration as much as with getting started. In addition, you may need to examine two other elements. First, people sometimes have difficulty working at any task for longer than a few minutes. If this is a recurrent problem, use a clock and a self-contract to keep yourself at the task for a set period. Start with a short period of time that is close to what you normally work. Then make a contract with yourself such as "I'm going to work straight through for the next 20 minutes before taking a break." Gradually increase the amount of time by adding 1 or 2 minutes each day. When you are able to concentrate on a task for at least an hour, consider yourself over the hump.

Second, some people try to work for too long at a single task. The problem of short-term concentration is that it does not provide for continuity and rhythm, especially in complex tasks. The problem with long-term concentration is that it tends to produce fatigue, lower motivation, and reduced mental efficiency. The way to deal with this is to distribute work sessions and alternate tasks. For example, you can reward yourself with a short break, say 10 minutes, for every hour you work. During this time, you might do some more menial work, return phone calls, or close your eyes and enjoy some favorite music. You might also switch tasks. The varying content can help keep motivation and interest at a higher level over longer periods.

A major problem in the normal work environment, as discussed earlier, is dealing with unscheduled interruptions. Post a "Do Not Disturb" sign, or make it clear what your study times are and keep them consistent. Avoid the notion that you have to have an open door policy. Be gentle but firm if people violate the Do Not Disturb sign. Also, do not feel guilty! You have a right to privacy to complete your work, and you can exercise a measure of control in that regard. If all else fails, consider using a second office such as a library study-cubicle.

Dealing with the chronic drop-in can be a problem, but there are some effective solutions. According to Rutherford (1978), every time you respond to drop-ins with idle, pleasant chatter, you sign an implicit or silent contract that encourages them to do it again. In effect, you give them a license to interrupt anytime they want. You can prevent this by advising the interrupter that you are in the middle of a project that needs to be completed. You can suggest that you both talk at your next scheduled break. If the behavior persists, you can ignore the person until he or she gets the hint. It is also appropriate to tell the person bluntly that the behavior is disruptive and that you do not appreciate visits during your study time.

Dealing with phone interruptions may be somewhat easier than dealing with face-to-face confrontation. One simple solution is to disconnect the phone during your study time. If someone really needs to talk with you, they will try later. Caller IDs and answering machines can also help. With caller ID, you can turn off the phone, and then check the new calls when you are ready for a break. You can return the calls you want and ignore the ones you want. Answering machines allow you to screen calls, but if left on at an audible level, they can be as disrupting as the phone call itself. If you take a call, ask how much time the call will require and either call back or set a time limit. Then set aside some time, perhaps one of your rest breaks, when you return calls and make some of your own calls.

Staying with It: Marking Time and Progress

Perhaps the most effective way to keep yourself at a task is to provide some tangible reward or marker for completion of a small step. You can do this by using a checklist of the total project with each step listed separately. You can then check off each step as it is finished. A daily "to do" list is valuable for just this reason. A project calendar can also provide valuable feedback.

HINTS FOR EFFECTIVE TIME MANAGEMENT

Many suggestions for better use of time do not conveniently fit into any of the preceding categories. The next few paragraphs present a potpourri of ideas that may prove helpful for one time management problem or another.

Internal Prime Time

Recall the concept of diurnal cycles and circadian rhythms. We each function on a slightly different internal clock that makes us more efficient at certain times. Know your **internal prime time,** when you work the best, and try to structure your work so you do the most demanding tasks in synchrony with your prime time.

Also, study your sleep habits. Many people sleep more than they need to. The norm is eight hours per night, but this standard may vary from six to nine hours. Evidence exists that sleep over nine or ten hours can have three bad results: Your overall metabolic rate may lower, leading to increased difficulty in maintaining a desirable weight; muscle tone may drop, leading to increased effort in carrying out normal tasks and reducing the ease with which you can exercise; and performance of the mental system may decrease due to lethargy.

If you observe that you are sleeping more than ten hours (the exception being when you are ill), a simple experiment will tell you whether you are sleeping more than necessary. Get up a half hour earlier for a few mornings. If you find you are no more tired at the end of the day and do not feel the need to go to bed earlier, you can probably get by without the half hour of sleep. You can repeat this process until you reach a point where you sleep enough but do not waste time sleeping. Even if you cut down, you should realize that you will not be cutting down on deep sleep, when the really important biological repair work is done. You will actually be reducing the amount of light sleep that occurs in the morning just before you are ready to wake up. On the other hand, if you are already sleeping less than six or seven hours, you probably should not cut down any further. Very few people can get by on less sleep than that without doing their bodies harm.

Reading for Professional Development

In many technical and professional fields, it is necessary to stick to a routine reading program in order to keep up with important developments. If you tried to read everything, you would be overwhelmed. But even trying to read the bare minimum is a struggle much of the time.

One problem is the habit of reading word for word. On the average, a person will complete college reading at the rate of about 350 words per minute. However, repeated reading of very technical information leads to the habit of slower reading, a habit that then is carried over to reading a newspaper or novel. One survey showed that managers were reading at a constant speed of about 250 words per minute, which did not change from one type of material to another (Heyel, 1979). At this rate, it takes anywhere from 1 to 3 minutes for each page of text. Even a 20-page article can consume an hour or more, far too much time to be able to keep up. But you do not have to read word for word to get what you need. This will be explained in a moment.

Speed-reading courses claim to be able to increase reading speed to thousands of words per minute. Be assured, though, that what is going on is not word-for-word reading! The visual system is physiologically incapable of processing information at that speed. These exaggerated claims have been shown to be based on a skimming procedure or on some systematic reading procedure (such as reading only the first and last sentence in each paragraph). The target most often cited for speed reading is from 600 to 1000 words per minute. Even at this rate, you would still not be able to keep up with your reading quotas.

There are ways to whittle the task to manageable size. First, be selective of what you read. If you have summary or review journals, you may be able to keep up on the high spots of your profession. From the summaries, identify articles or books that contain the detailed information most critical to maintaining and developing your skills.

Then, learn to read with an eye for the forest and not the trees. Develop the ability to scan material and pick out the basic details without reading the entire article. Most of the time, word-for-word reading is based on the fear that something important will be missed.

Some concepts from memory research can work in your favor. In general, much of the information you read is lost in the first 24 to 48 hours after reading. Only high spots, or story lines, are retained. Skimming is a way of detecting the gist from the outset. Also, if you are reading word for word, you are overriding one of the great powers of the mind—its ability to fill in gaps. You do not need to read all the prepositions, for example, because the mind will just assume they are there.

Another way of reducing reading time is to look for organizing themes in the author's style. Some authors provide the main idea at the beginning of a paragraph, elaborate in the middle, and summarize or provide transition at the end. Therefore, you can often obtain the most important information by reading just the first and last sentences of each paragraph. If material is highlighted in the middle, scan it on the way. Also, note other highlights, such as lists of essential points, and markers such as *first, second, third,* and *finally.*

Once Should Always Be Enough

Never handle paper more than once. How many times has a letter crossed your desk and you felt you did not have time to deal with it? Each time you pick it up, you follow the same sequence: Read it, think about it, decide what to do, decide not to do anything, wait until later, and repeat the sequence. Each time, you add delays and excess mental baggage. If you do this even twice for each piece of correspondence, you add as much as 25% to your workload. The work you could accomplish in eight hours will take you ten hours or more.

Downtime and Idling

If you are too busy for relaxation, socializing, and exercising, you are just too busy. Downtime is important as a change of both physical and mental pacing. It refreshes the body and revives the spirit. Too often, though, downtime is considered nonproductive, a waste of time. But the usual effect of downtime is that you are able to go back to work after idling and accomplish more in less time. It is important to note that being in good physical condition increases the percentage of prime-time working hours (Bliss, 1976).

On the other hand, continuing to work under pressure usually has a snowball effect. Job performance gradually goes down, though often so insidiously that the real reason is overlooked. The conclusion erroneously drawn is that more work and harder work is what is needed, and the snowball grows even bigger.

The idea is to attain a balance between the necessity of work and the value of idling. If you spend 18 hours in front of the tube for sports or soaps, you are probably overdoing the idling end. But allow yourself a minimum of 3 to 4 hours at least 2 or 3 times a week when you can shut everything out of your mind and let your mind rest. It may not be the most productive time of your life, but it can still contribute greatly to your overall satisfaction with life and work.

SUMMARY

In this chapter, we discussed some common student stressors including personal transitions and academic pressures. The major points made can be summarized as follows.

1. The most frequently reported personal stressors revolve around transitions to the university community and the consequent disruptions in family relations that typically occur.
2. Many students find that they experience significant periods of loneliness as the family members and friends they once counted on are no longer available, but new relationships have not yet matured to replace the disrupted relations.
3. Loneliness itself can lower psychological and physical well-being. Loneliness may be reduced or managed through both attitudinal and behavioral changes as discussed in the text.
4. Many students also struggle with managing money to meet their many social needs and academic obligations. Basic strategies were described including making money management a matter of study.

5. Academic stressors include test anxiety and time management. Text anxiety can be managed by learning the relaxation and desensitization skills described in earlier chapters.

6. Minority and international students often confront acculturation stressors in the academic environment. That is, the university culture often reflects a dominant Anglo-European mode of thinking, values, and code of conduct.

7. In addition, minority students often find themselves even more in the minority in college than they did in their home environs. This can lead to feelings of isolation, discrimination, and not belonging.

8. Time management is a core stress management skill. It seems especially important in a society that has become increasingly complex and fast-paced.

9. Time management was defined as the efficient use of our resources—in this case the resource of time—to help us meet our personal goals.

10. We identified seven major time traps, or ways that time may be wasted. These time traps were identified as confusion, indecision, diffusion, procrastination, avoidance, interruptions, and perfectionism.

11. Confusion stems from lack of a clear vision of where to go. The solution is to set clear goals for where you want to be in the next few months and the next few years.

12. Indecision is the inability to act decisively when required. Many difficulties in decision making stem from psychological factors—such as not being interested in the current type of work—that need to be resolved.

13. Diffusion means expending energy on so many activities that all efforts are less focused and efficient than they could otherwise be. The solution is to focus on the most important goals and learn to say no to demands that diffuse focus.

14. Procrastination is unnecessary delay in finishing a task. Careful analysis of the types of tasks that you keep putting off may reveal a pattern that can help to eliminate the problem.

15. Avoidance involves using a number of escape behaviors to avoid dealing with unpleasant duties.

16. Interruptions result from unscheduled drop-ins, mismanaged phone calls, and self-initiated stops and starts that detract from continuity on the job.

17. Perfectionism is compulsive overdoing beyond the point of value.

18. The major means of dealing with these errors in time management are setting goals and priorities within those goals.

19. Use cue control for the work environment to increase concentration and reduce interruptions. Batching and handling several routine chores at one time also will minimize interruptions.

20. Downtime, like the pause that refreshes, is important to maintaining mental and physical energy.

CRITICAL THINKING AND STUDY QUESTIONS

1. How do the personal and academic stressors listed in this chapter compare with your own personal list of the college stressors? You might consider doing an informal survey among friends and acquaintances and again compare your findings to the listed stressors.
2. If one of the stressors is personally relevant and needs to be managed better, how would you go about it in your particular university environment?
3. What are the resources at your university that could help students deal with some of these stressors? Are some of these resources relevant to your personal concerns? If so, how could you take advantage of them?
4. Why is time management such an important stress management skill? How may time management transcend the academic pressure cooker to serve well in later family and professional life?

KEY TERMS

battered mind syndrome	Pareto principle	test anxiety
indecision	perfectionism	time management
internal prime time	procrastination	(defined)
loneliness		

WEBSITES student survival skills

URL ADDRESS	SITE NAME & DESCRIPTION
http://members.aol.com/rslts/tmmap.html	Time-Management Guide
http://www.odos.uiuc.edu/Counseling_Center/brochure.htm	University of Illinois. Time management and overcoming procrastination
http://www.cmhc.com/guide/selfestm.htm	Self-esteem and Shyness Includes issues about assertiveness and loneliness, and links to related sites
http://www.shyness.com	The Shyness Home Page. An index to resources for shyness

CHAPTER 15

Behavioral Health Strategies:

Nutrition and Exercise

Running has given me a glimpse of the greatest freedom that a man can ever know, because it results in the simultaneous liberation of both body and mind.

ROGER BANNISTER

QUESTIONS

- How do diet and exercise relate to stress management?
- How does stress alter metabolism and eating behavior?
- What makes for a healthy diet?
- Is it possible to abuse vitamins with unhealthy consequences?
- How does the body's "set point" impact our efforts to lose or gain weight?
- What are the overall benefits of regular exercise?
- What rules of thumb should guide our weekly pattern of exercise?
- What are the major barriers to effective exercise?
- What precautions should be observed in beginning and maintaining an exercise program?
- What behavioral methods help people stick with an exercise program?

The value of exercise can hardly be underestimated, whether it is to maintain good health or to recover from some catastrophic health event. The story of Kelly Perkins is as informative in this regard as it is inspirational. At the age of 30, Perkins had about all a young woman could ask for in life, including good health with plenty of exercise (Perkins, 1997). She ran about 5 miles per day and spent time with her husband hiking and camping. Still, when she began to feel something was wrong, she went to her doctor for a checkup. After some persistence, but also to her shock and dismay, she discovered that she had an enlarged left ventricle. Further diagnosis revealed that a virus had damaged her heart (viral cardiomyopathy), leading to a rapid heart beat. Medication (30 pills per day) and an implanted defibrillator[1] helped to keep things under control for nearly 2 years, but then she took a turn for the worse.

In a short period of time, Perkins' condition deteriorated to such an extent that she had no hope short of a heart transplant. In November 1995, she became number one on the transplant wait list at the UCLA Medical Center. Within 24 hours, as fate would have it, she received the heart of another woman killed in a fall from a horse. The next few months still contained several crises for Kelly, including her body's attempt to reject the heart.

After nearly a 6-month battle, with her body now accommodating the heart and her weight slowly on the rise, she decided it was time to return to her fitness ways. What she accomplished in the next few months was astounding. She resumed hiking, not just as an end in itself, but as a prelude to a more taxing adventure—mountain climbing. Her return to mountain climbing began in August 1996 with a trip to Yosemite and a 17-mile 12-hour climb up Half Dome, an 8842-foot peak. Then, in September 1997, she tackled Mount Whitney, a mountain she had climbed years earlier at 25 years of age. At 14,495 feet, Mount Whitney is the nation's highest peak outside of Alaska. It took her 3 days to make the 22-mile trip, but when she stood on top at last, she knew that she had made the long road back to the fitness she wanted to claim. When asked what had helped her withstand the terrible stress from her years of uncertainty and failing health, she attributed it to the unwavering support of her husband and her faith in God.

STRESS AND HEALTH: LINKS TO NUTRITION AND EXERCISE

On the surface, nutrition and exercise may seem unrelated to stress. Yet a positive personal health program is as much a part of stress management as relaxation training, anxiety management, or cognitive restructuring.

Good health increases resistance to stress by improving a person's capacity for responding to demand. This is true whether the demands are challenging and exciting or threatening and anxiety provoking. Conversely, poor health places a load on the psychophysiological system, thus increasing vulnerability to stress. Beyond this, nutrition can alter mood and neural sensitivity, which in turn can change our reactions to stressors (Spring, Lieberman, Swope, & Garfield, 1986). Further, exercise may function to reduce stress (Crews & Landers, 1987), and it may serve as an antidepressant (Dubbert & Wilson, 1984). Often it provides a natural high (Clingman & Hilliard, 1987), and it may be a buffer against illness (Kobasa, Maddi, & Puccetti, 1982).

---

[1] A defibrillator is a device used to shock the heart to restore its natural rhythm.

UNHEALTHY BEHAVIORS: DIET AND SEDENTARY LIFESTYLES

Many statistics support the contention that Americans engage in a wide range of unhealthy behaviors, including smoking, overeating, improper diet, lack of exercise, and excessive use of drugs. For example, each year Americans take nearly 5 billion doses of tranquilizers to calm down. They take another 5 billion doses of barbiturates to unwind and sleep, and another 3 billion doses of amphetamines to perk up (Posner, 1982).

Although nearly 30 million Americans quit smoking in the decade between 1965 and 1975, largely through their own efforts (Schachter, 1982), approximately 25% of adults still smoke. Nearly 420,000 people die each year from smoking-related diseases (American Lung Association, 1997). In spite of an overall decline in smoking, there is a large increase in teenage girls and working women who now smoke. In addition, smokers are less likely to begin exercise programs and more likely to quit exercise programs than are nonsmokers (Martin & Dubbert, 1982).

In the ongoing battle of the bulge, we consume an excess of fats and do not take in enough carbohydrates. This contributes to increased frequency of obesity and coronary disease. Of the ten leading causes of death, diet is a contributing factor in five, including heart disease, cancers, strokes, diabetes, and atherosclerosis[2] (National Center for Health Statistics, 1988). In addition, we spend about $6 billion each year on packaged nutrients that may have adverse side effects.

Recent estimates suggest that nearly 34 million Americans, approximately one-fourth of the population, are overweight (McGinnis & Nestle, 1989). Obesity affects about 33% of adults, and the associated health care costs amount to nearly $68 billion per year (Rosenbaum, Leibel, & Hirsch, 1997). Although a Gallup poll in 1984 showed that approximately 59% of the adult population engaged in daily exercise—over twice the number in 1961 (Gallup, 1984)—the remaining 41% were probably active only at levels too low in intensity and frequency to provide for cardiovascular fitness (Herbert & Teague, 1989). One estimate is that nearly 12% of total deaths[3] each year are due to lack of regular exercise, and new data suggests that people may be reverting to more sedentary lifestyles again (American Heart Association, 1997). Approximately 50% of those who begin an exercise program drop out in less than a year (Kendzierski & Lamastro, 1988). Among those who exercise regularly, too many have an "Olympic" syndrome, going into exercise programs too fast and too hard and pushing themselves to limits far beyond what is necessary for good health.

The purpose of this chapter, then, is to provide basic principles to establish and maintain a good personal health program. There are many ways to construct such a program, but here we will focus on nutrition and exercise. Later in this chapter, we will discuss cognitive-behavioral self-control techniques, which can be used to change a variety of unhealthy behaviors.

---

[2]Of the remaining five, excessive alcohol consumption contributes to three—unintentional injuries (auto accidents, for example), suicide, and chronic liver disease.

[3]This translates in raw frequency to about 250,000 deaths per year.

EFFECTS OF STRESS ON METABOLISM AND DIET

Because stress has a general arousing effect on a person, it has the potential to change both energy expenditure and energy intake. First, stress increases the rate of metabolism, the rate at which the body changes food supplies into energy. This leads to increased levels of sugar, free fatty acids, and lactic acid in the blood (Niaura, Stoney, & Herbert, 1992). Stress also has indirect effects on metabolism due to the influence of the pituitary. These include changes in water balance, suppression of the immune system, and increased carbohydrate and protein metabolism. The net effect of stress is that the body uses energy at a faster rate.

The pattern of eating also may change. Whether a person will be affected in this way and how significantly his or her behavior will change depends on a variety of factors, such as learning, emotionality, and personality. Some learn that food is a means of escape when one is sad or depressed, whereas others learn that food is less desirable under these same conditions. The former may not only eat more, but may eat more frequently while under pressure. The latter may want to eat only subsistence meals or not want to eat at all.

When the typical stress response includes eating more and eating more frequently, the person will find weight control very difficult. The person may even reach weights that qualify as obesity. When the pattern is to eat less, especially to such extremes as going without food for days, the body may be depleted of energy reserves at an even faster rate. Any dramatic change in eating patterns should be a warning to look for stressful events at work, at school, or in the family.

EFFECTS OF DIET ON STRESS

Arousal can change metabolism and eating behavior, but dietary habits can also change sensitivity to stressors. In this sense, eating right is just as important as managing stress, because vulnerability to stress increases with poor diet. There are two ways in which this happens.

First, excess amounts of sugars deplete vitamins and minerals. This can have negative side effects, because vitamins and minerals are essential to keep body systems, especially the nervous system, working properly. Depletion of certain B vitamins (thiamine, niacin, and B12, for example) increases nervous system reactivity, irritability, and nervousness. In other words, you increase vulnerability to stressful events by taking in too many sweets.

Second, numerous foods commonly taken in large amounts have the potential to increase stress sensitivity. For example, coffee, cola, chocolate, and other products containing caffeine are frequently abused. Heller (1987) estimated that almost 200 over-the-counter drugs contain caffeine. "Cold-caffeine" colas are on their way to replacing coffee as the "wake up drink," and soft drink manufacturers have been in a market race to provide consumers with higher-caffeine versions of popular colas.

One cup of drip-brewed coffee contains approximately 100 to 150 mg of caffeine, while decaffeinated[4] coffee contains only 3 mg per 5-oz cup (Mayo Clinic, 1981). As

---

[4]Be careful not to use decaffeinated coffees processed with methylene chloride, because this process carries increased risk of cancer and may also cause side effects such as headaches. "Naturally" decaffeinated coffees use either ethyl acetate, a natural substance found in fruits and vegetables, or some combination of water and carbon dioxide or coffee oils to extract the caffeine.

little as 250 mg of caffeine can cause nervousness, insomnia, and headaches. It is now well known that caffeine acts as a stimulant to the central nervous system (Boulenger, Salem, Marangos, & Uhde, 1987). It tends to charge up the autonomic system, and it lowers thresholds for stress reactions (Lane, 1983). Stated in other terms, you are more likely to interpret an event as stressful if you take in large amounts of caffeine. Further, you are more likely to respond impulsively and intensely in stressful situations after taking in excess caffeine.

Research from Boulenger's group suggests that caffeine is an anxiogenic substance that is dose dependent. That is, caffeine induces clinically definable anxiety states when ingested at around 720 mg (Boulenger et al., 1987). It takes only five or six cups of coffee to reach this anxiety-inducing level. Although these dangers can occur with excessive use, the system apparently can handle lower levels with few or no negative side effects. Before proceeding to the next section, take time to respond to the nutrition and diet scales provided in Self-Study Exercise 15-1.

EATING RIGHT: BALANCING ENERGY INTAKE

Proper nutrition depends on eating the right foods in the right amounts. In 1988, the Surgeon General's office released a report that resulted from an intensive review of nutrition and health in America. The report contained five specific recommendations for all people.

1. *Fats and cholesterol:* Reduce the consumption of fat to no more than 20% of daily calories and cholesterol to less than 300 mg daily.
2. *Energy and weight control:* Work to reach a desirable body weight, then maintain that weight through both regulation of caloric intake and energy expenditure (exercise).
3. *Complex carbohydrates and fiber:* Increase intake of whole-grain foods, cereals, vegetables, and fruits so that about 50% of total calories come from complex carbohydrates.
4. *Sodium:* Reduce sodium intake by using foods low in sodium content and limiting the amount of salt added to foods at the table.
5. *Alcohol:* Take alcohol only in moderation (two drinks per day maximum, no matter what type of alcohol) to reduce the risk of chronic disease (McGinnis & Nestle, 1989).

Nutrition research has shown that the adult human body must have 46 nutrients to be healthy and stay healthy. To maintain a constant weight, the average woman needs about 1600 to 2400 calories, and the average man needs about 2300 to 3100 calories (Mayo Clinic, 1981, p. 270).[5] Table 15-1 shows the average energy needs with ranges for children and adults of different weights and heights. To obtain the 46 nutrients, normal adults need to average, *as a bare minimum,* about 1300 calories per day (Mirkin, 1983). For these reasons, there is danger in any diet that reduces to the extreme either the type or quantity of food, and such diets should be avoided.

---

[5]Nutrition research uses the term calorie without qualifying that it is the big C—the great calorie, or the kilocalorie—that is at issue. The kilocalorie is the amount of heat required to raise 1 kilogram of water 1 degree centigrade. For the remainder of this discussion, the term *calorie* will always refer to the great calorie, or kilocalorie.

SELF-STUDY EXERCISE 15-1

Health Behavior Profile for Nutrition and Diet

The following scale will help you compare your dietary practice to what is considered good practice. Instructions for scoring are provided at the end.

Circle the answer that most accurately describes your eating habits.

DAILY = once or more per day
FREQUENTLY = every week but not once per day
OCCASIONALLY = a few times each month but not once per week
SELDOM = no more than once per month

HOW OFTEN DO YOU:	SELDOM	OCCASIONALLY	FREQUENTLY	DAILY
1. Eat fruits, vegetables, fiber?	1	2	3	4
2. Drink five or more cups of coffee in a day?	4	3	2	1
3. Eat fats, red meats, dairy products?	4	3	2	1
4. Drink five or more soft drinks (diet or regular)?	4	3	2	1
5. Eat candies, sugars, pastries?	4	3	2	1
6. Take vitamin supplements?	4	3	2	1
7. Overeat at meals?	4	3	2	1
8. Eat between meals?	4	3	2	1
9. Eat while watching TV, reading, and so on?	4	3	2	1
10. Skip breakfast?	4	3	2	1
11. Skip lunch?	4	3	2	1
12. Skip dinner?	4	3	2	1
13. Use crash diets to lose weight?	4	3	2	1
14. Take diet pills?	4	3	2	1
15. Use amphetamines to lose weight?	4	3	2	1

After you have completed the scale, go back and add up the values listed in the boxes you circled. Then circle the point on the following scale that corresponds to your total score. A high score suggests that your eating habits are fairly good. On the other end, a low score indicates there is some risk in your eating habits. If you have a score in the High Risk region, look back at the items you checked that have values of 1 or 2. These items provide clues to areas where a change in diet and nutritional habits may be warranted.

```
Score sum   ..42.....45.....47.....48.....49.....51.....52.....53.....54..

              ←High risk→  |  ←Normal nutrition→  |  ←Excellent→

Percentile  ..10.....20.....30.....40.....50.....60.....70.....80.....90..
```

The average score on this scale is 49.2, and the median is 49.5. The median indicates that 50% of the respondents scored higher than 49.5, and 50% scored lower. The scale has a reliability of .695, which is acceptable for this type of scale. This scale is not intended to be a comprehensive nutrition assessment and is provided for instructional purposes only.

TABLE 15-1
Recommended daily energy (calorie) intake for children and adults

	AGE (YEARS)	WEIGHT (POUNDS)	HEIGHT (INCHES)	ENERGY NEEDS (CALORIES)
Youth	1–3	29	35	1300 (900–1800)
	4–6	44	44	1700 (1300–2300)
	7–10	62	52	2400 (1650–3300)
Males	11–14	99	62	2700 (2000–3700)
	15–18	145	69	2800 (2100–3900)
	19–22	154	70	2900 (2500–3300)
	23–50	154	70	2700 (2300–3100)
	51–75	154	70	2400 (2000–2800)
	76+	154	70	2050 (1650–2450)
Females	11–14	101	62	2200 (1500–3000)
	15–18	120	64	2100 (1200–3000)
	19–22	120	64	2100 (1700–2500)
	23–50	120	64	2300 (1600–2400)
	51–75	120	64	1800 (1400–2200)
	76+	120	64	1600 (1200–2000)
Pregnancy				+300
Nursing				+500

SOURCE: Adapted from Mayo Clinic, Committee on Dietetics (1981)

The guidelines provided here are for the so-called normal adult, and suggested caloric intake levels are averages. Children differ in their requirements, as do adults over 55 to 60 years of age and pregnant and nursing women. A person with a large frame or a strenuous job requires more calories than someone with a small frame or a less demanding job. Professional bikers, such as Lance Armstrong or Miguel Indurain, may consume as many as 10,000 calories per day while racing, and still lose weight. Illness also affects nutritional requirements. Finally, food intake does not have to exactly match the standard each day, but it should average out over a few days.

The 46 essential nutrients cover 6 categories: water, carbohydrates, 9 proteins, fat, 13 vitamins, and 21 minerals. Of these 6 categories, only carbohydrates, proteins, and fats contain calories. Calories provide the energy for internal processes, for muscular action, and for brain work. When taken in large amounts, calories are the culprits that make excess body weight. Carbohydrates are the least likely to add unwanted body weight, whereas fats are the worst offenders. Water, vitamins, and minerals are essential to keep the body functioning properly, but they do not contain calories.

We can meet most of our nutritional needs through natural food supplies. The challenge is to obtain a balance. We need to fit all the nutrients into a calorie count that still maintains desirable weight. The ideal diet should consist of about 50% carbohydrate calories, 30% protein calories, and 20% fat calories. About 80% of the carbohydrates should be complex, and not more than 10% of the fats should be saturated (Gershoff, 1990). Overall quality of the American diet has been improving across both different

TABLE 15-2

Comparison of calorie content for food groups and one abused drug

Carbohydrates	4 calories per gram
Protein	4 calories per gram
Fat	9 calories per gram
Alcohol	7 calories per gram

SOURCE: Data from Mayo Nutrition O@sis, 1997

socioeconomic and ethnic groups (Popkin, Siega-Riz, & Haines, 1996). Unfortunately, the average American diet is still out of balance, with 40% carbohydrates (with too many sugars), and about 20% protein. Although percent of fat calories has decreased to around 35%, Americans have increased food consumption so that more fat is being taken in and too much of that is saturated fats (Mayo, 1997b). To carry out an interactive diet analysis, use the web site noted in Self-Study Exercise 15-2.

SELF-STUDY EXERCISE 15-2

Internet Interactive Diet Analysis
http://dawp.futuresouth.com/cgi-bin/w3-msql/dawp.html

Carbohydrates: Filling Up, Not Fattening Up

Carbohydrates are complex food molecules made up of carbon, oxygen, and hydrogen—or more simply, sugars. There are single-molecule (simple) sugars called *mono-saccharides,* double-molecule sugars called *disaccharides,* and complex sugar molecules called *polysaccharides.* One simple sugar is glucose, the high-energy fuel in your bloodstream. Fruits and honey contain pure glucose that can pass directly into the bloodstream for fast energy. Foods such as bananas and oranges also contain simple sugars, but the sugars they contain must be converted to glucose for the body's use. Other sugars must be converted to glucose as well. Common table sugar[6] and milk are sources of double sugars, whereas corn, beans, and potatoes are sources of complex sugars. Simple sugars, such as those used in candies and table sugar, are empty calories with no nutritional value (Gershoff, 1990).

Carbohydrates provide the primary fuel for exercise, labor, and brain work. The brain depends on a continuous supply of glucose to work properly. It cannot reserve fuel for later use. This is why a good breakfast is important to start the day off right. If you do not eat in the morning, the brain does not have the immediate energy it needs to work properly. The muscles, though, can save glucose in a type of energy bank to withdraw when needed. In addition to providing quick energy, carbohydrates fill you up more quickly with fewer calories than any other food.

[6]Common table sugar is a disaccharide, a combination of two simple sugars, glucose and fructose.

Paradoxically, loading up on carbohydrates may not be the best practice early in the day. Tests have shown that people feel sleepier after a carbohydrate meal (breakfast or lunch) as compared with a protein meal. In addition, mental alertness as measured by a selective-attention task is lower for almost three hours after eating a high-carbohydrate meal. This effect is most intense in people over 40 who eat a high-carbohydrate lunch (Spring et al., 1986). It appears that carbohydrates have sedative-like effects related to tryptophan content and brain chemistry (Lieberman, Spring, & Garfield, 1986).

The complex carbohydrates, made from millions of sugar molecules, are typically high in fiber or cellulose content. Two characteristics of high-fiber foods make them valuable to a healthy diet. First, high-fiber foods do not break down in the digestive system as readily as other foods. The upper intestine cannot break down fiber at all. Since it cannot be broken down, fiber also cannot be absorbed in the body as worrisome weight. Second, fats bind to fiber and ride out as body waste. So when you eat a richly marbled steak, eat it with fiber to reduce the amount of fat that remains in the system.

Common foods containing carbohydrates are vegetables, fruits, and whole grains. However, appearance is not a good clue to fiber content. Lettuce is not as high in fiber as you might think from appearance, but peas are very high in fiber. For snacks, avoid potato chips with their high fat content, and eat apples, celery, or carrots instead. This will reduce hunger, provide energy, and add fiber to the digestive tract.

Still, be wary of exaggerated claims for the cholestrol-reducing nutritional value of high-fiber diets or foods such as oat brans. Adding any fiber to one's diet will reduce serum cholesterol levels (Swain, Rouse, Curley, & Sacks, 1990), but only because the fiber tends to replace fat in the diet. In other words, it is reduction in fat that is beneficial, not any intrinsic cholesterol-lowering properties of fiber itself. In addition, high-fiber diets can have some unpleasant gastrointestinal side effects, such as flatulence, cramping, and diarrhea.

The Proteins

Proteins may be the most overrated food in the American diet. While our bodies need only 8 or 9% protein calories to function properly (Gershoff, 1990), we usually consume more than the recommended 20%. Many people believe the myth that protein generates strength and that the best source of protein is meat. Strength comes through exercise, and the best source of energy for exercise comes from carbohydrates. The idea that a vegetarian must be inherently weaker than a "meat eater" is an unfortunate and inaccurate one.

Further, protein is *not* a source of quick energy. It has to be converted before it can be used. Although protein contains calories, it is the last food converted to energy after the carbohydrates and the fats. The body uses protein for energy only during periods of severe starvation or dieting.

Proteins are the basic building blocks for all body tissues. Antibodies and other parts of the immune system are proteins. Thus, proteins play an important role in protecting against disease (Gershoff, 1990). During periods of intense stress, illness, infection, and injury, the body may increase its demand for protein by as much as 100%. Intense exercise and bodybuilding may have the same effect (Gutlin & Kessler, 1983). Even the enzymes that regulate body functions are proteins.

The body uses 22 different amino acids to make proteins, manufacturing 13 of them internally. The remaining 9 amino acids have to come from diet. We usually obtain protein from animal sources such as poultry, eggs, fish, lean meat, cheese, and milk. Protein is also available from many plant sources, such as cereals, nuts, beans, and leafy vegetables. Still, you do not need to eat meat at all to obtain essential protein. You can get nearly all you need in two large glasses of milk (preferably low-fat milk) or in 12 ounces of corn and beans (Mirkin, 1983). Although Americans are moving toward lower-fat milk, there is an overall increase in demand for cheese products, which are high in milk fat.

For people who want meat in their diet, though, nutrition experts recommend that no more than two to three meals per week consist of red meat. The remaining meals should use white meats (chicken or turkey, for example) and especially fish. Eating fish is associated with lower overall risk for coronary heart disease (Daviglus et al., 1997). However, some seafoods, such as shrimp, are high in cholesterol, so do not assume that simply because it comes from the sea that a food is good for you.

Good Fats and Bad Fats

If proteins are the most overrated foods, fats may be the most misunderstood. We have developed a strong fear of fats because of their connection to obesity and coronary problems. Despite this fear, we continue to overuse, if not abuse, fats. Fats still make up about 45% of the American diet when the maximum should be about 20%. The average male should carry no more than 15% body fat, and the average female should carry no more than 25% body fat. Yet the average American carries much more fat, excess baggage that may have harmful effects. A 45-year-old male carrying 25 pounds of excess fat will have a life expectancy shortened by 25% (Mirkin, 1983). To determine your own risk, you can check your body mass index at the interactive website noted in Self-Study Exercise 15-3.

SELF-STUDY EXERCISE 15-3

Internet Interactive Body Mass Index Analysis
http://healthyweight.com/

Still, fats are essential to a healthy body and to survival. Fat is a storehouse of energy and fluids for the body to draw on whenever it needs. Fat converts to energy much more quickly than protein and is essential to vitamin transport. The immune system's ability to protect the body against viruses and bacteria also depends on fat. Finally, fat is one major way in which the body protects itself against cold.

Most of the danger from fat comes from the buildup of **yellow fat** on the body and from deposits of **cholesterol** in the bloodstream. Yellow fat is the reservoir of excess calories. The fatty tissue beneath the skin, such as the fold of fat around the waistline, is yellow fat.

Cholesterol is a lipid, chemically different from fats, but still a member of the same family. The liver manufactures cholesterol from excess calories, so cholesterol does not need to be eaten to meet body needs. It is, to correct some bad press, necessary for certain functions of the body. Cholesterol cannot move through the bloodstream by itself (Gershoff, 1990). For that, it needs carriers called lipoproteins. One lipoprotein is a good type of fat, whereas the other is bad fat. Good cholesterol is **high-density lipoprotein (HDL).** Bad cholesterol is **low-density lipoprotein (LDL).** HDL helps keep the arteries clean and elastic. By contrast, LDL embeds itself in the arterial walls, forming plaques.

This narrows and hardens the artery. Then the heart must work harder and at a higher pressure to force blood through the arteries.

HDLs are like high-tech garbage trucks that pick up cell cholesterol, compact it into a very small space, and deliver it to the liver without losing any of their load (Gershoff, 1990). They also act like street sweepers, picking up some, but not all, the droppings of LDLs. LDLs are more like open wagons. They do not compact their load, so they cannot carry as much cholesterol as HDLs. More importantly, LDLs are prone to accidents: They spill part of their loads. This dropped cholesterol stays in the bloodstream and accumulates. This is the building material for arterial plaques and blocked arteries.

One newly discovered LDL, Lipoprotein(a), may explain why some people are prone to heart attacks (Hajjar, Gavish, Breslow, & Nachman, 1989). Hajjar's research group found that some people appear to have a genetic disposition to produce more Lipoprotein(a). This lipoprotein does not respond to diet and so may contribute to the formation of plaques. Coronary attacks occur more frequently in connection with a high concentration of LDL. Persons with high HDL tend to have fewer attacks (Pekkanen et al., 1990).

Recent research showed that exercisers consistently carry more of their cholesterol as HDLs, the good kind, and less as LDLs, the bad kind. Lower LDLs following exercise are seen in children as well as adults (Craig, Bandini, Lichtenstein, Schaefer, & Dietz, 1996). Sedentary people carry more of their cholesterol as low-density lipoprotein (Gutlin & Kessler, 1983). One interesting note is that HDLs appear to be predicted by waist-to-hip ratio and not by sex or total body fat (Ostlund et al., 1990).

We consume fats in butter, oils such as those used in fast-food frying, salad dressings, ice cream, and fatty meats such as bacon. The best way to control problems associated with fats is to reduce their intake and maintain a regular exercise program.

Will the Really Good Fats Please Stand Up?

Just when we thought we knew what was safe to eat on our bread and potatoes, a new culprit has popped up—hydrogenated vegetable oils. These oils occur in margarines, margarine-based products, shortenings, and frying fats. The products themselves may be advertised as low in cholesterol, but the process of manufacturing them produces potentially harmful by-products.

Food processors and consumers like shortenings that have a certain firmness yet plasticity. To obtain this texture, the food industry has to hydrogenate the liquid oils. This makes the oil firm but leaves by-products called trans fatty acids. Recent research has shown that these trans fatty acids change the ratio of LDLs to HDLs in a harmful way; that is, they raise LDLs and lower HDLs (Mensink & Katan, 1990). The net effect is as harmful as that of a diet loaded with saturated fats. Mensink and Katan think the average intake of trans fatty acids is low enough that there is probably little danger. Still, they recommend that people at risk for atherosclerosis should avoid diets high in trans fatty acids.

VITAMINS: USE OR ABUSE AND ADDICTION?

In recent years, we have been bombarded with vitamin supplement diets and therapies that advocate taking megadoses of a particular vitamin. Marketing ploys have apparently worked well since the industry now has $6 billion in sales of vitamins per year (Mayo

Health O@sis, 1997c). The rationale for the vitamin supplements varies. One line of thinking derives from the age-old observation that vitamin deficiencies can cause extremely serious physical problems—pellagra and scurvy, for example. If a little supplement keeps this from happening, then a lot must be even better. This argument does not consider what vitamin poisoning can do to the body.

Another argument states that vitamin guidelines are minimums that do not consider variations in the size and health of the individual. Larger people and sick people need more vitamins. Therefore, as the argument goes, we should be looking at nothing less than an "average" allowance that must be larger than the minimums. Of course, this argument does not consider the vitamins obtained from daily food. A balanced diet can supply most of the vitamins needed at the level needed. If you then supplement your daily diet with a vitamin tablet that provides 100% of daily requirements, you may be taking close to twice the needed amount.

Perhaps the most difficult argument to refute is the one that says, "I was really sick with _____ , and I took _____ and got better right away." Fill in the blanks with "a cold" and "Vitamin C," and you have the argument made famous by Linus Pauling.

Unfortunately, this argument does not consider the placebo effect: If a person *believes* a treatment will be effective, it is more likely to be effective. This belief is often sufficient to summon the body's natural healing powers. A review of studies on Vitamin C and frequency and duration of colds did not show any practical significance and showed few statistically significant results. Among the best-designed studies (those with controls against the placebo effect), 50% show no significant results. The remaining, less

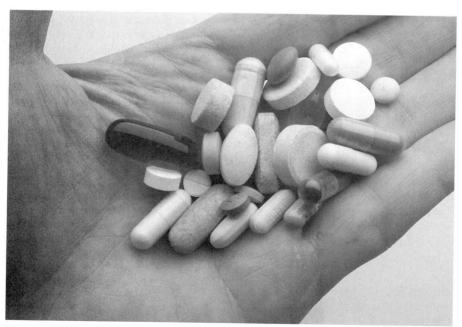

The vitamin industry presents a convincing case that daily intake of vitamins is a healthy choice, but abuse of vitamins also has negative consequences.

carefully designed, studies showed such small differences that they are scientifically meaningless (Marshall, 1983).

In contrast to the astounding publicity surrounding the alleged positive effects of vitamin megadoses, the public receives little warning about the potential dangers of vitamin overdose. Charles Marshall (1983) documented the hidden dangers of **vitamin abuse** by overdose. He noted that use of vitamin supplements has become a pattern of abuse based on the mistaken notion that more is better. This notion often combines with a false security that translates to: "I take so many vitamins I don't have to worry about the rest of my diet" (Marshall, 1983, pp. 20–21). He also noted that some vitamins have addictive properties. In support of this idea, users may encounter withdrawal symptoms if they reduce their dosage level or stop altogether. The remaining discussion summarizes a few of the dangerous **vitamin side effects** documented by Marshall.

Large doses of Vitamin A produce an immense array of negative effects. The list includes loss of appetite and weight loss, loss of hair, anemia, blurred vision, extreme drying and thickening of the skin, itching, dry and cracking lips, canker sores, increased brain and spinal fluid pressure with headache, irritability in children, and birth defects in children born to mothers who took megadoses of Vitamin A during pregnancy (Marshall, 1983).

There are no known toxic effects from the B-complex vitamins, although some unpleasant side effects may occur with too much niacin.

Vitamin C, much heralded for its ability to prevent, or at least reduce, colds and flu, is probably the most abused vitamin in American society. Although the recommended dietary allowance for Vitamin C is 60 mg for both men and women, average daily consumption is around 125 mg. Yet, based on advice from "experts," many people take 2000 to 4000 mg per day. The dangers from Vitamin C megadoses are extensive. The most common side effect is diarrhea. Other dangers include complications in pregnancy, spontaneous abortion, lowered sperm count, increased uric acid excretion, decreased tolerance for low oxygen levels, interference with urine tests for sugar and stool tests for blood, decreased resistance to bacterial infections and tumors, and damage to tooth enamel (Mirkin, 1983).

Overdoses of Vitamin D can cause loss of appetite, nausea, headaches, and depression. Long-term use may result in calcification of soft tissues and kidney failure. Excessive urination and diarrhea or constipation may occur. When the kidneys become involved, high blood pressure, increased levels of blood cholesterol, and heart damage may follow, with fatal results.

Americans spend approximately $100 million each year on Vitamin E. Some use of Vitamin E is justified as a well-known antioxidant that may reduce risk for cancer and heart disease, primarily among those whose diet is already deficient (Diaz, Frei, Vita, & Keaney, 1997). Otherwise, it is difficult to explain American's obsession with Vitamin E. One guess ties it to the myth of sexual virility. Early observations in laboratory rats showed that Vitamin E conferred increased sexual vitality and longevity. Researchers have not observed these effects in humans, and the studies with rats are far from convincing. Megadoses of Vitamin E result in elevated blood triglycerides in women and a reduction in thyroid hormone in both sexes. Laboratory studies of animals overdosed with Vitamin E show thyroid gland damage.

In addition to the potential dangers from megavitamin therapy, there are physiological and practical reasons for avoiding such excesses. Physiologically, the body acts like a reservoir that can hold only a certain amount of a vitamin before overflowing. For example, the body can hold only about 1500 mg of Vitamin C. If the body's reservoir is close to full (as it usually is) when you take a 1000-mg pill, the body does what any reservoir does—some old Vitamin C goes out with some new, and some stays in the body. The body absorbs about 500 mg of new Vitamin C. It loses about 500 mg in stools and another 500 mg in urine. Thus, the body balances its ledger sheet for Vitamin C. Practically, then, you are spending hard-earned money to pass stools and urine rich in Vitamin C.

In sum, megavitamin therapy does not have a stellar track record, and it can have dangerous side effects. The body cannot use the huge amounts of vitamins some people consume, which means that they are wasting large sums of money.

EATING LIGHT

Some people refer to this period as the age of diets and dieting. There are now dozens of diets on the market. Each one claims to have the secret to taking off and keeping off excess pounds. Millions of Americans now spend a combined $30 billion dollars each year trying to lose weight (Rosenbaum et al., 1997). In this section, I will discuss several issues to set dieting in perspective.

First, you should be skeptical about any diet program that emphasizes what goes in (calories) without discussing what goes out (energy expenditure through exercise). The key to weight reduction and maintenance is to balance the equation of input and output. Simply put, you must burn more calories than you take in. The way the body manages its resources, though, is much more subtle. The body tries to maintain a set-point that balances energy use and food intake to support body weight.

Set-Point Theory

Set-point theory comes from an impressive long-term research program led by Richard Keesey, among others. Keesey argued that food intake does not *directly* regulate body weight any more than activity does. Instead, the body regulates weight *indirectly* through the physiological mechanism of energy expenditure (Keesey & Powley, 1986). More precisely, the body has its own set-point—the exact weight at which there is an energy balance, when resting metabolism can be predicted from metabolic body size. This set-point represents a state of adaptation, a reference level of normal activity and normal food intake. Obesity resulting from overeating is an example of a maladaptive set-point. Once body weight is set, the body tries to maintain itself and resists deviations from the norm. If new input shows a change, the body takes action to restore the balance and maintain the set body weight.

Consider this example. Assume that an adult male has a stable body weight of 180 pounds. Further, imagine that he goes on a binge some night and eats a heavy meal with wine and a rich dessert. This excess caloric intake would push the body in the direction of weight gain. The body senses this caloric overload, however, and takes remedial action. It boots the metabolic rate, generates more heat, and burns calories at a faster rate. The result is that fewer calories remain to turn into body fat. Unfortunately, this small compensatory blessing for the overeater is also a great frustration for the dieter.

Suppose this person believes he is heavy and decides to go on a diet. Now, the body senses caloric deprivation and works to conserve energy. From a biological point of view, this makes sense. Imagine you were lost at sea in a boat with a limited amount of food and had no way of knowing when you might be rescued. You would voluntarily restrict the amount of food you ate. The body, in its infinite wisdom, would aid your efforts by shutting down, or attenuating, the basal metabolic rate.

In the same way, dieters trick the body into believing that it is in a state of deprivation. Reduced eating leads the body to conserve energy and preserve weight. Severe caloric restriction causes the body to conserve energy at an even greater rate. This is why dieters may "hit a wall" if they depend on diet alone. Note that it makes no difference whether the dieter is light or heavy to begin with. Conserving energy and maintaining the set-point weight occur equally in obese and normal-weight people.

This theory suggests that the most effective way to change weight is to reset the set-point. Increasing energy expenditure through a consistent exercise program forces the metabolic rate higher, resulting in a lower weight. Caloric intake can be at an even higher level, but the body will see itself as balanced within the exercise program and work to maintain this new balance.

Dieting Dangers

There are many dangers inherent in programs that focus solely or primarily on the input side. Probably no story has caught the dieting public off guard as much as the recent revelations that the darling of medical intervention in weight control, fen-phen, was itself the cause of valvular heart disease (Connolly et al., 1997). The argument used to justify combining the two drugs was that it allowed for lower doses with equal weight loss and allegedly fewer side effects. Unfortunately, no one ever bothered to test the interaction effects of the drugs, and in spite of the fact that the FDA had never approved the combined use of the drugs, nearly 18 million prescriptions were written in 1996 alone for this potent combination. The result now is at least 24 women with valvular heart disease—so severe in five cases that surgical interventions were needed. The outcome reminds us again of the old adage, "Buyer beware," especially with new treatments. The Internet now provides full access to consumers to obtain information for approved drugs. As always, an informed buyer is a wiser and probably happier buyer.

One danger comes in diets that reduce calories to the extreme. Such diets generally cannot provide balance in the six essential nutrients. Mirkin (1983) suggested that diets should never go below 1000 calories if you are not exercising and should stay above 1300 calories if you are.

Another danger in dieting is that it takes off muscle tissue, not fat. Ignoring exercise and emphasizing caloric intake is self-defeating. Exercising removes fat and tones muscle (Martin & Dubbert, 1982; van Dale & Saris, 1989). This improves body composition, which is important to health. Proper exercise effectively reduces weight and gets rid of yellow fat.

Yo-yo dieting (also called weight cycling) is a common problem among dieters today. Weight cycling often leads to feelings of shame, guilt, and frustration, but it appears that more serious psychiatric disturbances, such as depression, are not a likely consequence (Bartlett, Wadden, & Vogt, 1996; Foster, Wadden, Kendall, Stunkard, & Vogt, 1996). Yo-yo dieting is a sequence of dieting to lose weight, followed by a pattern of normal to overeating,[7] followed by weight gain. Regaining the weight often occurs with frustrating ease compared with the difficulty of getting rid of it. Recent research has shown why

---

[7]Binge eating may occur as well, but it is not a consistent finding in weight cycling research (Venditti, Wing, Jakicic, Butler, & Marcus, 1996).

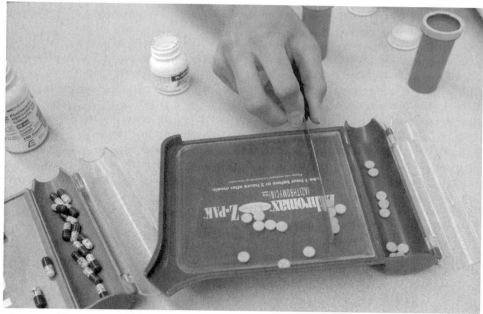

Mixing two weight-loss medications seemed a good idea at the time, but the consequences were fatal for some who developed heart valve problems.

yo-yo dieting leads so often to feelings of futility and failure. The practice may permanently *reduce* resting metabolic rate (RMR), the speed at which your body burns energy even while resting. Under these conditions, your body will convert more calories to body mass, even when you have reduced caloric intake. It is then more difficult to maintain weight at a desirable level (van Dale & Saris, 1989).

One body change may cause confusion at the beginning of a program that emphasizes weight loss through exercise. Muscles are denser than fat and thus weigh more than fat for the same volume. Although you burn off fat during exercise, you may not see an immediate change on the scales. You may even see a weight gain. Still, it is better to carry weight as conditioned muscle than as fat debris under your skin and in your blood. It is not weight per se but percentage of body fat that is dangerous.

To summarize, if you must diet, observe the following guidelines:

· Keep caloric intake above the minimum so you obtain all the essential food groups.
· Combine dieting with exercise that burns off more calories than you consume.
· Keep food intake balanced in the proportions of 50% or more carbohydrates, 30% protein, and 20% fats. If you cut anything further, it should be fats.
· Avoid diets that require dangerously low caloric intake.
· Avoid diets that completely eliminate one food group or that suggest excessive amounts of a particular food.
· Proceed only with great caution with a diet that depends on medications, especially experimental medication.
· Do not assume that vitamin supplements can replace carbohydrates, proteins, or fats. Vitamins contain no calories.

EXERCISE, HEALTH, AND STRESS

As noted at the outset, the benefits of exercise cannot be overemphasized, and the necessity cannot be underestimated. Before the dawn of the industrial-technological society, getting enough exercise was rarely an issue, and diet clinics were unnecessary. Daily life consisted of an incessant struggle for existence. Now, technology automates many chores that once demanded physical activity. This also removes any physical benefit. We automate changing TV channels, need portable phones, and think that escalators and elevators are essential. In this environment, it is little wonder that people are on the dieting treadmill. Even a low-calorie diet probably will result in weight gains, because energy expenditure does not use the calories. Before proceeding to the next section on the physical benefits of exercise, you should find it helpful to complete the health behavior profile for exercise provided in Self-Study Exercise 15-4.

Physical Benefits of Exercise

Physical exercise has a wide range of positive effects for the body. They include:

- Increased respiratory capacity
- Increased muscle tone (anaerobic)
- Increased strength in bones, ligaments, and tendons
- Physiological toughness with lower SNS base rate (Dienstbier, 1989)
- Improved cardiovascular functioning (aerobic) and reduced risk of heart disease (Haskell, 1987)
- Lower LDL cholesterol and triglyceride levels
- Increased levels of protective HDL cholesterol (Martin & Dubbert, 1982)
- Increased energy
- Improved sleep and reduced need for sleep (Horne, 1981)
- Increased rate of metabolism, both resting and active
- Reduced body weight and improved fat metabolism
- Reduced risk of injury from slips, falls, and so forth
- Slower aging process (Harris, Frankel, & Harris, 1977)

These benefits are not just for adults; they apply equally to children and adolescents (Klesges et al., 1990).

Mental Benefits of Exercise

Many athletes report several mental benefits that come with physical activity. One benefit is **runner's euphoria,** a feeling of elation and spiritual ecstasy or transcendence. It can be so powerful that many people run to achieve the same state again. Short of a peak experience, exercise still has many other psychosocial benefits:

- Increased feelings of self-control, independence, and self-sufficiency
- Increased self-confidence
- Improved body image and self-esteem
- Mental change of pace from the pressures of work, even when work is physical
- Improved mental functioning, alertness, and efficiency (Tomporowski & Ellis, 1986)
- Emotional catharsis, or cleansing, of tensions from interpersonal conflict and job stress

SELF-STUDY EXERCISE 15-4

Health Behavior Profile for Exercise

This profile is intended to help you determine the adequacy of your current physical activities and/or exercise program. Read the instructions before completing the profile. Instructions for scoring are given at the end along with the necessary information on how to interpret your own score.

Indicate the level of your participation in any of the listed activities by circling the appropriate boxes below.

AEROBIC = four or more times per week
FREQUENTLY = two or three times per week
WEEKLY = about once per week
MONTHLY = about once per month
NEVER = almost never

HOW OFTEN DO YOU PARTICIPATE IN:

	NEVER	MONTHLY	WEEKLY	FREQUENTLY	AEROBIC
1. Swimming	0	1	2	3	4
2. Walking (1 mile per day)	0	1	2	3	4
3. Hiking or backpacking	0	1	2	3	4
4. Gardening	0	1	2	3	4
5. Bicycling	0	1	2	3	4
6. Calisthenics, aerobics, dance exercise	0	1	2	3	4
7. Racquetball, tennis	0	1	2	3	4
8. Canoeing or boating	0	1	2	3	4
9. Water or snow skiing	0	1	2	3	4
10. Hunting or fishing	0	1	2	3	4
11. Golfing	0	1	2	3	4
12. Team sports	0	1	2	3	4
13. Running (5 or more miles per week)	0	1	2	3	4
14. Other physical exercise	0	1	2	3	4

After answering all 14 questions, *sum* the values in all the circled boxes. Then, *count* all the boxes with the value of 1 or more. *Divide* the *sum* by the *count*. This is your *aerobic index*. Finally, locate your aerobic index on the scale below. A low aerobic index suggests that you are not getting enough exercise. A high aerobic index suggests that your pattern of exercise is fairly good. If you have a score at the high-risk end of the scale, you should think about how to begin a consistent exercise program that will place you in the normal, if not excellent, range.

Aerobic Index	. .1.00. .1.25. .1.50. .1.75. .2.00. .2.50. .3.00. .3.50. .4.00. .
	←High risk→ ⎮ ←Normal exercise→ ⎮ ←Excellent→
Percentile	. . .20. . .30. . .40. . .50. . .60. . .70. . .80. . .90. . .100. .

- Reduced levels of stress (Crews & Landers, 1987)
- Relief from mild depressions (Morgan & Goldston, 1987)

We must not assume, however, that these are simple effects. For example, one research team observed the typical association between fitness from aerobic exercise and cardiovascular fitness (Czajkowski et al, 1990). The team used an anger temperament scale in their study. This follows other observations suggesting that negative affect plays a significant role in the coronary-prone profile. Physically fit subjects did report lower levels of anger than those not as fit. Yet when they analyzed the relation between exercise and cardiovascular fitness, controlling for angry temperament, the relationship all but disappeared. It appears, then, that dispositional anger may offset or reduce the positive effects of exercise.

PREPARING FOR EXERCISE

Preparing for exercise can be as important as the exercise itself. Think of each exercise session as divided into three distinct periods: **warm-up,** exercise, and cool-down. Whatever the sport, schedule a 10- to 20-minute warm-up period before the main workout. During this time, do some easy stretching and limbering routines. The goal is to bring your body temperature up slowly and get your muscles ready for more demanding activity. If bicycling, set an easy pace for the first mile or two before increasing the pace. If running, do light calisthenics or the equivalent before starting. Never start at full speed.

When you finish exercising, allow 10 to 20 minutes for cooling off. The longer and harder the workout, the longer you need for cooling down. Taking a brisk walk may be enough, but you can use light calisthenics as well. If you do not cool down properly, the muscles may become congested with increased blood flow. Ketones, or poisons, build up in the blood, producing pain and discomfort, such as in cramps.

It is preferable to think of an exercise program as a developmental process. Begin with light exercise during short sessions. As your fitness improves, you can increase the intensity and the length of the sessions. Later, exercise should be viewed primarily as a **maintenance** strategy, not a continuous improvement strategy. Avoid the idea that you have to lift more weights, play more racquetball games, run more miles, or run faster miles. Continuous progress is ultimately impossible. You will reach a plateau sometime and will find you can go no farther. Consider switching to a maintenance strategy before exercise burn-out occurs, but at a point where you are comfortable with your fitness level and exercise is still enjoyable. As others have pointed out, fitness is not a ribbon you win in competition; it is a road you travel all your life. After reaching speed, you do not keep accelerating.

EXERCISING FOR FITNESS

A few important rules should guide your exercise program. First, exercise programs should aim for aerobic fitness more than strength, but do not overlook anaerobic exercise as a possible activity. **Aerobic fitness** means "the ability to take in, transport, and utilize oxygen" (Sharkey, 1984, p. 3). Building muscle strength through bodybuilding routines is acceptable if a hard body is your main goal, but you should still use some exercise that builds cardiovascular fitness. Bodybuilding routines are, for the most part, **anaerobic,** or done without air. They involve high work output but produce lactic acid and eventually muscle fatigue that limits how long the exercise can last (Tomporowski & Ellis, 1986). Anaerobic programs do not do *as much* for cardiovascular fitness as aerobic programs, but anaerobic exercise may still bring some cardiovascular benefits.

Second, to achieve aerobic improvement, four factors may vary: frequency, type, duration, and intensity of exercise. How effective your exercise program is over the short run and how well you maintain it over the long haul depends on the interaction of these four factors.

How Often to Exercise?

The rule is to exercise at least three—and preferably four—times each week, from 30 to 45 minutes each time, to obtain **aerobic** improvement. Based on the fact that the half-life of exercise is 72 hours, anything less than three times weekly may result in more losses in the off days than you gain on exercise days. Anything more than this may wear down your body. When this happens, you feel increasing fatigue and may lose motivation for exercise. If you absolutely must exercise more than four times per week, do what professional athletes do. Schedule major workouts on an every-other-day basis, and schedule light workouts on the off days. You might even use a different type of exercise (cross train) on the off days to provide variety and maintain motivation.

What Exercise Is Best?

Many books detail specific forms of exercise and provide some assessment of their adequacy. In this section, we will discuss the most important findings. Whatever exercise you choose, it should fit sensibly into your lifestyle and be within reach of your physical capacities.

One method of rating different types of exercise uses the number of calories burned in one hour. Table 15-3, a typical caloric expenditure table, contains some interesting information. For example, note that rapid walking burns more calories than even swimming or running. The moral is simple: You do not have to engage in extremely intense and demanding sports, such as marathons, to achieve aerobic fitness. Any activity that burns from about 200 to 300 calories per hour is sufficient if you do it consistently three or four times per week.

Also note that just walking slowly burns about 200 calories per hour. Moderate aerobic exercise is about 300 calories per hour. Using this as the norm, there are many activities that can provide adequate aerobic fitness. For example, a brisk 2-mile walk at approximately 3 miles per hour is adequate for most people. Even the steps in your home, apartment, classroom buildings, or work site can be viewed as opportunities for exercise. There are no equipment expenses, no club memberships and fees, no embarrassment, no competition, and little worry about overdoing.

The prevailing opinion is that running, bicycling, swimming, or aerobic exercise classes are the most beneficial. Home-based treadmills and exercise machines provide adequate exercise where time and access are problems. Even the common jump rope provides a simple yet excellent aerobic exercise. It is cheap. It can be done anywhere, and it can be varied in intensity and length of time. Another simple exercise, similar to the "step-up" test for cardiovascular fitness, can be done on stairs. Just step up two or three steps, back down, and repeat. Doing this at a continuous pace for just 15 minutes is equivalent to a 3-mile slow walk.

TABLE 15-3
Energy expenditure per hour during different types of activity for a 70-kilogram man

FORM OF ACTIVITY	CALORIES PER HOUR
Sleeping	65
Awake, lying still	77
Sitting at rest	100
Standing relaxed	105
Dressing and undressing	118
Tailoring	135
Typewriting rapidly	140
Light exercise	170
Walking slowly (2.6 miles per hour)	200
Carpentry, metal working, industrial painting	240
Active exercise	290
Severe exercise	450
Sawing wood	480
Swimming	500
Running (5.3 miles per hour)	570
Very severe exercise	600
Walking very fast (5.3 miles per hour)	650
Walking up stairs	1100

SOURCE: Adapted from Guyton (1977)

How Long Should an Exercise Session Last?

You can obtain aerobic fitness by increasing the length or intensity of the workout or both. Very severe workouts can be dangerous, though, for a variety of reasons. You are more likely to have muscle strains or tears, ankle sprains, and other injuries as the intensity of the workout increases. You should never try intense workouts at the start of an exercise program. This can cause serious injuries and even heart attacks. The wiser course is to use slightly longer, moderately demanding workouts.

To understand how long and how intense exercise should be, it may help to examine the goal of exercise. To be fit means three things: Muscles have strength and tone to carry on work; lungs have the capacity to take in air to supply the heart and muscles; and the heart can increase its capacity (beats and volume) to meet the demands of work and exercise. Anaerobic exercise helps strengthen and tone muscles but only aerobic exercise meets all three criteria for fitness.

Consider these facts about the lungs and heart. The average adult has a resting heart rate around 70 to 75 beats per minute (bpm). A finely conditioned athlete has a resting pulse of 60 bpm, sometimes even lower. Miguel Indurain was reported to have a resting heart rate of from around 40 to 45, and Lange Armstrong a resting heart rate around 39. A person with a sedentary lifestyle is more likely to have a resting pulse around 80 to 90 bpm. In addition, a sedentary person's heart cannot respond to demand as readily as the tuned heart. This difference between the conditioned and the "deconditioned" heart means more wear and tear for the unfit person's heart. The untuned heart must beat about 30,000 more times each day compared to the tuned heart!

TABLE 15-4
Maximum heart rate (by age) with maximum and minimum training heart rates for aerobic fitness

AGE	MAXIMUM HEART RATE	RANGE	MAXIMUM TRAINING RATE	MINIMUM TRAINING RATE
10	210	200-220	168	126
15	205	195-215	164	123
20	200	190-210	160	120
25	195	185-205	156	117
30	190	180-200	152	114
35	185	175-195	148	111
40	180	170-190	144	108
45	175	165-185	140	105
50	170	160-180	136	102
55	165	155-175	132	99
60	160	150-170	128	96
70	150	140-160	120	90
80	140	130-150	112	84

Note. The range given for the maximum heart rate is provided as an indication of individual variability. The upper limit may be safely reached by individuals in better condition, but *the lower limit may be the upper limit of safety for those not in good condition.* Also, the high- and low-range concept should be carried over to both the maximum and minimum training rates. To do this, multiply the range values by 80% for maximum training rate and by 60% for minimum training rate.

Under workload, the heart can beat much faster than the 70-bpm average. It can beat as fast as 200-plus beats per minute. The ability to engage in work with minimum strain depends on how much the heart rate can be raised and sustained over time. Aerobic exercise gradually increases the rate at which your heart can work. As an added benefit, it gradually decreases the resting pulse, so your heart does not have to work as hard even when it is resting. The risk for coronary disease declines as exercise increases up to a maximum of 3000 calories per week of exercise (Haskell, 1987). For perspective, a 3000-calorie expenditure in one week would be equal to jogging 4 hours 15 minutes at a 5-mph rate, or about 21 miles total for the week.

The rule is that exercise should increase heart rate between 60% and 80% of the maximum capacity for your age. The maximum capacity can be obtained by taking 220 minus your age. If exercise does not increase heart rate above 60%, or about 114 bpm for the 30-year-old ($220 - 30 = 190 \times .6 = 114$ bpm), little or no progress will be made toward aerobic fitness. If you are 30 years old, the upper limit for aerobic exercise is about 152 bpm ($220 - 30 = 190 \times .8 = 152$ bpm). Table 15–4 provides calculated maximum heart rates for different ages with the minimum and maximum ranges for aerobic exercise. Also, note that the value for each age is the *average* for that age. Depending on several factors, the value you should use may vary more than 10 bpm more or less than the listed value. These ranges also appear in the table.

You can achieve adequate fitness from a 1-hour workout of moderate intensity that includes warm-up and cool-down. The real benefit for cardiovascular improvement, though, comes from the 20 to 30 minutes in the middle, when the heart rate accelerates above its normal resting rate. The quality of the exercise determines how much the heart rate accelerates. Low-intensity aerobic effort is when heart rate reaches only the minimum (115 bpm for the 30-year-old). Moderate-intensity aerobic effort occurs when the heart rate accelerates above the minimum but not above about 70% (between 115 and 135 bpm). Heart rates between 70% and 80% reflect a high-intensity aerobic effort.

How Hard to Exercise: The "No Pain, No Gain" Myth

How hard you should exercise depends on your goals and your current physical condition. Although some exertion is necessary to develop fitness, too much exertion can be physically damaging. This is especially true in the early stages of exercise. If your goal is to achieve and maintain an adequate level of fitness, then moderate workouts are all you need. If you are a born competitor, in search of excellence and the chance to prove just how good you are, a more strenuous level of exercise may be warranted. Still, do not depend on the competition motive to sustain a long-term exercise program. Attitudes that emphasize competition may be the single biggest barrier to getting more people into safe but adequate exercise programs.

Work into exercise slowly if you are out of shape. Typically, it will require several weeks of low-intensity exercise and several more weeks of moderate exercise before the body can profit from strenuous workouts. Research in hydraulic-circuit exercises (similar to the popular Nautilus machines) also suggests that you can alternate rest and exercise periods across a wide range (from 5 to 40 minutes) and still experience positive effects on oxygen uptake (Ballor et al., 1989). This suggests that there is little merit in exercising to the point of pain, burning, or nausea simply because of an arbitrary time line for exercise.

Far too much emphasis is placed on competition and the notion of "no pain, no gain." The Olympic syndrome mentioned earlier is the idea that the exercise, to be useful, must lead to the pinnacle of success. That may be acceptable for the athletically gifted young, but for the average adult, a more modest and attainable goal should suffice. Exercise should be fun, and it does not have to be painful to be helpful. This should be clear, since either a brisk walk or 30 minutes of moderate aerobic exercise is sufficient for cardiovascular fitness. Even a daily 5-minute, 100-calorie workout is sufficient to provide some progress to aerobic fitness. After a few weeks, move into the 300-calorie range, and later, even higher if you wish. If you are exercising in part to control weight, then workouts should be in the 300-calorie range, but workouts that push the limit are not as conducive to fat burning as are more moderate workouts. For example, biking at closer to the 60% level will burn fat off faster than constantly pushing it to the 80% level or higher.

BARRIERS TO EFFECTIVE EXERCISE

Given the proven benefits of exercise, it may seem surprising that more people do not exercise regularly. This has led researchers to examine the role of attitudes in exercise. Attitudes toward exercise may predict interest in exercise, but they do not seem to predict whether a person will stick with a program (Kendzierski & Lamastro, 1988). Many attitudes keep people from exercise. Two such attitudes are society's obsession with competition and the Olympic syndrome, as already noted. Another attitudinal barrier is the perception of lack of need. This is the person who says, "I'm in as good shape as anyone else, if not better." While that may be partially true, it is no excuse to avoid regular exercise. You need exercise no matter how fit you feel.

There is also the excuse that exercise programs cost too much. As noted before, several exercises cost virtually nothing, yet they provide adequate physical conditioning. Another excuse is that exercise takes too much time or competes with more important activities. Consider these facts. The 3 or 4 hours per week needed for physical health is less than 4% of total waking time. It is much less than the average time spent watching TV. Even TV time can be used for calisthenics, jumping rope, or riding an exercise bicycle.

Some people feel they will be embarrassed if they go to an exercise class or take up a competitive sport. There are several ways around this. Get a friend who is in about the same shape to exercise with you. In a Jazzercise class, for example, remember that many people there may have taken the classes before and are there now to maintain fitness. You should not even compare yourself with them. Often you will find more support and encouragement for trying than anything else.

Another attitudinal barrier is that some people think exercise takes place only in a gym. It is as though one must be in a health center, dressed in exercise fashions, working out on a universal gym, to be engaged in exercise. In reality, exercise can take place in many different settings, in everyday clothes, and with no high-tech equipment. You can exercise in your office building by going up and down stairs repeatedly or on the job if your work involves climbing, lifting, and kneeling. Frequently repeated activities that emulate calisthenics can help tone the body even if you don't do them fast enough to improve aerobic fitness. If the exercise does not provide heart rate acceleration to aerobic levels, you may still need some exercise outside work.

Finally, some people tend to exaggerate a failure and use it as an excuse to quit. There will be setbacks in any exercise program and times when you do not feel well, when you cannot run as far or as fast. These should be considered part of the process. Most of all, you should keep a flexible attitude toward exercise. Allow exercise to vary with mood and condition, but keep on exercising.

THE EXERCISER: A PSYCHOLOGICAL PROFILE

Several personal characteristics may correlate with beginning an exercise program and sticking to it. These include self-efficacy, self-motivation, and self-schemata. You may recall that self-efficacy is a self-schema about personal competency and mastery. It is the belief or expectation that one has the skills to act appropriately and successfully in certain situations. Exercise seems to greatly enhance self-efficacy (Cameron & Best, 1987). Conversely, the perception of lack of self-efficacy may be a major stumbling block to beginning an exercise program. This suggests that exercisers have both accurate and positive judgments of self-efficacy. We will discuss the practical implications of this later in this chapter.

The desire to change body image and improve health is an important motive (Gillett, 1988). Exercisers also possess a degree of self-motivation that carries them through tough times (Martin & Dubbert, 1982). They do not seem to require external prompts to keep them interested and involved. People with low self-motivation drop out of exercise programs more frequently than self-motivators.

Clingman and Hilliard (1987) have studied the super-adherer and constructed a personality profile. The super-adherer is one who is doggedly determined to exercise, who sets high exercise goals, and who wants to be competitive in his or her chosen sport. The profile includes motivation to achieve combined with endurance and dominance. Clingman and Hilliard also noted that certain personality traits fit an individual to a sport. For example, swimmers were not as aggressive as cyclists or triathletes. Runners were more autonomous than any other athletes tested, and cyclists were the most aggressive.

According to Deborah Kendzierski (1990), exercisers have self-schemata that include exercise in many ways. Self-schemata are cognitive structures that include generalizations about the self and important aspects of self. Individuals with exercise schemata use more exercise activity words to describe themselves. They recall more exercise events and behaviors in their past. They are more likely to be involved in exercise programs than people with nonexercise-oriented self-schemata.

MARATHON RUNNING: THE MYTH OF CORONARY IMMUNITY

Space does not permit more than a brief statement about the unfortunate myth that if you can run a marathon, you will acquire immunity to coronary. The myth is unfortunate, because many people pursued the dream of immunity too fast and too hard, with too much pain and sometimes with unnecessary death. The deaths of several runners who were in peak condition shattered the notion of coronary immunity. The most celebrated case is the death of Jim Fixx (1977), the author of a popular book on running. Yet vulnerability to coronary disease results from several factors, including genetic endowment, diet, and exercise. Exercise itself does not reverse the effects of genetic endowment. It may help someone at risk to live a healthier and higher-quality life, but it does not remove risk altogether.

EXERCISING FOR WEIGHT CONTROL

As noted earlier, exercise can be an important asset to a weight loss program. Attempts to reduce weight that do not include exercise are generally less effective, if not doomed to failure. Exercise speeds up a sluggish metabolism, causing the body to burn calories faster. This effect continues beyond the period of activity. The body burns calories about 10% faster up to six hours beyond the exercise (Mirkin, 1983). Even during sleep, metabolism is slightly higher than it would be if you did not exercise!

PRECAUTIONS FOR EXERCISE PROGRAMS

There are a few precautions to consider before starting an exercise program. First, people over 35 years of age should obtain a thorough medical exam if they have not been on a regular exercise schedule for a while. The longer it has been since you last exercised, the more crucial this precaution is. The exam probably should include a routine physical and a stress test. You should not hide the purpose of the exam from your physi-

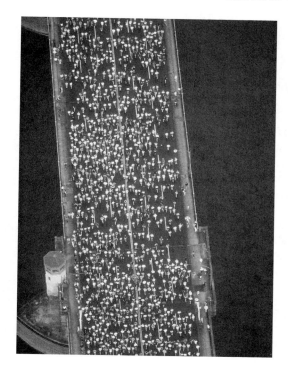

At one time, an unfortunate myth circulated that being able to run a marathon would confer immunity to coronary attacks. This is untrue—this extreme form of exercise is not even necessary to maintain or improve coronary health.

cian, so that the best medical judgement can work in your favor. This is a case where ignorance is not bliss, but potentially dangerous to you.

Overweight people should set modest goals, especially at the beginning. Recognize that high-intensity exercise programs are not necessary to achieve satisfactory weight loss or aerobic fitness (Gillett, 1988). Remember to use warm-up and cool-down periods before and after exercise. Finally, make sure you take in both enough fluids and calories to sustain physical exercise. Lack of either can produce physical problems during exercise and increase fatigue.

BEHAVIORAL SELF-CONTROL: PRINCIPLES FOR STICKING WITH IT

Behavioral psychologists have studied issues of self-control to help us understand better how we can accomplish what we set out to do. Self-control principles have emerged from many clinical studies designed to help people do the very things discussed in this chapter—reduce weight and engage in consistent exercise. At the same time, the ideas presented here can be extended to cover a variety of other unhealthy behaviors, such as smoking.

Set Attainable Goals

There are two factors to this principle. First, you need to know exactly where you want to go with your program. If you want to lose 25 pounds or exercise 3 times per week each week of the year, make that goal absolutely clear. Setting fuzzy goals like "I want to look better" or "I want to get in shape" do not specify how you can get there.

Then you need to make sure you can get there. Don't try to lose 50 pounds if you only need to lose 25. Also, don't try to run a 4-minute mile or a 2-hour marathon. These are goals difficult enough for the professionals. Be happy, then, even with modest achievements.

Allow for Success and Build Self-Efficacy

The practical implication of research on self-efficacy is that one should arrange for success in behavioral control, even if that success is modest. As you attain success, your perception of self-efficacy is likely to increase. With increases in self-efficacy, you are more likely to keep after your goals, and even more success is likely.

Break Long-Range Goals Down into Short-Term Goals

In addition to deciding where you want to go, set goals that mark progress for the trip there. Do not think in terms of losing 25 pounds or running a marathon. Think instead of losing 2 pounds per week or of running a 3-mile race. This way, you can divide a big trip into smaller parts, and you can more easily chart your progress. Then you will be more likely to stay motivated and keep at the program because you can see you are making gains.

Provide for Observable Progress Reports

It is important that you see your progress. In behavioral terms, this is **self-monitoring.** There are many ways to count or measure behavior. You can count frequency of repetitions in an exercise routine. You can time how long it takes you to bicycle a certain distance. A daily log can be checked to show the exercise you carried out. You can keep a caloric intake and weight record each day. A caloric record is more effective than just a weigh record (Cameron & Best, 1987). A record of eating behavior should record what you eat in calories, when you eat, what other activities are going on while eating, and people present.

A popular, easy way to record behavior change is to use a **calendar for self-observation.** Often, it is helpful to translate the calendar record to a simple chart or graph. You receive positive feedback by seeing your progress. Also, you can see patterns (weight gains over the weekend that slow progress) or detect problem areas in your program. Most exercise and diet programs use some type of chart for this purpose.

Making the chart public or semipublic can help you maintain motivation. A public chart becomes almost a contract with the viewers that you will succeed. You draw on powerful sources of social approval as you progress and gentle reproof when you let down. The chart does not have to be public in the literal sense, but it might be visible to people in your office or to your inner circle of friends.

Provide Yourself with Tangible Rewards

When you meet certain short-term goals, you ought to reward yourself. One way is to set aside a small amount of money to buy something personal, a nice piece of clothing or compact disk to add to your collection. In formal terms, this is a **contingency contract.**

In addition to rewards, you should agree on fines for failure to meet goals. Say you want to lose a pound each week for a month. The positive reward will be a sweater you have had your eye on for a while. If you do not meet your goal, the money will go to something that you really do not like–support of a politician or organization that you cannot stand.

Identify and Control Environmental Stimuli

An important part of self-control is recognizing environmental events that support bad habits (Cameron & Best, 1987). A chart of eating habits may reveal heavy eating when you are alone. A similar analysis may show continual snacking while watching TV.

The rule is to change the environment in a way that reverses the relationship. For example, you could use behavioral restrictions. Eat only in the kitchen, and do not move the TV into the kitchen to bypass the rule! Do not keep tempting, fattening snacks on the shelves. If you find that you do not exercise after you get home because of distractions, take your workout gear to work or school with you. Some people schedule a walk as part of their lunch break. Others take a longer break to go to the local health club and work out. This can be an excellent idea; it serves as a change of pace and recharges you for the balance of the day. Other people schedule a workout on their way home. Any of these strategies may break the pattern of negative stimulus control at home.

Make the Routine Habit-Forming

Whatever exercise you choose, get into a routine and stay with it. When a person's schedule gets tight, typically the first thing to go is exercise. Resist this temptation, especially early in your program. If you work out consistently for long enough, even a few weeks, you should find that consistency is habit-forming. You may even feel tension if you disrupt the new habit.

Use Nonproductive Time for Double-Timing

Some people complain that they do not have time for exercise, yet they spend hours watching TV. Turn nonproductive time into fitness time. You could do calisthenics, skip rope, or cycle and never miss a heartbeat of *ER* or *Monday Night Football*. Also, you could watch a Jazzercise class on TV and exercise with it. Then you could relax when you watch TV at other times.

Perhaps you use quiet times at home to read or keep up with correspondence. You can still take breaks for fitness exercises. You may find that your mind continues to work on issues and problems while exercising. A novel solution may occur to you during exercise, and you can return to your work energized in two ways.

One word of caution is in order. Many people have only a few leisure hours available. If you watch TV sparingly and for specific reasons, such as self-development or just relaxation, do not feel guilty about using TV-watching for that purpose. Instead, look for ways to free some other part of your schedule to provide the time you need for fitness.

Preventing Relapse

Emphasizing the things that will draw you to success is one part of the battle. The other part is thinking about the things that will prevent your falling back into the old unhealthy behaviors. There are several means to prevent relapse, including social support from friends or family or both, flexibility in goal setting for exercise, and use of cognitive strategies while exercising (Martin et al., 1984). Spouse involvement is especially useful in weight-loss programs and may be useful in exercise programs as well (Brownell, Marlatt,

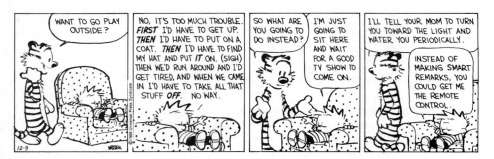

Calvin and Hobbes © 1989 Watterson. Dist. by Universal Press Syndicate. Reprinted with permission. All rights reserved.

Lichtenstein, & Wilson, 1986). Group exercise can aid adherence, especially when there is strong group cohesiveness (Carron, Widmeyer, & Brawley, 1988).

Marlatt's research team provided guidelines for using distraction-based cognitive strategies (Brownell et al., 1986). Negative cognitions occur when one dwells on body sensations—fatigue in the legs while biking, sore feet while running. A distraction-based program suggests that you think about the beauty of the day, pleasant smells from the woods, or flowers growing along the path. This provides positive, supportive internal feedback that sustains your motivation to exercise. Such strategies appear to lead to higher adherence to a training program (Martin et al., 1984).

SUMMARY

In this chapter, we have discussed basic elements of sound nutrition, diet, and exercise. The general principles have been clearly established by a solid line of research over the past quarter-century. The following points were among the core concepts introduced in the text.

1. A complete stress management program will consider the ways in which a good diet and exercise program can improve our ability to cope. Poor diet can "de-tune" the nervous system, leaving us more vulnerable to jitters and irritability. Lack of exercise can lead to increased loads on the body that make it more difficult to confront stressors.
2. Although Americans and most Europeans have been making improvements in lifestyle, there is still a large percentage of the population that lives a sedentary lifestyle and indulges in fatty goods.
3. Try to balance your diet with more carbohydrates and fewer proteins and fats; the percentages should be about 50%, 30%, and 20%, respectively.
4. A well-balanced diet will also have a good blend of high-fiber foods, since fiber helps remove fat, helps you feel full, and reduces the tendency to overeat.

5. Reduce the amount of saturated fats, sugars, and salt. At the same, do not overdo the reduction. This is one area where you should not and cannot apply the rule that if a little reduction is good, a big reduction must be even better. We need a certain amount of each of the foods for a healthy body.

6. Avoid taking megadoses of vitamins. Your body cannot absorb excess vitamins, and typically you get almost all you need from a good diet. Taking megadoses of vitamins is simply passing off expensive vitamins in urine and stools.

7. If you feel you need to diet for health reasons, plan a diet program around an exercise program. This is the most effective way to lose weight, because exercise will help you burn off more calories even when you are not exercising.

8. Exercise also allows you to eat more of what you want to eat, meaning that any diet you need will be less severe and easier to stay on.

9. Avoid diets that go to the extreme either in reducing calories to a very low amount or by excluding one kind of food. Keep the calorie count above 1300, especially while exercising.

10. Do not try to lose huge amounts of weight at a time; this could be very dangerous. Think instead in terms of a program in which you lose, at most, about one pound per week. Then, think in terms of maintaining an altered eating lifestyle, coupled with exercise, after you reach your weight loss goal.

11. In choosing a fitness program, consider an exercise that fits your physical capabilities and meshes comfortably with your professional and family patterns. Exercise does not have to be painful, expensive, excessively time-consuming, or glamorous to provide benefits.

12. Once you have selected an appropriate exercise and set a schedule, make that schedule habitual. Always do some warm-up exercises before commencing hard workouts, and be careful to cool down slowly.

13. The most intense exercise should raise your heart rate to somewhere between 70% and 80% of your resting heart rate, but a good fat burning exercise program will work closer to the 60% level.

14. Avoid the Olympic syndrome, and remember that there is a limit to what you can do. Also, avoid the notion that you must always be improving. After you have reached an adequate level of fitness, shift your program to one of maintenance.

CRITICAL THINKING AND STUDY QUESTIONS

1. How does your current diet compare to the guidelines described in the text? What if any changes should you make in order to have a more optimal diet?

2. Why is it ill-advised to take mega-doses of vitamins? Do you currently take some vitamin in large quantities? If so, have you carefully investigated whether the dosage level you are taking does or is not expected to have negative consequences?

3. How does your current activity level compare to the guidelines? What could you do to make your weekly exercise program more effective?

4. Why is it important to avoid extremes in diet programs?

KEY TERMS

aerobic exercise

aerobic fitness (defined)

anaerobic exercise

calendar for self-
     observation

cholesterol

contingency contract

dieting dangers

exercise for maintenance

exercise for warm-up

high-density lipoprotein
     (HDL)

low-density lipoprotein
     (LDL)

runner's euphoria

self-monitoring

set-point theory

vitamin abuse

vitamin side effects

yellow fat

WEBSITES behavioral health strategies

URL ADDRESS	SITE NAME & DESCRIPTION
http://primusweb.com/fitnesspartner	☆Excellent fitness and nutrition site with many online materials as well as excellent links
http://www.arfa.org/index.htm	American Running and Fitness Association
http://www.fda.gov/	U.S. Food and Drug Administration. Access to information on approved drugs and other health information
http://www.eatright.org	American Dietetic Association
http://www.pharminfo.com/	☆Pharmaceutical Information Network. Great data source for the layperson as well as the professional
http://www.nalusda.gov/fnic/dga/dguide95.html	U.S. Department of Agriculture. Dietary guidelines

Relaxation Instructions

Preparation

At least for the first few weeks, go over the mechanics of what you are to do just before each relaxation session. Review the instructions for the proper sequence of relaxation of muscle groups and make the final arrangements you prefer in regard to phone, music, lighting, and so on. If you are using taped relaxation instructions, make sure the recorder is adjusted for proper volume (a little on the soft side is preferable) and set at the right place to begin. Attention to these little details can make for a much smoother and easier relaxation period. Obviously, as you progress in your practice, more and more of these details will become like second nature to you. Then relaxation will have become a useful tool requiring little effort for its use.

Getting Started with Relaxation

The following instructions are for the first few relaxation sessions. Subsequently, the instructions are abbreviated and shortcuts taken to produce relaxation faster. These techniques will be discussed later. To begin, *read through the instructions entirely once before trying to actually relax*. The instructions for self-direction are written in indented blocks. Some comments are interspersed that will enable you to understand why you are being asked to do certain things.

During the first reading, you may try some of the tension-relaxation cycles just to get a feel for what it is like. But do not count your first run-through as a relaxation session! After reading through once, get in your chair, turn the lights down low, put on your background music—whatever you have decided on for your setting and preparation—and go through the procedure to relax. You will soon find that there is a logic to the progression, which will come in handy for further sessions. Further instructions for timing and other matters will be provided as needed.

You may want to record the instructions on tape in your own voice. This will allow you to concentrate on relaxing instead of worrying about what the next instruction is. Should you decide to do this, just read the instructions given and elaborate or extend where necessary as you are putting it on tape. You may paraphrase the instructions to some extent. Pronouns can be changed and sequences extended for the number of repetitions required. As long as the sense is the same, the words used do not make a difference. (More will be said about ways to handle the instructions at the end of the appendix.)

Instructions for Relaxation

What you are going to do for the next few minutes is study the difference between tension and relaxation in a number of your muscles. In the process you should begin to feel more and more relaxed. At the end, you should experience a comfortable heaviness in your body and have a feeling of easy peacefulness.

Remove any tight fitting clothes first. Loosen ties, belts, or any other articles of clothing that are snug. Take off your shoes. Also remove any tight-fitting jewelry such as watches, rings, or necklaces. Get comfortably situated in your chair. Put your arms on the arms of the chair with your palms down and hands open over the end of the chair's arms. Sit back in the chair and let your head fall gently onto your chest. Close your eyes. Let your legs lie comfortably apart on a stool or the leg support of your recliner. Do not cross your legs regardless of the type of chair you are using. If your chair is not a recliner and you do not have a footstool available, place your feet a few inches apart on the floor and let your arms lie across your thighs with your hands in your lap. (For self-guided or self-taped instructions, begin here. Use only those sections that are indented and elaborate or extend them as necessary.)

> Now take a few deep breaths: Hold each breath for a few seconds, and then let each breath out fully and completely. As you breathe in, you will notice some tension in your chest and diaphragm. As you breathe out, you will notice a sense of relaxing, almost of going limp. Relaxing feels good and comfortable and it would be nice if the feeling could be kept. But as you breathe in deeply again you feel the same tension as before, especially as you hold it for a moment. Let the breath out again, completely, and feel the pleasant relaxing sensation of letting go. Try it one more time. Dwell for just a moment on the sense of relaxation as you let the breath out.

> Try to maintain that sense of relaxation in your chest and diaphragm for a moment. As you breathe from now on, just breathe easily and naturally, almost as though you were napping.

> Concentrate for a moment on your right arm [left arm if you are left-handed]. Now flex your biceps as though you were showing off your muscles. Notice how it feels.

It may be easiest to do this by just pushing your elbow into the arm of the chair. Also, by doing it this way, you do not actually have to raise your arm from the chair.

> Flex it as tight as you can and hold it [about 10 seconds]. As you hold, study the sensation of tension. Notice how unpleasant it can be. Now let it go all at once. Let your arm go completely limp. Relax! And study the contrast. Notice how different it is from tension. Store the contrast in your mind even as you are studying it. One more time: Tense your bicep and hold it. Observe the feeling of tightness. Tune in to the signal of tension in your muscle. Then let it go. Completely relaxed. If someone picked your arm up and turned it loose, it would simply drop to your side. There is no tension at all. It feels so good. One more time. *Tense; hold; observe; relax; and observe.*

We are going to repeat this same sequence now for several other muscle groups. You will notice a general progression from the head down, with the exception of this first arm-hand sequence. The arm-hand sequence is done first because it is easy to experience the difference between tension and relaxation in these muscle groups. Also, note the pattern for each muscle group: Tense; hold; observe; relax; and observe. The cycles will be *approximately 10–15 seconds for the tension segments and 15–20 seconds for the relaxation segments, or roughly 30 seconds per cycle, with just slightly more time devoted to the relaxation than to the tension.* In normal practice, especially in the early stages, you should *do about 3 repetitions for each muscle group.* Later on, it will not be necessary to do as many. But hold fairly strictly to the time limits and repetitions for now.

Breathe deeply for a moment, hold, let it out. Relax. Your arm is relaxed also. Now do the other arm. Tense your bicep. Recognize the presence of tension in your arm even as the rest of your body is mostly relaxed. Hold and then release. Tune in to the pleasant sensation of relaxation. Repeat again. *Tense; hold; observe; relax; and observe.* And once more. Now both of your arms are relaxed and you continue to breathe in a calm and easy fashion.

Note the instruction "Repeat again" with the abbreviated sequence. If you are putting these instructions on tape, this is your signal to extend or elaborate the instructions to cover additional repetitions.

While the arms may not be involved frequently in tension patterns, your fingers and your palms often indicate the presence of stress. Your palms can sweat, your fingers can start to lock up, or your fists may clench during stress. The palms have long been recognized as indicators of emotionality, and this fact is capitalized on in the so-called lie-detector test. Athletes frequently try a variety of measures to relieve their hands of tension in order to be able to perform better.

Breathe deeply again. As you breathe out say to yourself, "Relax." And let it go all at once. Your arms are still relaxed. Clench your right fist [left if you are left-handed]. Hold it for a moment and observe the tightness. Notice the sensation of tension. Put that sensation in your memory. Now let your fist go completely loose, relaxed. Your fingers could not hold anything even if you tried. Once more, notice the difference in the sensations. Observe the pleasant heaviness of the hand when all the tension is gone. Clench your fist again, tight, very tight. Hold it for just a few seconds and study the sensation. Then let it go. All at once and completely. Study the contrast. Feel how good the relaxation is. Once more. *Tense; hold; observe; relax; observe.*

From this point on, I will give you the muscle group, some abbreviated instructions, and any special things to look for. But I will not repeat the extended instructions for each of the repetitions. Instead, you will see a bracketed statement that is some variation on the theme such as this: [Repeat the tension-relaxation cycle twice more.] This tells you where to repeat the instructions. To emphasize, *for each muscle group, repeat the tension-relaxation cycle three times.* Carry out the study and observation for each segment of tension and relaxation with diligence. It is through this means that you begin to feel the difference between relaxed and tense muscles. It is the beginning of being able to hear your muscles telling you that tension is present.

The next set of muscles is the shoulder muscle group. These muscles very frequently tense under stress, such as during driving or intense periods of concentration. They may roll up in a knot or just ache as though they have been overworked. But they will hurt. Shoulder muscle tension, if not relieved quickly, may also spread to the neck and back and additionally contribute to a headache.

> Take a deep breathe now, and hold it for a moment. Then say to yourself, "Relax," as you let the air out of your lungs completely. Now tighten up the shoulder muscle as tight as you can get it.

You may have to experiment with different ways of doing this. A slight rolling forward and upward of the shoulder may work best.

> Hold the tension for a moment and study the feeling. Then let your shoulder simply slump. Let all the tension go out of it. Study the difference and enjoy the feeling of relaxation. [Repeat this with the same shoulder two more times.] Next, do the other shoulder in the same way. At all times take care to notice the difference between relaxation and tension. [Repeat this with the alternate shoulder two more times.]
> Continue to keep all the parts of the body relaxed that you have relaxed to this point—the arms, the hands, the shoulders. Take another deep breath and hold it for a moment. Again release it as you are saying to yourself, "Relax." Enjoy the feeling of relaxation as it settles more and more over your whole body.

Now you are going to relax the neck muscles. They may become tense apart from the shoulder muscles, which you just relaxed. More often than not, neck muscles are tense when mental pressures are high. Neck muscle tension is also associated with severe forms of headache. Later on you will want to make mental connections to any experiences of neck muscle tension from the past. This will help you to spot conditions in your environment that are putting pressure on you. To tense your neck muscle:

> Flex your head backward, as though you were pulling down on the back of your skull with your neck. [You may even feel a slight amount of pain right at the base of the skull if you pull hard enough. Do not pull so hard that you strain something!] As you tense the neck muscles, again study the feeling of tightness. Hold it for about 10 seconds. Now release all the tension. Let your head fall gently back onto your chest and enjoy the feeling of relief from letting the tension go. Just enjoy relaxing for a few seconds, and observe the difference. [Repeat the neck tension and relaxation cycle two more times.] Continue at all times to breath easily and naturally. When you are done, scan the rest of your body to see if any parts seem tense. Do not do anything about it right now, just make a mental note of it. But *if any part of the body that you have relaxed before has become tense again, go back quickly and relax that part again.*

It may take you a little while to feel comfortable with this request—that is, trying to keep the rest of the body relaxed while you are concentrating on one part of the body and tensing it. But you will get used to it after a while. Also, it is important to start developing a sense of what it means to scan the body. Perhaps an analogy will help.

Many people have a type of CB radio that is only a receiver, but a special type of receiver. The radio actually scans up to 40 channels used by police, fire chiefs, sheriffs, ambulance personnel, and people who are just into CB radio. The scanner electronically runs through all 40 channels as fast as it can in some systematic fashion. When it is done scanning channels, it does it all over again. It is actually looking for action, a radio signal, some sign that someone somewhere is talking. You need to develop a sense of scanning your body in the same way. It should become like an internal sixth sense that automatically scans the muscle groups from one to the other and then *locks in* on any muscle group when a signal, tension, is found. It may be the most important talking your body does.

Now, concentrate on the forehead muscles. These muscles are referred to in medicine as the frontalis muscles. They wrinkle when you frown. They tighten when you are under pressure. Some clinicians believe that tension in the frontalis muscle group is associated with one form of headache, the tension headache. One high-tech solution to this problem is biofeedback.

Biofeedback in the treatment of tension headaches teaches how to relax the frontalis muscles. Overall, the clinical tests that have pitted biofeedback against relaxation find that the gains in symptomatic relief are largely a result of the relaxation itself. But some people experience difficulty trying to learn relaxation through the PMR procedure. They seem to need the visual picture that electronic feedback provides to learn how to relax. Biofeedback serves as an ally, helping people learn how to relax and how to "read" body signals of tension. It makes little difference, practically speaking, whether you learn to relax through PMR or through biofeedback. The outcome is the same. Once the skill of reading body tension has been developed, you can use this body information to help with a variety of coping procedures.

If you suffer from tension headaches, pay attention to this muscle group and learn how to relax it, through PMR or through biofeedback. If your headaches are of a different variety (vascular pressure instead of muscular tension), they may not respond to relaxation training as readily as to other types of training, including biofeedback. For now just concentrate on the contrast between tension and relief in this muscle group.

> Wrinkle up your forehead. Squint your eyes if you wish. It can help you feel the tension. You will feel your scalp tighten at the same time. Do not worry about any of these other tensions. Just treat them all as though they belong to one group. Hold the tension. Look at the tension. Turn your mind's eye up and look at it. Then let it go. Completely relaxed. Forehead, scalp, and eyes—all are relaxed. Study the difference. Enjoy the feeling of relaxation. [Repeat the cycle two more times, each time paying attention to difference in the feelings.]

Now we will move to the jaws and tongue. Both of these muscles can be treated independently. I prefer to work only with the jaw muscles for a variety of reasons. If you find yourself having any difficulty achieving complete relaxation of the face, you may want to give the tongue special attention. This is usually done by rolling the tongue up to about the middle of the roof of the mouth. Then, just like doing an isometric exercise, you can push against the roof of the mouth and feel the tightness come into the tongue. Relaxing is merely letting the tongue fall back to its natural resting place in the mouth.

The jaw muscles are frequently involved when stress is occurring. For example, during anger many people clench their jaws. In a slender-cheeked person, one can see the ropelike muscle stand out on the side of the cheek when the jaw is clenched. In some cases of chronic stress, certain people will develop a *tic*, a condition in which a particular muscle group (usually in the jaw or cheek area) twitches convulsively. Tension may be relieved in these muscle groups through the use of relaxation training.

Again, take a deep breath. Hold it. Let it out, saying "Relax" at the same time. Clench your jaws by biting down just as though you were chewing on a stick. Hold it for a moment. Study the sensations, the tightness going all the way up to the ears, the cheeks swelling out as the muscles tighten. Now let it go. Quickly, completely, let the jaw relax. You do not have to open your mouth for the jaws to relax. Just let all the tension go. Observe the difference again between this comfortable easy feeling and the tightness you felt before. [Repeat the tension relaxation cycle twice more.]

Continue relaxing. Enjoy the feeling. Now, take a very deep breath and hold it for a few seconds. Notice the tightness in your chest and diaphragm. Try not to tighten your stomach as you are breathing in. Now, say "Relax" to yourself as you let your breath go. Your whole body just seems to go into relaxation with the release. Try it once more. Breathe deeply. *Tense; hold; observe; relax; observe.* And once more. Breathe deeply; hold; study; relax; and study. Just let the relaxation take hold. You really do not have to do much to relax. It just comes when you let tension go.

Go on breathing easily and naturally for a few moments. While you are coasting, quickly scan your body. Do you notice any muscle tension anywhere? Are your arms still relaxed? Your hands? Your neck and shoulder muscles? Your forehead, eyes, and jaws? If not, quickly relax them again. All of your body is sinking into a pleasant state of heaviness, as though you couldn't lift a finger if you wanted to. Continue to scan and relax and drift and enjoy for a moment longer.

Now, it is time to turn attention to your stomach. Try to pull your stomach in to itself; shrink it by pulling in the muscles around it. It feels somewhat like it does when you have a *knot* in it. It is not all that comfortable. Hold the tightness for a moment and notice the sensations that occur. Try to link up to times when your stomach has been literally tied in knots and see how similar it is. Now, let it go. Let all the tightness, all the tension out. Observe. . . . Feel. . . . Enjoy for a moment. [Repeat the cycle twice.]

Few problems are as distressing as lower back pain. When the pain is of a chronic variety, going on and on without end, it becomes almost unbearable. A variety of conditions may produce or relate to lower back pain. Some people seem to be more prone to express the results of stress through tension in the lower back than in other parts of their bodies. For this reason, it is a good idea to include the lower back as a specific part of your relaxation exercises.

One word of caution is in order. Be very careful if you have had any history of back disorders or have had back surgery! It would be wise to obtain clearance from your physician before engaging in any strenuous back tensing. If permission has been given to proceed or you feel comfortable in going ahead on your own, at the least move into the back tension exercises somewhat gingerly until you are confident that you are not going to produce undue strain.

It is sometimes difficult to get a very good feeling of the pull in the lower back muscles from the prescribed means of producing tension. The instructions given here suggest arching the back—in other words, bending forward, pulling the shoulders slightly in, and making the small of your back stick out relative to the rest of the back. If you find that you are not getting any strong sensation from this technique, you may want to try some alternative approaches. One is to try to roll the back muscles toward each other just as you might roll your shoulders back and toward each other to produce tension there. One problem with this technique is that rolling the muscles may put tension into the stomach at the same time you are putting tension into the back. The arched back approach tends to put less tension into the stomach and more pure pull into the back muscles. This is something you will need to experiment with until you find what is right for you.

Concentrate now on your lower back. Arch your back and feel the pull of the muscles along the spine. Hold this tension for a few seconds. Notice the feeling. Try not to tense the stomach area, if at all possible, while tensing the back muscles. Now let yourself settle back, release the arch in your back, and notice the feeling of relaxation settling into your back. Enjoy the pleasant feeling for a few seconds, and once again arch your back, study the sensations of tightness, and release. [Repeat one more time.] Each time you let go, try to get a picture in your mind of the muscles letting go and relaxing.

Continue to breathe calmly and easily. Keep your head resting gently on your chest. And squeeze your buttocks together, just as though you were trying to shut off your sphincter muscle. You may feel your hips and sphincter all tighten up together. That's all right. Hold for a few seconds while you tune in to the signals of tightness. Now let the muscle tension go. Relax and observe. Pay attention to the difference. [And repeat the cycle twice.]

Now concentrate on your legs, starting with the thighs. Do just your right thigh first [left if you prefer]. Tighten the large muscles on the back of your legs. Think of it as though you were pushing against something, as though you were climbing a mountain or a set of steps. Pull your upper leg muscles as tight as you can without tightening your calves, feet, and toes. And study the feeling. Hold it for a few seconds. Now let go. Study the contrast, how pleasant the relief is. Feel the difference. [Then repeat the cycle two more times. Then do the same thing three times with your left thigh, or your right thigh if you started with the left.]

Now, attend to the calves and feet. Again, just concentrate on your right leg [left if preferred]. Pull your foot toward your body, tightening your calf muscle as you do. Be careful not to pull so hard that you start a cramp in the muscle. Hold it for a moment and notice how it feels. Then let the tension go. Just let it loose all at once. And notice the difference. For a moment, let the relaxation settle on you and enjoy the comfortable heaviness throughout your body and in your leg. [Tense and relax two more times for the right leg. Then tense and relax three times for the left leg.]

Every part of your body is relaxed. Breathe easily, peacefully. And feel how good it feels when the body is completely relaxed. Without stirring or changing positions, scan your entire body. Tune in to any signs of tension anywhere. If any parts have tension, relax them again. Take a deep breath and hold it for a short while. Then let it go and say to yourself, "Relax." Drift for a moment and feel the pleasant sensation of having all the tension drained out of your body. Take some time [about one or two minutes] to experience this feeling of relaxing.

Now I am going to count backward from three to one. On the count of one, I want you to open your eyes slowly, raise your head, and just as though you were waking up from a nap, reach your arms over your head and stretch.

Three. . .two. . .one. And you are done with your first relaxation session.

Preparing Your Own Relaxation Instructions

In general, there are four basic methods of presenting the instructions. First, you could try to recall the gist of the instructions and *think* yourself through the entire relaxation exercise without any external prompts. In some ways, this is the preferred technique because then you can take relaxation with you to the office or on the road wherever you are. You want the technique to be something very private, even in public. You want to be able to relax in the board meeting, on the plane, or at the church bazaar. If you have the procedure as an internally controlled routine, this is possible. Try to persevere with this internal-control procedure through the first week or two. You should find the routine becoming virtually habitual. You may even come to *see* with the mind's eye your muscles relaxing in the prescribed sequence. That is, you will be able to relax without thinking specifically about each and every muscle, without having to tell yourself verbally each and every instructional set. This is the ideal, the goal to which you should aspire. Any of the other techniques suggested below should be regarded as intermediate steps to be used only in the early stages and abandoned as soon as possible.

As a second alternative, you can have someone read the instructions for you the first few times. This will relieve you of the need to concentrate on both the sequence and the relaxing. It will free you to tune in on the differing sensations of relaxation and tension. You will probably acquire an incidental feel for the sequence and the logic of the procedure just by being guided through it by spouse or friend. In a short time, you will probably sense that the external prompts are no longer necessary and you will very naturally move to the optimal situation described in the first method.

The third approach is to tape the instructions in your own voice on a cassette recorder. Once you have put the instructions on tape, you are free to concentrate on the relaxation exercises without undue worry about what should come next. In addition, should you decide to have a friend handle the instructions initially, your friend may not always be available. The taped instructions provide you with a backup. Also, you might use relaxation for a period of time and then let it go for a while. When you return to it, you might feel rusty. A taped set of instructions can help you get back in the groove very quickly and efficiently.

Fourth, you could buy a commercially prepared tape that gives the complete instructional sequence. Several publishing companies offer tapes of this variety, ranging from very inexpensive to quite expensive.

Instructions for Reducing the Steps by Grouping Muscles

You should have a good working knowledge of the basic instructions and sequence for relaxing. In fact, you may have already weaned yourself from whatever instructional prompts—tapes or friend—you were using early in your practice. If so, all you need for this new step is to *read* the instructions with the very slight modifications suggested below. If you are still dependent on a tape or friend to give the instructions to you, then you may want to set up an alternate tape, or provide your friend with a new listing of the instructions following the suggested modifications. Remember that each session starts with the deep breathing exercise before going into the first tension-relaxation cycle.

Now I want you to take a few deep breaths, hold each breath for a few seconds, and then let each breath out fully and completely. As you breathe in, you will notice some tension in your chest and diaphragm. As you breathe out, you will notice a sense of relaxing, almost going limp. Relaxing feels good and comfortable and it would be nice if the feeling could be kept. But as you breathe in deeply again, you feel the same tension as before, especially as you hold it for a moment. Let the breath out again, completely, and feel the pleasant relaxing sensation of letting go. Try it one more time. Dwell for just a moment on the sense of relaxation as you let this breath out.

Try to maintain that relaxation in your chest and diaphragm. As you breathe from now on, breathe easily and naturally, almost as though you were napping.

Concentrate for a moment on both your arms. How do they feel? Flex the biceps on both your arms as though you were showing off your muscles.

Flex them as tight as you can and hold [for about 10 seconds]. As you keep both biceps flexed, notice the sensation of tension. Notice how unpleasant it can be. Now let it go all at once. Let your arms go completely limp. Relax! And study the contrast. Notice how different it is from tension. Store the contrast in your mind even as you are studying it. One more time. Tense your biceps and hold the tension. Observe the feeling of tightness. Tune in to the signal of tension in your muscles. Then let it go. Become completely relaxed. If someone picked your arms up and let them loose, they would simply drop to your side. There is no tension at all. It feels so good. One more time: *tense; hold; observe; relax; and observe.*

Notice what has changed in the instructions. Instead of telling yourself to relax only the preferred arm, you tell yourself to relax both arms. This grouping of muscles can be done all the way through the instructions you have learned. For each of the eight steps listed in the chart, simply modify the instructions accordingly. Otherwise, the instructions remain the same, as will be shown. Continue the same pattern: tense, hold, observe, relax, and observe.

For the sake of simplicity, I have used the generic word *relax.* You should note that the particular word, however, is relatively unimportant. Select a word that is of significance to you. It may be better to actually use some other word than *relax* because of the frequency with which that word is used in everyday communication. Your personal cue word can be very secret, very unique. Whatever you select as that word, however, use it consistently. Simply substitute it in the instructions anytime you read "Relax."

Cue-Controlled Relaxation Instructions

Breathe in deeply. Hold the breath for approximately 10 seconds. Then let the breath out completely as you are saying your personal cue word. Also, as you say the cue word, let your entire body go limp. Go immediately into a state of deep relaxation. It may help to form a mental picture of your whole body going limp, as though you are seeing yourself at the end of one of your regular relaxation sessions. Take a moment to evaluate subjectively how good and deep the feeling of relaxation is.

Do this from about 15 to 20 times, but no more. Now for the important part: At any time during the 15 or more cycles, should you feel that your relaxation is even 50 to 75% as good and deep as you have been getting through the tension-relaxation cycles, congratulate yourself and count the session a success. Complete the minimum of 15 cycles and go on relaxing for your normal length of time.

If you are not able to get relaxed to the 50 to 75% level, stop after the 20th cycle. Then *wait until the next relaxation period to try the deep breathing-cue word-relaxation cycle again by itself.* But before you quit, go back to the usual tension-relaxation cycle and get the fullest depth of relaxation possible. Then enjoy your normal period of relaxing. Remember that you should always use the breathing–cue-word cycles a few times in your tension-relaxation cycles as you have been taught from the beginning.

References

Abella, R., & Heslin, R. (1984, May). *Health locus of control, values, and the behavior of family and friends: An integrated approach to understanding preventive health behavior.* Paper presented at the Midwestern Psychological Association Conference, Chicago.

Abramson, L. Y., Seligman, M. E. P., & Teasdale, J. D. (1978). Learned helplessness in humans: Critique and reformulation. *Journal of Abnormal Psychology, 87,* 49–74.

Adams, J. H., Hayes, J., & Hopson, B. (1976). *Transition: Understanding and managing personal change.* London: Martin Robertson.

Ader, R. (1983). Developmental psychoneuroimmunology. *Developmental Psychobiology, 16,* 251–267.

Ader, R., Cohen, N., & Felten, D. L. (1987). Brain, behavior, and immunity. *Brain, Behavior, and Immunity, 1,* 1–6.

Adler, J. (1997, June 2). Road rage: We're driven to destruction. *Newsweek, 129*(22), 70.

Aldwin, C. M. (1994). *Stress, coping, and development: An integrative perspective.* New York: Guilford.

Alexander, C. N., Robinson, P., Orme-Johnson, D. W., Schneider, R. H., & Walton, K. G. (1994). The effects of transcendental meditation compared to other methods of relaxation and meditation in reducing risk factors, morbidity, and mortality. *Homeostasis, 35,* 243–263.

Alexander, F. (1939). Emotional factors in essential hypertension. *Psychosomatic Medicine, 1,* 173–179.

Alexander, F. (1950). *Psychosomatic medicine: Its principles and applications.* New York: Norton.

Allport, G. (1937). *Personality: A psychological interpretation.* New York: Henry Holt.

Allport, G. W. (1961). *Pattern and growth in personality.* New York: Holt, Rinehart & Winston.

Allred, K., & Smith, T. W. (1989). The hardy personality: Cognitive and physiological responses to evaluative threat. *Journal of Personality and Social Psychology, 56,* 257–266.

Alster, K. B. (1989). *The holistic health movement.* Tuscaloosa: The University of Alabama Press.

Alterman, A. I., & Tarter, R. E. (1983). The transmission of psychological vulnerability: Implications for alcoholism etiology. *The Journal of Nervous and Mental Disease, 171,* 147–154.

Altmaier, E. M., Ross, S. L., Leary, M. R., & Thornbrough, M. (1982). Matching stress inoculation's treatment components to clients' anxiety mode. *Journal of Counseling Psychology, 29,* 331–334.

Amato, P. R. (1996). A prospective study of divorce and parent-child relationships. *Journal of Marriage and the Family, 58,* 356–365.

Amato, P. R., & Keith, B. (1991). Parental divorce and the well-being of children: A meta-analysis. *Psychological Bulletin, 110,* 26–46.

American Heart Association. (1997). Physical activity and cardiovascular health fact sheet. Retrieved March 21, 1997, from the World Wide Web: http://www.amhrt.org/heartscore97/PAfact.html.

American Lung Association. (1997). American Lung Association fact sheet—Smoking cessation resources. Retrieved April 4, 1997, from the World Wide Web: http://www.lungusa.org.

American Psychiatric Association. (1994). *Diagnostic and statistical manual of mental disorders* (4th ed.). Washington, DC: Author.

Anand, B. K., Chhina, G. S., & Singh, B. (1961a). Some aspects of electroencephalographic studies in Yogis. *Electroencephalography and Clinical Neurophysiology, 13,* 452–456.

Anand, B. K., Chhina, G. S., & Singh, B. (1961b). Studies on Shri Ramananda Yogi during his stay in an air-tight box. *Indian Journal of Medical Research, 49,* 82–89.

Anastasi, A. (1988). *Psychological testing* (6th ed.). New York: Macmillan.

Anderson, J. R. (1990). *Cognitive psychology and its implications* (3rd ed.). New York: W. H. Freeman.

Anderson, N. B., Lawrence, R. S., & Olson, T. W. (1981). Within-subject analysis of autogenic training and cognitive coping training in the treatment of tension headache pain. *Journal of Behavior Therapy and Experimental Psychiatry, 12,* 219–223.

Anderson, R. N., Kochanek, K. D., & Murphy, S. L. (1997). Report of final mortality statistics, 1995. *Monthly Vital Statistics Report, 45*(11), Suppl. 2, Table 7.

Aneshensel, C. S. (1992). Social stress: Theory and research. *Annual Review of Sociology, 18,* 15–38.

Angell, M. (1985). Disease as a reflection of the psyche. *The New England Journal of Medicine, 312,* 1570–1572.

Associated Press. (1997, October 16). Road rage 101: Driver's ed teacher attacks motorist. *The Forum,* A1.

Apao, W. K., & Damon, A. M. (1982). Locus of control and the quantity-frequency index of alcohol use. *Journal of Studies on Alcohol, 43,* 233–239.

Arbeit, J. M. (1990). Molecules, cancer, and the surgeon. *Annals of Surgery, 212,* 3–13.

Armstrong, M. S., & Vaughan, K. (1996). An orienting response model of eye movement desensitization. *Journal of Behavior Therapy & Experimental Psychiatry, 27,* 21–32.

Aslan, S., Nelson, L., Carruthers, M., & Lader, M. (1981). Stress and age effects on catecholamines in normal subjects. *Journal of Psychosomatic Research, 25,* 33–41.

Assael, M., Naor, S., Pecht, M., Trainin, N., & Samuel, D. (1981). *Correlation between emotional reaction to loss of loved object and lymphocyte response to mitogenic stimulation in women.* Paper presented at the Sixth World Congress of the International College of Psychosomatic Medicine, Quebec, Canada.

Averill, J. R. (1973). Personal control over aversive stimuli and its relationship to stress. *Psychological Bulletin, 80,* 286–303.

Ax, A. F. (1953). The physiological differentiation of fear and anger in humans. *Psychosomatic Medicine, 15,* 433–442.

Baekeland, F., & Lundwall, L. (1975). Dropping out of treatment: A critical review. *Psychological Bulletin, 82,* 738–783.

Bagchi, B. K., & Wenger, M. A. (1957). Electrophysiological correlates of some Yogi exercises. *EEG Clinical Neurophysiology* (Supplement No. 7), 132–149.

Ballor, D. L., Becque, M. D., Marks, C. R., Nau, K. L., & Katch, V. L. (1989). Physiological responses to nine different exercise: Rest protocols. *Medicine and Science in Sports and Exercise, 21,* 90–95.

Bandura, A. (1973). *Aggression: A social learning analysis.* Englewood Cliffs, NJ: Prentice-Hall.

Bandura, A. (1977). Self-efficacy: Toward a unifying theory of behavioral change. *Psychological Review, 84,* 191–215.

Bandura, A. (1989). Human agency in social cognitive theory. *American Psychologist, 44,* 1175–1184.

Bandura, A., Reese, L., & Adams, N. E. (1982). Microanalysis of action and fear arousal as a function of differential levels of perceived self-efficacy. *Journal of Personality and Social Psychology, 43,* 5–21.

Barker, R. G. (1968). *Ecological psychology: Concepts and methods for studying the environment of human behavior.* Stanford, CA: Stanford University Press.

Barofsky, I. (1981). Issues and approaches to the psychosocial assessment of the cancer patient. In C. K. Prokop & L. A. Bradley (Eds.), *Medical psychology: Contributions to behavioral medicine* (pp. 55–65). New York: Academic Press.

Baron, R. M., & Needel, S. R. (1980). Toward an understanding of the differences in the responses of humans and other animals to density. *Psychological Review, 87,* 320–326.

Bartlett, F. C. (1932). *Remembering: A study in experimental and social psychology.* London: Cambridge University Press.

Bartlett, S. J., Wadden, T. A., & Vogt, R. A. (1996). Psychosocial consequences of weight cycling. *Journal of Consulting and Clinical Psychology, 64,* 587–592.

Bartrop, R. W., Lazarus, L., Luckhurst, E., Kiloh, L. G., & Penny, R. (1977). Depressed lymphocyte function after bereavement. *Lancet, 1,* 834–836.

Batchelor, W. F. (1984). AIDS: A public health and psychological emergency. *American Psychologist, 39,* 1279–1284.

Batchelor, W. F. (1988). AIDS 1988: The science and limits of science. *American Psychologist, 43,* 853–858.

Baum, A. (1990). Stress, intrusive imagery, and chronic stress. *Health Psychology, 9,* 653–675.

Baum, A., Fleming, R., & Singer, J. (1983). Coping with victimization by technological disaster. *Journal of Social Issues, 39,* 117–138.

Baum, A., & Koman, S. (1976). Differential response to anticipated crowding: Psychological effects of social and spatial density. *Journal of Personality and Social Psychology, 34,* 526–536.

Baum, A., Singer, J. E., & Baum, C. S. (1981). Stress and the environment. *Journal of Social Issues, 37,* 4–35.

Baum, A., & Valins, S. (1979). Architectural mediation of residential density and control: Crowding and the regulation of social contact. In L. Berkowitz (Ed.), *Advances in experimental social psychology* (Vol. 12, pp. 131–175). New York: Academic Press.

Beehr, T. A., & Newman, J. E. (1978). Job stress, employee health, and organizational effectiveness: A facet analysis, model, and literature review. *Personnel Psychology, 31,* 655–699.

Behanan, K. T. (1964). *Yoga: A scientific evaluation.* New York: Dover.

Bellack, A. S., & Hersen, M. (Eds.). (1988). *Behavioral assessment: A practical handbook* (3rd ed.). New York: Pergamon.

Belsky, J. (1980). Child maltreatment: An ecological integration. *American Psychologist, 35,* 320–335.

Benson, H. (1975). *The relaxation response.* New York: Avon.

Berg, W. E., & Johnson, R. (1979). Assessing the impact of victimization: Acquisition of the victim role among elderly and female victims. In W. H. Parsonage (Ed.), *Perspectives on victimology* (pp. 58–71). Newbury Park, CA: Sage.

Berkowitz, L. (1990). On the formation and regulation of anger and aggression: A cognitive-neoassociationistic analysis. *American Psychologist, 45,* 494–503.

Bernstein, D. A., & Borkovec, T. D. (1978). *Progressive relaxation training: A manual for the helping professions.* Champaign, IL: Research Press.

Berntson, G. G., Cacioppo, J. T., & Quigley, K. S. (1991). Autonomic determinism: The modes of autonomic control, the doctrine of autonomic space, and the laws of autonomic constraint. *Psychological Review, 98,* 459–487.

Bexton, W. H., Heron, W., & Scott, T. H. (1954). Effects of decreased variation in the sensory environment. *Canadian Journal of Psychology, 8,* 70–76.

Blai, B. (1989). Health consequences of loneliness: A review of the literature. *Journal of the American College of Health, 37,* 162–167.

Blanchard, E. B., Andrasik, F., Neff, D. F., Arena, J. G., Ahles, T. A., Jurish, S. E., Pallmeyer, T. P., Saunders, N. L., Teders, S. J., Barron, K. D., & Rodichok, L. D. (1982). Biofeedback and relaxation training with three kinds of headache: Treatment effects and their prediction. *Journal of Consulting and Clinical Psychology, 50,* 562–575.

Blanchard, E. B., Appelbaum, K. A., Guarnieri, P., Neff, D. F., Andrasik, F., Jaccard, J., & Barron, K. D. (1988). Two studies of the long-term follow-up of minimal therapist contact treatments of vascular and tension headache. *Journal of Consulting and Clinical Psychology, 56,* 427–432.

Blanchard, E. B., & Haynes, M. R. (1975). Biofeedback treatment of a case of Raynaud's disease. *Journal of Behavior Therapy & Experimental Psychiatry, 6,* 230–234.

Blanchard, E. B., McCoy, G. C., Berger, M., Musso, A., Pallmeyer, T. R., Gerardi, R. J., Gerardi, M. A., & Pangburn, L. (1989). A controlled comparison of thermal biofeedback and relaxation training in the treatment of essential hypertension: IV. Prediction of short-term clinical outcome. *Behavior Therapy, 20,* 405–415.

Blanchard, E. B., McCoy, G. C., Musso, A., Gerardi, M. A., Pallmeyer, T. R., Gerardi, R. J., Cotch, P. A., Siracusa, K., & Andrasik, F. (1986). A controlled comparison of thermal biofeedback and relaxation training in the treatment of essential hypertension: I. Short-term and long-term outcome. *Behavior Therapy, 17,* 563–579.

Blanchard, E. B., Schwarz, S. R., & Radnitz, C. R. (1987). Psychological assessment and treatment of irritable bowel syndrome. *Behavior Modification, 11,* 348–372.

Blechman, E. A., & Brownell, K. D. (Eds.). (1988). *Handbook of behavioral medicine for women.* New York: Pergamon.

Blessing, W. W., Sved, A. F., & Reis, D. J. (1982). Destruction of noradrenergic neurons in rabbit brainstem elevates plasma vasopressin, causing hypertension. *Science, 217,* 661–663.

Bliss, E. C. (1976). *Getting things done: The ABCs of time management.* New York: Scribner's.

Bloom, B. L., Asher, S. J., & White, S. W. (1978). Marital disruption as a stressor: A review and analysis. *Psychological Bulletin, 85,* 867–894.

Bloomfield, H. H., Cain, M. R., Jaffe, D. T., & Kory, R. B. (1975). *TM: Discovering inner energy and overcoming stress.* New York: Dell.

Blum, K., Noble, E. P., Sheridan, P. J., & Finley, O. (1991). Association of the A1 allele of the D-sub-2 dopamine receptor gene with severe alcoholism. *Alcohol, 8,* 409–416.

Blumberg, M. (1974). Psychopathology of the abusing parent. *American Journal of Psychotherapy, 28,* 21–29.

Blumenthal, J. A., Barefoot, J., Burg, M. M., & Williams, R. B. (1987). Psychological correlates of hostility among patients undergoing coronary angiography. *British Journal of Medical Psychology, 60,* 349–355.

Boerstler, R. W. (1986). Meditation and the dying process. *Journal of Humanistic Psychology, 26,* 104–124.

Bolger, N., & Zuckerman, A. (1995). A framework for studying personality in the stress process. *Journal of Personality and Social Psychology, 69,* 890–902.

Booth, G. (1969). General and organ-specific object relationships in cancer. *Annals of the New York Academy of Sciences, 164,* 568–577.

Booth-Kewley, S., & Friedman, H. S. (1987). Psychological predictors of heart disease: A quantitative review. *Psychological Bulletin, 101,* 343–362.

Booth-Kewley, S., & Vickers, R. R., Jr. (1994). Associations between major domains of personality and health behavior. *Journal of Personality, 62,* 281–298.

Boss, P. G. (1988). *Family stress management.* Newbury Park, CA: Sage.

Bost, J. M. (1984). Retaining students on academic probation: Effects of time management peer counseling on students' grades. *Journal of Learning Skills, 3,* 38–43.

Boulenger, J. R., Salem, N., Marangos, R. J., & Uhde, T. W. (1987). Plasma adenosine levels: Measurement in humans and relationship to the anxiogenic effects of caffeine. *Psychiatry Research, 21,* 247–255.

Brady, J. V., Porter, R. W., Conrad, D. G., & Mason, J. W. (1958). Avoidance behavior and the development of gastroduodenal ulcers. *Journal of the Experimental Analysis of Behavior, 1,* 69–72.

Branson, S. M., & Craig, K. D. (1988). Children's spontaneous strategies for coping with pain: A review of the literature. *Canadian Journal of Behavioural Science, 20,* 402–412.

Bremner, J. D., Southwick, S. M., & Charney, D. S. (1995). Etiological factors in the development of posttraumatic stress disorder. In C. M. Mazure (Ed.), *Does stress cause psychiatric illness?* (pp. 149–185). Washington, DC: American Psychiatric Press.

Brenner, A. (1984). *Helping children cope with stress.* Lexington, MA: Lexington Books.

Brenner, M. H. (1973). *Mental illness and the economy.* Cambridge, MA: Harvard University Press.

Brent, R. L. (1972). *The god-men of India.* London: Allen Lane.

Brett, J. F., Brief, A. P., Burke, M. J., George, J. M., & Webster, J. (1990). Negative affectivity and the reporting of stressful life events. *Health Psychology, 9,* 57–68.

Brewin, C. R. (1988). Explanation and adaptation in adversity. In S. Fisher & J. Reason (Eds.), *Handbook of life stress, cognition and health* (pp. 423–439). New York: Wiley.

Bridge, T. P. (1988). AIDS and HIV CNS disease: A neuropsychiatric disorder. In T. P. Bridge, A. F. Mirsky, & F. K. Goodwin (Eds.), *Psychological, neuropsychiatric, and substance abuse aspects of AIDS* (pp. 1–13). New York: Raven Press.

Brod, C. (1982). Managing technostress: Optimizing the use of computer technology. *Personnel Journal, 61,* 753–757.

Brod, C. (1988). *Technostress: Human cost of the computer revolution.* Reading, MA: Addison-Wesley.

Bronzaft, A. L., & McCarthy, D. P. (1975). The effects of elevated train noise on reading ability. *Environment and Behavior, 7,* 517–527.

Brooks, J. (1981). The fear of crime in the United States. In B. Galaway & J. Hudson (Eds.), *Perspectives on crime victims* (pp. 90–92). St. Louis, MO: C. V. Mosby.

Brooks, J. S., & Scarano, T. (1985). Transcendental meditation in the treatment of post-Vietnam adjustment. *Journal of Consulting and Development, 64,* 212–215.

Brownell, K. D., Marlatt, G. A., Lichtenstein, E., & Wilson, G. T. (1986). Understanding and preventing relapse. *American Psychologist, 41,* 765–782.

Bruning, N. S., & Frew, D. R. (1987). Effects of exercise, relaxation, and management skills training on physiological stress indicators: A field experiment. *Journal of Applied Psychology, 72,* 515–521.

Budzynski, T., Stoyva, J., & Adler, C. (1970). Feedback-induced muscle relaxation: Application to tension headache. *Journal of Behavior Therapy & Experimental Psychiatry, 4,* 205–211.

Budzynski, T. H., Stoyva, J. M., Adler, C. S., & Mullaney, D. J. (1973). EMG biofeedback and tension headache: A controlled outcome study. *Psychosomatic Medicine, 35,* 484–496.

Bulman, R. J., & Wortman, C. B. (1977). Attribution of blame and coping in the "real world": Severe accident victims react to their lot. *Journal of Personality and Social Psychology, 35,* 351–363.

Bureau of Justice. (1997). *Violent crime rate trends.* Retrieved November 1997 from the World Wide Web: http://www.ojp.usdoj.gov/bjs.

Burgess, A. W. (1983). Rape trauma syndrome. *Behavioral Sciences and the Law, 1,* 97–113.

Burish, T. G. (1981). EMG biofeedback in the treatment of stress-related disorders. In C. K. Prokop & L. A. Bradley (Eds.), *Medical psychology: Contributions to behavioral medicine* (pp. 395–421). New York: Academic Press.

Burish, T. G., Vasterling, J. J., Carey, M. R., Matt, D. A., & Krozely, M. G. (1988). Posttreatment use of relaxation training by cancer patients. *The Hospice Journal, 4,* 1–8.

Burke, R. J. (1986). Occupational and life stress and the family: Conceptual frameworks and research findings. *International Review of Applied Psychology, 35,* 347–368.

Burny, A. (1986, May). More and better trans-activation. *Nature, 321,* 378.

Burstein, A. G., & Loucks, S. (1982). The psychologist as health care clinician. In T. Millon, C. Green, & R. Meagher (Eds.), *Handbook of clinical health psychology* (pp. 175–189). New York: Plenum.

Buss, A. H., & Plomin, R. (1975). *A temperament theory of personality development.* New York: Wiley.

Byrne, D., & Clore, G. L. (1970). A reinforcement model of evaluative responses. *Personality: An International Journal, 1,* 103–128.

Calnan, M. W., & Moss, S. (1984). The Health Belief Model and compliance with education given at a class in breast self-examination. *Journal of Health and Social Behavior, 25,* 198–210.

Cameron, R., & Best, J. A. (1987). Promoting adherence to health behavior change interventions: Recent findings from behavioral research. *Patient Education and Counseling, 10,* 139–154.

Camp, D. E., Klesges, R. C., & Relyea, G. (1993). The relationship between body weight concerns and adolescent smoking. *Health Psychology, 12,* 24–32.

Campbell, J. M., Amerikaner, M., Swank, P., & Vincent, K. (1989). The relationship between the Hardiness Test and the Personal Orientation Inventory. *Journal of Research in Personality, 23,* 373–380.

Cannon, W. B. (1932). *The wisdom of the body.* New York: Norton.

Caplan, G., & Killilea, M. (1976). *Support systems and mutual help: Multidisciplinary explorations.* New York: Grune & Stratton.

Capra, E. (1982). *The turning point.* New York: Simon & Schuster.

Carlson, C. R., & Hoyle, R. H. (1993). Efficacy of abbreviated progressive muscle relaxation training: A quantitative review of behavioral medicine research. *Journal of Consulting and Clinical Psychology, 61,* 1059–1067.

Carroll, L. (1966). *Alice's adventures in wonderland.* New York: Macmillan. (Original work published 1865).

Carron, A. V., Widmeyer, W. N., & Brawley, L. R. (1988). Group cohesion and individual adherence to physical activity. *Journal of Sport and Exercise Psychology, 10,* 127–138.

Carton, J. S., & Schweitzer, J. B. (1996). Use of a token economy to increase compliance during hemodialysis. *Journal of Applied Behavior Analysis, 29,* 111–113.

Carver, C. S. (1989). How should multifaceted personality constructs be tested? Issues illustrated by self-monitoring, attributional style, and hardiness. *Journal of Personality and Social Psychology, 56,* 577–585.

Carver, C. S., & Scheier, M. F. (1981). *Attention and self-regulation: A control-theory approach to human behavior.* New York: Springer-Verlag.

Carver, C. S., & Scheier, M. F. (1982). Control theory: A useful conceptual framework for personality-social, clinical, and health psychology. *Psychological Bulletin, 92,* 111–135.

Centers for Disease Control. (1992, May 22). Discomfort from environmental tobacco smoke among employees at worksites with minimal smoking restrictions—United States, 1988. *MMWR—Mortality and Morbidity Weekly Reports, 41,* 351–354.

Centers for Disease Control. (1992, September 18). Tobacco, alcohol, and other drug use among high school students—United States, 1991. *MMWR—Mortality and Morbidity Weekly Reports, 41,* 698–703.

Centers for Disease Control. (1996, September 6). Physical violence and injuries in intimate relationships—New York, Behavioral Risk Factor Surveillance System, 1994. *MMWR—Mortality and Morbidity Weekly Reports, 44,* 765–767.

Centers for Disease Control and Prevention. (1997a). *HIV/AIDS surveillance report, 9*(1), 1–37.

Centers for Disease Control and Prevention. (1997b). *Suicide in the United States.* Found at http://www.cdc.gov/ncipc/dvp/suifacts.htm.

Chapman, S. L. (1986). A review and clinical perspective on the use of EMG and thermal biofeedback for chronic headaches. *Pain, 27,* 1–43.

Charlesworth, E. A., Murphy, S., & Beutler, L. E. (1981). Stress management skill for nursing students, *Journal of Clinical Psychology, 37,* 284–290.

Clark, J. M., & Paivio, A. (1989). Observational and theoretical terms in psychology: A cognitive perspective on scientific language. *American Psychologist, 44,* 500–512.

Cline, D. W., & Westman, J. C. (1971). The impact of divorce on the family. *Child Psychiatry and Human Development, 2,* 135–139.

Clingman, J. M., & Hilliard, D. V. (1987). Some personality characteristics of the superadherer: Following those who go beyond fitness. *Journal of Sport Behavior, 10,* 123–136.

Cobb, S. (1974). Physiological changes in men whose jobs were abolished. *Journal of Psychosomatic Research, 18,* 245–258.

Cobb, S. (1976). Social support as a moderator of life stress. *Psychosomatic Medicine, 38,* 300–314.

Cockerham, W. C. (1982). *Medical sociology* (2nd ed.). Englewood Cliffs, NJ: Prentice-Hall.

Coffin, J., Haase, A., Levy, J. A., Mautagnier, L., Oroszlan, S., Teich, N., et al. (1986). What to call the AIDS virus? *Nature 321,* 10.

Cohen, L., & Roth, S. (1984). Coping with abortion. *Journal of Human Stress, 10,* 140–145.

Cohen, R. A., Williamson, D. A., Monguillot, J. E., Hutchinson, R. C., Gottlieb, J., & Waters, W. E. (1983). Psychophysiological response patterns in vascular and muscle-contraction headaches. *Journal of Behavioral Medicine, 6,* 93–107.

Cohen, S. (1988). Psychosocial models of the role of social support in the etiology of physical disease. *Health Psychology, 7,* 269–297.

Cohen, S., Evans, G. W., Krantz, D. S., & Stokols, D. (1980). Physiological, motivational, and cognitive effects of aircraft noise on children: Moving from the laboratory to the field. *American Psychologist, 35,* 231–243.

Cohen, S., Kessler, R. C., & Gordon, L. U. (Eds.). (1995). *Measuring stress: A guide for health and social scientists.* New York: Oxford University Press.

Cohen, S., & Syme, S. L. (Eds.). (1985). *Social support and health.* New York: Academic.

Cohen, S., Tyrrell, D. A. J., & Smith, A. P. (1991). Psychological stress and susceptibility to the common cold. *The New England Journal of Medicine, 325,* 606–612.

Cohen, S., & Wills, T. A. (1985). Stress, social support, and the buffering hypothesis. *Psychological Bulletin, 98,* 310–357.

Coile, D. C., & Miller, N. E. (1984). How radical animal activists try to mislead humane people. *American Psychologist, 39,* 700–701.

Colletta, N. D. (1983). Stressful lives: The situation of divorced mothers and their children. *Journal of Divorce, 6,* 19–31.

Conger, R., Burgess, R., & Barrett, C. (1979). Child abuse related to life change and perceptions of illness: Some preliminary findings. *Family Coordinator, 28,* 73–78.

Conger, R. D., & Elder, G. H., Jr. (1994). *Families in troubled times: Adapting to change in rural America.* New York: A. de Gruyter.

Connolly, H. M., Crary, J. L., McGoon, M. D., Hensrud, D. D., Edwards, B. S., Edwards, W. D., & Schaff, H. V. (1997). Valvular heart disease associated with fenfluramine-phentermine. *New England Journal of Medicine, 337,* 581–588.

Contrada, R. J. (1989). Type A behavior, personality hardiness, and cardiovascular responses to stress. *Journal of Personality and Social Psychology, 57,* 895–903.

Cook, T. D., & Campbell, D. T. (1979). *Quasi-experimentation: Design and analysis issues for field settings.* Chicago: Rand McNally.

Cooper, C. L. (1983). Identifying stressors at work: Recent research developments. *Journal of Psychosomatic Research, 27,* 369–376.

Cordes, C. L., & Dougherty, T. W. (1993). A review and an integration of research on job burnout. *Academy of Management Review, 18,* 621–656.

Cotler, S. B., & Guerra, J. J. (1980). *Assertion training.* Champaign, IL: Research Press.

Coyne, J. C., & Holroyd, K. (1982). Stress, coping, and illness: A transactional perspective. In T. Millon, C. Green, & R. Meagher, *Handbook of clinical health psychology* (pp. 103–127). New York: Plenum.

Coyne, J. C., & Lazarus, R. S. (1980). Cognitive style, stress perception, and coping. In I. L. Kutash, L. B. Schlesinger, & Associates (Eds.), *Handbook on stress and anxiety* (pp. 144–158). San Francisco: Jossey-Bass.

Crabbe, J. C., Belknap, J. K., & Buck, K. J. (1995). Genetic animal models of alcohol and drug abuse. *Science, 264,* 1715–1723.

Craig, S. B., Bandini, L. G., Lichtenstein, A. H., Schaefer, E. J., & Dietz, W. H. (1996). The impact of physical activity on lipids, lipoproteins, and blood pressure in preadolescent girls. *Pediatrics, 98,* 389–395.

Cramer, S. H., Keitel, M. A., & Rossberg, R. H. (1986). The family and employed mothers. *International Journal of Family Psychiatry, 7,* 17–34.

Crawford, A. N. (1996). Stigma associated with AIDS: A meta-analysis. *Journal of Applied Social Psychology, 26,* 398–416.

Crews, D. J., & Landers, D. M. (1987). A meta-analytic review of aerobic fitness and reactivity to psychosocial stressors. *Medicine and Science in Sports and Exercise, 19,* S114–S120.

Crump, J. H. (1979). Review of stress in air traffic control: Its measurement and effects. *Aviation, Space, and Environmental Medicine, 50,* 243–248.

Cullen, M. R., Cherniack, M. G., & Rosenstock, L. (1990a). Occupational medicine [First of two parts]. *The New England Journal of Medicine, 322,* 594–601.

Cullen, M. R., Cherniack, M. G., & Rosenstock, L. (1990b). Occupational medicine [Second of two parts]. *The New England Journal of Medicine, 322,* 675–683.

Cunningham, A. J. (1985). The influence of mind on cancer. *Canadian Psychology, 26,* 13–29.

Curran, D. (1987). *Stress and the healthy family.* San Francisco: Harper & Row.

Czajkowski, S. M., Hindelang, R. D., Dembroski, T. M., Mayerson, S. E., Parks, E. B., & Holland, J. C. (1990). Aerobic fitness, psychological characteristics, and cardiovascular reactivity to stress. *Health Psychology, 9,* 676–692.

Czeisler, C. A., Johnson, M. P., Duffy, J. F., Brown, E. N., Ronda, J. M., & Kronauer, R. E. (1990). Exposure to bright light and darkness to treat physiologic maladaptation to night work. *The New England Journal of Medicine, 322,* 1253–1259.

Dahrendorf, R. (1979). *Lebenschancen.* Frankfurt G. M.: Suhrkamp. Cited in H. Strassei & S. Randall (1981), *An introduction to theories of social change.* London: Routledge & Kegan Paul.

Dan, A. J., Pinsof, D. A., & Riggs, L. L. (1995). Sexual harassment as an occupational hazard in nursing. *Basic and Applied Social Psychology, 17,* 563–580.

Dantzer, R., & Kelley, K. W. (1989). Stress and immunity: An integrated view of relationships between the brain and the immune system. *Life Sciences, 44,* 1995–2008.

Dattore, P. J., Shontz, R. C., & Coyne, L. (1980). Premorbid personality differentiation of cancer and noncancer groups: A test of the hypothesis of cancer proneness. *Journal of Consulting and Clinical Psychology, 48,* 388–394.

David, D., Mellman, T. A., Mendoza, L. M., Kulick-Bell, R., Ironson, G., & Schneiderman, N. (1996). Psychiatric morbidity following Hurricane Andrew. *Journal of Traumatic Stress, 9,* 607–612.

Daviglus, M. L., Stamler, J., Orencia, A. J., Dyer, A. R., Liu, K., Greenland, P., Walsh, M. K., Morris, D., & Shekelle, R. B. (1997). Fish consumption and the 30-year risk of fatal myocardial infarction. *The New England Journal of Medicine, 336,* 1046–1053.

Dawson, D. A. (1994). Heavy drinking and the risk of occupational injury. *Accident Analysis and Prevention, 26,* 655–665.

de Kloet, E. R., Oitzl, M. S., & Joëls, M. (1993). Functional implications of brain corticosteroid receptor diversity. *Cellular and Molecular Neurobiology, 13,* 433–455.

de Young, M. (1982). *The sexual victimization of children.* Jefferson, NC: McFarland.

Decker, T. W., Williams, J. M., & Hall, D. (1982). Preventive training in management of stress for reduction of physiological symptoms through increased cognitive and behavioral controls. *Psychological Reports, 50,* 1327–1334.

Delmonte, M. M. (1984). Meditation practice as related to occupational stress, health and productivity. *Perceptual and Motor Skills, 59,* 581–582.

Dembroski, T. M., & Costa, P. (1987). Coronary prone behavior: Components of the Type A pattern and hostility. *Journal of Personality, 55,* 211–235.

Department of Labor. (1997). *The North American occupational safety and health week: United States fact sheet.* Retrieved November 1, 1997, from the World Wide Web: http://www.dol.gov/dol/ilab/public/usfacts.htm.

Desivilya, H. S., Gal, R., & Ayalon, O. (1996). Extent of victimization, traumatic stress symptoms, and adjustment of terrorist assault survivors: A long-term follow-up. *Journal of Traumatic Stress, 9,* 881–889.

Diamond, S. (1985, May 19). Warren Anderson: A public crisis, a personal ordeal. *The New York Times,* Section 3, pp. 1F, 8F.

Diaz, M. N., Frei, B., Vita, J. A., & Keaney, J. F. (1997). Antioxidants and atherosclerotic heart disease. *The New England Journal of Medicine, 337,* 408–416.

Dienstbier, R. A. (1989). Arousal and physiological toughness: Implications for mental and physical health. *Psychological Review, 96,* 84–100.

DiIulio, J. J., Jr. (1997). Deadly divorce: Divorce can be hazardous to your health. *National Review, 49*(6), 39–41.

Dillbeck, M. C., Aron, A. P., & Dillbeck, S. L. (1979, November). The Transcendental Meditation program as an educational technology: Research and applications. *Educational Technology, 19,* 7–13.

Dillbeck, M. C., & Orme-Johnson, D. W. (1987). Physiological differences between transcendental meditation and rest. *American Psychologist, 42,* 879–880.

Dimsdale, J. E. (1988). A perspective on Type A behavior and coronary disease. *The New England Journal of Medicine, 318,* 110–112.

Dingle, G. A., & Oei, T. P. S. (1997). Is alcohol a cofactor of HIV and AIDS? Evidence from immunological and behavioral studies. *Psychological Bulletin, 122,* 56–71.

Dix, T. (1991). The affective organization of parenting: Adaptive and maladaptive processes. *Psychological Bulletin, 110,* 3–25.

Dodge, D. L., & Martin, W. T. (1970). *Social stress and chronic illness.* Notre Dame, IN: University of Notre Dame Press.

Dohrenwend, B. S., & Dohrenwend, B. R. (1982). Some issues in research on stressful life events. In T. Millon, C. Green, & R. Meagher (Eds.), *Handbook of clinical health psychology* (pp. 91–102). New York: Plenum.

Donham, G. W., Ludenia, K., Sands, M. M., & Holzer, P. D. (1983). Personality correlates of health locus of control with medical inpatients. *Psychological Reports, 52,* 659–666.

Donovan, D. M., Marlatt, G. A., & Salzberg, P. M. (1983). Drinking behavior, personality factors and high-risk driving: A review and theoretical formulation. *Journal of Studies on Alcohol, 44,* 395–428.

Dooley, D., & Catalano, R. (1984). The epidemiology of economic stress. *American Journal of Community Psychology, 12,* 387–409.

Dressler, W. W. (1994). Social status and the health of families: A model. *Social Science & Medicine, 39,* 1605–1613.

Druss, R. G., & Douglas, C. J. (1988). Adaptive responses to illness and disability: Healthy denial. *General Hospital Psychiatry, 10,* 163–168.

Dubbert, R. M., & Wilson, G. T. (1984). Goal-setting and spouse involvement in the treatment of obesity. *Behavior Research and Therapy, 22,* 227–242.

Dull, V. T., & Skokan, L. A. (1995). A cognitive model of religion's influence on health. *Journal of Social Issues, 51*, 49–64.

Dunn, T. M., Schwartz, M., Hatfield, R. W., & Wiegele, M. (1996). Measuring effectiveness of eye movement desensitization and reprocessing (EMDR) in non-clinical anxiety: A multi-subject, yoked-control design. *Journal of Behavior Therapy & Experimental Psychiatry, 27*, 231–239.

Durkheim, E. (1951). *Suicide: A study in sociology.* New York: Free Press.

Dush, D. M., Hirt, M. L., & Schroeder, H. (1983). Self-statement modification with adults: A meta-analysis. *Psychological Bulletin, 94*, 408–422.

Dutton, D., & Painter, S. L. (1981). Traumatic bonding: The development of emotional attachments in battered women and other relationships of intermittent abuse. *Victimology: An International Journal, 6*, 139–155.

Edwards, J. R. (1992). A cybernetic theory of stress, coping, and well-being in organizations. *Academy of Management Review, 17*, 238–274.

Egeland, B., & Brunquell, D. (1979). An at-risk approach to the study of child abuse: Some preliminary findings. *Journal of the American Academy of Child Psychiatry, 18*, 219–235.

Elkind, D. (1994). *Ties that stress: The new family imbalance.* Cambridge, MA: Harvard.

Ellickson, P. L., & Hays, R. D. (1992). On becoming involved with drugs: Modeling adolescent drug use over time. *Health Psychology, 11*, 377–385.

Ellis, A. (1962). *Reason and emotion in psychotherapy.* New York: Stuart.

Emery, R. E. (1989). Family violence. *American Psychologist, 44*, 321–328.

Engel, B. T., Glasgow, M. S., & Gaarder, K. R. (1983). Behavioral treatment of high blood pressure: III. Follow-up results and treatment recommendations. *Psychosomatic Medicine, 45*, 23–29.

Engel, G. L. (1977). The need for a new medical model: A challenge for biomedicine. *Science, 196*, 129–136.

Everly, G. S., Jr., & Girdano, D. A. (1980). *The stress mess solution.* Bowie, MD: Robert J. Brady.

Facts on File. (1993, April 8). Americans seen losing healthy habits. *Facts on File, 53*, 249–250.

Facts on File. (1994, October 20). Single-parent children tallied. *Facts on File, 54*, 772.

Facts on File. (1995, August 31). Divorce rate at all-time high. *Facts on File, 53*, 639.

Faris, R., & Dunham, H. W. (1939). *Mental disorders in urban areas.* Chicago: University of Chicago Press.

Farrar, D. J., Locke, S. E., & Kantrowitz, F. G. (1995). Chronic fatigue syndrome 1: Etiology and pathogenesis. *Behavioral Medicine, 21*, 5–16.

Farrell, D., & Stamm, C. L. (1988). Meta-analysis of the correlates of employee absence. *Human Relations, 41*, 211–227.

Fauci, A. S., Pantaleo, G., Stanley, S., & Weissman, D. (1996). Immunopathologenic mechanisms of HIV infection. *Annals of Internal Medicine, 124*, 654–663.

Federal Office of Road Safety. (1994). *Alcohol controls and drunk driving: The social context* (p. 31). Canberra: Australian Government Printing Service.

Ferguson, W. E. (1981). Gifted adolescents, stress, and life changes. *Adolescence, 16*, 973–985.

Fernandez, E., & Turk, D. C. (1989). The utility of cognitive coping strategies for altering pain perception: A meta-analysis. *Pain, 38*, 123–135.

Ferner, J. D. (1980). *Successful time management.* New York: Wiley.

Fielding, J. E., & Phenow, K. J. (1988). Health effects of involuntary smoking. *The New England Journal of Medicine, 319*, 1452–1460.

Figley, C. R. (1993). Coping with stressors on the home front. *Journal of Social Issues, 49,* 51–71.

Fisher, C. D. (1985). Social support and adjustment to work: A longitudinal study. *Journal of Management, 11,* 39–53.

Fisher, J. D., Bell, P. A., & Baum, A. (1984). *Environmental psychology* (2nd. ed.). New York: Holt, Rinehart & Winston.

Fisher, S. (1988). Life stress, control strategies and the risk of disease: A psychobiological model. In S. Fisher & J. Reason (Eds.), *Handbook of Life Stress, Cognition and Health* (pp. 561–602). New York: Wiley.

Fixx, J. E. (1977). *The complete book of running.* New York: Random House.

Fleming, J. S., & Courtney, B. E. (1984). The dimensionality of self-esteem: II. Hierarchical facet model for revised measurement scales. *Journal of Personality and Social Psychology, 46,* 404–421.

Fleming, R., Baum, A., Gisriel, M. M., & Gatchel, R. J. (1982). Mediating influences of social support on stress at Three Mile Island. *Journal of Human Stress, 8,* 14–22.

Foerster, K. (1984). Supportive psychotherapy combined with autogenous training in acute leukemic patients under isolation therapy. *Psychotherapy and Psychosomatics, 41,* 100–105.

Foley, F. W., Bedell, J. R., LaRocca, N. G., Scheiriberg, L. C., & Reznikoff, M. (1987). Efficacy of stress-inoculation training in coping with multiple sclerosis. *Journal of Consulting and Clinical Psychology, 55,* 919–922.

Folkman, S., & Lazarus, R. S. (1980). An analysis of coping in a middle-aged community sample. *Journal of Health and Social Behavior, 21,* 219–239.

Folkman, S., Schaefer, C., & Lazarus, R. S. (1979). Cognitive processes as mediators of stress and coping. In V. Hamilton & D. M. Warburton (Eds.), *Human stress and cognition: An information processing approach* (pp. 265–298). New York: Wiley.

Folkman, S., Chesney, M. A., Pollack, L., & Phillips, C. (1992). Stress, coping, and high-risk sexual behavior. *Health Psychology, 11,* 218–222.

Ford, D. H. (1990). Positive health and living systems frameworks. *American Psychologist, 45,* 980–981.

Forssman, H., & Thuwe, I. (1966). One hundred and twenty children born after application for therapeutic abortion refused. *Acta Psychiatry Scandinavia, 42,* 71–88.

Fosson, A. (1988). Family violence. In S. Fisher & J. Reason (Eds.), *Handbook of life stress, cognition, and health* (pp. 161–174). New York: Wiley.

Foster, G. D., Wadden, T. A., Kendall, P. C., Stunkard, A. J., & Vogt, R. A. (1996). Psychological effects of weight loss and regain: A prospective evaluation. *Journal of Consulting and Clinical Psychology, 64,* 752–757.

Frazier, P. A., & Schauben, L. J. (1994). Stressful life events and psychological adjustment among female college students. *Measurement and Evaluation in Counseling and Development, 27,* 280–292.

Free, C. (1997, September 1). Make their day: Fury at the wheel turns frustrated drivers into outlaw Dirty Harrys with a rage for revenge. *People Weekly, 48*(9), 59–60.

Freedman, J. L. (1975). *Crowding and behavior.* San Francisco: W. H. Freeman.

Freedman, R. R., Ianni, R., & Wenig, P. (1983). Behavioral treatment of Raynaud's disease. *Journal of Consulting and Clinical Psychology, 51,* 539–549.

French, J. R. P., Caplan, R. D., & Van Harrison, R. (1982). *The mechanisms of job stress and strain.* New York: Wiley.

Freud, S. (1966). *The psychopathology of everyday life* (A. Tyson, Trans.). New York: Norton.

Friedland, G. H., Saltzman, B. R., Rogers, M. F., Kahl, P. A., Lesser, M. L., Mayers, M. M., & Klein, R. S. (1986). Lack of transmission of HTLV-III/LAV infection to household contacts of patients with AIDS or AIDS-related complex with oral candidiasis. *The New England Journal of Medicine, 314,* 344–349.

Friedman, H. S., & Booth-Kewley, S. (1987). The "disease-prone personality": A meta-analytic view of the construct. *American Psychologist, 42,* 539–555.

Friedman, L., Bliwise, D. L., Yesavage, J. A., & Salom, S. R. (1991). A preliminary study comparing sleep restriction and relaxation treatments for insomnia in older adults. *Journal of Gerontology, 46,* 1–8.

Friedman, M., & Rosenman, R. H. (1974). *Type A behavior and your heart.* New York: Knopf.

Friedman, M., Thoresen, C. E., Gill, J. J., Ulmer, D., Powell, L. H., Price, V. A., Brown, B., Thompson, L., Rabin, D. D., Breall, W. S., Bourg, E., Levy, R., & Dixon, T. (1994). Alteration of Type A behavior and its effect on cardiac recurrences in postmyocardial infarction patients: Summary results of the recurrent coronary prevention project. In A. Steptoe & J. Wardle (Eds.), *Psychosocial processes and health: A reader* (pp. 478–506). Cambridge: Cambridge University Press.

Fry, P. S. (1995). Perfectionism, humor, and optimism as moderators of health outcomes and determinants of coping styles of women executives. *Genetic, Social, and General Psychology Monographs, 121,* 213–245.

Fuller, G. D. (1977). *Biofeedback: Methods and procedures in clinical practice.* San Francisco: Biofeedback Press.

Fuller, J. L., & Thompson, W. R. (1978). *Foundations of behavior genetics.* St. Louis, MO: Mosby.

Galaway, B., & Hudson, J. (Eds.). (1981). *Perspectives on crime victims.* St. Louis, MO: Mosby.

Gallup, G., Jr. (1984). *The Gallup poll: Public opinion 1984.* Wilmington, DE: Scholarly Resources.

Garneski, N., & Deikstra, R. F. W. (1997). Child sexual abuse and emotional and behavioral problems in adolescence: Gender differences. *Journal of the American Academy of Child and Adolescent Psychiatry, 36,* 323–329.

Garron, D. C., & Leavitt, R. (1983). Chronic low back pain and depression. *Journal of Clinical Psychology, 39,* 486–493.

Gebhardt, D. L., & Crump, C. E. (1990). Employee fitness and wellness programs in the workplace. *American Psychologist, 45,* 262–272.

Geer, B. W., McKechnie, S. W., Heinstra, P. W. H., & Pyka, M. J. (1991). Heritable variation in ethanol tolerance and its association with biochemical traits in *Drosophila melanogaster. Evolution, 45,* 1107–1119.

Gelles, R. J. (1985). Family violence. *Annual Review of Sociology, 11,* 347–367.

Gelles, R. J., & Straus, M. A. (1979). Determinants of violence in the family: Toward a theoretical integration. In W. R. Burr, R. Hill, F. I. Nye, & R. L. Reiss (Eds.), *Contemporary theories about the family* (Vol. 1, pp. 549–581). New York: Free Press.

George, F. R. (1987). Genetic and environmental factors in ethanol self-administration. *Pharmacology, Biochemistry and Behavior, 27,* 379–384.

George, F. R. (1988). Genetic tools in the study of drug self-administration. *Alcoholism: Clinical and Experimental Research, 12,* 586–590.

George, F. R. (1990). Genetic approaches to studying drug abuse: Correlates of drug self-administration. *Alcohol, 7,* 207–211.

Gershoff, S. (1990). *The Tufts University guide to total nutrition.* New York: Harper & Row.

Gibbs, L. M. (1983). Community response to an emergency situation: Psychological destruction and the Love Canal. *American Journal of Community Psychology, 11,* 116–125.

Gibson, V. M. (1993). Stress in the workplace: A hidden cost factor. *HR Focus, 70*(1), 15.

Giesbrecht, N., & Dick, R. (1993). Societal norms and risk-taking behavior: Inter-cultural comparisons of casualties and alcohol consumption. *Addiction, 88,* 867–876.

Gillett, R. A. (1988). Self-reported factors influencing exercise adherence in overweight women. *Nursing Research, 37,* 25–29.

Ginsburg, H., & Opper, S. (1979). *Piaget's theory of intellectual development* (2nd ed.). Englewood Cliffs, NJ: Prentice-Hall.

Girdano, D. A., & Everly, G. S. (1979). *Controlling stress and tension: A holistic approach.* Englewood Cliffs, NJ: Prentice-Hall.

Glass, D. C. (1977). Stress, behavior patterns, and coronary disease. *American Scientist, 65,* 177–187.

Glass, G. V. (1976). Primary, secondary, and meta-analysis of research. *Educational Researchers, 5,* 3–8.

Gleick, E. (1996, April 15). Living with nightmares. *Time, 147*(16), 60–64.

Gold, P. W., Goodwin, F. K., & Chrousos, G. P. (1988a). Clinical and biochemical manifestations of depression: Relation to the neurobiology of stress [First of two parts]. *The New England Journal of Medicine, 319,* 348–353.

Gold, P. W., Goodwin, F. K., & Chrousos, G. P. (1988b). Clinical and biochemical manifestations of depression: Relation to the neurobiology of stress [Second of two parts]. *The New England Journal of Medicine, 319,* 413–420.

Goldband, S. (1980). Stimulus specificity of physiological response to stress and the Type A coronary-prone behavior pattern. *Journal of Personality and Social Psychology, 39,* 670–679.

Goldstein, D. S. (1995). Stress as a scientific idea: A homeostatic theory of stress and distress. *Homeostasis, 36,* 177–215.

Goldstein, I. B. (1981). Assessment of hypertension. In C. K. Prokop & L. A. Bradley (Eds.), *Medical psychology: Contributions to behavioral medicine* (pp. 37–54). New York: Academic Press.

Gray, G. P., & Rottmann, L. H. (1988). Perceptions of stress in undergraduate college students. *The Journal of College and University Student Housing, 18,* 14–20.

Green, E. E., Green, A. M., & Walters, E. D. (1972). Biofeedback for mind-body self-regulation: Healing and creativity. *Fields Within Fields ... Within Fields, 5,* 131–144.

Green, E. E., Green, A. M., Walters, E. D., Sargent, J. D., & Meyer, R. G. (1973). *Autogenic feedback training.* Topeka, KS: The Menninger Foundation.

Green, R. G. (1985). Stress and accidents. *Aviation, Space, and Environmental Medicine, 56,* 638–641.

Greenberg, E. R., Baron, J. A., Stukel, T. A., Stevens, M. M., Mandel, J. S., Spencer, S. K., Elias, P. M., Lowe, N., Nierenberg, D. W., Bayrd, G., Vance, J. C., Freeman, D. H., Jr., Clendenning, W. E., Kwan, T., & the Skin Cancer Prevention Study Group. (1990). A clinical trial of beta carotene to prevent basal-cell and squamous-cell cancers of the skin. *The New England Journal of Medicine, 323,* 789–795.

Greenberg, W., & Shapiro, D. (1987). The effects of caffeine and stress on blood pressure in individuals with and without a family history of hypertension. *Psychophysiology, 24,* 151–156.

Greene, W. C. (1991). The molecular biology of Human Immunodeficiency Virus Type 1 infection. *The New England Journal of Medicine, 324,* 308–317.

Greer, S., & Morris, T. (1975). Psychological attributes of women who develop breast cancer: A controlled study. *Journal of Psychosomatic Research, 19,* 147–153.

Grimm, L. G., & Yarnold, R. R. (1984). Performance standards and the Type A behavior pattern. *Cognitive Therapy and Research, 8,* 59–66.

Grobbee, D. E., Rimm, E. B., Giovannucci, E., Colditz, G., Stampfer, M., & Willett, W. (1990). Coffee, caffeine, and cardiovascular disease in men. *The New England Journal of Medicine, 323,* 1026–1032.

Grossman, S. (1973). *Essentials of physiological psychology.* New York: Wiley.

Groth, A. N., & Burgess, A. W. (1977). Motivational intent in the sexual assault of children. *Criminal Justice and Behavior, 4,* 253–264.

Grych, J. H., & Fincham, R. D. (1990). Marital conflict and children's adjustment: A cognitive-contextual framework. *Psychological Bulletin, 108,* 267–290.

Gutlin, B., & Kessler, G. (1983). *The high energy factor.* New York: Random House.

Guyton, A. C. (1977). *Basic human physiology: Normal function and mechanisms of disease.* Philadelphia: Saunders.

Hafen, B. Q., Karren, K. J., Frandsen, K. J., & Smith, N. L. (1996). *Mind/body health* (Chap. 13). Boston: Allyn & Bacon.

Hajjar, K. A., Gavish, D., Breslow, J. L., & Nachman, R. L. (1989). Lipoprotein(a) modulation of endothelial cell surface fibrinolysis and its potential role in atherosclerosis. *Nature, 339,* 303–305.

Hall, H. R. (1982–1983). Hypnosis and the immune system: A review with implications for cancer and the psychology of healing. *American Journal of Clinical Hypnosis, 25,* 92–103.

Hall, R. L., Hesselbrock, V. M., & Stabenau, J. R. (1983). Familial distribution of alcohol use: 1. Assortative mating in the parents of alcoholics. *Behavior Genetics, 13,* 361–372.

Hamilton, V. (1979). "Personality" and stress. In V. Hamilton & D. M. Warburton (Eds.), *Human stress and cognition: An information processing approach* (pp. 67–114). New York: Wiley.

Hammen, C., Marks, T., Mayol, A., & deMayo, R. (1985). Depressive self-schemas, life stress, and vulnerability to depression. *Journal of Abnormal Psychology, 94,* 308–319.

Hannah, T. E. (1988). Hardiness and health behavior: The role of health concern as a moderator variable. *Behavioral Medicine, 14,* 59–63.

Hannah, T. E., & Morrissey, C. (1987). Correlates of psychological hardiness in Canadian adolescents. *The Journal of Social Psychology, 127,* 339–344.

Hanson, R. G. (1986). *The joy of stress.* Fairway, KS: Andrews, McMeel & Parker.

Hargie, O. (Ed.). (1986). *A handbook of communication skills.* New York: New York University Press.

Harris, R., Frankel, L. J., & Harris, S. (Eds.). (1977). *Guide to fitness after fifty.* New York: Plenum.

Hart, R. H. (1970). The concept of APS: Air Pollution Syndrome(s). *Journal of the South Carolina Medical Association, 66,* 71–73.

Hartwell, T. D., Steele, P., French, M. T., Potter, F. J., Rodman, N. F., & Zarkin, G. A. (1996). Aiding troubled employees: The prevalence, cost, and characteristics of employee assistance programs in the United States. *American Journal of Public Health, 86,* 804–808.

Haskell, W. L. (1987). Developing an activity plan for improving health. In W. R. Morgan & S. E. Goldston (Eds.), *Exercise and mental health* (pp. 37–55). Washington, DC: Hemisphere.

Hatch, J. P., & Riley, P. (1986). Growth and development of biofeedback: A bibliographic analysis. *Biofeedback and Self-Regulation, 10,* 289–299.

Hays, R. B., Turner, H., & Coates, T. J. (1992). Social support, AIDS-related symptoms, and depression among gay men. *Journal of Consulting and Clinical Psychology, 60,* 463–469.

Heatherington, E. M., Cox, M., & Cox, R. (1976). Divorced fathers. *Family Coordinator, 25,* 417–428.

Heatherington, E. M., Cox, M., & Cox, R. (1977). The aftermath of divorce. In J. H. Stevens, Jr., & M. Matthews (Eds.), *Mother-child, father-child relations* (pp. 149–176). Washington, DC: National Association for the Education of Young Children.

Heatherington, E. M., Stanley-Hagan, M., & Anderson, E. R. (1989). Marital transitions: A child's perspective. *American Psychologist, 44,* 303–312.

Hegel, M. T., Abel, G. G., Etscheidt, M., Cohen-Cole, S., & Wilmer, C. I. (1989). Behavioral treatment of angina-like chest pain in patients with hyperventilation syndrome. *Journal of Behavior Therapy and Experimental Psychiatry, 20,* 31–39.

Heide, F. J., & Borkovec, T. D. (1983). Relaxation-induced anxiety: Paradoxical anxiety enhancement due to relaxation training. *Journal of Consulting and Clinical Psychology, 51,* 171–182.

Heimberg, R. G. (1989). Cognitive and behavioral treatments for social phobia: A critical analysis. *Clinical Psychology Review, 9,* 107–128.

Heller, J. (1987). What do we know about the risks of caffeine consumption in pregnancy? *British Journal of Addiction, 82,* 885–889.

Heninger, G. R. (1995). Neuroimmunolgy of stress. In M. J. Friedman, D. S. Charnery, & A. Y. Deutch (Eds.), *Neurobiological and clinical consequences of stress: From normal adaptation to PTSD* (pp. 381–401). Philadelphia: Lippincott-Raven.

Henningfield, J. E., & Woodson, P. P. (1989). Dose-related actions of nicotine on behavior and physiology: Review and implications for replacement therapy for nicotine dependence. *Journal of Substance Abuse, 1,* 301–317.

Hepburn, J. R., & Monti, D. J. (1979). Victimization, fear of crime, and adaptive responses among high school students. In W. H. Parsonage, *Perspectives on victimology* (pp. 121–132). Newbury Park, CA: Sage.

Herbert, L., & Teague, M. L. (1989). Exercise adherence and older adults: A theoretical perspective. *Activities, Adaptation, and Aging, 13,* 91–105.

Herbert, T. B., & Cohen, S. (1993). Stress and immunity in humans: A meta-analytic review. *Psychosomatic Medicine, 55,* 364–379.

Herek, G. M., & Glunt, E. K. (1988). An epidemic of stigma: Public reactions to AIDS, *American Psychologist, 43,* 886–891.

Herman, C., Blanchard, E. B., & Flor, H. (1997). Biofeedback treatment for pediatric migraine: Prediction of treatment outcome. *Journal of Counsulting and Clinical Psychology, 65,* 611–616.

Herman, C., Kim, M., & Blanchard, E. B. (1995). Behavioral and prophylactic pharmacological intervention studies of pediatric migraine: An exploratory meta-analysis. *Pain, 60,* 239–256.

Heyel, C. (1979). *Getting results with time management* (2nd ed.). New York: American Management Association.

Higgins, N. C. (1986). Occupational stress and working women: The effectiveness of two stress reduction programs. *Journal of Vocational Behavior, 29,* 66–78.

Hildebrand, J. F. (1986). Mutual help for spouses whose partners are employed in stressful occupations. *Journal for Specialists in Group Work, 11*(1), 80–84.

Hill, R. (1949). *Families under stress.* New York: Harper & Row.

Hindelang, M. J., Gottfredson, M. R., & Garofalo, J. (1978). *Victims of personal crime: An empirical foundation for a theory of personal victimization.* Cambridge, MA: Ballinger.

Hinkle, L. E. (1974a). The concept of "stress" in the biological and social sciences. *International Journal of Psychiatry in Medicine, 5,* 335–357.

Hinkle, L. E. (1974b). The effect of exposure to culture change, social change, and changes in interpersonal relationships on health. In B. S. Dohrenwend & B. R. Dohrenwend (Eds.), *Stressful life events: Their nature and effect* (pp. 9–44). New York: Wiley.

Hobfoll, S. (1989). Conservation of resources: A new attempt at conceptualizing stress. *American Psychologist, 44,* 513–524.

Hoenig, J. (1968). Medical research on Yoga, *Confinia Psychiatrica, 11,* 69–89.

Holahan, C. J. (1986). Environmental psychology. *Annual Review of Psychology, 37,* 381–407.

Hollingshead, A. B., & Redlich, F. C. (1958). *Social class and mental illness: A community study.* New York: Wiley.

Holmes, D. S. (1981). The use of biofeedback for treating patients with migraine headaches, Raynaud's disease, and hypertension: A critical evaluation. In C. K. Prokop & L. A. Bradley (Eds.), *Medical psychology: Contributions to behavioral medicine* (pp. 423–437). New York: Academic Press.

Holmes, D. S., Solomon, S., Cappo, B. M., & Greenberg, J. L. (1983). Effects of transcendental meditation versus resting on physiological and subjective arousal. *Journal of Personality and Social Psychology, 44,* 1245–1252.

Holmes, T. H., & Masuda, M. (1974). Life change and illness susceptibility. In B. S. Dohrenwend & B. R. Dohrenwend (Eds.), *Stressful life events: Their nature and effect* (pp. 45–72). New York: Wiley.

Holmes, T. H., & Rahe, R. H. (1967). The social readjustment rating scale. *Psychosomatic Medicine, 11,* 213–218.

Hopkins, B. L., Conard, R. J., Dangel, R. E., Fitch, H. G., Smith, M. J., & Anger, W. K. (1986). Behavioral technology for reducing occupational exposures to styrene. *Journal of Applied Behavior Analysis, 19,* 3–11.

Horn, J. D., Feldman, H. M., & Ploof, D. L. (1995). Parent and professional perceptions about stress and coping strategies during a child's lengthy hospitalization. *Social Work in Pediatrics, 21,* 107–127.

Horne, J. A. (1981). The effects of exercise upon sleep: A critical review. *Biological Psychology, 12,* 241–290.

Horowitz, M. J. (1979). Psychological response to serious life events. In V. Hamilton & D. M. Warburton (Eds.), *Human stress and cognition: An information processing approach* (pp. 235–263). New York: Wiley.

House, J. S. (1987). Chronic stress and chronic disease in life and work: Conceptual and methodological issues. *Work & Stress, 1,* 129–134.

Howard, J. H., Cunningham, D. A., & Rechnitzer, P. A. (1976). Health patterns associated with Type A behavior: A managerial population. *Journal of Human Stress, 2,* 24–31.

Hull, J. G., van Treuren, R. R., & Propsom, R. M. (1988). Attributional style and the components of hardiness. *Personality and Social Psychology Bulletin, 14,* 505–513.

Ilgen, D. R. (1990). Health issues at work: Opportunities for industrial/organizational psychology. *American Psychologist, 45,* 273–283.

Information technology revolution: Boon or bane? (1997, January–February). *The Futurist, 31,* 10–15.

Institute of Medicine (United States). (1979). *Healthy people: The Surgeon General's report on health promotion and disease prevention.* (Government Document No. HE20.2:H34/5). Rockville, MD: U.S. Government Printing Office.

Irvine, J., Lyle, R. C., & Allon, R. (1982). Type A personality as psychopathology: Personality correlates and an abbreviated scoring system. *Journal of Psychosomatic Research, 26,* 183–189.

Irwin, J., & Livnat, S. (1987). Behavioral influences on the immune system: Stress and conditioning. *Progress in Neuro-Psychopharmacology and Biological Psychiatry, 11,* 137–143.

Ivancevich, J. M., Matteson, M. T., Freedman, S. M., & Phillips, J. S. (1990). Worksite stress management interventions. *American Psychologist, 45,* 252–261.

Jaccard, J., & Becker, M. A. (1997). *Statistics for the behavioral sciences* (3rd ed.). Pacific Grove, CA: Brooks/Cole.

Jackson, J. O. (1994, October 10). The cruel sea: The Baltic ferry *Estonia* sinks with the loss of more than 900 lives. *Time, 144*(15), 52–53.

Jacobs, G. A., Quevillon, R. P., & Stricherz, M. (1990). Lessons from the aftermath of Flight 232: Practical considerations for the mental health profession's response to air disasters. *American Psychologist, 45,* 1329–1335.

Jacobsen, P. B., Bovbjerg, D. H., & Redd, W. H. (1993). Anticipatory anxiety in women receiving chemotherapy for breast cancer. *Health Psychology, 12,* 469–475.

Jacobson, E. (1938). *Progressive relaxation* (2nd ed.). Chicago: University of Chicago Press.

JAMA. (1996). Integration of behavioral and relaxation approaches into the treatment of chronic pain and insomnia. *JAMA, The Journal of the American Medical Association, 276,* 313–318.

Janis, I. L. (1982). *Stress, attitudes, and decisions.* New York: Praeger.

Janis, I. L. (1983). The role of social support in adherence to stressful decisions. *American Psychologist, 38,* 143–160.

Janoff-Bulman, R. (1988). Victims of violence. In S. Fisher & J. Reason (Eds.), *Handbook of life stress, cognition and health* (pp. 101–113). New York: Wiley.

Jason, L. A., Ji, P. Y., Anes, M. D., & Birkhead, S. H. (1991). Active enforcement of cigarette control laws in the prevention of cigarette sales to minors. *JAMA, Journal of the American Medical Association, 266,* 3159–3161.

Jemmott, J. B. (1985). Psychoneuroimmunology: The new frontier. *American Behavioral Scientist, 28,* 497–509.

Jenkins, C. D., Zyzanski, S. J., & Rosenman, R. H. (1965). *Jenkins Activity Survey.* New York: The Psychological Corporation.

Jevning, R., Wallace, R. K., & Beidebach, M. (1992). The physiology of meditation: A review. A wakeful hypometabolic integrated response. *Neuroscience and Biobehavioral Reviews, 16,* 415–424.

Job, R. F. S. (1988). Community response to noise: A review of factors influencing the relationship between noise exposure and reaction. *Journal of the Acoustical Society of America, 83,* 991–1001.

Johansson, G., Aronsson, G., & Lindstrom, B. O. (1976). *Social psychological and neuroendocrine stress reactions in highly mechanized work* (Report No. 488). Stockholm, Sweden: University of Stockholm, Department of Psychology.

John, E. R. (1967). *Mechanisms of memory.* New York: Academic Press.

Johnson, B. T. (1989). *DSTAT software for the meta-analytic review of research literatures.* Hillsdale, NJ: Lawrence Erlbaum Associates.

Johnson, D. (1990). Animal rights and human lives. Time for scientists to right the balance. *Psychological Science, 1,* 213–214.

Jorgensen, R. S., & Houston, B. K. (1989). Reporting of life events, family history of hypertension, and cardiovascular activity at rest and during psychological stress. *Biological Psychology, 28,* 135–148.

Jorgensen, R. S., Johnson, B. T., Kolodziej, M. E., & Schreer, G. E. (1996). Elevated blood pressure and personality: A meta-analytic review. *Psychological Bulletin, 120,* 293–320.

Joseph, S., Yule, W., Williams, R., & Hodgkinson, P. (1993). Increased substance use in survivors of the *Herald of Free Enterprise* disaster. *British Journal of Medical Psychology, 66,* 185–191.

Kabat-Zinn, J., Lipworth, L., & Burney, R. (1985). The clinical use of mindfulness meditation for the self-regulation of chronic pain. *Journal of Behavioral Medicine, 8,* 163–190.

Kagan, A. (1974). Psychosocial factors in disease: Hypotheses and future research. In E. K. E. Gunderson & R. H. Rahe (Eds.), *Life stress and illness* (pp. 41–57). Springfield, IL: Charles C. Thomas.

Kamiya, J. (1969). Operant control of the EEG alpha rhythm and some of its reported effects on consciousness. In C. T. Tart (Ed.), *Altered states of consciousness* (pp. 519–529). Garden City, NY: Anchor Books.

Kanner, A. D., Coyne, J. C., Schaefer, C., & Lazarus, R. S. (1981). Comparison of two modes of stress measurement: Daily hassles and uplifts versus major life events. *Journal of Behavioral Medicine, 4,* 1–39.

Kaplan, R. M. (1990). Behavior as the central outcome in health care. *American Psychologist, 45,* 1211–1220.

Kapleau, R. (Ed.). (1966). *The three pillars of Zen.* New York: Harper & Row.

Karlin, R. A., Katz, S., Epstein, Y., & Woolfolk, R. (1979). The use of therapeutic interventions to reduce crowding-related arousal: A preliminary investigation. *Environmental Psychology and Nonverbal Behavior, 3,* 219–227.

Karoly, P. (1985). *Measurement strategies in health psychology.* New York: Wiley.

Karoly, P. (Ed.). (1988). *Handbook of child health assessment: Biopsychosocial perspectives.* New York: Wiley.

Kasamatsu, A., & Hirai, T. (1963). Science of zazen. *Psychologia, 6,* 86–91.

Kasl, S. V., & Cobb, S. (1966). Health behavior, illness behavior, and sick-role behavior: II. Sick-role behavior. *Archives of Environmental Health, 12,* 531–541.

Kasl, S. V., & Cooper, C. L. (1987). *Stress and health: Issues in research methodology.* New York: Wiley.

Kater, D. (1985). Management strategies for dual-career couples. *Journal of Career Development, 12,* 75–80.

Katz, J., Ackerman, P., Rothwax, R., Sachar, E. J., Weiner, H., Hellman, L., & Gallagher, T. R. (1970). Psychoendocrine aspects of cancer of the breast. *Psychosomatic Medicine, 32,* 1–18.

Katzell, R. A., & Thompson, D. E. (1990). Work motivation: Theory and practice. *American Psychologist, 45,* 144–153.

Keesey, R. E., & Powley, T. L. (1986). The regulation of body weight. *Annual Review of Psychology, 37,* 109–133.

Keita, G. P., & Jones, J. M. (1990). Reducing adverse reaction to stress in the workplace. *American Psychologist, 45,* 1137–1141.

Keller, S. E., Weiss, J. M., Schleifer, S. J., Miller, N. E., & Stein, M. (1981). Suppression of immunity by stress: Effect of a graded series of stressors on lymphocyte stimulation in the rat. *Science, 213,* 1397–1400.

Kelly, G. A. (1955). *The psychology of personal constructs* (Vols. 1 and 2). New York: Norton.

Kendzierski, D. (1990). Exercise self-schemata: Cognitive and behavioral correlates. *Health Psychology, 9,* 69–82.

Kendzierski, D., & Lamastro, V. D. (1988). Reconsidering the role of attitudes in exercise behavior: A decision theoretic approach. *Journal of Applied Social Psychology, 18,* 737–759.

Kessler, R. C., & Essex, M. (1982). Marital status and depression: The importance of coping resources. *Social Forces, 61,* 484–507.

Kiecolt-Glaser, J. K., Fisher, L. D., Ogrocki, R., Stout, J. C., Speicher, B. S., & Glaser, R. (1985). Marital quality, marital disruption, and immune function. *Psychosomatic Medicine, 40,* 13–34.

Kiecolt-Glaser, J. K., & Glaser, R. (1988). Psychological influences on immunity: Implications for AIDS. *American Psychologist, 43,* 892–898.

Kiecolt-Glaser, J. K., Glaser, R., Williger, D., Stout, J., Messick, G., Sheppard, S., Ricker, D., Romisher, S. C., Briner, W., Bonnell, G., & Donnerberg, R. (1985). Psychosocial enhancement of immunocompetence in a geriatric population. *Health Psychology, 4,* 25–41.

King, A. C., Winett, R. A., & Lovett, S. B. (1986). Enhancing coping behaviors in at-risk populations: The effects of time-management instruction and social support in women from dual-earner families. *Behavior Therapy, 17,* 57–66.

Kirkham, M. A., Schilling, R. F., Norelius, K., & Schinke, S. P. (1986). Developing coping styles and social support networks: An intervention outcome study with mothers of handicapped children. *Child: Care, Health and Development, 12,* 313–323.

Kirscht, J. R., Haefner, D. R., Kegeles, S. S., & Rosenstock, I. M. (1966). A national study of health beliefs. *Journal of Health and Human Behavior, 7,* 248–254.

Kissen, D. M. (1967). Psychosocial factors, personality and lung cancer in men aged 55–64. *British Journal of Medical Psychology, 40,* 29–43.

Klein, D. M. (1983). Family problem solving and family stress. *Marriage and Family Review, 6,* 85–112.

Klein, M., & Stern, L. (1971). Low birth weight and the battered child syndrome. *American Journal of Diseases of Childhood, 122,* 15–18.

Kleinbaum, D. G., Kupper, L. L., & Morgenstern, H. (1982). *Epidemiologic research: Principles and quantitative methods.* New York: Van Nostrand Reinhold.

Klesges, R. C., Eck, L. H., Hanson, C. L., Haddock, C. K., & Klesges, L. M. (1990). Effects of obesity, social interactions, and physical environment on physical activity in preschoolers. *Health Psychology, 9,* 435–449.

Klingman, A. (1985). Mass inoculation in a community: The effect of primary prevention of stress reactions. *American Journal of Community Psychology, 13,* 323–332.

Knapp, T. W. (1982). Treating migraine by training in temporal artery vasoconstriction and/or cognitive behavioral coping: A one-year follow-up. *Journal of Psychosomatic Research, 26,* 551–557.

Kobasa, S. C. (1979a). Personality and resistance to illness. *American Journal of Community Psychology, 7,* 413–423.

Kobasa, S. C. (1979b). Stressful life events, personality and health: An inquiry into hardiness. *Journal of Personality and Social Psychology, 37,* 1–11.

Kobasa, S. C. (1982). Commitment and coping in stress resistance among lawyers. *Journal of Personality and Social Psychology, 42,* 707–717.

Kobasa, S. C., Maddi, S. R., & Puccetti, M. C. (1982). Personality and exercise as buffers in the stress-illness relationship. *Journal of Behavioral Medicine, 5,* 391–404.

Koller, M. (1996). Occupational health services for shift and night workers. *Applied Ergonomics, 27,* 31–37.

Konecni, V. J., Libuser, L., Morton, H., & Ebbesen, E. B. (1975). Effects of a violation of personal space on escape and helping responses. *Journal of Experimental Social Psychology, 11,* 288–299.

Koopman, C., Classen, C., Cardeña, E., & Spiegel, D. (1995). When disaster strikes, acute stress disorder may follow. *Journal of Traumatic Stress, 8,* 29–46.

Koopman, C., Classen, C., & Spiegel, D. (1996). Dissociative responses in the immediate aftermath of the Oakland/Berkeley firestorm. *Journal of Traumatic Stress, 9,* 521–540.

Kozoll, C. E. (1982). *Time management for educators.* Bloomington, IN: Phi Delta Kappa Educational Foundation.

Krantz, D. S., & Raisen, S. E. (1988). Environmental stress, reactivity and ischaemic heart disease. *British Journal of Medical Psychology, 61,* 3–16.

Krinsky, N. I. (1989). Carotenoids and cancer in animal models. *The Journal of Nutrition, 119,* 123–126.

Kuller, L., Neaton, J., Caggiula, A., & Falvo-Gerard, L. (1980). Primary prevention of heart attacks: The Multiple Risk Factor Intervention Trial. *American Journal of Epidemiology, 112,* 185–199.

Kutash, I. L., Schlesinger, L. B., & Associates (Eds.). (1980). *Handbook on stress and anxiety.* San Francisco: Jossey-Bass.

LaGreca, A. M., Silverman, W. K., Vernberg, E. M., & Prinstein, M. J. (1996). Symptoms of post-traumatic stress in children after Hurricane Andrew: A prospective study. *Journal of Consulting and Clinical Psychology, 64,* 712–723.

Lambert, C. E., & Lambert, V. A. (1987). Hardiness: Its development and relevance to nursing. *Image: Journal of Nursing Scholarship, 19,* 92–95.

Lane, J. D. (1983). Caffeine and cardiovascular responses to stress. *Psychosomatic Medicine, 45,* 447–451.

Latack, J. C., Kinicki, A. J., & Prussia, G. E. (1995). An integrative process model of coping with job loss. *Academy of Management Review, 20,* 311–342.

Lazarus, R. S. (1991). Progress on a cognitive-motivational-relational theory of emotion. *American Psychologist, 46,* 819–834.

Lazarus, R. S. (1993). Why we should think of stress as a subset of emotion. In L. Goldberger & S. Breznitz (Eds.), *Handbook of stress: Theoretical and clinical aspects* (pp. 21–39). New York: Free Press.

Lazarus, R. S., & Launier, R. (1978). Stress-related transactions between person and environment. In L. A. Pervin & M. Lewis (Eds.), *Perspectives in interactional psychology* (pp. 287–327). New York: Plenum.

Le, A. D. (1990). Factors regulating ethanol tolerance. *Annals of Medicine, 22,* 265–268.

Leach, J. (1995). Psychological first-aid. A practical aide-memoire. *Aviation, Space, and Environmental Medicine, 66,* 668–674.

Leadbeater, B. J., Blatt, S. J., & Quinlan, D. M. (1995). Gender-linked vulnerabilities to depressive symptoms, stress, and problem behaviors in adolescents. *Journal of Research on Adolescence, 5,* 1–29.

Leak, G. K., & Williams, D. E. (1989). Relationship between social interest, alienation, and psychological hardiness. *Individual Psychology, 45,* 369–375.

Leavy, R. L. (1983). Social support and psychological disorder: A review. *Journal of Community Psychology, 11,* 3–21.

LeBoeuf, M. (1979). *Working smart.* New York: McGraw-Hill.

Lee, C. (1989). The clinical aspects of AIDS/HIV. In R. Miller & R. Bor, *AIDS: A guide to clinical counseling* (pp. 29–34). London: Science Press.

Lee, R. T., & Ashforth, B. E. (1996). A meta-analytic examination of the correlates of the three dimensions of job burnout. *Journal of Applied Psychology, 81,* 123–133.

Lefcourt, H. M. (1976). *Locus of control: Current trends in theory and research.* Hillsdale, NJ: Lawrence Erlbaum Associates.

Leigh, J. P., Markowitz, S. B., & Landrigan, P. J. (1997). Occupational injury and illness in the United States: Estimates of costs, morbidity, and mortality. *Archives of Internal Medicine, 157,* 1557–1568.

Lerner, M. J., & Matthews, G. (1967). Reactions to suffering of others under conditions of indirect responsibility. *Journal of Personality and Social Psychology, 5,* 319–325.

Lerner, M. J., & Simmons, C. (1966). Observer's reaction to the "innocent victim": Compassion or rejection? *Journal of Personality and Social Psychology, 4,* 203–210.

Levav, I., Friedlander, Y., Kark, J. D., & Peritz, E. (1988). An epidemiologic study of mortality among bereaved parents. *The New England Journal of Medicine, 319,* 457–461.

Levi, L. (1990). Occupational stress: Spice of life or kiss of death? *American Psychologist, 45,* 1142–1145.

Levin, J. S., & Puchalski, C. M. (1997). Religion and spirituality in medicine: Research and education. *JAMA, Journal of the American Medical Association, 278,* 792–793.

Levy, S. M., & Wise, B. D. (1987). Psychosocial risk factors, natural immunity, and cancer progression: Implications for intervention. *Current Psychological Research and Reviews, 6,* 229–243.

Lewin, K. (1948). *Resolving social conflicts.* New York: Harper & Row.

Lieberman, H. R., Spring, B. J., & Garfield, G. S. (1986). The behavioral effects of food constituents: Strategies used in studies of amino acids, protein, carbohydrate and caffeine. *Nutrition Reviews: Diet and Behavior, 44,* 61–70.

Liebert, R. M., & Spiegler, M. D. (1994). *Personality: Strategies and issues* (7th ed.). Pacific Grove, CA: Brooks/Cole.

Liebman, M. (1979). *Neuroanatomy made easy and understandable.* Baltimore: University Park Press.

Light, R. (1973). Abuse and neglected children in America: A study of alternative policies. *Harvard Educational Review, 43,* 556–598.

Light, R. J., & Pillemer, D. B. (1984). *Summing up: The science of reviewing research.* Cambridge, MA: Harvard University Press.

Lilienfeld, A. M., & Lilienfeld, D. E. (1980). *Foundations of epidemiology* (2nd. ed.). New York: Oxford University Press.

Lilienfeld, S. O. (1996). EMDR treatment: Less than meets the eye? *Skeptical Inquirer, 20*(1), 25–31.

Lintel, A. G. (1980). Physiological anxiety responses in transcendental meditators and non-meditators. *Perceptual and Motor Skills, 50,* 295–300.

Lloyd, G. G., & Cawley, R. H. (1983). Distress or illness? A study of psychological symptoms after myocardial infarction. *British Journal of Psychiatry, 142,* 120–125.

Locke, S. E., Hurst, M. W., Heisel, J. S., et al. (1978, April). *The influence of stress on the immune response.* Annual Meeting of the American Psychosomatic Society, Washington, DC.

Lohr, J. M., Kleinknecht, R. A., Tolin, D. F., & Barrett, R. H. (1995). The empirical status of the clinical application of eye movement desensitization and reprocessing. *Journal of Behavior Therapy & Experimental Psychiatry, 26,* 285–302.

Lovallo, W. R., & Pishkin, V. (1980). A psychophysiological comparison of Type A and B men exposed to failure and uncontrollable noise. *Psychophysiology, 17,* 29–36.

Lowenthal, B. (1987). Stress factors and their alleviation in parents of high-risk pre-term infants. *The Exceptional Child, 34,* 21–30.

Ludenia, K., & Donham, G. W. (1983). Dental outpatients: Health locus of control correlates. *Journal of Clinical Psychology, 39,* 854–858.

Lukins, R., Davan, I. G. P., & Drummond, P. D. (1997). A cognitive behavioural approach to preventing anxiety during magnetic resonance imaging. *Journal of Behavior Therapy & Experimental Psychiatry, 28,* 97–104.

Lundberg, U. (1976). Urban commuting: Crowdedness and catecholamine excretion. *Journal of Human Stress, 2,* 26–32.

Lustman, P. J., & Sowa, C. J. (1983). Comparative efficacy of biofeedback and stress inoculation for stress reduction. *Journal of Clinical Psychology, 39,* 191–197.

Luthe, W. (1969). *Autogenic therapy.* New York: Grune & Stratton.

Luthe, W., & Blumberger, S. R. (1977). Autogenic therapy. In E. D. Wittkower & H. Warries (Eds.), *Psychosomatic medicine: Its clinical applications* (pp. 146–165). New York: Harper & Row.

Lystad, M. H. (1985). Human response to mass emergencies: A review of mental health research. *Emotional First Aid, 2,* 5–18.

Macewen, K. E., & Barling, J. (1988). Interrole conflict, family support and marital adjustment of employed mothers: A short term, longitudinal study. *Journal of Organizational Behavior, 9,* 241–250.

Maclean's. (1996, July 1). The changing family. *Maclean's, 109*(27), 23.

Mader, T. E., & Mader, D. C. (1990). *Understanding one another: Communicating interpersonally.* Dubuque, IA: William C. Brown.

Mandell, W., Eaton, W. W., Anthony, J. C., & Garrison, R. (1992). Alcoholism and occupations: A review and analysis of 104 occupations. *Alcoholism: Clinical and Experimental Research, 16,* 734–746.

Manne, S. L., Redd, W. H., Jacobsen, P. B., Gorfinkle, K., Schorr, O., & Rapkin, B. (1990). Behavioral intervention to reduce child and parent distress during venipuncture. *Journal of Consulting and Clinical Psychology, 58,* 565–572.

Marsh, R. (Ed.). (1988). *Eye to eye: How people interact.* Topsfield, MA: Salem House.

Marshall, C. W. (1983). *Vitamins and minerals: Help or harm?* Philadelphia: George E. Stickley.

Martin, B. (1981). *A sociology of contemporary cultural change.* New York: St. Martin's Press.

Martin, J. E., & Dubbert, R. M. (1982). Exercise applications and promotion in behavioral medicine: Current status and future directions. *Journal of Consulting and Clinical Psychology, 50,* 1004–1017.

Martin, J. E., Dubbert, R. M., Katell, A. D., Thompson, J. K., Raczynski, J. R., Lake, M., et al. (1984). Behavioral control of exercise in sedentary adults: Studies 1 through 6. *Journal of Consulting and Clinical Psychology, 52,* 795–811.

Martin, R. A., & Lefcourt, H. M. (1983). Sense of humor as a moderator of the relation between stressors and moods. *Journal of Personality and Social Psychology, 45,* 1313–1324.

Martinez, R. (1997, July 17). Statement of the Honorable Ricardo Martinez, M.D. Administrator National Highway Traffic Safety Administration before the Subcommittee on Surface Transportation Committee on Transportation and Infrastructure, U.S. House of Representative. Retrieved March 8, 1998, from the World Wide Web: http://www.nhtsa.dot.gov/nhtsa/announce/testimony/aggres2.html.

Martocchio, J. J., & O'Leary, A. M. (1989). Sex differences in occupational stress: A meta-analytic review. *Journal of Applied Psychology, 74,* 495–501.

Matarazzo, J. D. (1986). Computerized clinical psychological test interpretations: Unvalidated plus all mean and no sigma. *American Psychologist, 41,* 14–24.

Matheny, K. B., Aycock, D. W., Pugh, J. L., Curlette, W. L., & Silva-Cannella, K. A. (1986). Stress coping: A qualitative and quantitative synthesis with implications for treatment. *Counseling Psychologist, 14,* 499–549.

Matthews, K. A., Glass, D. C., Rosenman, R. H., & Bortner, R. W. (1977). Competitive drive, Pattern A and coronary heart disease: A further analysis of some data from the Western Collaborative Group Study. *Journal of Chronic Diseases, 30,* 489–498.

Mayo Clinic, Committee on Dietetics (Ed.). (1981). *Mayo Clinic diet manual.* Philadelphia: Saunders.

Mayo Health O@sis. (1997a). *Facts about calories.* Retrieved December 1, 1997, from the World Wide Web: http://www.mayo.ivi.com.

Mayo Health O@sis. (1997b). *Healthy People 2000: America's nutrition check-up.* Retrieved December 1, 1997, from the World Wide Web: http://www.mayo.ivi.com.

Mayo Health O@sis. (1997c). *Vitamin and nutritional supplements.* Retrieved December 1, 1997, from the World Wide Web: http://www.mayo.ivi.com.

McCaffrey, R. J., & Blanchard, E. B. (1985). Area review: Hypertension. *Annals of Behavioral Medicine, 7,* 5–12.

McCauley, J., Kern, D. E., Kolodner, K., Dill, L., Schroeder, A. F., DeChant, H. K., Ryden, J., Derogatis, L. R., & Bass, E. B. (1997). Clinical characteristics of women with a history of childhood abuse: Unhealed wounds. *JAMA, The Journal of the American Medical Association, 277,* 1362–1368.

McClelland, D. C. (1989). Motivational factors in health and disease. *American Psychologist, 44,* 675–683.

McConalogue, T. (1984). Developing the skill of time management. *Leadership and Organization Development Journal, 5,* 25–27.

McCrae, R. R., & Costa, P. T., Jr. (1987). Validation of the five-factor model of personality across instruments and observers. *Journal of Personality and Social Psychology, 52,* 81–90.

McCubbin, H. I., & Patterson, J. M. (1983). The family stress process: The double ABCX model of adjustment and adaptation. *Marriage and Family Review, 6,* 7–37.

McCubbin, H. I., Joy, C. B., Cauble, A. E., Comeau, J. K., Patterson, J. M., & Needle, R. H. (1980). Family stress and coping: A decade review. *Journal of Marriage and the Family, 42,* 855–871.

McCubbin, J. A., Wilson, J. F., Bruehl, S., Ibarra, P., Carlson, C. R., Norton, J. A., & Colclough, G. W. (1996). Relaxation training and opioid inhibition of blood pressure response to stress. *Journal of Consulting and Clinical Psychology, 64,* 593–601.

McDaniel, J. S., Musselman, D. L., Porter, M. R., Reed, D. A., & Nemeroff, C. B. (1995). Depression in patients with cancer: Diagnosis, biology, and treatment. *Archives of General Psychiatry, 52,* 89–99.

McFarlane, A. C. (1988). The phenomenology of posttraumatic stress disorders following natural disaster. *The Journal of Nervous and Mental Disease, 176,* 22–29.

McGinnis, J. M., & Nestle, M. (1989). The Surgeon General's report on nutrition and health: Policy implications and implementation strategies. *American Journal of Clinical Nutrition, 49,* 23–28.

McGrath, P. (1997, January 27). The Web: Infotopia or marketplace? *Newsweek, 129*(4), 82–84.

McLaughlin, M., Cormier, L. S., & Cormier, W. H. (1988). Relation between coping strategies and distress, stress, and marital adjustment of multiple-role women. *Journal of Counseling Psychology, 35,* 187–193.

McLeod, B. (1984, October). In the wake of disaster. *Psychology Today, 18*(10), 54–57.

Mechanic, D. (1966). Response factors in illness: The study of illness behavior. *Social Psychiatry, 1,* 11–20.

Medalie, J. H., & Goldbourt, U. (1976). Angina pectoris among 10,000 men: II. Psychosocial and other risk factors as evidenced by a multivariate analysis of a five year incidence study. *American Journal of Medicine, 60,* 910–921.

Mehrabian, A., & Russell, J. A. (1974). *An approach to environmental psychology.* Cambridge, MA: MIT Press.

Meichenbaum, D. (1977). *Cognitive-behavior modification: An integrative approach.* New York: Plenum.

Meichenbaum, D., & Jaremko, M. E. (1983). *Stress reduction and prevention.* New York: Plenum.

Melamed, B. G., & Siegel, L. J. (1975). Reduction of anxiety in children facing surgery by modeling. *Journal of Consulting and Clinical Psychology, 43,* 511–521.

Melton, C. E., Smith, R. C., McKenzie, J. M., Wicks, S. M., & Saldivar, J. T. (1977). *Stress in air traffic personnel: Low-density towers and flight service stations* (FAA Office of Aviation Medicine Report No. AM-77-23). Washington, DC: U.S. Government Printing Office.

Melzack, R., & Wall, R. (1965). Pain mechanisms: A new theory. *Science, 50,* 971–979.

Memmler, R. L., & Wood, D. L. (1977). *The human body in health and disease* (4th ed.). Philadelphia: Lippincott.

Menaghan, E. (1982). Assessing the impact of family transitions on marital experience. In H. I. McCubbin, A. E. Cauble, & J. M. Patterson (Eds.), *Family stress, coping and social support* (pp. 90–108). Springfield, IL: Charles C. Thomas.

Menaghan, E. G. (1983). Individual coping efforts: Moderators of the relationship between life stress and mental health outcomes. In H. B. Kaplan (Ed.), *Psychosocial stress: Trends in theory and research* (pp. 157–191). New York: Academic Press.

Mensink, R. R., & Katan, M. B. (1990). Effect of dietary trans fatty acids on high density and low density lipoprotein cholesterol levels in healthy subjects. *The New England Journal of Medicine, 323,* 439–445.

Metcalfe, J., & Jacobs, W. J. (1996). A "hot-system/cool-system" view of memory under stress. *PTSD Research Quarterly, 7*(2), 1–7.

Michelson, D., Licinio, J., & Gold, P. W. (1995). Mediation of the stress response by the hypothalamic-pituitary-adrenal axis. In M. J. Friedman, D. S. Charney, & A. Y. Deutch (Eds.), *Neurobiological and clinical consequences of stress: From Normal Adaptation to PTSD* (pp. 225–238). Philadelphia: Lippincott-Raven.

Miller, N. E. (1944). Experimental studies in conflict. In J. McV. Hunt (Ed.), *Personality and the behavior disorders* (Vol. 1, pp. 431–465). New York: Ronald Press.

Miller, N. E. (1969). Learning of visceral and glandular responses. *Science, 163,* 434–445.

Miller, N. E. (1985). The value of behavioral research on animals. *American Psychologist, 40,* 423–440.

Miller, T. Q., Smith, T. W., Turner, C. W., Guijarro, M. L., & Hallet, A. J. (1996). A meta-analytic review of research on hostility and physical health. *Psychological Bulletin, 119,* 322–348.

Millon, T. (1982). On the nature of clinical health psychology. In T. Millon, C. Green, & R. Meagher (Eds.), *Handbook of clinical health psychology* (pp. 1–27). New York: Plenum.

Mirkin, G. (1983). *Getting thin.* Boston: Little, Brown.

Mishel, M. H. (1984). Perceived uncertainty and stress in illness. *Research in Nursing and Health, 7,* 163–171.

Mitchell, R. E., Cronkite, R. C., & Moos, R. H. (1983). Stress, coping, and depression among married couples. *Journal of Abnormal Psychology, 92,* 433–448.

Moch, M. K., Bartunek, J., & Brass, D. J. (1979). Structure, task characteristics, and experienced role stress in organizations employing complex technology. *Organizational Behavior and Human Performance, 24,* 258–268.

Moran, E. F. (1981). Human adaptation to arctic zones. *Annual Review of Anthropology, 10,* 1–25.

Morgan, W. R., & Goldston, S. E. (Eds.). (1987). *Exercise and mental health.* Washington, DC: Hemisphere.

Morin, S. E., Charles, K. A., & Malyon, A. K. (1984). The psychological impact of AIDS on gay men. *American Psychologist, 39,* 1288.

Morrison, A. M., & von Glinow, M. A. (1990). Women and minorities in management. *American Psychologist, 45,* 200–208.

Morrison, E. R., & Paffenbarger, R. A. (1981). Epidemiological aspects of biobehavior in the etiology of cancer: A critical review. In S. M. Weiss, J. A. Herd, & B. H. Fox (Eds.), *Perspectives on behavioral medicine* (pp. 135–161). New York: Academic Press.

Mueser, K. T., Yarnold, P. R., & Bryant, E. B. (1987). Type A behaviour and time urgency: Perception of time adjectives. *British Journal of Medical Psychology, 60,* 267–269.

Muldoon, L. (Ed.). (1979). *Incest: Confronting the silent crime.* St. Paul, MN: Minnesota Program for Victims of Sexual Assault.

Murphy, L. R. (1984). Occupational stress management: A review and appraisal. *Journal of Occupational Psychology, 57,* 1–15.

Murphy, S. A. (1984). Stress levels and health status of victims of a natural disaster. *Research in Nursing and Health, 7,* 205–215.

Nack, W. (1986, February 26). This case was one for the books. *Sports Illustrated,* 34–42.

Nagy, S., & Nix, C. L. (1989). Relations between preventive health behavior and hardiness. *Psychological Reports, 65,* 339–345.

Naisbitt, J. (1982). *Megatrends: Ten new directions transforming our lives.* New York: Warner Books.

Nakano, K. (1989). Intervening variables of stress, hassles, and health. *Japanese Psychological Research, 31,* 143–148.

National Center for Health Statistics. (1988). Monthly vital statistics report, 37, 1–10.

National Clearinghouse on Child Abuse and Neglect. (1997). *What is child maltreatment?* Retrieved November 1997 from the World Wide Web: http://www.calib.com/nccanch/pubs/whatis.htm.

Neiman, L. (1988). A critical review of resiliency literature and its relevance to homeless children. *Children's Environments Quarterly, 5,* 17–25.

Neisser, U. (1976). *Cognition and reality: Principles and implications of cognitive psychology.* New York: W. H. Freeman.

Nelson, P. D. (1974). Comment. In E. K. E. Gunderson & R. H. Rahe (Eds.), *Life stress and illness* (pp. 79–89). Springfield, IL: Charles C. Thomas.

Nerviano, V. J., & Gross, H. W. (1983). Personality types of alcoholics on objective inventories: A review. *Journal of Studies on Alcohol, 44,* 837–851.

Niaura, R., Stoney, C. M., & Herbert, P. N. (1992). Lipids in psychological research: The last decade. *Biological Psychology, 34,* 1–43.

Nilles, J. M., Carlson, F. R., Jr., Gray, R., & Honneman, G. J. (1976). *The telecommunications transportation tradeoff.* New York: Wiley.

Norman, P., Collins, S., Conner, M., Martin, R., & Rance, J. (1995). Attributions, cognitions, and coping styles: Teleworkers' reactions to work-related problems. *Journal of Applied Social Psychology, 25,* 117–128.

Nossal, G. J. V. (1987). The basic components of the immune system. *The New England Journal of Medicine, 316,* 1320–1325.

Nouwen, A., & Bush, C. (1984). The relationship between paraspinal EMG and chronic low back pain. *Pain, 20,* 109–123.

Novaco, R. W. (1977). A stress inoculation approach to anger management in the training of law enforcement officers. *American Journal of Community Psychology, 5,* 327–346.

O'Leary, A. (1985). Self-efficacy and health. *Behaviour Research and Therapy, 23,* 437–451.

O'Leary, K. D., & Borkovec, T. D. (1978). Conceptual, methodological, and ethical problems of placebo groups in psychotherapy research. *American Psychologist, 33,* 821–830.

Orman, M. C. (1991). *The 14 day stress cure.* Houston: Breakthru Publishing.

Orzek, A. M. (1985). The child's cognitive processing of sexual abuse. *Child and Adolescent Psychotherapy, 2,* 110–114.

Ostlund, R. E., Staten, M., Kohrt, W. M., Schultz, J., & Malley, M. (1990). The ratio of waist-to-hip circumference, plasma insulin level, and glucose intolerance as independent predictors of the HDL2 cholesterol level in older adults. *The New England Journal of Medicine, 322,* 229–234.

Pagano, R. R., Rose, R. M., Stivers, R. M., & Warrenburg, S. (1976). Sleep during transcendental meditation. *Science, 191,* 308–309.

Parsons, R. A. (1988). Behavior, stress, and variability. *Behavior Genetics, 18,* 293–308.

Parsons, T. (1951). *The social system.* New York: Free Press.

Patrick, V., & Patrick, W. K. (1981). Cyclone '78 in Sri Lanka—The mental health trail. *British Journal of Psychiatry, 138,* 210–216.

Patterson, G. (1977). A performance theory for coercive family interaction. In R. B. Cairns (Ed.), *The analysis of social interactions: Methods, issues, and illustrations* (pp. 119–162). Hillsdale, NJ: Lawrence Erlbaum Associates.

Patterson, J. M. (1989). The family stress model: The family adjustment and adaptation response. In C. N. Ramsey, Jr. (Ed.), *Family systems in medicine* (pp. 95–118). New York: Guilford.

Patterson, J. M., & Garwick, A. W. (1994). Levels of meaning in family stress theory. *Family Process, 33,* 287–304.

Pearlin, L. I., Lieberman, M., Menaghan, E., & Mullan, J. (1981). The stress process. *Journal of Health and Social Behavior, 22,* 337–356.

Pearlin, L. I., & Schooler, C. (1978). The structure of coping. *Journal of Health and Social Behavior, 19,* 2–21.

Pekkanen, J., Linn, S., Heiss, G., Suchindran, C. M., Leon, A., Rifkind, B. M., & Tyroler, H. A. (1990). Ten-year mortality from cardiovascular disease in relation to cholesterol level among men with and without preexisting cardiovascular disease. *The New England Journal of Medicine, 322,* 1700–1707.

Pelletier, K. (1977). *Mind as healer, mind as slayer: A holistic approach to preventing stress disorders.* New York: Delacorte/Delta.

Pennebaker, J. W., & Newtson, D. (1983). Observation of a unique event: The psychological impact of the Mount Saint Helens volcano. *New Directions for Methodology of Social and Behavioral Sciences, 15,* 93–109.

Pepper, S. C. (1942). *World hypotheses.* Berkeley: University of California Press.

Perkins, K., with Bernstein, N. (1997, April). A new heart put me back on top. *McCall's,* April 1997, 66, 68, 70–71.

Peter, L. J. (1969). *The Peter principle.* New York: Morrow.

Peters, M. F., & Massey, G. (1983). Mundane extreme environmental stress in family stress theories: The case of black families in white America. In H. I. McCubbin, M. B. Sussman, & J. M. Patterson (Eds.), *Social stress and the family* (pp. 193–218). New York: Haworth Press.

Peterson, C., & Seligman, M. E. P. (1984). Causal explanations as a risk factor for depression: Theory and evidence. *Psychological Review, 91,* 347–374.

Peterson, C., & Seligman, M. E. P. (1987). Explanatory style and illness. *Journal of Personality, 55,* 237–265.

Peterson, C., Seligman, M. E. P., & Vaillant, G. E. (1988). Pessimistic explanatory style is a risk factor for physical illness: A thirty-five-year longitudinal study. *Journal of Personality and Social Psychology, 55,* 23–27.

Peterson, L., & Harbeck, C. (1988). *The pediatric psychologist.* Champaign, IL: Research Press.

Phares, E. J. (1976). *Locus of control in personality.* Morristown, NJ: General Learning Press.

Pinel, J. P. J. (1993). *Biopsychology* (2nd ed.). Boston: Allyn & Bacon.

Pinkerton, S., Hughes, H., & Wenrich, W. W. (1982). *Behavioral medicine: Clinical applications.* New York: Wiley.

Plaut, S. M., & Friedman, S. B. (1981). Psychosocial factors, stress, and disease processes. In R. Ader (Ed.), *Psychoneuroimmunology* (pp. 3–29). New York: Academic Press.

Pletcher, B. A. (1978). *Saleswoman: A guide to career success.* Homewood, IL: Dow Jones-Irwin.

Pollock, S. E. (1989). The hardiness characteristic: A motivating factor in adaptation. *Advances in Nursing Science, 11,* 53–62.

Pons, T. P., Garraghty, P. E., Ommaya, A. K., Kaas, J. H., Taub, E., & Mishkin, M. (1991). Massive cortical reorganization after sensory deafferentation in adult macaques. *Science, 252,* 1857–1861.

Popkin, B. M., Siega-Riz, A. M., & Haines, P. S. (1996). A comparison of dietary trends among racial and socioeconomic groups in the United States. *The New England Journal of Medicine, 335,* 716–720.

Porjesz, B., & Begleiter, H. (1982). Evoked brain potential deficits in alcoholism and aging. *Alcoholism: Clinical and Experimental Research, 6,* 53–63.

Posner, M. J. (1982). *Executive essentials.* New York: Avon Books.

Puente, A. E., & Beiman, I. (1980). The effects of behavior therapy, self-relaxation, and transcendental meditation on cardiovascular stress response. *Journal of Clinical Psychology, 36,* 291–295.

Quarantelli, E. L., & Dynes, R. R. (1977). Response to social crisis and disaster. *Annual Review of Sociology, 3,* 23–49.

Quinn, R. R., & Staines, G. L. (1979). *The 1977 quality of employment survey.* Ann Arbor: Survey Research Center, University of Michigan.

Rabkin, J. G., & Struening, E. L. (1976a). Life events, stress, and illness. *Science, 194,* 1013–1020.

Rabkin, J. G., & Struening, E. L. (1976b). Social change, stress, and illness: A selective literature review. *Psychoanalysis and Contemporary Science, 5,* 573–624.

Ragland, D. R., & Brand, R. J. (1988). Type A behavior and mortality from coronary heart disease. *The New England Journal of Medicine, 318,* 65–69.

Rahe, R. H. (1974). Life change and subsequent illness reports. In E. K. E. Gunderson & R. H. Rahe (Eds.), *Life stress and illness* (pp. 58–78). Springfield, IL: Charles C. Thomas.

Rahe, R. H., & Arthur, R. J. (1978). Life change and illness studies: Past history and future directions. *Journal of Human Stress, 4,* 3–15.

Rajecki, R., Lamb, M., & Obmascher, R. (1978). Toward a general theory of infantile attachment: A comparative review of aspects of the social bond. *The Behavioral and Brain Sciences, 3,* 417–464.

Ralston, D. A., Anthony, W. P., & Gustafson, D. J. (1985). Employees may love flextime, but what does it do to the organization's productivity? *Journal of Applied Psychology, 70,* 272–279.

Ray, C., Jefferies, S., & Weir, W. R. C. (1995). Life-events and the course of chronic fatigue syndrome. *British Journal of Medical Psychology, 68,* 323–331.

Rhodewalt, F., & Zone, J. B. (1989). Appraisal of life-change, depression, and illness in hardy and nonhardy women. *Journal of Personality and Social Psychology, 56,* 81–88.

Riad, J. K., & Norris, F. H. (1996). The influence of relocation on the environmental, social, and psychological stress experienced by disaster victims. *Environment and Behavior, 28,* 163–182.

Rich, V. L., & Rich, A. R. (1987). Personality hardiness and burnout in female staff nurses. *Image: Journal of Nursing Scholarship, 19,* 63–66.

Richmond, J. B., & Beardslee, W. R. (1988). Resiliency: Research and practical implications for pediatricians. *Journal of Developmental and Behavioral Pediatrics, 9,* 157–163.

Richmond, V. P., McCroskey, J. C., & Payne, S. K. (1987). *Nonverbal behavior in interpersonal relations.* Englewood Cliffs, NJ: Prentice-Hall.

Riscalla, L. M. (1983). A holistic concept of the immune system. *Journal of the American Society of Psychosomatic Dentistry and Medicine 30,* 97–101.

Roberts, J. T. (1993). Psychosocial effects of workplace hazardous exposures: Theoretical synthesis and preliminary findings. *Social Problems, 40,* 74–89.

Rodin, J., & Baum, A. (1978). Crowding and helplessness: Potential consequences of density and loss of control. In A. Baum & Y. Epstein (Eds.), *Human response to crowding* (pp. 390–401). Hillsdale, NJ: Lawrence Erlbaum Associates.

Rodin, J., & Salovey, P. (1989). Health psychology. *Annual Review of Psychology, 40,* 533–579.

Rodriquez, N., Ryan, S., Vande Kemp, H., & Foy, D. W. (1997). Posttraumatic stress disorder in adult female survivors of childhood sexual abuse: A comparison study. *Journal of Consulting and Clinical Psychology, 65,* 53–59.

Rofes, E. E. (Ed.). (1982). *The kids' book of divorce: By, for and about kids.* New York: Vintage Books.

Rohner, R. (1975). Parental acceptance-rejection and personality: A universalistic approach to behavioral science. In R. W. Brislin, S. Bochner, & W. J. Lonner (Eds.), *Cross-cultural perspectives on learning* (pp. 251–269). New York: Halsted.

Roque, G. M., & Roberts, M. C. (1989). A replication of the use of public posting in traffic speed control. *Journal of Applied Behavior Analysis, 22,* 325–330.

Rose, G. D., & Carlson, J. G. (1987). The behavioral treatment of Raynaud's disease: A review. *Biofeedback and Self-regulation, 12,* 257–272.

Rosen, L. N. (1995). Life events and symptomatic recovery of army spouses following Operation Desert Storm. *Behavioral Medicine, 21,* 131–139.

Rosen, T. J., Terry, N. S., & Leventhal, H. (1982). The role of esteem and coping in response to a threat communication. *Journal of Research in Personality, 16,* 90–107.

Rosenbaum, M., Leibel, R., & Hirsch, J. (1997). Obesity. *The New England Journal of Medicine, 337,* 396–407.

Rosenhan, D. L., & Seligman, M. E. P. (1989). *Abnormal psychology* (2nd ed.). New York: Norton.

Rosenman, R. H. (1993). Relationships of the Type A Behavior Pattern with coronary heart disease. In L. Goldberger & S. Breznitz (Eds.), *Handbook of stress: Theoretical and clinical aspects* (pp. 449–476). New York: Free Press.

Rosenman, R. H., & Friedman, M. (1974). Neurogenic factors in pathogenesis of coronary heart disease. *Medical Clinics of North America, 58,* 269–279.

Rosenman, R. H., & Friedman, M. (1977). Modifying Type A behaviour pattern. *Journal of Psychosomatic Research, 21,* 323–331.

Rosenman, R. H., Friedman, M., Straus, R., Jenkins, C. D., Zyzanski, S. J., & Wurm, M. (1970). Coronary heart disease in the Western Collaborative Group Study: A follow-up experience of $4\frac{1}{2}$ years. *Journal of Chronic Disease, 23,* 173–190.

Rosenman, R. H., Friedman, M., Straus, R., Wurm, M., Kositcheck, R., Hahn, W., & Verthessen, N. T. (1964). A predictive study of coronary heart disease: The Western Collaborative Group Study. *Journal of the American Medical Association, 189,* 15–22.

Rosenstock, I. M. (1966). Why people use health services. *Milbank Memorial Fund Quarterly, 44,* 94–124.

Rosenstock, I. M., Strecher, V. J., & Becker, M. H. (1988). Social learning theory and the Health Belief Model. *Health Education Quarterly, 15,* 175–183.

Rosenthal, R. (1966). *Experimenter effects in behavioral research.* New York: Appleton-Century-Crofts.

Rosenthal, R., & Rosnow, R. L. (1991). *Essentials of behavioral research: Methods and data analysis* (2nd ed.). New York: McGraw-Hill.

Rossouw, J. E. (1990). The value of lowering cholesterol after myocardial infarction. *The New England Journal of Medicine, 323,* 1112–1119.

Rotter, J. B. (1966). Generalized expectancies for internal versus external control of reinforcement. *Psychological Monographs, 80.*

Rotter, J. B. (1990). Internal versus external control of reinforcement: A case history of a variable. *American Psychologist, 45,* 489–493.

Rounsaville, B. (1978). Theories of marital violence: Evidence from a study of battered women. *Victimology: An International Journal, 3,* 11–31.

Rousseau, D. M. (1978). Relationship of work to nonwork. *Journal of Applied Psychology, 63,* 513–517.

Rozanksi, A., Bairey, C. N., Krantz, D. S., Friedman, J., Resser, K. J., Morell, M., et al. (1988). Mental stress and the induction of silent myocardial ischemia in patients with coronary artery disease. *The New England Journal of Medicine, 318,* 1005–1012.

Rubin, R. T. (1974). Biochemical and neuroendocrine responses to severe psychological stress. In E. K. E. Gunderson & R. H. Rahe (Eds.), *Life stress and illness* (pp. 227–241). Springfield, IL: Charles C. Thomas.

Rudolph, K. D., Dennig, M. D., & Weisz, J. R. (1995). Determinants and consequences of children's coping in the medical setting: Conceptualization, review, and critique. *Psychological Bulletin, 118,* 328–357.

Rutherford, R. D. (1978). *Administrative timepower: Meeting the time challenge of the busy secretary/staff assistant/manager team.* Austin, TX: Learning Concepts.

Saile, H., Burgmeier, R., & Schmidt, L. R. (1988). A meta-analysis of studies on psychological preparation of children facing medical procedures. *Psychology and Health, 2,* 107–132.

Sakai, M., & Takeichi, M. (1996). Two cases of panic disorder treated with autogenic training and in vivo exposure without medication. *Psychiatry & Clinical Neuroscience, 50,* 335–336.

Salvendy, G. (1982). Human-computer communications with special reference to technological developments, occupational stress and educational needs. *Ergonomics, 25,* 435–447.

Sandhu, D. S. (1995). An examination of the psychological needs of the international students: Implications for counselling and psychotherapy. *International Journal for the Advancement of Counselling, 17,* 229–239.

Sauter, S. L., Murphy, L. R., & Hurrell, J. J. (1990). Prevention of work-related psychological disorders. *American Psychologist, 45,* 1146–1158.

Sawrey, W. L., & Weiss, J. D. (1956). An experimental method of producing gastric ulcers. *Journal of Comparative and Physiological Psychiatry, 49,* 269.

Schachter, S. (1982). Recidivism and self-cure of smoking and obesity. *American Psychologist, 37,* 436–444.

Schafer, S. (1977). *Victimology: The victim and his criminal.* Reston, VA: Reston.

Schank, R. C., & Abelson, R. (1977). *Scripts, plans, goals, and understanding.* Hillsdale, NJ: Lawrence Erlbaum Associates.

Schatzkin, A., Jones, Y., Hoover, R. N., Taylor, P. R., Brinton, L. A., Ziegler, R. G., Harvey, E. B., Carter, C., Licitra, L. M., Dufour, M. C., & Larson, D. B. (1987). Alcohol consumption and breast cancer in the epidemiologic follow-up study of the first national health and nutrition examination survey. *The New England Journal of Medicine, 316,* 1169–1173.

Scheier, M., & Carver, C. S. (1987). Dispositional optimism and physical well-being: The influence of generalized outcome expectancies on health. *Journal of Personality, 55,* 169–210.

Scheier, M., Weintraub, J. K., & Carver, C. S. (1986). Coping with stress: Divergent strategies of optimists and pessimists. *Journal of Personality and Social Psychology, 51,* 1257–1264.

Schill, I., & O'Laughlin, S. (1984). Humor preference and coping with stress. *Psychological Reports, 55,* 309–310.

Schlesinger, B. (1969). The one-parent family in perspective. In B. Schlesinger (Ed.), *The one-parent family: Perspectives and annotated bibliography* (pp. 3–12). Toronto, Canada: University of Toronto Press.

Schmelzer, R. V., Schmelzer, C. D., Figler, R. A., & Brozo, W. G. (1987). Using the critical incident technique to determine reasons for success and failure of university students. *Journal of College Student Personnel, 28,* 261–266.

Schneider, A. L., & Schneider, P. R. (1981). Victim assistance programs: An overview. In B. Galaway & J. Hudson (Eds.), *Perspectives on crime victims* (pp. 364–373). St. Louis, MO: Mosby.

Schneider, C. J. (1987). Cost effectiveness of biofeedback and behavioral medicine treatments: A review of the literature. *Biofeedback and Self-Regulation, 12,* 71–92.

Schroeder, D. H., & Costa, P. T. (1984, May). *Do stressful life events influence objectively mea-sured health? A prospective evaluation.* Paper presented at the Midwestern Psychological Association Annual Conference, Chicago.

Schultz, B. J., & Saklofske, D. H. (1983). Relationship between social support and selected measures of psychological well-being. *Psychological Review, 53,* 847–850.

Schultz, J., & Luthe, W. (1959). *Autogenic training: A psychophysiological approach to psy-chotherapy.* New York: Grune & Stratton.

Schwartz, G. E. (1982). Testing the biopsychosocial model: The ultimate challenge facing be-havioral medicine? *Journal of Consulting and Clinical Psychology, 50,* 1040–1053.

Schwartz, G. E. (1983). Disregulation theory and disease: Applications to the repression/cerebral disconnection/cardiovascular disorder hypothesis. *International Re-view of Applied Psychology, 32,* 95–118.

Scrignar, C. B. (1983). *Stress strategies: The treatment of the anxiety disorders.* New York: Karger.

Seeman, J. (1989). Toward a model of positive health. *American Psychologist, 44,* 1099–1109.

Seligmann, M., Chess, L., Fahey, J. L., Fauci, A. S., Lachmann, R. J., L'Age-Stehr, J., et al. (1984). AIDS—An immunologic reevaluation. *The New England Journal of Medicine, 311,* 1286–1292.

Seligman, M. E. P. (1975). *Helplessness.* San Francisco: W. H. Freeman.

Selye, H. (1956). *The stress of life.* New York: McGraw-Hill.

Selye, H. (1974). *Stress without distress.* Philadelphia: Lippincott.

Selye, H. (1976). *Stress in health and disease.* Reading, MA: Butterworth.

Selye, H. (1979). The stress concept and some of its implications. In V. Hamilton & D. M. War-burton (Eds.), *Human stress and cognition: An information processing approach* (pp. 11–32). New York: Wiley.

Selye, H. (1980). The stress concept today. In I. L. Kutash, L. B. Schlesinger, & Associates (Eds.), *Handbook on stress and anxiety* (pp. 127–143). San Francisco: Jossey-Bass.

Selye, H. (1993). History of the stress concept. In L. Goldberger & S. Breznitz (Eds.), *Hand-book of stress: Theoretical and clinical aspects* (pp. 7–17). New York: Free Press.

Shapiro, D. H., & Zifferblatt, S. M. (1976). Zen meditation and behavioral self-control: Similar-ities, differences, and clinical applications. *American Psychologist, 31,* 519–532.

Shapiro, F. (1995). *Eye movement desensitization and reprocessing: Basic principles, protocols and procedures.* New York: Guilford Press.

Shapiro, F. (1996). Eye movement desensitization and reprocessing (EMDR): Evaluation of controlled PTSD research. *Journal of Behavior Therapy & Experimental Psychiatry, 27,* 209–218.

Shapiro, J. (1983). Family reactions and coping strategies in response to the physically ill or handicapped child: A review. *Social Science and Medicine, 17,* 913–931.

Sharkey, B. J. (1984). *Physiology of fitness: Prescribing exercise for fitness, weight control, and health* (2nd ed.). Champaign, IL: Human Kinetics.

Shavit, Y., Lewis, J. W., Terman, G. W., Gale, R. P., & Liebeskind, J. C. (1984). Opioid peptides mediate the suppressive effect of stress on natural killer cell cytotoxicity. *Science, 223,* 188–190.

Shekelle, R. B., Gale, M., Ostfeld, A. M., & Paul, O. (1983). Hostility, risk of coronary heart dis-ease, and mortality. *Psychosomatic Medicine, 45,* 109–114.

Shiffman, S., Fischer, L. A., Paty, J. A., Gnys, M., Hickcox, M., & Kassel, J. D. (1994). Drinking and smoking: A field study of their association. *Annals of Behavior Medicine, 16,* 203–209.

Shumaker, S. A., & Hill, D. R. (1991). Gender differences in social support and physical health. *Health Psychology, 10,* 102–111.

Siegel, J. M., & Steele, C. M. (1980). Environmental distraction and interpersonal judgments. *British Journal of Social and Clinical Psychology, 19,* 23–32.

Silver, B. V., & Blanchard, E. B. (1978). Biofeedback and relaxation training in the treatment of psychophysiological disorders: Or are the machines really necessary? *Journal of Behavioral Medicine, 2,* 217–239.

Simkins, L. (1982). Biofeedback: Clinically valid or oversold? *Psychological Record, 32,* 3–17.

Simonton, O. C., & Simonton, S. (1975). Belief systems and management of the emotional aspects of malignancy. *Journal of Transpersonal Psychology, 7,* 29–47.

Singer, R., & Rutenfranz, J. (1971). Attitudes of air traffic controllers at Frankfurt Airport towards work and the working environment. *Ergonomics, 14,* 633–639.

Situ, Y., Austin, T., & Liu, W. (1995). Coping with anomic stress: Chinese students in the USA. *Deviant Behavior: An Interdisciplinary Journal, 16,* 127–149.

Sklar, L. S., & Anisman, H. (1980). Social stress influences tumor growth. *Psychosomatic Medicine, 42,* 347–365.

Slavin, L. A., Rainer, K. L., McCreary, M. L., & Gowda, K. K. (1991). Toward a multicultural model of the stress process. *Journal of Counseling & Development, 70,* 156–163.

Smart, J. F., & Smart, D. W. (1995). Acculturative stress of Hispanics: Loss and challenge. *Journal of Counseling & Development, 73,* 390–396.

Smith, J. C. (1988). Steps toward a cognitive-behavioral model of relaxation. *Biofeedback and Self-Regulation, 13,* 307–329.

Smith, M. S., & Womack, W. M. (1987). Stress management techniques in childhood and adolescence: Relaxation training, meditation, hypnosis, and biofeedback: Appropriate clinical applications. *Clinical Pediatrics, 26,* 581–585.

Smith, S. L. (1984). Significant research findings in the etiology of child abuse. *Social Casework, 65,* 665–683.

Smith, S. M., & Hanson, R. (1975). Interpersonal relationships and childrearing practices in 214 parents of battered children. *British Journal of Psychiatry, 127,* 513–525.

Sobel, D. S. (1979). *Ways of health: Holistic approaches to ancient and contemporary medicine.* New York: Harcourt Brace Jovanovich.

Soll, A. H. (1990). Pathogenesis of peptic ulcer and implications for therapy. *The New England Journal of Medicine, 322,* 909–916.

Solomon, L. J., & Rothblum, E. D. (1984). Academic procrastination: Frequency and cognitive-behavioral correlates. *Journal of Counseling Psychology, 31,* 504–510.

Sorbi, M., & Tellegen, B. (1988). Stress-coping in migraine. *Social Science and Medicine, 26,* 351–358.

Sparacino, J., Ronchi, D., Brenner, M., Kuhn, J. W., & Flesch, A. L. (1982). Psychological correlates of blood pressure: A closer examination of hostility, anxiety, and engagement. *Nursing Research, 31,* 143–149.

Spector, P. E. (1986). Perceived control by employees: A meta-analysis of studies concerning autonomy and participation at work. *Human Relations, 39,* 1005–1016.

Spector, P. E., Dwyer, D. J., & Jex, S. M. (1988). Relation of job stressors to affective, health, and performance outcomes: A comparison of multiple data sources. *Journal of Applied Psychology, 73,* 11–19.

Spielberger, C. D. (1966). Theory and research on anxiety. In C. D. Spielberger (Ed.), *Anxiety and behavior* (pp. 1–22). New York: Academic Press.

Spielberger, C. D., & Jacobs, G. A. (1982). Personality and smoking behavior. *Journal of Personality Assessment, 46,* 396–403.

Spielman, A. J., Saskin, P., & Thorpy, M. J. (1987). Treatment of chronic insomnia by restriction of time in bed. *Sleep, 10,* 45–56.

Spring, B. J., Lieberman, H. R., Swope, G., & Garfield, G. S. (1986). Effects of carbohydrates on mood and behavior. *Nutrition Reviews: Diet and Behavior 44,* 51–60.

Srole, L., Langner, T. S., Michael, S. T., Opler, M. K., & Rennie, T. A. C. (1962). *Mental health in the metropolis.* New York: McGraw-Hill.

Stacy, A. W., Sussman, S., Dent, C. W., Burton, D., & Flay, B. R. (1992). Moderators of peer social influence in adolescent smoking. *Personality and Social Psychology Bulletin, 18,* 163–172.

Steele, C. M., & Josephs, R. A. (1990). Alcohol myopia: Its prized and dangerous effects. *American Psychologist, 45,* 921–933.

Steinmetz, S. K. (1977). The use of force for resolving family conflict: The training ground for abuse. *The Family Coordinator, 26,* 19–26.

Stephens, G. J. (1980). *Pathophysiology for health practitioners.* New York: Macmillan.

Stern, R. M., & Ray, W. J. (1977). *Biofeedback: Potential and limits.* Lincoln: University of Nebraska Press.

Stevens, M. J., & Pfost, K. S. (1984). Stress management interventions. *Journal of College Student Personnel, 25,* 269–270.

Stokols, D. (1980). Instrumental and spiritual views of people-environment relations. *American Psychologist, 45,* 641–646.

Stokols, D., & Novaco, R. (1981). Transportation and well-being: An ecological perspective. In I. Altman, J. R. Wohlwill, & R. B. Evertt (Eds.), *Transportation and behavior* (pp. 85–130). New York: Plenum.

Stone, A., Cox, D. S., Valdimarsdottir, H., Jandorf, L., & Neale, J. M. (1987). Evidence that secretary IgA Antibody is associated with daily mood. *Journal of Personality and Social Psychology, 52,* 988–993.

Stone, A. A., & Shiffman, S. (1994). Ecological Momentary Assessment (EMA) in behavioral medicine. *Annals of Behavior Medicine, 16,* 199–202.

Stoney, C. M., Davis, M. C., & Matthews, K. A. (1987). Sex differences in physiological responses to stress and in coronary heart disease: A causal link? *Psychophysiology, 24,* 127–131.

Stout, N. A., Jenkins, E. L., & Pizatella, T. J. (1996). Occupational injury mortality rates in the United States: Changes from 1980 to 1989. *The American Journal of Public Health, 86,* 73–79.

Stoyva, J. M., & Carlson, J. G. (1993). A coping/rest model of relaxation and stress management. In L. Goldberger & S. Breznitz (Eds.), *Handbook of stress: Theoretical and clinical aspects* (pp. 724–756). New York: Free Press.

Straus, M. A. (1977). Sociological perspective on the prevention and treatment of wifebeating. In M. Roy (Ed.), *Battered women: A psychosociological study of domestic violence* (pp. 194–239). New York: Van Nostrand Reinhold.

Straus, M. A., Gelles, R. J., & Steinmetz, S. K. (1980). *Behind closed doors: Violence in the American family.* Garden City, NY: Doubleday/Anchor.

Strickland, B. (1989). Internal-external control expectancies: From contingency to creativity. *American Psychologist, 44,* 1–12.

Suls, J., & Fletcher, B. (1985). The relative efficacy of avoidant and nonavoidant coping strategies: A meta-analysis. *Health Psychology, 4,* 249–288.

Suls, J., & Mullen, B. (1981). Life events, perceived control and illness: The role of uncertainty. *Journal of Human Stress, 7,* 30–34.

Swain, J. E., Rouse, I. L., Curley, C. B., & Sacks, F. M. (1990). Comparison of the effects of oat bran and low-fiber wheat on serum lipoprotein levels and blood pressure. *The New England Journal of Medicine, 322,* 147–152.

Sytkowski, R. A., Kannel, W. B., & D'Agostino, R. B. (1990). Changes in risk factors and the decline in mortality from cardiovascular disease. *The New England Journal of Medicine, 322,* 1635–1641.

Taiminen, T. J., & Tuominen, T. (1996). Psychological responses to a marine disaster during a recoil phase: Experiences from the *Estonia* shipwreck. *British Journal of Medical Psychology, 69,* 147–153.

Tanaka, M., Kohno, Y., Nakagawa, R., Ida, Y., Takeda, S., Nagasaki, N., & Noda, Y. (1983). Regional characteristics of stress-induced increases in brain noradrenaline release in rats. *Pharmacology, Biochemistry and Behavior, 19,* 543–547.

Taylor, A. L., & Fishman, L. M. (1988). Corticotropin-releasing hormone. *The New England Journal of Medicine, 319,* 213–222.

Taylor, C. B., & Fortmann, S. R. (1983). Essential hypertension. *Psychosomatics, 24,* 433–448.

Taylor, P., Abrams, D., & Hewstone, M. (1988). Cancer, stress and personality: A correlational investigation of life-events, repression-sensitization and locus of control. *British Journal of Medical Psychology, 61,* 179–183.

Taylor, S. (1996). Meta-analysis of cognitive-behavioral treatments for social phobia. *Journal of Behavior Therapy & Experimental Psychiatry, 27,* 1–9.

Taylor, S. E. (1983). Adjustment to threatening events: A theory of cognitive adaptation. *American Psychologist, 38,* 1161–1173.

Taylor, S. E. (1997). Health psychology: What is an unhealthy environment and how does it get under the skin? *Annual Review of Psychology, 48,* 411–447.

ter Kulle, M. M., Spinhoven, P., Linssen, A. C., & van Houwelingen, H. C. (1996). Cognitive coping and appraisal processes in the treatment of chronic headaches. *Pain, 64,* 257–264.

Teshima, H., Kubo, C., Kihara, H., Imada, Y., Nagata, S., Ago, Y., & Ikemi, Y. (1982). Psychosomatic aspects of skin diseases from the standpoint of immunology. *Psychotherapy and Psychosomatics, 37,* 165–175.

Thackray, R. J. (1981). The stress of boredom and monotony: A consideration of the evidence. *Psychosomatic Medicine, 43,* 165–176.

Thomas, A., Chess, S., & Birch, H. (1970). The origin of personality. *Scientific American, 223,* 102–109.

Thomas, M. R., Rapp, M. S., & Gentles, W. M. (1979). An inexpensive automated desensitization procedure for clinical application. *Journal of Behavior Therapy and Experimental Psychiatry, 10,* 317–321.

Throll, D. A. (1982). Transcendental meditation and progressive relaxation: Their physiological effects. *Journal of Clinical Psychology, 38,* 522–530.

Toffler, A. (1970). *Future shock.* New York: Bantam Books.

Toffler, A. (1980). *The third wave.* New York: Bantam Books.

Tomporowski, R. D., & Ellis, N. R. (1986). Effects of exercise on cognitive processes: A review. *Psychological Bulletin, 99,* 338–346.

Tooley, K. M. (1977). The young child as victim of sibling attack. *Social Casework, 58,* 25–28.

Topf, M. (1989). Sensitivity to noise, personality hardiness, and noise-induced stress in critical care nurses. *Environment and Behavior, 21,* 717–733.

Trent, J. T., Smith, A. L., & Wood, D. L. (1994). Telecommuting: Stress and social support. *Psychological Reports, 74,* 1312–1314.

Tryon, G. S. (1979). A review and critique of thought stopping research. *Journal of Behavior Therapy & Experimental Psychiatry, 10,* 189–192.

Turk, D. C., Meichenbaum, D. H., & Berman, W. H. (1979). Application of biofeedback for the regulation of pain: A critical review. *Psychological Bulletin, 86,* 1322–1338.

Turkington, C. (1985, April). Farmers strain to hold the line as crisis uproots mental health. *APA Monitor 16,* pp. 1, 26, 27, 38.

Turnage, J. J. (1990). The challenge of new workplace technology for psychology. *American Psychologist, 45,* 171–178.

Turner, R. J. (1983). Direct, indirect, and moderating effects of social support on psychological distress and associated conditions. In H. B. Kaplan (Ed.), *Psychosocial stress: Trends in theory and research* (pp. 105–155). New York: Academic Press.

Tyrrell, J. (1992). Sources of stress among psychology undergraduates. *The Irish Journal of Psychology, 13,* 184–192.

U.S. Department of Commerce, Bureau of the Census. (1979). *Statistical Abstract of the United States* (100th ed.). Washington, DC: U.S. Government Printing Office.

U. S. Department of Health and Human Services. (1997). Child maltreatment 1995: Reports from the states to the National Child Abuse and Neglect Data System. Washington, D. C.: U. S. Government Printing Office.

U. S. Department of Health and Human Services (NIOSH). (1997). The effects of workplace hazards on male reproductive health. Retrieved October 31, 1997, from the World Wide Web: http://www.cdc.gov/niosh/malrepro.html.

Uttal, W. R. (1978). *The psychobiology of mind.* Hillsdale, NJ: Lawrence Erlbaum Associates.

Vaillant, G. E. (1977). *Adaptation to life.* Boston: Little, Brown.

Valentino, R. J., Drolet, G., & Aston-Jones, G. (1995). Central nervous system noradrenergic-peptide interactions. In M. J. Friedman, D. S. Charnery, & A. Y. Deutch (Eds.), *Neurobiological and clinical consequences of stress: From normal adaptation to PTSD* (pp. 33–72). Philadelphia: Lippincott-Raven.

van Dale, D., & Saris, W. H. M. (1989). Repetitive weight loss and weight regain: Effects on weight reduction, resting metabolic rate, and lipolytic activity before and after exercise and/or diet treatment. *American Journal of Clinical Nutrition, 49,* 409–416.

van Doornen, L. J. R. (1980). The Coronary Risk Personality: Psychological and psychophysiological aspects. *Psychotherapy and Psychosomatics, 34,* 204–215.

van Egeren, L. E., Fabrega, H., & Thornton, D. W. (1983). Electrocardiographic effects of social stress on coronary-prone (Type A) individuals. *Psychosomatic Medicine, 45,* 195–203.

Vázquez, L. A., & García-Vázquez, E. (1995). Variables of success and stress with Mexican American students. *College Student Journal, 29,* 221–226.

Venditti, E. M., Wing, R. R., Jakicic, J. M., Butler, B. A., & Marcus, M. D. (1996). Weight cycling, psychological health, and binge eating in obese women. *Journal of Consulting and Clinical Psychology, 64,* 400–405.

Veniga, R. L., & Spradley, J. R. (1981). *The work/STRESS connection.* Boston: Little, Brown.

Vest, J., Cohen, W., & Tharp, M. (1997, June 2). Road rage: Tailgating, give the finger, outright violence. *U. S. News & World Report, 122*(21), 24–28.

Vickers, R. R., Jr., & Hervig, L. K. (1984). *Health behaviors: Empirical consistency and theoretical significance of subdomains* (Tech. Rep. 84-14). San Diego: Naval Health Research Center.

Vlisides, C. E., Eddy, J. P., & Mozie, D. (1994). Stress and stressors: Definition, identification and strategy for higher education constitutents. *College Student Journal, 28,* 123–124.

von Bertalanffy, L. (1968). General system theory—A critical review. In W. Buckley (Ed.), *Modern systems research for the behavioral scientist* (pp. 11–30). Chicago: Aldine.

Walker, A. (1985). Reconceptualizing family stress. *Journal of Marriage and the Family, 47,* 827–837.

Wallace, R. K., & Benson, H. (1972). The physiology of meditation. *Scientific American, 226,* 84–90.

Wallerstein, J. S., & Kelly, J. B. (1980). *Surviving the breakup: How children and parents cope with divorce.* New York: Basic Books.

Walsh, R., Dale, A., & Anderson, D. E. (1977). Comparison of biofeedback, pulse wave velocity and progressive relaxation in essential hypertensives. *Perceptual and Motor Skills, 44,* 839–843.

Walster, E. (1966). Assignment of responsibility for an accident. *Journal of Personality and Social Psychology, 3,* 73–79.

Walter, H., Hofman, A., Vaughan, R. D., & Wynder, E. L. (1988). Modification of risk factors for coronary disease: Five-year results of a school-based intervention trial. *The New England Journal of Medicine 318,* 1093–1100.

Ward, M. M., Mefford, I. N., Parker, S. D., Chesney, M. A., Taylor, C. B., Keegan, D. L., & Barchas, J. D. (1983). Epinephrine and norepinephrine responses in continuously collected human plasma to a series of stressors. *Psychosomatic Medicine, 45,* 471–486.

Watanabe, Y., Halberg, F., Cornelissen, G., Saito, Y., Fukuda, K., Otsuka, K., & Kikuchi, T. (1996). Chronobiometric assessment of autogenic training effects upon blood pressure and heart rate. *Perceptual Motor Skills, 83,* 1395–1410.

Watson, J. B., & Rayner, R. (1920). Conditioned emotional reactions. *Journal of Experimental Psychology, 3,* 1–14.

Watzl, B., & Watson, R. R. (1992). Role of alcohol abuse in nutritional immunosuppression. *The Journal of Nutrition, 122,* 733–737.

Webber, R. A. (1972). *Time and management.* New York: Van Nostrand Reinhold.

Webster's New Twentieth Century Dictionary, unabridged (2nd ed.). (1979). New York: Simon & Schuster.

Weiss, J. M. (1968). Effects of coping responses on stress. *Journal of Comparative Physiological Psychology, 65,* 251–260.

Weiss, J. M. (1971). Effects of coping behavior in different warning signal conditions on stress pathology in rats. *Journal of Comparative Physiological Psychology, 77,* 1–13.

Weiss, K. B., Gergen, P. J., & Hodgson, T. A. (1992). An economic evaluation of asthma in the United States. *The New England Journal of Medicine, 326,* 862–866.

Wenger, M. A., & Bagchi, B. K. (1961). Studies of autonomic function in practitioners of Yoga in India. *Behavioral Science, 6,* 312–323.

Werner, E. E. (1984). Resilient children. *Young Children, 40,* 68–72.

West, D. J., Horan, J. J., & Games, P. A. (1984). Component analysis of occupational stress inoculation applied to registered nurses in an acute care hospital setting. *Journal of Counseling Psychology, 31,* 209–218.

Wiedenfeld, S. A., O'Leary, A., Bandura, A., Brown, S., Levine, S., & Raske, K. (1990). Impact of perceived self-efficacy in coping with stressors on components of the immune system. *Journal of Personality and Social Psychology, 59,* 1082–1094.

Wiener, N. (1954). *The human use of human beings: Cybernetics and society.* Garden City, NY: Doubleday/Anchor.

Wiener, N. (1961). *Cybernetics* (2nd ed.). Cambridge, MA: MIT Press.

Wilkinson, H. (1996). Marriage deserves another try. *New Statesman, 126*(4320), 10.

Williams, R. B. (1995). Somatic consequences of stress. In M. J. Friedman, D. S. Charnery, & A. Y. Deutch (Eds.), *Neurobiological and clinical consequences of stress: From normal adaptation to PTSD* (pp. 403–412). Philadelphia: Lippincott-Raven.

Wills, T. A., & Langner, T. S. (1980). Socioeconomic status and stress. In I. L. Kutash, L. B. Schlesinger, & Associates (Eds.), *Handbook on stress and anxiety* (pp. 159–173). San Francisco: Jossey-Bass.

Wilson, B. R. A. (1989). Cardiovascular risk reduction. *International Psychologist, 29,* 49–54.

Wilson, D. L., Silver, S. M., Covi, W. G., & Foster, S. (1996). Eye movement desensitization and reprocessing: Effectiveness and autonomic correlates. *Journal of Behavior Therapy & Experimental Psychiatry, 27,* 219–229.

Winfield, I. (1983). Counselling with biofeedback: A review. *British Journal of Guidance and Counselling, 11,* 46–51.

Witmer, J. M., Rich, C., Barcikowski, R. S., & Mague, J. C. (1983). Psychosocial characteristics mediating the stress response: An exploratory study. *The Personnel and Guidance Journal, 62,* 73–77.

Wohlwill, J. F. (1974). Human adaptation to levels of environmental stimulation. *Human Ecology, 2,* 127–147.

Wolfe, J., & Proctor, S. P. (1996). The Persian Gulf War: New findings on traumatic exposure and stress. *PTSD Research Quarterly, 7*(1), 1–8.

Wolpe, J. (1958). *Psychotherapy by reciprocal inhibition.* Stanford, CA: Stanford University Press.

Wright, L. (1988). The Type A behavior pattern and coronary artery disease. *American Psychologist, 43,* 2–14.

Wyatt, G. E. (1995). The prevalence and context of sexual harassment among African American and white American women. *Journal of Interpersonal Violence, 10,* 309–321.

Yablin, B. A. (1986). Maximizing the disabled adolescent: Family challenges and coping techniques. *International Journal of Adolescent Medicine and Health, 2,* 223–231.

Yarnold, R. R., & Grimm, L. G. (1982a, May). *Interpersonal dominance and coronary-prone behavior.* Paper presented at the 3rd Annual Meeting of the Society of Behavioral Medicine, Chicago.

Yarnold, R. R., & Grimm, L. G. (1982b). Time urgency among coronary-prone individuals. *Journal of Abnormal Psychology, 91,* 175–177.

Yerkes, R. M., & Dodson, J. D. (1908). The relation of strength of stimulus to rapidity of habit formation. *Journal of Comparative and Neurological Psychology, 18,* 459–482.

Young, T. J., Ekeler, W. J., Sawyer, R. M., & Prichard, K. W. (1994). Black student subcultures in American universities: Acculturation stress and cultural conflict. *College Student Journal, 28,* 504–508.

Zautra, A., & Sandler, I. (1983). Life event needs assessments: Two models for measuring preventable mental health problems. *Prevention in Human Services, 2,* 35–58.

Zedeck, S., & Mosier, K. L. (1990). Work in the family and employing organization. *American Psychologist, 45,* 240–251.

Zich, J., & Temoshok, L. (1987). Perceptions of social support in men with AIDS and ARC: Relationships with distress and hardiness. *Journal of Applied Social Psychology, 17,* 193–215.

Zinsmeister, K. (1997, February). Divorce's toll on children. *Current, N390,* 29–33.

Zuckerman, M. (1971). Dimensions of sensation seeking. *Journal of Consulting and Clinical Psychology, 36,* 35–52.

Zuker, E. (1983). *Mastering assertiveness skills: Power and positive influence at work.* New York: American Management Association.

Zullow, H. M., Oettingen, G., Peterson, C., & Seligman, M. E. P. (1988). Pessimistic explanatory style in the historical record. *American Psychologist, 43,* 673–682.

Subject Index

Name Index